Health
the basics

Seventh Canadian Edition

Health
the basics

Rebecca J. Donatelle
Oregon State University

Amanda Froehlich Chow
University of Saskatchewan

Angela M. Kolen-Thompson
St. Francis Xavier University

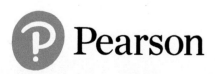

EDITORIAL DIRECTOR: Claudine O'Donnell
ACQUISITIONS EDITOR: Cathleen Sullivan
MARKETING MANAGER: Jordana Caplan Luth
PROGRAM MANAGER: Kamilah Reid-Burrell
PROJECT MANAGER: Andrea Falkenberg
MANAGER OF CONTENT DEVELOPMENT: Suzanne Schaan
DEVELOPMENTAL EDITOR: Toni Chahley
MEDIA EDITOR: Tamara Capar
MEDIA DEVELOPER: Kelli Cadet

PRODUCTION SERVICES: Cenveo® Publisher Services
PERMISSIONS PROJECT MANAGER: Joanne Tang
PHOTO PERMISSIONS RESEARCH: Aptara
TEXT PERMISSIONS RESEARCH: Aptara
COVER AND INTERIOR DESIGNER: Anthony Leung
COVER IMAGE: Hero Images/Getty Images
VICE-PRESIDENT, CROSS MEDIA AND PUBLISHING SERVICES: Gary Bennett

Pearson Canada Inc., 26 Prince Andrew Place, Don Mills, Ontario M3C 2T8.

978-0-13-429939-6

5   18

Library and Archives Canada Cataloguing in Publication

Donatelle, Rebecca J., 1950-, author
    Health : the basics / Rebecca J. Donatelle (Oregon State University), Amanda Froehlich Chow (University of Saskatchewan), Angela M. Kolen-Thompson (St. Francis Xavier University). – Seventh Canadian edition.

Includes bibliographical references and index.
ISBN 978-0-13-429939-6 (hardback)

    1. Health--Textbooks. I. Chow, Amanda Froehlich, author II. Kolen-Thompson, Angela M., author III. Title.

RA776.D65 2017   613   C2016-905584-1

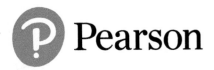

BRIEF CONTENTS

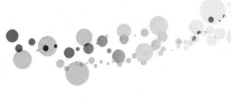

CONTENTS

PREFACE

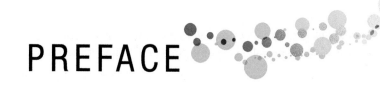

A LETTER TO OUR READERS

Dear Readers,

We are pleased to present you with the seventh Canadian edition of *Health: The Basics*. Please know that we revised this textbook with you in mind—you, the postsecondary student.

Some of the health challenges you face today are different than when we entered university years ago. However, some are the same—managing stress, eating well, being physically active, protecting yourself from sexually trans-mitted infections, using the health-care system wisely, to name a few similarities.

Although we likely now know more about what it takes to live healthily, we also seem to face more challenges in doing so. We know we should be physically active, and we are well aware of the importance of eating a balanced diet—focusing on vegetables and fruits—each day, and yet many of us cannot manage to do either. Some of us choose to drive short distances when walking or cycling would be a healthier—and the more environmentally friendly—option. Many believe that we must work out to benefit from physical activity. Food choices can be perplexing, especially given the abundance and availability of fast and convenient foods; media and advertising messages convince us that such foods will save us time.

Many of us also have an "all-or-nothing" way of thinking. In other words, we may not recognize that each lifestyle choice—whether physical or mental—is important and contributes to our overall health and wellness. Further, our health results from a culmination of many factors and influences with each playing its own role. Sometimes we think of and manage only the components related to our physical health, neglecting our social, emotional, intellectual, and spiritual dimensions.

You may be studying Human Kinetics or Kinesiology, Physical Education, Nursing, Health Sciences, Business, or General Arts or Science. Regardless of your program of study, we invite you to engage with this textbook, your classmates, and your professor. Please read and think about how each opening scenario, introductory section, and detailed presentation of various Canadian statistics is relevant to you. How does each topic apply to you? Do you invest time thinking about a particular topic? Why or why not?

We challenge you to question the choices you make and the attitudes you have toward your health and wellness. Are they the best for you, for right now? How can you make better decisions? When will you make better choices? We also encourage you to question contemporary thinking about many health issues; for example, binge drinking. Why is it socially acceptable and expected to drink heavily in your college and university years? You might also query the societal and media pressures regarding body image. Why do we expect men and women to look a certain way? Why do we judge people based upon how they look? Question contemporary thinking about many issues, not just those we bring up here.

We encourage you to read and to reflect deeply. Learning can only happen with reflection. Further, we urge you to ask questions that will help you to better understand yourself, questions that will help you to better understand health and wellness, questions that will encourage you to choose more wisely now while you are a student and later when you are not.

Finally, we suggest you approach this textbook with a sense of optimism and hopefulness, as well as an oppor-tunity to be selfish. Reading this textbook, participating in class, and completing your assignments provide you with the chance to think about yourself and what is best for you and your health. As you read through this book, you will understand why we suggest you have a sense of optimism and hopefulness—that is a choice we all make.

Wishing you all the best and success in your studies!

Sunshine and smiles,
Angie and Amanda

In developing *Health: The Basics*, we listened to the comments and concerns of Canadian personal health educators and learned that we share the following goals for a personal health textbook:

- To prepare students to lead healthy lives, now and in the future, by providing knowledge, tools, and strategies to make responsible and appropriate decisions regarding their health.
- To include "high-interest" topics not always included in health texts, such as multicultural and sex-specific perspectives on health.
- To include current Canadian research, material, and statistics.
- To recognize that students learn in many ways and require strong pedagogical elements to help them synthesize information and build healthy attitudes and behaviours.
- To include practical, real-life applications to encourage students to think critically about their health and to apply the material to their own lives.
- To encourage self-awareness, integrity, respect, self-responsibility, and gratitude in the reader.

INSIDE THE BOOK

- **Decision making through critical thinking** is the cornerstone of every chapter, beginning with the introduction of the **DECIDE model for decision making**, **Prochaska and DiClemente's Stages of Change model**, and various behaviour change techniques in Chapter 1.
- **Personal reflection**, a hallmark feature woven throughout, includes *Consider This* . . . scenarios and reflective questions, *Student Health* and *Point of View* boxed features, and *Taking Charge* sections with the opportunity to *Assess Yourself* at the end of each chapter.
- An overriding **philosophy of self-responsibility**, including a better understanding and self-awareness behind the reasons why we do what we do (or do not do) in regards to our health and wellness, appears throughout each section of this book.
- Each part of the textbook concludes with **Focus On**, a three- to five-page feature that provides additional information on an engaging topic relevant to university and college students and their health.
- **Coverage of sex issues in health** is integrated throughout the text. Topics include sex bias in mental health treatment; women and heart disease; and how sex and gender roles can affect stress, stress management, and a person's ultimate health status.
- Updated references in APA format help the reader connect more easily to the research and to the thinking that leads to making better choices regarding his or her health.
- Each chapter applies a **pedagogical framework** that stresses building health skills consistently. Students can personalize each chapter through the *Student Health* and *Point of View* textboxes within each chapter, as well as through the *Assess Yourself* and *Taking Charge* boxes at the end of each chapter.

NEW TO THE SEVENTH CANADIAN EDITION

Building on a strong foundation, the seventh Canadian edition of *Health: The Basics* continues to reflect and exemplify self-awareness, integrity, respect, self-responsibility, and gratitude. Key changes to each chapter include the following:

Chapter 1 features a new figure illustrating the Socio Ecological Model. Updated figures illustrating the leading causes of death in Canada have also been incorporated.

We have incorporated updated information about volunteer rates, mental illness, and depression in Canada into **Chapter 2**. Also included is updated information on LGBT Youth and Suicide prevention. A new section discusses what happens when mood disorder and substance use disorders mix.

Chapter 3 includes updated and clarified material on the general adaptation syndrome (GAS). In addition, information and statistics on technostress have been updated.

The introduction to **Chapter 4** has been heavily revised and reframed and now incorporates material on physical literacy. There is an updated and revised section on physical activity for health, and a new discussion talks about doctors prescribing physical activity for treating and preventing disease. The section on identifying your physical fitness goals and designing your physical fitness program has been revised, and a new exercise called the "your movement journey" (physical activity and physical literacy in your life so far) has been incorporated.

New to **Chapter 5** is the *First Nations, Inuit, and Métis Food Guide*, including a new table with estimated daily calorie needs. This chapter also includes a completely revised section on carbohydrates, and a new section on choosing organic or locally grown foods, and the slow food movement.

Chapter 6 includes updated statistics and discussion of overweight and obesity in Canada

Chapter 7 includes updates to the discussion and terminology related to gender and sex, including an updated gender differences diagram. Selected activities have been updated to incorporate social orientation, and a new figure on gender-specific communication patterns has been added. This chapter also includes an updated and revised discussion of sexual orientation.

Chapter 8 incorporates updated statistics and information on paternal health and sperm damage.

Chapter 9 includes updated material on gambling addiction.

In **Chapter 10** information on alcohol use and Low Risk Drinking Guidelines have been updated. Material on alcohol sales by province has also been updated. New figures have been added that illustrate reported heavy drinking by age, the physiological and behavioural effects of increased blood alcohol concentration, and compare a healthy liver to a cirrhotic liver. A new figure and example of the use of the decision support framework have been incorporated. Information on smoking rates in Canada has been updated, and a new Student Health Today box dealing with the dangers of e-cigarettes and a new application activity has been added.

Chapter 11 includes updates to material on use of illicit drugs in Canada and self-reported use of marijuana.

Clarified and updated material on heart disease and heart function have been added to **Chapter 12**. Updated information on cancer incidence and mortality, including updated information on the incidences of specific types of cancer has been incorporated, and a new figure on the geographic distribution of new cancer cases across Canada has been added. We have also added new figures on the percent distribution of estimated new cancer cases, by sex, and the process of metastasis.

New to **Chapter 13** is a figure illustrating the epidemiological triad of disease. A number of updates have been made to the chapter including updated information on worldwide rates of tuberculosis, instances of hepatitis C in Canada, and instances of death from measles worldwide. Updated information on the instances of chlamydia in Canada and the rate of gonorrhoea in Canada has also been included, along with updated information regarding HIV/AIDS.

Updated and revised material on overpopulation and fertility is presented in **Chapter 14**, along with a new figure illustrating global fertility rates by region.

Chapter 15, features new figures illustrating homicide rates by province and female homicide rates by Indigenous group. Updated information on youth violence, domestic violence, violence against children, and violence against older adults are also include, along with an updated figure illustrating suicide rates by sex and age group. Lastly, a new figure illustrating incidents of elder abuse has been added.

New to **Chapter 16** is the introduction to section on self-care. Material on the number of physicians and nurses in Canada has been updated, and a new section has been added on complementary and alternative medicine.

Chapter 17 has been revised to include an updated discussion of the proportion of Canadians who are 65 years of age or older. Moreover, a new figure illustrates the normal effects of aging on the body.

HALLMARK PEDAGOGICAL FEATURES

In addition to the features noted above, *Health: The Basics* continues to employ the following pedagogical features.

- **Learning Objectives:** Each chapter begins with learning outcomes that provide a learning path of the important topics covered within the chapter.

- **Consider This . . . Chapter-Opening Scenarios:** These practical, real-life scenarios introduce concepts covered in the chapter and can be a springboard to stimulating discussions. End-of-Chapter Application Exercises provide further discussion of the topic.

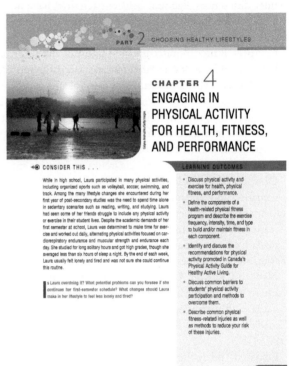

- **Point of View boxes:** Each chapter features a *Point of View* box that offers perspectives on a controversial health issue and provokes students to consider where they stand.

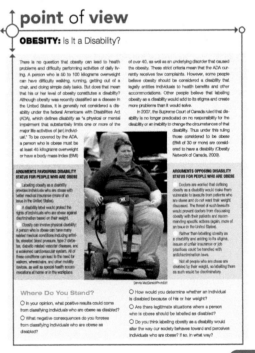

- **Student Health Today boxes:** A *Student Health Today* box stimulates critical and personal thinking through the presentation of a student-related issue relevant to the chapter's topic.

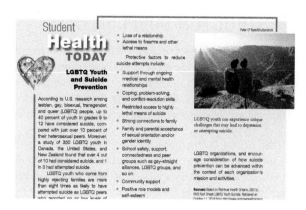

Student Health TODAY

LGBTQ Youth and Suicide Prevention

According to U.S. research among lesbian, gay, bisexual, transgender, and queer (LGBTQ) people, up to 40 percent of youth in grades 9 to 12 have considered suicide, compared with just over 10 percent of their heterosexual peers. Moreover, a study of 350 LGBTQ youth in Canada, the United States, and New Zealand found that over 4 out of 10 had considered suicide, and 1 in 3 had attempted suicide.

LGBTQ youth who come from highly rejecting families are more than eight times as likely to have attempted suicide as LGBTQ peers who reported no or low levels of

- Loss of a relationship
- Access to firearms and other lethal means

Protective factors to reduce suicide attempts include:
- Support through ongoing medical and mental health relationships
- Coping, problem-solving, and conflict-resolution skills
- Restricted access to highly lethal means of suicide
- Strong connections to family
- Family and parental acceptance of sexual orientation and/or gender identity
- School safety, support, connectedness and peer groups such as gay-straight alliances, LGBTQ groups, and so on
- Community support
- Positive role models and self-esteem

LGBTQ youth can experience unique challenges that may lead to depression or attempting suicide.

LGBTQ organizations, and encourage consideration of how suicide prevention can be advanced within the context of each organization's mission and activities.

Sources: Based on Rainbow Health Ontario, (2013). RHO Fact Sheet: LGBTQ Youth Suicide. Retrieved on October 11, 2016 from http://www.rainbowhealthontario.ca

- **Assess Yourself:** Every chapter and *Focus On* feature ends by encouraging the reader to "take charge" of his or her health. These textboxes include *Assess Yourself* questionnaires, a personal self-assessment tool.

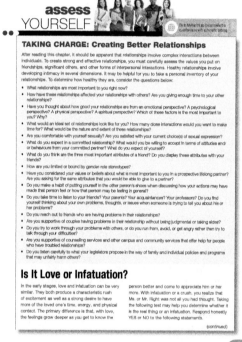

assess YOURSELF

Go to MyHealthLab to complete the questionnaire with automatic scoring.

TAKING CHARGE: Creating Better Relationships

After reading this chapter, it should be apparent that relationships involve complex interactions between individuals. To create strong and effective relationships, you must carefully assess the values you put on friendships, significant others, and other forms of interpersonal interactions. Healthy relationships involve developing intimacy in several dimensions. It may be helpful for you to take a personal inventory of your relationships. To determine how healthy they are, consider the questions below:

- What relationships are most important to you right now?
- How have these relationships affected your relationships with others? Are you giving enough time to your other relationships?
- Have you thought about how good your relationships are from an emotional perspective? A psychological perspective? A physical perspective? A spiritual perspective? Which of these factors is the most important to you? Why?
- What would an ideal set of relationships look like for you? How many close interactions would you want to make time for? What would be the nature and extent of these relationships?
- Are you comfortable with yourself sexually? Are you satisfied with your current choice(s) of sexual expression?
- What do you expect in a committed relationship? What would you be willing to accept in terms of attitudes and/or behaviours from your committed partner? What do you expect of yourself?
- What do you think are the three most important attributes of a friend? Do you display these attributes with your friends?
- How are you limited or bound by gender-role stereotypes?
- Have you considered your values or beliefs about what is most important to you in a prospective lifelong partner? Are you asking for the same attributes that you would be able to give to a partner?
- Do you make a habit of putting yourself in the other person's shoes when discussing how your actions may have made that person feel or how that person may be feeling in general?
- Do you take time to listen to your friends? Your parents? Your acquaintances? Your professors? Do you find yourself thinking about your own problems, thoughts, or issues when someone is trying to tell you about his or her problems?
- Do you reach out to friends who are having problems in their relationships?
- Are you supportive of couples having problems in their relationship without being judgmental or taking sides?
- Do you try to work through your problems with others, or do you run from, avoid, or get angry rather than try to talk through your difficulties?
- Are you supportive of counselling services and other campus and community services that offer help for people who have troubled relationships?
- Do you listen carefully to what your legislators propose in the way of family and individual policies and programs that may unfairly harm others?

Is It Love or Infatuation?

In the early stages, love and infatuation can be very similar. They both produce a characteristic rush of excitement as well as a strong desire to have more of the loved one's time, energy, and physical contact. The primary difference is that, with love, the feelings grow deeper as you get to know the person better and come to appreciate him or her more. With infatuation or a crush, you realize that Ms. or Mr. Right was not all you had thought. Taking the following test may help you determine whether it is the real thing or an infatuation. Respond honestly YES or NO to the following statements.

(continued)

- **Running Glossary of Key Terms:** Key terms are boldfaced in the text and defined in the margins on the page where they first appear.

- **Discussion Questions:** These questions encourage critical thinking about important concepts presented from a variety of angles.

- **Focus On:** After the last chapter of each part, these three- to five-page features present in-depth information relevant to the topic(s) of the section, including spiritual health, body image, STIs, sleep, diabetes, and financial health.

focus On Diabetes

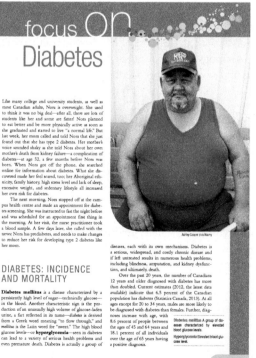

Like many college and university students, as well as most Canadian adults, Nora is overweight. She used to think it was no big deal—after all, there are lots of students like her and some are fatter! Nora planned to eat better and be more physically active as soon as she graduated and started to live "a normal life." But last week, her mom called and told Nora that she just found out that she has type 2 diabetes. Her mother's voice sounded shaky as she told Nora about her own mother's death from kidney failure—a complication of diabetes—at age 52, a few months before Nora was born. When Nora got off the phone, she searched online for information about diabetes. What she discovered made her feel scared, too; her Aboriginal ethnicity, family history, high stress level and lack of sleep, excessive weight, and sedentary lifestyle all increased her own risk for diabetes.

The next morning, Nora stopped off at the campus health centre and made an appointment for diabetes screening. She was instructed to fast the night before and was scheduled for an appointment first thing in the morning. At her visit, the nurse practitioner took a blood sample. A few days later, she called with the news: Nora has prediabetes, and needs to make changes to reduce her risk for developing type 2 diabetes like her mom.

Ashley Cooper (rics)/Alamy

DIABETES: INCIDENCE AND MORTALITY

Diabetes mellitus is a disease characterized by a persistently high level of sugar—technically glucose—in the blood. Another characteristic sign is the production of an unusually high volume of glucose-laden urine, a fact reflected in its name—*diabetes* is derived from a Greek word meaning "to flow through," and *mellitus* is the Latin word for "sweet." The high blood glucose levels—or **hyperglycemia**—seen in diabetes can lead to a variety of serious health problems and even premature death. Diabetes is actually a group of

diseases, each with its own mechanisms. Diabetes is a serious, widespread, and costly chronic disease and if left untreated results in numerous health problems, including blindness, amputation, and kidney dysfunction, and ultimately, death.

Over the past 20 years, the number of Canadians 12 years and older diagnosed with diabetes has more than doubled. Current estimates (2012, the latest data available) indicate that 6.5 percent of the Canadian population has diabetes (Statistics Canada, 2013). At all ages except for 20 to 34 years, males are more likely to be diagnosed with diabetes than females. Further, diagnoses increase with age, with 8.6 percent of people between the ages of 45 and 64 years and 18.1 percent of all individuals over the age of 65 years having a positive diagnosis.

Diabetes mellitus A group of diseases characterized by elevated blood glucose levels.

Hyperglycemia Elevated blood glucose level.

INSTRUCTOR SUPPLEMENTS

Designed to facilitate lecture preparation and learning, a comprehensive set of ancillary material accompanies *Health: The Basics,* Seventh Canadian Edition. These instructor supplements are available for download from a password-protected section of Pearson Canada's online catalogue (http://www.pearsoncanada.ca/highered). Navigate to your book's catalogue page to view a list of those supplements that are available. Speak to your local Pearson sales representative for details and access.

Instructor's Manual

This comprehensive manual, filled with material to enhance the course, includes chapter outlines; discussion questions; student activities including individual, community, and diverse population/nontraditional categories; and additional references for further information.

Computerized Test Bank

Pearson's computerized test banks allow instructors to filter and select questions to create quizzes, tests, or homework. Instructors can revise questions or add their own, and can choose print or online options. These questions are also available in Microsoft Word format.

PowerPoint Slides

Every chapter features a Microsoft PowerPoint® slide deck that highlights, illuminates, and builds on key concepts for lecture or online delivery. Educators can tailor each deck to their specifications.

Image Libraries

Image libraries help with the creation of vibrant lecture presentations. Most figures, tables, charts, photos, and *Assess Yourself* features from the text are provided in electronic format, organized by chapter for convenience. These images can be imported easily into Microsoft PowerPoint®.

Learning Solutions Managers

Pearson's Learning Solutions Managers work with faculty and campus course designers to ensure that Pearson technology products, assessment tools, and online course materials are tailored to meet your specific needs. This highly qualified team is dedicated to helping schools take full advantage of a wide range of educational resources, by assisting in the integration of a variety of instructional materials and media formats. Your local Pearson Canada sales representative can provide you with more details on this service program.

MasteringHealth

MasteringHealth (www.masteringhealthandnutrition.com or www.pearsonmastering.com) is an online homework, tutorial, and assessment product designed to improve student performance. MasteringHealth coaches students through the toughest health topics. A variety of Coaching Activities guide students through key health concepts with interactive mini-lessons, complete with hints and wrong-answer feedback. Reading Quizzes ensure students have completed the assigned reading before class. ABC News videos stimulate classroom discussions and include multiple-choice questions with feedback for students. Assignable Behaviour Change Video Quiz and Which Path Would You Take? activities ensure students complete and reflect on behaviour change and health choices. NutriTools in the nutrition chapter allow students to combine and experiment with different food options and learn firsthand how to build healthier meals. MP3 Tutor Sessions relate to chapter content and come with multiple-choice questions that provide wrong-answer feedback. Learning Catalytics provides open-ended questions students can answer in real time. MasteringHealth also includes the Behavior Change Log Book.

Pearson eText

The Pearson eText gives students access to their textbook anytime, anywhere. In addition to note taking, highlighting, and bookmarking, the Pearson eText offers interactive and sharing features. Instructors can share their comments or highlights, and students can add their own, creating a tight community of learners within the class.

STUDENT SUPPLEMENTS

The Study Area of MasteringHealth

The Study Area of MasteringHealth™ is organized by learning areas. Read It houses the Pearson eText as well as the Chapter Objectives and up-to-date health news. *See It* includes ABC News videos and the Behaviour Change videos. *Hear It* contains MP3 Tutor Session files and audio-based case studies. *Do It* contains the choose-your-own-adventure-style Interactive Behaviour Change Activities—Which Path Would You Take?, interactive NutriTools activities, critical-thinking Points of View questions, and Web links. *Review It* contains Practice Quizzes for each chapter, Flashcards, and Glossary. *Live It* will help jump-start students' behaviour change projects with interactive Assess Yourself Worksheets and resources to plan change.

ACKNOWLEDGMENTS

We thank the following people at Pearson Canada for their part in the seventh Canadian edition of *Health: The Basics:* executive acquisitions editor Cathleen Sullivan; marketing manager Jordanna Caplan Luth; developmental editor Toni Chahley; program manager Kamilah Reid-Burrell; production manager Andrea Falkenberg; senior designer Anthony Leung; copy editor Ruth Chernia; and proofreader Cat Haggert. We gratefully acknowledge the contribution of our technical reviewer Kerry-Anne Hogan of the University of Ottawa and Queen's University.

We also thank the following reviewers whose helpful feedback helped shape this new edition:

Brant Bradley, St. Lawrence College

Frank Christinck, Algonquin College

Michelle Cundari, Canadore College

Tara Dinyer, Mohawk College

Shaun Ferguson, Confederation College

Pam Fitch, Algonquin College

Paula Fletcher, Wilfrid Laurier University

David Harper, University of the Fraser Valley

Ken Kustiak, MacEwan University

Robin Laking, Georgian College

Emilio Landolfi, University of the Fraser Valley

Katherine McLeod, University of Regina

Robin Milhausen University of Guelph

Chris Perkins, Lambton College

And our thanks to the reviewers whose feedback helped shape the fifth and sixth Canadian editions:

Brenda Bruner, Queen's University

Penny Deck, Simon Fraser University

Cathy Deyo, College of New Caledonia

Joe Ellis, Sir Sanford Fleming College

Celine Homsy, John Abbott College

Gareth R. Jones, University of British Columbia

Jennifer Kuk, York University

Emilio Landolfi, University of the Fraser Valley

Patty McCrodan, Camosun College

Linda McDevitt, Algonquin College

Mary McKenna, University of New Brunswick

Chris Perkins, Lambton College

Michelle Meuller, University of Alberta

Rick Muldoon, St. Clair College

Tien Nguyen, University of Ottawa

Noel Quinn, Sheridan College

Mandana Salijegheh, Simon Fraser University

Deanna Schick, Trinity Western University

Tammy Whitaker-Campbell, Brock University

Sanni Yaya, University of Ottawa

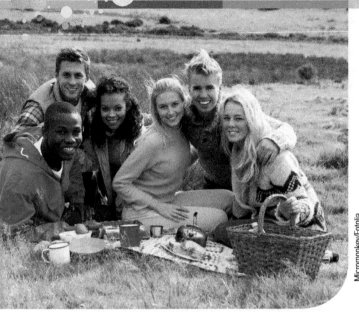

Micromonkey/Fotolia

CHAPTER 1
DISCOVERING YOUR PERSONAL RHYTHM FOR HEALTHY LIVING

◄◉ CONSIDER THIS . . .

Jonah is a 22-year-old, fourth-year university student who engages in very little physical activity, eats a lot of fast food, and is 20 kilograms overweight. A sensitive, caring young man, he has many close friends and volunteers at various agencies that help people in need. He enjoys nature and the inner peace he derives from sitting on the beach listening to the rolling surf or a quiet night by a campfire in the wilderness. He is a strong advocate for social justice and the preservation of the environment.

Camesha is a 19-year-old, first-year university student who lives off campus. She tries to eat well most of the time, thinks she is fat, and walks two to four kilometres per day. She is shy and has not made many friends since coming to university. During a typical day, she goes to class, studies, watches TV or a movie, texts with her high-school friends and family, and spends time on Facebook. She likes cycling and usually rides each weekend on her own.

D o you know people similar to either Jonah or Camesha? Who do you think is healthier? Why? What factors might contribute to their current attitudes and behaviours regarding their health? What actions might you suggest to help them achieve a more balanced "healthstyle" or one that is more in rhythm with what they are doing?

LEARNING OUTCOMES

- Identify and define the seven dimensions of health and wellness.

- Discuss the goals and objectives of the Pan-Canadian Healthy Living Strategy.

- List the lifestyle behaviours related to living longer.

- Compare and contrast behaviour-change techniques that identify not only when, but how and why to change.

- Describe the role of decision making in making behaviour changes.

f you and your close friends listed the most important things in your lives, you might be surprised by what the others have to say. Some would likely include family, love, financial security, significant others, and happiness. Others might list health. Raised on a steady stream of clichés and slogans—"If you have your health, you have everything," "Be all that you can be," "Use it or lose it," "Just do it!"—most of us readily acknowledge that good health is desirable. However, many of us struggle to define health, let alone good health. What does it mean to be healthy? How do you 'get' healthy? How can you maintain and enhance the positive attitudes and behaviours you already have toward your health and wellness? How can you change your not-so-good, health-detracting attitudes and behaviours?

This text provides you with health information consistent with making positive lifestyle decisions that support who you are and what you want to be. You can learn how to change your attitudes and behaviours to not only reduce your risk for many physical and mental health issues, but equally, or even more importantly, to positively influence how you feel right now. For the risk factors beyond your control, you can learn to react, adapt, and make optimal use of the resources available to you to create the best situation for you. Further, by making informed, rational decisions, you will be able to improve the quality—and quantity—of your life.

WHAT IS HEALTH?

Although we use the term *health* widely, few people understand the broad scope of the word. For some, health simply means the antithesis of sickness or to be without disease. To others, it means being in good physical shape or having the ability to resist disease and illnesses. Still others include in the terms *wellness* or *well-being* a wide array of factors that lead to positive health status. Why all the definitions? Partly because of the different perceptions of an increasingly enlightened view of health that has evolved over time. As our understanding of illness has improved, so has our ability to understand the many nuances of health.

Health and Sickness: Defined by Extremes

Before the late 1800s, people viewed health simply as the absence of diseases. A person was healthy if he or she was not suffering from a life-threatening infectious disease. When deadly epidemics such as bubonic plague, pneumonic plague, influenza, tuberculosis, and cholera killed millions of

Mortality Death rate.

Morbidity Illness rate.

people, survivors were considered healthy and congratulated themselves on their good fortune. In the late 1800s and early 1900s, researchers discovered that the victims of these epidemics were not simply people who were unhealthy but rather victims of microorganisms found in contaminated water, air, and human waste. Public health officials moved swiftly to sanitize the environment, and, as a result, many people began to think of health as good hygiene. Practices such as sanitary disposal of wastes, hand washing, and other behaviours that promoted hygiene then became the harbingers of good health.

Health: More Than Not Being Sick

Once scientists learned about the microorganisms that caused infectious diseases, dramatic changes occurred in the sickness profile of the Canadian population. In the early 1900s, the leading causes of death were infectious diseases such as tuberculosis, pneumonia, and influenza, and the average life expectancy at birth was only 58.8 years for men and 60.6 years for women (Statistics Canada, 1997). Improved sanitation brought about remarkable changes in life expectancy, and the development of vaccines and antibiotics added years to the average life span. According to **mortality** (death rate) statistics, people live longer now than at any other time in our history. Further, **morbidity** (illness) rates indicate that people are also sick less often from the common infectious diseases that devastated previous generations. Today, because most childhood diseases are curable and multiple public health efforts are aimed at reducing the spread of infectious diseases, many people are living well into their 70s, 80s, and even 90s. The average Canadian child born between 2007 and 2009 (the latest data available) has a life expectancy of 81.1 years—78.8 years for men and 83.3 years for women (Statistics Canada, 2012). There are approximately 5825 persons in Canada over the age of 100 (Statistics Canada, 2011). Also, the gender gap is slowly decreasing as men's life

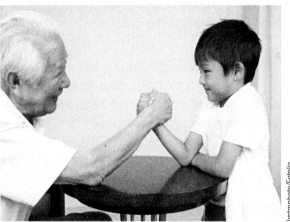

Good health refers to more than living long; it also means living well.

lmtmphoto/Fotolia

expectancy increases at a greater rate than women's (Statistics Canada, 2012). However, although fewer people are dying from infections caused by bacteria, the number of people dying from chronic diseases continues to rise. Scientists have expressed concern that children born today may live a shorter life span than their parents, most likely because of higher rates of obesity (Daniels, 2006; Franks et al., 2010).

Just because we are living longer and not getting sick as often does not necessarily mean we are healthier. Further, there is more to enjoying life than simply prolonging it by doing whatever it takes to avoid disease or delay its onset. Quality of life is important too; living for the moment, making healthier choices, and feeling good now.

The World Health Organization (WHO), whose objective is "the attainment by all peoples of the highest possible level of health"[*] (Beckington, 1975), defined **health** as ". . . complete physical, mental, and social well-being, not merely the absence of disease or infirmity" (World Health Organization, 1947). For the first time, health was defined as more than the absence of disease or a vital statistic indicating low mortality or morbidity rates. Although there is recognition given to factors beyond physical health with the inclusion of mental, social, occupational, environmental, and spiritual contributions to quality and quantity of life, some critics still argue that health is more than what is listed in the WHO's definition. Regardless of the various components included, health can be limited by income, education, occupation, access to medical care, environmental pollution, age, and sex. Since education is considered a determinant of health, increasing your knowledge may bring you one step closer to obtaining an optimal level of health.

FIGURE 1.1

The Dimensions of Health and the Wellness Continuum

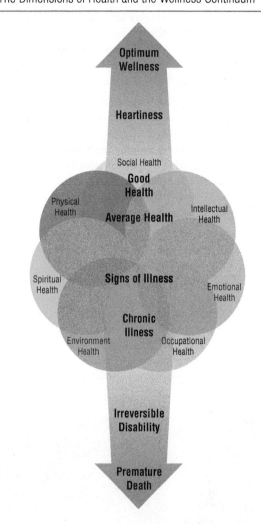

Health as Wellness: Putting Quality into Years

Biologist and philosopher Rene Dubos provided a multi-dimensional definition of health, noting that it "involves social, emotional, mental, spiritual, and biological fitness on the part of the individual, which results from adaptations to the environment" (Dubos, 1968). The concept of adaptability or the ability to successfully cope with life's ups and downs is a key element of this definition. In recent decades, the term **wellness** has become popular. It includes the previously mentioned elements and implies as well that there are levels to obtain in each category: to achieve a high level of wellness, a person attempts to move progressively higher on a continuum of positive health indicators. Today, *health* and *wellness* are often used interchangeably to refer to the dynamic, ever-changing process of trying to achieve one's individual potential in each of the interrelated dimensions. These dimensions typically include those presented in Figure 1.1.

- **Physical health.** Includes physical characteristics such as body size and shape, sensory acuity, susceptibility to disease and disorders, body functioning, and recuperative ability. The definition also encompasses the ability to perform activities of daily living, such as getting out of bed in the morning, bending to tie shoes, and shoulder checking while driving. To obtain optimal physical health, you need to make good choices regarding your physical activity; dietary intake; sleep, alcohol, and tobacco consumption; and health care.

> **Health** Dynamic, ever-changing process of trying to achieve individual potential in the physical, social, intellectual, occupational, emotional, environmental, and spiritual dimensions.

> **Wellness** Similar to health, a dynamic, ever-changing process in which a person attempts to reach his or her potential in each of health's components.

[*] From "Our mission, our work," http://www.searo.who.int/about/mission/en/. Published by World Health Organization, © 2016.

- **Social health.** Refers to the capacity for satisfying interpersonal relationships, interacting with others, and adapting to various social situations. It also includes communication skills and other daily activities. To obtain optimal social health, you make choices regarding the social activities you engage in, becoming a better communicator—listener and speaker—and thinking before you speak.

- **Intellectual health.** Refers to the ability to think clearly, reason objectively, analyze critically, and use brain power effectively to meet life's challenges. It includes learning from successes and failures and making responsible decisions. To obtain optimal intellectual health, you should learn from the mistakes you have made, think before you act, manage your time well, and so on.

- **Occupational health.** Refers to the satisfaction a person gets from his or her career or stage of career development. It also involves attaining and maintaining a satisfying balance between work and leisure. Part of obtaining optimal occupational health involves choosing a career that will fulfill you rather than simply provide a paycheque. As a student, you should view this dimension in terms of the satisfaction you experience as a result of your education in preparation for your future career.

- **Emotional health.** Refers to the "feeling" or emotional component of health and the ability to effectively and appropriately express those feelings. Feelings of self-esteem, self-confidence, self-efficacy, trust, love, and others are part of emotional health. To obtain optimal emotional health, you should learn how to express your feelings or emotions effectively, limit your worrying, and be receptive to change.

- **Environmental health.** Refers to an appreciation of the external environment and the role individuals play in maintaining, preserving, protecting, and improving it. Biophilia specifically refers to the instinctive bond between people and their environment (Barbiero, Berto, & Pasini, 2011). It also includes a student's personal studying environment—the desk, room, lighting, noise level, comfortable emotional atmosphere, and so on. To obtain optimal environmental health, make choices regarding personal use as well as responsibility for advocating to others regarding preserving the environment.

- **Spiritual health.** Your spirit refers to the deepest or innermost part of you, the part that provides meaning, purpose, transcendence, connectedness and energy to your life (Polzer Casarez & Engebretson, 2012). We draw strength and hope from spirituality. It is through understanding our spiritual selves that we know who we are, what we value, and what our specific purpose is. Spiritual health may or may not involve a belief in a supreme being, or a specified way of living prescribed by a particular religion. Regardless of whether you believe in a higher entity, spiritual health relates to your personal relationships with others and/or being at peace with nature. Reflecting about who you are and who you want to be, your values and beliefs, and whether or not the choices you make reflect your values and beliefs is part of obtaining optimal spiritual health.

Whether the term used is *health,* or *wellness,* or *health and wellness,* the focus is on personal attitudes and behaviours to achieve optimal well-being within a realistic framework of individual potential. In Figure 1.1, in addition to the dimensions of health and wellness, there is a continuum from illness to optimal well-being. Where you are on this continuum may vary slightly from day to day, week to week, month to month, and year to year. That said, if you persist in your attempts to change attitudes and behaviours to reduce risk and/or improve health, your chances of remaining on the positive end of the continuum greatly increase. Each of us must try to achieve this optimal level of being in a sometimes hostile environment, and come to terms with obstacles by focusing on our positive attributes whenever possible, changing what negative aspects we

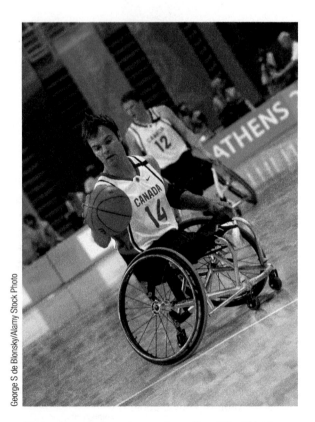

George S de Blonsky/Alamy Stock Photo

Having the motivation to improve the quality of life within the framework of your unique capabilities and limitations is part of achieving optimal health and wellness.

can, and learning to recognize and manage the aspects we cannot change.

Individuals who are well take an honest look at their capabilities and limitations and make an effort to change that which is not at its optimum and is within their control. They attempt to achieve a sense of rhythm in each dimension of health and wellness in efforts to attain or maintain a positive position on the imaginary wellness continuum. Many people believe wellness can best be achieved by adopting a holistic approach in which emphasis is placed on integrating mind, body, and spirit in a rhythmic interplay such that they experience optimal health and wellness in each phase of their lives. The disability component of the wellness continuum in Figure 1.1 does not imply that a person with a physical and/or intellectual disability is unwell and cannot achieve wellness. Individuals with disabilities can be healthy in all aspects of wellness—within their potential, recognizing physical and/or intellectual limitations. In contrast, a person who spends hours in front of a mirror lifting weights to perfect the size and shape of each muscle may be less healthy in the other aspects of wellness—even though he or she has no limitations regarding his or her physical and intellectual capacity.

Typically, the closer you get to your potential in the seven components of wellness, the healthier you are. Keep in mind that optimal health and wellness is not a static state that one achieves, but rather a dynamic state with various challenges and supports arising during various stages of your life. These supports and challenges to your health and wellness can in fact happen on a daily, weekly, monthly, and yearly basis. As such, try to perceive your health and wellness in a continual flux where you continuously work on making the best choices to find a rhythm and flow for living your best in the moment while recognizing the influence of your choices on your future health and wellness.

Complete the 'How Healthy Are You?' questionnaire at the end of this chapter to get a better perspective of your capacity and potential in each of the wellness dimensions discussed in this section.

Health Promotion: Helping You Stay Healthy

In discussions of health and wellness, the term **health promotion** is often used. Health promotion generally refers to all efforts made to encourage healthy behaviours with a goal of improving the health of an individual or population (World Health Organization, 2013). Health promotion requires educational, organizational, environmental, political, and financial supports to help individuals and groups build positive health attitudes and behaviours and to change negative ones. In other words, health promotion does not just involve telling people

FIGURE 1.2
Socio Ecological Model

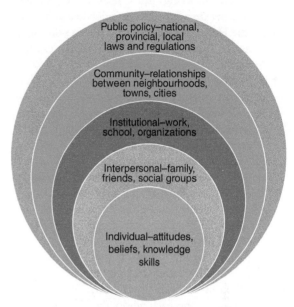

Source: McLeroy, K. R., Bibeau, D., Steckler, A., & Glanz, K. (1988). An Ecological Perspective on Health Promotion Programs. *Health Education & Behavior, 15*(4), 351–377. http://doi.org/10.1177/109019818801500401.

to lose weight and to eat better. Efforts are also made to promote learning (*educational supports*), provide programs and services that encourage participation (*organizational supports*), establish rules governing attitudes and behaviours and supporting decisions to change (*environmental policies and supports*), and provide monetary incentives or disincentives to motivate them toward healthful decision making (*financial supports or barriers*). These supports are not independent, but rather crosscutting and must deal with many of the same issues, including gender inequity, poverty, and the social determinants of health in the efforts made at health promotion (Gould, Fleming, & Parker, 2012). Thus our health is influenced by multilevel factors in the environments where we work, live, and play. Figure 1.2 depicts the multiple levels of factors that can interact to influence our health

In short, health promotion enhances the likelihood that, once a person decides to change a behaviour, conditions are optimal for successful implementation of that change. In health promotion, healthy people at risk for disease are identified and efforts are made to motivate them to improve their health. Further, various health promotion efforts encourage those whose health and wellness are already sound to maintain and improve their relevant health-enhancing activities for immediate and long-term health.

Health promotion Various efforts aimed at encouraging individuals and communities to make healthier choices.

An example of health promotion is the *Integrated Pan-Canadian Healthy Living Strategy 2005* (ACPHHS, 2006). This strategy is the result of an extensive, deeply involved and involving pan-Canadian consultation process. Rather than focusing on individual behaviour change, the Healthy Living Strategy takes a population health approach, recognizing that sustainable changes in individual behaviours are difficult to achieve without addressing living and working conditions. Thus, one of the key elements of the Strategy is to recognize and address linkages between lifestyle choices and the surrounding social, economic, and environmental influences (ACPHHS, 2006). Actions proposed through this Strategy should improve the health status and health outcomes of the Canadian population (ACPHHS, 2006). Further, the proposed actions, if implemented, should reduce the current burden and contribute to the efficiency and sustainability of Canada's universal health-care delivery system.

Through "healthy living targets" the Strategy emphasizes healthy eating and physical activity, and their relationship to healthy weight. As mentioned, a population health approach guides the Healthy Living Strategy. Using this approach, healthy living refers to the attitudes and behaviours that improve or maintain the health of the entire population and its subgroups (ACPHHS, 2006). When this approach is applied to individuals, healthy living refers to enhancing healthy behaviours, making healthy choices, and living in healthy ways. At all levels, the social, economic, political, cultural, and environmental conditions must be supportive of healthy living.

The Strategy has since been supported and enhanced through the creation and implementation of two more federal, provincial, and territorial government initiatives (Public Health Agency of Canada, 2010). The first is the "Declaration on Prevention and Promotion" in which the Ministers of Health and Healthy Living/Promotion agreed to work together to prioritize health promotion and the prevention of disease and injury. The second is "Curbing Childhood Obesity: A Federal, Provincial, and Territorial Framework for Action to Promote Healthy Weights" (Public Health Agency of Canada, 2011a). The focus of this initiative, as noted in the title, is to reduce childhood obesity by creating environments that support physical activity and healthy eating, identifying and addressing risk for obesity early, and increasing the availability and accessibility of healthy foods (Public Health Agency of Canada, 2011a).

Whether we use the term *health* or *wellness*, we are talking about a person's overall responses to the everyday challenges of living. An occasional dip into the ice cream bucket, a missed walk, an outburst of anger, or other deviations from optimal behaviours should not be viewed as major failures in attaining or maintaining your health and wellness. In fact, the ability to recognize that each of us is an imperfect being trying to adapt in an imperfect world signals individual well-being. Further, living life means that you savour some less healthy foods in smaller quantities, infrequently, and that there are times when your usual level of physical activity is not possible or you get a short night's sleep. This means that it is your *overall* approach or rhythmical interplay of healthy eating, physical activity, and other lifestyle habits that is of greater importance than any one element in that approach, and this should be your focus in your efforts to attain and maintain optimal health and wellness.

We must also remember to be tolerant of others trying to improve their health. We need to be supportive, understanding, and nonjudgmental in our interactions with those attempting to make positive changes to their lifestyle. Further, health bashing—intolerance or negative feelings, words, or actions aimed at people who fail to meet our expectations of healthy attitudes and behaviours—indicates deficiencies in our personal intellectual, mental, social, and spiritual dimensions of health.

Prevention: The Key to Future Health

Prevention means taking action now to avoid becoming sick or less well later. Getting immunized against diseases such as polio, measles, mumps, and hepatitis; not smoking or chewing tobacco; practising safer sex; eating well; engaging in regular physical activity; and taking other preventive measures constitute **primary prevention**—actions designed to prevent health problems. This would include programming which provides opportunities for children to engage in health promoting behaviours. For example, school breakfast programs or The Good Food Box, a community based initiative that provides fresh fruits and vegetable at an affordable price. **Secondary prevention** refers to the early recognition of a health issue and intervention to eliminate or reduce it before an even more serious illness develops. Modifying your dietary intake and physical activity levels in response to elevated blood-cholesterol or blood-glucose is an example of secondary prevention.

At least two-thirds of deaths in Canada are a result of cardiovascular diseases, cancer, type 2 diabetes, and respiratory diseases (Public Health Agency of Canada, 2011b; World Health Organization, 2013). These chronic diseases share common preventable risk factors: physical inactivity, poor dietary intake, and tobacco use. Further, these risk factors are influenced

Primary prevention Actions designed to reduce the chances of a health issue arising, or perhaps to delay the age at which it occurs.

Secondary prevention Intervention early in the development of a health problem to reduce symptoms or to halt or at the least delay its progression.

by income, employment, education, geographic isolation, and social exclusion. Common sense suggests that health promotion dollars should focus on the primary and secondary prevention of these and other lifestyle-related diseases. However, government money is primarily allocated for research and **tertiary prevention**—that is, treatment or rehabilitation efforts made after a person has become sick. (This is clearly a misnomer, since tertiary prevention is not really prevention at all, but rather a response *after* illness has developed.) In addition, although the intent of tertiary prevention is to prevent the further development or progression of the disease (for example, chemotherapy and radiation therapy for individuals with cancer, or coronary bypass surgery for people with cardiovascular disease), it is more costly and less effective in promoting health than primary and secondary prevention.

SEX DIFFERENCES

Although much of male and female anatomy is the same, it is clear that many major medical differences exist. Many diseases—osteoporosis, arthritis, headaches, thyroid disease, lupus, and Alzheimer's disease, for example—are far more common in women than in men. Heart disease, high blood pressure, and stroke are more common in men—at least until women reach menopause. About 8 percent of the population is affected by autoimmune diseases, but 78 percent of those affected are women (Medicinenet.com, n.d.). Further, diseases may manifest differently in women than in men—for example, symptoms of a heart attack in women are more vague than in men. Finally, although women live longer than men, they do not necessarily have a better quality of life (Miller, 1994).

Sex bias has been identified as a serious weakness in medical research. In one study that reviewed medical journals in Canada and the United States, four factors reflecting bias were identified: androcentricity, overgeneralization, gender insensitivity, and double standards (Eichler, Reisman, & Borins, 1992; Ruiz & Verbrugge, 1997). *Androcentricity* refers to viewing the world from a male perspective. *Overgeneralization* occurs when a study explores issues for one sex and generalizes the findings to both sexes. (The same thing can be said for age bias—that is, conducting research on 20-year-olds and applying the results to all adults.) In the past, studies that examined the precise effects of a drug or treatment did not include women because researchers did not want to deal with potential issues related to hormonal fluctuations. *Sex insensitivity* means overlooking sex as an important variable. An example of sex insensitivity is research on symptoms of heart disease in men and women where the data

from both sexes is analyzed in combination, disregarding potential similarities and differences. When differences do not exist between men and women, the data can be collapsed and analyzed together; otherwise, sex should be a controlled variable with the data analyzed separately. The term *double standards* refers to the "evaluation, treatment or measurement of the identical behaviours, traits or situations by different means" (Eichler, Reisman, & Borins, 1992). In 1996, a policy on clinical trials stated that if the product is likely to be used by women, then the testing must also be done on women. There has been increasing pressure placed on government to provide a more balanced approach to funding women's health programs. One example of increased activism is in the area of breast cancer. In Canada, one in nine women will be diagnosed with breast cancer and one in 29 will die from it (Canadian Cancer Society, 2013), yet it was not until the mid-1990s that any significant amount of research was conducted on the causes, treatments, and social and psychological concerns of women diagnosed with it.

IMPROVING YOUR HEALTH

Benefits of Achieving Optimal Health

Figure 1.3 provides an overview of the leading causes of death in Canada. Cancer is now the leading cause of mortality (death) for men and women (Statistics Canada, 2012), though in the past, heart disease was the leading cause of death in men and women. This change is likely due to the improvements in medical technology regarding diagnosis and treatment of various heart diseases. (See Chapter 12 for more details.)

While you cannot change your genetic history, and you may have little control over the medical services available in your area, you can influence your present and future health status by the attitudes and behaviours you choose today. Changing your lifestyle to improve your health status will not only lead to improved quality of life today but also reduced risk for cancer, cardiovascular disease, and other major chronic diseases. Although the reduction of risk for disease is a laudable reason for making lifestyle changes, this reason seldom resonates with young people—after all, a disease you may get when you are 50, 60, or 70 years old does not seem to matter as much when you are 18 to 22 years of age! The following reasons may resonate with you as to why you should focus on your health today:

- greater energy levels and increased capacity for and interest in having fun

Tertiary prevention Treatment or rehabilitation efforts aimed at limiting the effects of a disease.

FIGURE 1.3

Leading Causes of Death Among Adults in Canada, 2012

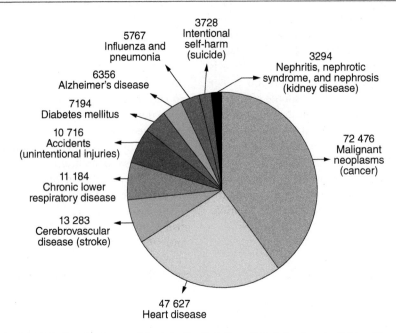

3728
Intentional
self-harm
(suicide)

5767
Influenza and
pneumonia

6356
Alzheimer's disease

7194
Diabetes mellitus

10 716
Accidents
(unintentional injuries)

11 184
Chronic lower
respiratory disease

13 283
Cerebrovascular
disease (stroke)

47 627
Heart disease

3294
Nephritis, nephrotic
syndrome, and nephrosis
(kidney disease)

72 476
Malignant
neoplasms
(cancer)

Source: Data from Table 102-0561. "Leading Causes of Death by Sex (Both Sexes)" Statistics Canada. Retrieved from www5.statcan .gc.ca/cansim/a26?lang=eng&id=1020561.

- a stronger immune system, which enhances your ability to fight infections, including the flu and common cold
- improved self-confidence, self-concept and self-esteem, and self-efficacy
- enhanced relationships with others due to better communication and "quality" time
- better sleep; longer and more restful sleep
- increased ability to handle the physical and mental reactions to stress
- a reduced reliance on the health-care system
- improved cardiovascular functioning, thus an enhanced capacity to be physically active
- increased muscle tone, strength, flexibility, and endurance, which results in ease of movement, improved physical appearance, and self-esteem
- a more positive outlook on life, fewer negative thoughts, and an ability to view life as challenging and see negative events as opportunities for growth
- improved environmental sensitivity, responsibility, and behaviours
- enhanced levels of spiritual health, awareness, and feelings of oneness with yourself, others, and the environment

Preparing for Behaviour Change

While it is easy to list things that one *should* do and even things that one may really *want* to do, behaviour change is not easy. It does not matter where you are on the health and wellness continuum, you can start wherever you are at and make changes to improve your health today. The key is to decide what needs to change, determine the actions necessary to make the change, set up a plan of action, put the plan into action, and then reinforce and maintain the plan. First, it is important to take a closer look at the factors that may contribute to your current health attitudes and behaviours.

In regard to behaviour change, Mark Twain said "habit is habit, and not to be flung out the window by anyone, but coaxed downstairs a step at a time." In other words, changing your attitudes and behaviours into healthier ones is a time-consuming and difficult process. The chance of successfully changing attitudes and behaviours improves when you make gradual changes that give you time to unlearn negative patterns and substitute positive ones. We have not yet developed a foolproof method for effectively changing attitudes and behaviours, and it may be, in fact, that different approaches work effectively for different individuals. To understand how the process of behaviour change

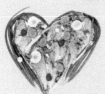
works, we must first identify specific behaviour patterns and try to understand the reasons for them.

Factors Influencing Behaviour Change

Figure 1.4 identifies three categories of factors involved in your attitudes, behaviours, and behaviour-change decisions.

Predisposing Factors

Our life experiences, knowledge, cultural and ethnic inheritance, and current beliefs and values are *predisposing factors*. These are factors that are likely to lead to a particular behaviour. These factors that predispose you to certain attitudes and behaviours include your age, sex, ethnicity, income, family, education, environment, and access to health care. For example, if your parents smoked, you are 90 percent more likely to start smoking than someone whose parents did not. However, it may only be the mothers' smoking behaviour that has an impact on their adolescent children's smoking behaviour (Harakeh, Scholte, & Vermulst, 2010). It should also be noted that the family influence on smoking behaviour also relates to family poverty as well as family processes such as monitoring and bonding (Hill et al., 2005). It is further estimated that if your peers smoke, you are 80 percent more likely to smoke than someone whose friends do not. A discerning factor here is whether this effect is due to peer influence or peer selection (Scherrer et al., 2012).

Enabling Factors

Skills or abilities; physical, mental, and intellectual capabilities; and resources and accessible facilities that make health decisions more convenient or difficult are *enabling factors*. Positive enablers encourage you to carry through on your intentions. Negative enablers work against your intentions to change. For example, if you would like to join a local fitness centre and

FIGURE 1.4

Factors That Influence Your Behaviour-Change Decisions

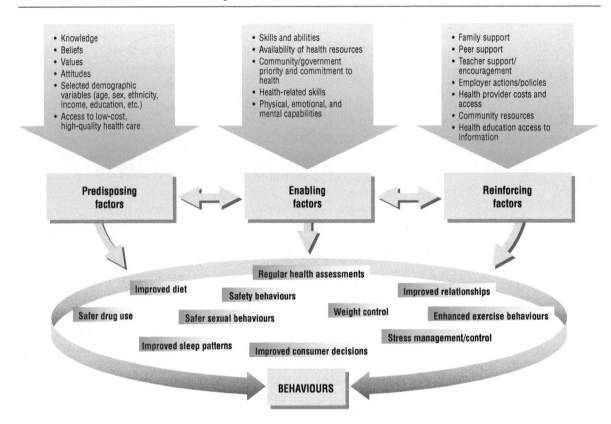

discover that the closest one is 10 kilometres away and the membership fee is $1000, these factors may deter you from joining. On the other hand, if your school's fitness centre is in the midst of campus, open from 6 a.m. until midnight, and has a reduced rate for students, these positive enablers might convince you to use it. Identifying the positive and negative enabling factors and devising alternative plans when the negative factors outweigh the positive ones is part of the necessary planning for behavioural change.

Reinforcing Factors

Reinforcing factors refer to the support and encouragement or discouragement that come from significant others or situations in your life that enable a particular behaviour. For example, if you decide you want to reduce the amount you drink and your friends continually pressure you to drink more when you are partying with them, you may be tempted to keep drinking rather than keep within the limits you set for yourself. In other words, your drinking behaviour is reinforced, rather than the change in drinking behaviours you wanted to make. If, however, your friends do not pressure you to drink, but rather rely

on you at the end of the party to drive them home, your behaviour change has been positively reinforced. Strict laws against drinking and driving, as well as various efforts on most campuses to raise awareness regarding the risks of binge drinking, may also reinforce your choice to drink less. Reinforcing factors that may influence you toward positive or negative behaviours include money, popularity, support and appreciation from friends, and family interest and enthusiasm for what you are doing.

The way you reward or punish yourself for your successes and failures may affect your chances of adopting healthy behaviours. Learning to accept small failures or setbacks and to concentrate on your successes—regardless of how small they are—may foster further successes. Berating yourself because you ate a bag of chips, argued with a friend, or did not jog when planned can create an internal environment in which failure becomes inevitable. Telling yourself that you are worth the extra time and effort and giving yourself a pat on the back for small accomplishments is an often-overlooked factor in successfully changing your attitudes and behaviours. We often need to remind ourselves about how good it feels when we make positive efforts and enact our choices to live better.

It is not our intent to blame you or make you feel guilty if you realize that some of your health attitudes and behaviours are not as good for your health and wellness as they could be. We also recognize—as should you—that all the variables that affect health are not within your control. Our goal is to help you realize which factors are within your control and to help you to make better decisions regarding those factors—to maintain or improve your current health and to prevent premature ill-health.

Making changes in your health behaviours requires careful thinking and planning rather than following easy, one-step recipes. In fact, lasting behaviour changes require careful thought, individual analysis, and considerable effort. Changing beliefs, attitudes, values, and behaviours that have been part of your life for a long time is difficult. Even the most strong-willed, disciplined people discover that willpower alone is not enough to get them through the changes needed to make lifelong behaviour changes.

Wanting to change is a prerequisite of the change process, as is recognizing the need to change, but there is much more to the process than motivation. Motivation must be combined with common sense, commitment, and a realistic understanding of how best to move forward with your plan for change. *Readiness* is the state of being that precedes behaviour change. People who are ready to change possess or develop the knowledge, attitudes, skills, and internal and external resources that make change a likely reality. For someone to be ready for change, certain basic steps and adjustments in thinking must occur as described in the following section.

Understanding When to Change vs. What to Change?

Have you ever come up with a great New Year's (or Monday-morning) resolution about something you are going to "do differently" only to have your good intention forgotten or ignored a few days later? As most people discover, changing established attitudes and behaviours is not an easy task. Much of what we do is influenced by a number of variables, including our history, reward systems, values, and culture. You have been doing the same sorts of things for years, and these behaviours become a part of who you are. Thus, changing that part of you will not be easy. Finding out where you are and how ready you are to change may help you in doing so.

Stages of Change, Transtheoretical Model

A number of theories or models are used to explain the behaviour change process. One of these is the Stages of Change or Transtheoretical model created by Prochaska

and DiClemente (1983). Developed from research on smoking cessation and drug and alcohol addiction, the Stages of Change model has been applied to a wide range of health behaviours, including HIV prevention, physical activity, and healthier eating. Essentially, the Stages of Change model asks

1. Are you ready for change?
2. Where are you in terms of readiness to change?

This probably sounds a bit familiar to you; the Stages of Change model indicates that the readier you are to change and the greater your motivation to change, the more likely it is that you will succeed at change. From their research, Prochaska and DiClemente (1983) concluded that an individual proceeds through distinctive stages. These stages are

1. **Precontemplation.** People in the precontemplation stage have no intention at the moment of changing. They likely are not even aware of a need to change. They may also have tried to change a behaviour before and given up.

> *Strategies for Change:* Sometimes a few frank yet kind words may be enough to help people in this stage to take a closer look at themselves. Improving knowledge by recommending readings or making tactful suggestions may help people in the precontemplation stage consider a need for change.

> *For example:* If you are not physically active, you might need to learn about the risks of inactivity and the benefits of regular physical activity. You should also consider the concerns you have—all of them regarding your participation in physical activity. Your goal at this stage is simply to *recognize* there is a need to become more physically active.

2. **Contemplation.** In this phase, people recognize that they need to change and are thinking about making a change. This acknowledgment of a need to change usually results from increased awareness, often due to input from family and friends or access to information or increased knowledge. People can languish in this stage for years, realizing that they have a problem, but lacking the time, energy, motivation, or knowledge to make the change.

> *Strategies for Change:* Often, people in this stage need a little push to get them thinking more seriously about the need to change. This may come in the form of further increasing awareness of the benefits of becoming more physically active (for example, more energy to accomplish more in a day), buying a helpful gift (such as a low-fat cookbook), sharing articles about a particular problem, or inviting them to go with you to hear a speaker on a related topic. People often need time to think about a course of action or to build the skills

needed to change. Your assistance can help them move off the point of indecision.

For example: At this stage, you may need to consider the obstacles or barriers to you becoming more physically active. You should also consider the benefits of an active lifestyle. You may even commit to *when* you will start to become more active and what steps you need to take to get ready to be active.

3. **Preparation.** Most people at this point are close to taking action. They know they need to change; they have been thinking about it and are ready to come up with a plan. Rather than thinking about why they cannot make the change right now, they have started to focus on what they can do to move into the action phase—to actually becoming more active.

Strategies for Change: People in the preparation stage benefit from a few simple guidelines: setting realistic goals (short and long term), learning about what is available and accessible to them, and coming up with a written plan. It may also be useful to identify factors that have enabled success or served as a barrier to success in the past, and modify them where possible.

For example: Once again, focus on the obstacles or barriers to you becoming more physically active. This time, think specifically about what has hindered you in the past. Plan when and where you will be active. Ensure you have the appropriate footwear and clothing. Set short- and long-term goals (for example, in the first week, I will walk twice to work; at the end of the year, I will run five kilometres). Focus on the positive, you can do it!

4. **Action.** In this stage, people actually make the change. Success comes to those prepared for change, specifically if you have considered alternatives, engaged social support, and made a realistic plan of action, you are more ready than those who have given change little thought.

Strategies for Change: Publicly stating the desire to change helps ensure success. Encourage friends making a change to share their plans with you. Offer to help, and try to remove potential obstacles from their intended action plan. Social support and the buddy system can provide a good source of motivation.

For example: At this stage, you do the physical activity you planned. Be positive, stay focused, and consider unexpected challenges to prepare for them.

5. **Maintenance.** Maintenance requires vigilance, attention to detail, and long-term commitment. Many people reach a goal, only to relax and slip back into the undesired behaviours. In this stage, it is important to be aware of the potential for relapses and develop strategies for dealing with such challenges. Common causes of relapse include no longer planning for the change, overconfidence, daily temptations, stress or emotional distractions, and self-deprecation.

Strategies for Change: During maintenance, continue taking the same actions that led to success in the first place. Find fun and creative ways to maintain positive behaviours. This is where a willing and caring support group can be vital. Knowing where on campus to turn for help when you do not have a close support network is also helpful.

For example: Praise and reward yourself for your current success. Continue to plan for your physical activities. Focus on *how* you have achieved success. Again, consider unexpected challenges to your physical activity participation and prepare for them.

6. **Termination.** Although some do not believe this stage actually exists and that a person may always have to put effort into continuing with his or her new behaviour, others believe that there is a point at which the behaviour becomes ingrained and is the "new" habit. In other words, the new behaviour becomes a part of daily living.

For example: At this point, you simply are physically active each and every day; you naturally look for ways to include physical activity in your daily life in addition to "working out."

7. **Relapse.** This is another stage that may or may not really exist. Relapse refers to the times when one does not continue with the behaviour change. Perhaps you were regularly physically active all term and then when final exams approached, you missed your daily swim for a week or two. Some may give up their new behaviour at this point, thinking they have failed. At this stage, it is important to learn from what happened, and accept that there are real reasons that lead to you not being able to keep up with your plan. Return to your plan and learn from your relapse in efforts to not allow that to happen again.

For example: During reading week, you decide to travel to an all-inclusive resort to enjoy some time away from the books. While away on your seven-day vacation, you do little more than lounge in the sun reading. When you return, choose to be physically active again; get back into the routine you had prior to your vacation. Do not let a day or two go by before getting back into it. Next time you go on vacation, think about how you can include physical activity. You could walk along the beach, swim lengths in the pool or ocean, play beach volleyball, dance, and so on.

Your Beliefs and Attitudes

Even if you know why and when you should make a specific behaviour change, your beliefs and attitudes about the value of your actions in making a difference (that is, whether or not making this change will have an impact) will significantly affect what you do. We assume that when rational people realize there is a risk in what they are doing, they will act to reduce that risk. But this is not necessarily true. Consider the number of people who smoke, fail to manage their stress response, consume high-fat diets, are inactive, and act in other less healthy ways. We all know better, but our "knowing" is often disconnected from our "doing." In other words, knowledge does not equal behaviours. Why not? Two strong influences on our actions are beliefs and attitudes.

A **belief** is an appraisal of the relationship between some object, action, or idea (for example, smoking) and some attribute of that object, action, or idea (for example, smoking is expensive, and smelly, and causes cancer—or, it is a sexy, cool, adult activity). Beliefs develop either from direct experience (for example, you become winded going up several flights of stairs from your smoking) or from secondhand experience or knowledge conveyed by other people (for example, if you see your grandfather, a pack-a-day smoker, die of lung cancer or emphysema) (DiMatteo, 1994). Although most of us have a general idea of what constitutes a belief, we may be a bit uncertain about what constitutes an attitude. We often hear or make such comments as "He has a rotten attitude," or "She needs an attitude adjustment," but may not be able to define *attitude*. An **attitude** is a relatively stable set of beliefs, feelings, and behavioural tendencies in relation to something or someone.

Do Beliefs and Attitudes Influence Behaviours?

It seems logical to conclude that your beliefs will influence your behaviours. If you believe (make the appraisal) that taking drugs (an action) is harmful for you (an attribute of that action), you will choose not to use drugs. If you believe that drinking and driving are incompatible, you will choose not to drink and drive. Or will you? Psychologists studying the relationship between beliefs and health behaviours determined that although beliefs may subtly influence behaviours, they may not actually cause people to change them. The **health belief model (HBM)** explains how beliefs may or may not influence subsequent behaviours (see Figure 1.5). According to this widely accepted model,

Belief Appraisal of the relationship between some object, action, or idea and some attribute of that object, action, or idea.

Attitude Relatively stable set of beliefs, feelings, and behavioural tendencies in relation to something or someone.

Health belief model (HBM) Model for explaining how our beliefs about our health may influence our attitudes and behaviours regarding our health and wellness.

FIGURE 1.5
Health Belief Model

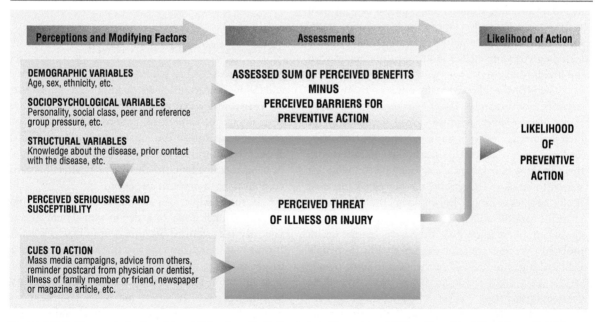

Source: Adapted by permission from Edward P. Sarafino, *Health Psychology: Biopsychosocial Interactions*, John Wiley & Sons, © 1990 by John Wiley & Sons.

several factors must support a belief in order for your behaviour to be affected (Sarafino, 1990):

- **Perceived seriousness of the health problem.** First, you consider how severe the medical and social consequences would be if the health problem were to develop or be left untreated. The more serious you believe the effects will be, the more likely you are to take action. For example, cancer is the leading cause of death for Canadians; therefore, you may perceive cancer as a serious health problem, one that you will make choices to avoid.

- **Perceived susceptibility to the health problem.** Another factor you consider is the likelihood that you will develop the health problem. If you perceive yourself as more likely to develop the health problem, you are more likely to take preventive action. For example, if your mother and sister were recently diagnosed with breast cancer, you are likely to consider yourself highly susceptible to breast cancer too and thus are more likely to adapt your behaviours accordingly.

- **Cues to action.** For some, when you are reminded or told about a potential health problem, you are more likely to take preventive action. For example, if your doctor tells you that your blood sugar levels are indicative of a prediabetic state, that may be the cue you need to eat better and become more physically active to prevent full-blown type 2 diabetes.

Three other factors are also linked to your perceived risk for health problems: *demographic variables,* including age, sex, ethnicity, and cultural background; *sociopsychological variables,* including personality traits, social class, and social pressure; and *structural variables,* including your knowledge about or prior contact with the health issue.

The HBM is followed many times every day. Take smokers, for example. Older smokers are likely to know other smokers who developed serious heart or lung diseases as a result of smoking. They are thus more likely to perceive a threat to their health connected with their smoking behaviour than a young person who just started to smoke. The greater the perceived threat of health problems caused by smoking, the greater the chance a person will quit smoking. However, many chronic smokers know that they have serious health problems, yet they continue to smoke. Why do people fail to take actions to avoid further harm? Some people do not believe that they will be affected by a severe problem—they act as if they have some kind of immunity—and thus are unlikely to change their behaviours. In some cases, they think that, even if they get cancer or have a heart attack, the health-care system and latest technologic developments will be able to take care of them. For these individuals, a cue such as a personal scare with heart disease, such as a mild heart attack, may be the cue needed to push them into action.

It may be particularly difficult for young people like you to believe in the importance of making healthier choices right now, as heart disease, cancer, type 2 diabetes, and other chronic diseases are a long way off. Further, this model focuses on making lifestyle choices to prevent illness or disease rather than making healthy lifestyle choices to feel better NOW. It is possible that if the focus is on feeling better today, feeling more energetic and capable of doing all you want to do (and any of the other things listed previously in this chapter), that young people may consider making lifestyle changes.

Other factors from the HBM that affect the likelihood of behaviour change are assessments about whether the benefits outweigh the costs and whether proposed actions will actually make a difference (that is, reduce risk and improve health). If you are addicted to nicotine, the thought of quitting may not be acceptable to you, and if you enjoy smoking too much, you will probably keep smoking—particularly if the consequences will not be felt for some time and the pleasure is instant. Similarly, you are not likely to make the effort to do something (for example, go for a jog) if you do not feel the health-related benefits right away. Most times, the health benefits take time to be felt. This is another challenge, since you are more likely to continue with a change in behaviour if your actions result in more immediate positive feedback.

Your Intentions to Change

Your attitudes tend to reflect your emotional responses and follow from your beliefs. According to the **theory of reasoned action**, your behaviours result from your intentions to perform actions. An intention is a result of your attitude toward an action and your beliefs about what others may want you to do (Bishop, 1994). A behavioural intention, then, is a written or stated commitment to perform an action.

If, for example, you are out of shape and struggle to get as much done in a day as you would like to, you may take steps to become more physically active. If your best friend also tells you that you really do need to get in shape and you value this person's opinion, your intention to become more physically active will become stronger. In brief, the more consistent and powerful your attitudes about an action, and the more you are influenced by others to take that action, the greater your intention to do so will grow. Further,

Theory of reasoned action Model for explaining the importance of our intentions in regard to our behaviours.

point of view

PROMOTING HEALTH TO COLLEGE AND UNIVERSITY STUDENTS: Short- or Long-term Focus?

When you think of your health and what motivates you to make the decisions you do, what first comes to mind? Be honest. Are your choices made based upon immediate gratification? Do you think about how your choices influence your health in the short- or long-term? It may be useful for you to better understand what motivates you regarding the decisions you make on a daily basis that influence your everyday health, as well as the potential influence of these decisions in the long-term if continued.

Consider something like choosing to be physically active—whether it is to go for a walk alone or with a friend, 'work out' in your campus facilities, play Frisbee with your roommates, or something else, which of the following better address your motivations to do so?

SHORT-TERM

- have fun
- reduce stress
- spend time with friends
- take a break from studying
- burn calories, to maintain weight
- sleep better at night
- feel better about yourself

LONG-TERM

- reduce risk for heart disease
- reduce risk for cancer
- reduce risk for type 2 diabetes
- maintain fitness for independent living in older age
- reduce risk of depression
- reduce risk of other chronic diseases

If you are not currently physically active on a regular basis, you might also look at these two lists and think about which is more likely to motivate you to decide to become more physically active NOW.

Health promotion efforts should be tailored to meet individual and specific needs at the point in time when the decision is being made. Chances are that you do not consider the long-term health implications of not being physically active as a primary motivator to become or continue to be physically active. It is likely that you do not perceive yourself as susceptible to the various chronic diseases for which risk is reduced. Until you perceive yourself as susceptible, you are not likely to be motivated for long-term health reasons. However, if you perceive the short-term reasons to be physically active as important, and perceive a lack of them in yourself, then you are more likely to be become physically active as a result.

the more you verbalize your commitment to the action, the more likely it is that you will do it.

Significant Others as Change Agents

Many people are highly influenced by the approval or disapproval (real or imagined) of close friends and loved ones and of the social and cultural groups to which they belong. Such influences can offer support for health actions, making healthy behaviours more possible to attain; they can also affect behaviours negatively, interfering with even the best intentions of making a positive change.

Your Family

For most of you, from the time you were born, your parents influenced your behaviours by giving you strong cues about which actions were socially acceptable and which were not. Brushing your teeth, bathing, wearing

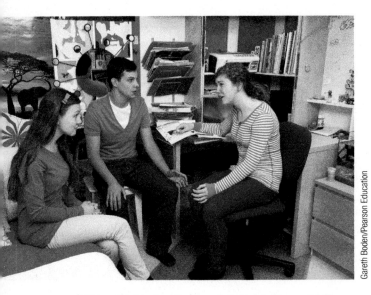

Gareth Boden/Pearson Education

Talking with friends or family can help you clarify your thinking about behaviours you want to change and provide ongoing support as you attempt to reach your goals.

deodorant, and chewing food with your mouth closed were probably behaviours that your family instilled in you long ago. Your family culture influences your food choices, your religious and political beliefs, and your other values and actions. If you deviated from your family's norms, a family member probably let you know fairly quickly.

Good family units share unconditional love and trust, dedication to the healthy development of all family members, and a commitment to working out difficulties. When a loving family unit does not exist, when it does not provide for basic human needs, or when dysfunctional individuals try to build a family under the influence of drugs or alcohol, it becomes difficult for a child to learn positive health behaviours. Healthy behaviours get their start in healthy homes; less healthy homes breed less healthy habits. Healthy families provide the foundation for a clear and necessary understanding of how to make solid decisions that lead to better health.

The Influence of Others

Just as your family influenced your actions during your childhood, now your friends, teachers/coaches, and significant others influence your behaviours as you grow older. Most of us desire to fit the "norm" and avoid hassles in our daily interactions with others. If you deviate from the actions expected in your hometown, among your friends, or in your peer group, you may suffer ostracism, strange looks, and other negative social consequences. Understanding the subtle and not-so-subtle ways in which other people influence your actions may be another important step in the process of changing your behaviours.

How others influence our behaviour choices is also explained in the *theory of planned behaviour* (Ajzen, 1991). This theory outlines three reasons for how you choose to act:

- **Your attitudes toward the behaviour**—for example, what you think about the positive or negative effects of your actions and the importance of each.

- **Your level of perceived behavioural control,** or your beliefs about the constraints and opportunities you might have concerning the behaviour. More specifically, how much control you think you have over the particular behaviour you want to change.

- **Your subjective norms,** or whether or not you think your actions will be approved of by the people important to you.

For example, if you want to become more physically active and reduce your risk for type 2 diabetes, you may develop strong intentions to attend an exercise program (*attitudes* toward the behaviour). Intentions are powerful indicators of successful behaviour change. If there is a convenient, affordable fitness centre near you, and if the schedule for exercise classes works for you, you will be more motivated and believe you can make the change (*control beliefs*). Finally, if your friends offer encouragement (*subjective norms*), you are more likely to remain motivated to change your behaviours. On the other hand, if you perceive that your friends do not approve of you going to an exercise class, or if the fitness centre is inconvenient (for instance, it is far away or has restricted hours of operation) or expensive, you may quickly lose your motivation. The opinions of key people play a powerful role in your motivation to change behaviours.

The influence of others can serve as a powerful social support for positive behaviour changes. Influential others can also play a role in your not-so-good health behaviours as you may also be influenced to drink too much, party too hard, eat too much, or engage in other negative actions because you do not want to be left out or because you fear criticism or being different. Learning to understand the subtle and not-so-subtle ways in which your family, friends, and others have influenced and continue to influence your behaviours is an important step toward making positive changes.

If you are part of an abusive relationship, having friends you trust and confide in can give you the strength to walk away—to change your behaviours. Someone who accepts you unconditionally and is there for you is a powerful asset to help deal with life's challenges regardless of what they are. The more social support you have, and the closer the relationship or social bonds, the greater the chances that you will be able to deal with crises in healthy ways. If you expand your social

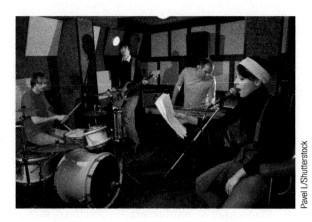

The support and encouragement of friends with similar interests will strengthen your commitment to develop and maintain positive health behaviours.

Pavel L/Shutterstock

support network to include counsellors, spiritual advisers, and others, you will further increase your likelihood of success. Whom would you call if you were stranded in the middle of a cold, snowy night on a remote road? Who would get out bed, without question, to come and get you? Surprisingly, many people have no one to call under any circumstances, let alone when they are in crisis. The importance of cultivating and maintaining close ties is an important part of overall health.

BEHAVIOUR CHANGE TECHNIQUES

Once you analyze the factors influencing your current behaviours, as well as the factors that may influence the direction and potential success of the behaviour change you are considering, you must decide which of several possible behaviour change techniques will work best for you.

Shaping: Developing New Behaviours in Small Steps

Regardless of how motivated and committed you are to change, some behaviours are difficult to change immediately because they require several smaller steps/goals to reach the ultimate goal. Thus, to reach your goal, you may need to take a number of individual steps, each designed to change one small part of the overall behaviour. This process is known as **shaping**.

For example, suppose you have been physically inactive for a long time. You decide that you want to

become more physically active and physically fit. Your long-term goal is to run almost every day and be able to complete a fun run of 5 kilometres in your community this coming summer. You realize that it is not wise—and it will hurt—to simply start running, so you decide to build up your physical fitness gradually and come up with a plan. During week 1, you will walk for 20 minutes every other day at a moderate pace. During week 2, you will walk on 5 days. In week 3, you will walk on 6 days. In week 4, you will walk for 20 minutes every day of the week. Then, in week 5, you will increase your walking time to 25 minutes on alternate days, but still walk for 7 days. Gradually, you will increase the time you walk, while maintaining a frequency of 6 or 7 days per week until you are ready to alternate walking and jogging. You may start with alternating 1 minute of walking with 1 minute of jogging, then 1 minute walking and 2 minutes jogging. These gradual steps—and more like them—will help you reach your goal.

Whatever the desired behaviour change, shaping involves:

- starting slowly to prevent or limit undue stress
- keeping the steps small and realistic/achievable
- being flexible/adaptable and ready to change if the original plan is not working
- refusing to skip steps or to move to the next step until the previous step has been mastered—or feels comfortable; your current lifestyle behaviours did not develop overnight, so they will not change overnight.
- rewarding yourself for meeting short- and long-term goals; these rewards should also be part of healthy living.

Visualizing: The Imagined Rehearsal

Mental practice and rehearsal can help in the behaviour change process. Athletes and others often use a technique called **imagined rehearsal** to reach their goals. By visualizing their planned action ahead of time, they are better prepared—and able—when they actually engage in the imagined behaviour. For example, suppose you want to ask a classmate out on a date. Imagine the setting (walking together to class). Then, in your mind and out loud, practise what you want to say ("I hear there is a dance on Friday night and I was wondering if . . ."). Mentally anticipate different responses ("Oh, I would love to, but . . ." or "That sounds like fun . . .") and what you will say in response ("That's okay, maybe another time," or "How about I text you later about

Shaping Using a series of small steps to reach a particular goal gradually.

Imagined rehearsal Practising a skill or behaviour through mental imagery.

it?"). Careful mental and verbal imagined rehearsal will greatly improve your likelihood of success.

Modelling

Modelling, or learning behaviours by carefully observing other people, is one of the most effective strategies for changing behaviours. If you carefully observe behaviours you admire, and isolate their components, you can model the steps of your behaviour-change strategy on a proven success. For example if you have trouble talking to people you do not know very well, one of the easiest ways for you to improve your communication skills is to observe someone whose communication skills you admire. Do they talk or listen more? How do they listen? What do they do when listening? How do people respond to them? What makes them good communicators? What is their body language like? Thus, when you observe the behaviours you admire and isolate their components, you can model the steps in your behaviour change based on a proven success.

Controlling the Situation

Sometimes, putting yourself in the right setting or with the right group of people will positively influence your behaviours directly or indirectly. Many situations and occasions trigger similar behaviours in different people. For example, in libraries, churches, and museums, most people talk softly. Few people laugh at funerals. The term **situational inducement** refers to an attempt to influence a behaviour by using situations and occasions structured to exert control over that behaviour. If you are trying to reduce the fat in your diet, an example could be choosing to eat at a vegetarian restaurant rather than a fast-food chain or choose lighter options such as a salad with toppings and dressing on the side.

Reinforcement

When there is **positive reinforcement**, it is likely that you will continue with a behaviour. Each of us is motivated by different reinforcers, so while a special T-shirt may be a positive reinforcer for young adults entering a fun run, it may not be for someone who dislikes message-bearing T-shirts, or for someone with

a drawer full of them. Most positive reinforcers can be classified under five headings:

- **Consumable reinforcers** are edibles such as candy, cookies, drinks, or gourmet meals. You should be careful with these reinforces as most often these reinforcers should only be consumed in moderation. Further, using food for rewards may set you up for challenges with your eating (see Chapter 6).
- **Activity reinforcers** are opportunities to participate in a fun run, go on a vacation, go swimming, or do something else enjoyable.
- **Manipulative reinforcers** are incentives such as lower rent in exchange for mowing the lawn or the promise of a better grade for doing an extra-credit project.
- **Possessional reinforcers** are tangible rewards such as a new laptop, dress, or sports car.
- **Social reinforcers** are such things as loving looks, affectionate hugs, and praise.

Changing Self-Talk

Self-talk, or the way you think and talk to yourself, also plays a role in your attempts at behaviour change. Rational-emotive therapy, Meichenbaum's self-instructional method, and blocking or thought stopping are examples of self-talk.

Rational-Emotive Therapy

This form of cognitive therapy or self-directed behaviour change is based on the premise that a close connection exists between what you say to yourself and how you feel. Rational-emotive therapy is a form of cognitive behaviour therapy that is action-oriented. During this therapy, you will be taught to identify, challenge, and replace your self-defeating thoughts and beliefs into more positive and healthier thoughts (DiGiuseppe, 2010).

Meichenbaum's Self-Instructional Methods

In Meichenbaum's behavioural therapy, you are encouraged to give *self-instructions* ("Slow down, don't rush") and *positive affirmations* ("My speech is going fine—I am almost done!") to yourself instead of thinking self-defeating thoughts ("I am talking too fast—my speech is terrible") when a situation seems to be getting out of control (Hatzigeorgiadis et al., 2011). Meichenbaum is perhaps best known for a process known as *stress inoculation,* in which clients are subjected to extreme stressors in a laboratory

Modelling Learning specific behaviours by watching others perform them.

Situational inducement Attempts to influence a behaviour by using situations and occasions structured to exert control over that behaviour.

Positive reinforcement Presenting something positive following a behaviour being reinforced.

environment. Before a stressful event (e.g., going to the doctor), clients practise individual coping skills (e.g., deep breathing exercises) and self-instructions (e.g., "I will feel better once I know what is causing my pain"). Meichenbaum demonstrated that clients who practised coping techniques and self-instruction were less likely to resort to negative behaviours in stressful situations.

Blocking or Thought Stopping

By purposely blocking or stopping negative thoughts, a person can concentrate on taking positive steps toward necessary behaviour change. For example, suppose you are preoccupied with your former partner, who recently left you for someone else. In blocking or thought stopping, you consciously stop thinking about the situation and force yourself to think about something more pleasant (for example, dinner tomorrow with your best friend). By refusing to dwell on negative images and by forcing yourself to focus elsewhere, you can save wasted energy, time, and emotional resources and move on to positive change.

MAKING BEHAVIOUR CHANGE

Self-Assessment: Antecedents and Consequences

Behaviours, thoughts, and feelings always occur in a context—the situation. Situations can be divided into two components: the events that come before a behaviour and those that come after it. *Antecedents* are the setting events for a behaviour; they cue or stimulate a person to act in certain ways. Antecedents can be physical events, thoughts, emotions, or the actions of other people. *Consequences*—the results of behaviours—affect whether a person will repeat a behaviour (Watson & Tharpe, 1993). Consequences also include physical events, thoughts, emotions, or the actions of other people.

Learning to recognize the antecedents of your behaviours and acting to modify them is one method of changing them. A diary noting your undesirable behaviours and the settings in which they occur can be useful. For example, if you are gaining weight, keep a diary of when, where, why, how, and with whom you eat. If you are eating chips while studying, you may need to study in the library, where food is not allowed, or not have that kind of snack available in your house. If you eat more when you are angry, upset, depressed, or stressed, try to deal directly with your stressors or engage in an alternative activity, such as going for a

walk or swim. The positive consequences of these changes will be that you will maintain your weight and feel better about yourself.

Analyzing the Behaviours You Want to Change

Successful behaviour change requires a careful assessment of exactly what it is that you want to change. All too often we berate ourselves by using generalities: "I am not a good person; I am lousy to my friends; I need to be a better person." Becoming a better person is a lofty goal, but difficult to define and measure. Before you can begin to change a negative behaviour, you must take a hard look at its specifics. Determining the specific behaviours you would like to change—as opposed to the general problem—will allow you to set clear goals for change. What are you doing that makes you a lousy friend? Are you gossiping about your friends? Are you lying to them? Have you been a "taker" rather than a "giver" in the friendship? Or are you really a good friend most of the time? What specifically do you do that makes you a not-so-good friend?

If the problem is gossiping, you can analyze your behaviour using the following:

- *Frequency.* How often do you gossip? In every conversation, once per day, less frequently?
- *Duration.* Have you been gossiping about your friend for a long period of time? A few weeks, a few months? Over the years?
- *Seriousness.* Is your gossiping idle chatter/sharing information, or are you really trying to injure the other person? What are the consequences for you? For your friend? For your friendship? For the person listening to you?
- *Basis for the problem behaviour.* Is your gossip based on facts, on your perceptions of facts, or on deliberate embellishments of facts? Are you trying to make yourself look or feel better? To discredit your friend?
- *Antecedents.* What kinds of situations trigger your gossiping? Do some settings or people bring out the gossip in you more than others? Why are you talking behind your friend's back?

Decision Making: Choices for Change

Once the background work is done, including the assessment of the antecedents and consequences to the behaviour you want to change, you next need to decide what to do when faced with choices that will assist or distract you from your intentions to change. Decision making is a skill you must consciously develop. Choosing among alternatives is difficult when you are consciously and unconsciously pressured by internal and external influences. For example, "just saying no" is, of course, one choice when you are handed a glass of beer or wine at a party. However, if you are trying desperately to fit in, if people with whom you identify all drink, or if you like the taste of beer or wine, the decision becomes harder. By practising the following decision-making skills prior to having that drink put into your hands, you will increase your chances of making the choice you really want to make. This set of skills, referred to by the acronym DECIDE, can be applied to many decision-making situations (Based on The Stanford DECIDE Drug Education Curriculum).[*]

D *Decide in advance what the problem is.* By defining the problem in advance, you will have time to determine how important it is. If you decide that you do not want to drink, or that drinking in certain situations puts you at risk, you will have your basic criteria for acting in specific situations.

E *Explore the alternatives.* List the possible alternatives, ranging from not drinking to drinking heavily and the various stages in between. If any of these alternatives is unacceptable to you, cross it off and work with those remaining.

C *Consider the consequences.* Think about each of the alternatives remaining. What are the possible positive and negative consequences of each? Think about what will probably happen, not just what may happen in the best and worst scenarios. How risky is each alternative? Are the consequences of losing the friendship of this particular group as serious as the risk of drinking heavily and getting into trouble sexually or drinking and driving? Or getting into a fight with someone? Is there another alternative that could reduce your risks?

I *Identify your values.* Your beliefs and feelings about certain behaviours represent your values, which then influence your behaviours. When choosing to drink or not to drink in a social setting, or when choosing how much to drink, you should base your choice on your values.

D *Decide and take action.* If you have seriously thought about the first four DECIDE components and determined that it is okay to have one or two drinks over the course of the evening and that is your absolute limit, this may be a reasonable decision for you. Then you must take action based upon this decision—you must actively take measures to ensure you stick to your limit.

E *Evaluate the consequences.* A key component of the decision-making process is a careful look backward at your decision, the decision-making process followed, and your resulting behaviours, how you felt about them, and whether you want to do anything differently in the future. You may add alternatives at the second step, for instance. The secret to success is to think about the problem in advance, consider your values and desires, and anticipate the choices you will likely face.

---

[*] Based on The Stanford DECIDE Drug Education Curriculum.

assess YOURSELF

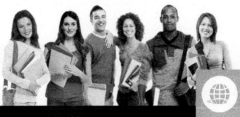

Go to MasteringHealth to complete this questionnaire with automatic scoring

TAKING CHARGE

From the information presented in this chapter, you should realize that your health and wellness include many dimensions and that changing your behaviours is a complicated, multifaceted process requiring commitment, personal insight, and knowledge. It is not likely that you can "just do it"—few of us can, at least not on the first try. As you continue to read this book, you will find that each chapter lists specific activities that enable you to choose to adopt or maintain healthy behaviours. Complete the following questionnaire and respond to the questions posed. In evaluating your current state of health and wellness, as well as considering your attitudes, values, and behaviours, you can decide whether or not there are any changes required to your lifestyle for you to achieve rhythm in your health and wellness.

How Healthy Are You?

Although many of us know we could be making better decisions that would lead to better health, we often do not recognize some of the poorer choices we make. Rate your health status in each of the following dimensions by circling the number of the response that best describes you. Honest responses will help you to determine where you most need to enact change.

After completing this section, how healthy do you think you are? Which area(s), if any, do you think you should work on improving? Respond to the following questions regarding each dimension of health by circling the number for the response that best describes you.

Rate yourself

	Very Unhealthy	Somewhat Unhealthy	Somewhat Healthy	Very Healthy
Physical Health	1	2	3	4
Social Health	1	2	3	4
Emotional Health	1	2	3	4
Environmental Health	1	2	3	4
Spiritual Health	1	2	3	4
Intellectual Health	1	2	3	4
Occupational Health	1	2	3	4

1 Physical Health

	Rarely, If Ever	Sometimes	Most of the Time	Always
1. I maintain a healthy weight.	1	2	3	4
2. I engage in moderate to vigorous physical activities such as brisk walking, jogging, swimming, or running for at least 150 minutes per week.	1	2	3	4
3. I do exercises designed to strengthen my muscles and joints as well as those to maintain my flexibility.	1	2	3	4
4. I follow Eating Well with Canada's Food Guide, obtaining the minimum serving in each food group on an almost daily basis.	1	2	3	4
5. I reduce my intake of excessive fat, salt, and sugars.	1	2	3	4
6. I get 7–8 hours of sleep each night.	1	2	3	4

(continued)

	Rarely, If Ever	Sometimes	Most of the Time	Always
7. My immune system is strong and I am able to avoid most infectious diseases, and when sick my body heals itself quickly	1	2	3	4
8. I do not use tobacco products.	1	2	3	4
9. I have lots of energy and can get through the day without being overly tired.	1	2	3	4
10. I listen to my body; when there is something wrong, I seek professional advice.	1	2	3	4

2 Social Health

	Rarely, If Ever	Sometimes	Most of the Time	Always
1. When I meet people, I feel good about the impression I make on them.	1	2	3	4
2. I am open, honest, and get along well with other people.	1	2	3	4
3. I participate in a wide variety of social activities and enjoy being with people who are different from me.	1	2	3	4
4. I try to be a "better person" and work on behaviours that have caused problems in my interactions with others.	1	2	3	4
5. I get along well with the members of my family.	1	2	3	4
6. I am a good listener.	1	2	3	4
7. I am open and accessible to a loving and responsible relationship.	1	2	3	4
8. I have someone I can talk to about my private feelings.	1	2	3	4
9. I consider the feelings of others and do not act in hurtful or selfish ways.	1	2	3	4
10. I consider how what I say might be perceived by others before I speak.	1	2	3	4

3 Emotional Health

	Rarely, If Ever	Sometimes	Most of the Time	Always
1. I find it easy to laugh about things that happen in my life.	1	2	3	4
2. I avoid using alcohol as a means of helping me forget my problems.	1	2	3	4
3. I can express my feelings without feeling silly.	1	2	3	4
4. When I am angry, I try to let others know in non-confrontational and non-hurtful ways.	1	2	3	4
5. I am a chronic worrier and tend to be suspicious of others.	4	3	2	1
6. I recognize when I am stressed and take steps to relax through physical activity, quiet time, or other activities.	1	2	3	4
7. I feel good about myself and believe others like me for who I am.	1	2	3	4
8. When I am upset, I talk to others and actively try to work through my problems.	1	2	3	4
9. I am flexible and adapt or adjust to change in a positive way.	1	2	3	4
10. My friends regard me as a stable, emotionally well-adjusted person.	1	2	3	4

4 Environmental Health

	Rarely, If Ever	Sometimes	Most of the Time	Always
1. I am concerned about environmental pollution and actively try to preserve and protect natural resources.	1	2	3	4
2. I report people who intentionally hurt the environment.	1	2	3	4
3. I recycle my garbage.	1	2	3	4
4. I reuse plastic and paper bags and tin foil.	1	2	3	4
5. I vote for pro-environmental candidates in municipal, provincial, and federal elections.	1	2	3	4
6. I write my elected leaders about environmental concerns.	1	2	3	4
7. I consider the amount of product packaging before I make a purchase.	1	2	3	4
8. I try to buy products that are recyclable.	1	2	3	4
9. I use both sides of the paper when taking class notes or doing assignments.	1	2	3	4
10. I try to reduce the amount of water I use when I brush my teeth, shave, or bathe.	1	2	3	4

5 Spiritual Health

	Rarely, If Ever	Sometimes	Most of the Time	Always
1. I believe life is a precious gift that should be nurtured.	1	2	3	4
2. I take time to enjoy nature and the beauty around me.	1	2	3	4
3. I take time alone to think about what is important in life—who I am, what I value, where I fit in, and where I am going.	1	2	3	4
4. I have faith in a greater power, be it a divinity, nature, the connectedness of all living things, or something else.	1	2	3	4
5. I engage in acts of caring and goodwill without expecting anything in return.	1	2	3	4
6. I feel sorrow for those who are suffering and try to help them through difficult times.	1	2	3	4
7. I feel confident that I have touched the lives of others in a positive way.	1	2	3	4
8. I work for peace in my interpersonal relationships, in my community, and in the world at large.	1	2	3	4
9. I am content with who I am.	1	2	3	4
10. I go for the gusto and experience life to the fullest.	1	2	3	4

6 Intellectual Health

	Rarely, If Ever	Sometimes	Most of the Time	Always
1. I tend to let my emotions get the better of me and I act without thinking.	4	3	2	1
2. I learn from my mistakes by responding differently the next time.	1	2	3	4
3. I follow directions or recommended guidelines and act in ways likely to keep myself and others safe.	1	2	3	4
4. I consider alternatives or the pros and cons before making decisions.	1	2	3	4

(continued)

	Rarely, If Ever	Sometimes	Most of the Time	Always
5. I am alert and ready to respond to life's challenges in ways that reflect thought and sound judgment.	1	2	3	4
6. I tend to act impulsively without thinking about the consequences.	4	3	2	1
7. I actively try to learn what I can about products and services before making decisions about them.	1	2	3	4
8. I manage my time well, rather than allowing time to manage me.	1	2	3	4
9. My friends and family trust my judgment.	1	2	3	4
10. I think about my self-talk (the things I tell myself) and then examine the real evidence for my perceptions and feelings.	1	2	3	4

7 Occupational Health

	Rarely, If Ever	Sometimes	Most of the Time	Always
(Students should consider the stage of career development they are at or the satisfaction they are deriving from their education.)				
1. I am happy with my career choice.	1	2	3	4
2. I look forward to work.	1	2	3	4
3. My work responsibilities are consistent with my values.	1	2	3	4
4. The advantages in my career are consistent with my values.	1	2	3	4
5. I am happy with the rhythm between my work, family, and play time.	1	2	3	4
6. I am happy with the amount of control I have in my work.	1	2	3	4
7. My work gives me personal satisfaction and stimulation.	1	2	3	4
8. I am happy with the professional and personal growth provided by my job.	1	2	3	4
9. I feel my work allows me to make a difference in the world.	1	2	3	4
10. My work contributes positively to my overall well-being.	1	2	3	4

Personal Checklist

Now, total your scores in each of the health dimensions and compare them to the ideal score. Which areas do you need to work on? How does your score compare with how you rated yourself in the first part of the questionnaire?

	Top Possible Score	Your Score
Physical Health	40	_____
Social Health	40	_____
Emotional Health	40	_____
Environmental Health	40	_____
Spiritual Health	40	_____
Intellectual Health	40	_____
Occupational Health	40	_____

What Do Your Scores Mean?

Scores of 36–40: Outstanding! Your answers show you are aware of the importance of this component of your health. More important, you are putting your knowledge to work by practising good health attitudes and habits. As long as you continue to do so, this component will not pose a serious health risk. It is likely that you are a role model for your family, friends, and classmates.

Scores of 30–35: Your health practices in this area are good, but there is room for improvement. Look again at the items where you scored one or two points. What changes could you make to improve your score? Even a small change in attitude and behaviour can help you achieve better health.

Scores of 20–30: Your health risks are showing! Do you need more information about the risks you are facing and why it is important for you to change these attitudes and behaviours? Perhaps you need help in deciding how to make the changes you desire. In either case, you can learn more from this book, from your professor, and from your student health services.

Scores below 20: You may be taking serious and unnecessary risks with your health. Perhaps you are not aware of the risks and what to do about them. Perhaps you are not sure what lifestyle attitudes and behaviours lead to good health and wellness. In this book, you will find the information you need to attain and maintain optimal health and wellness.

Source: Adapted from the U.S. Health and Human Services, "Health Style: A Self Test." Public Health Service, 1981.

Are You Ready?

To understand the Stages of Change model, try the following activity:

- Write down one health behaviour you would consider changing. Just the fact that you are aware of it puts you in the contemplative stage. Now take it a bit further.

- How serious are you about the change? Are you ready to make this change? Are you in a healthy mental state? Is this change for you or to please someone else?

- What are the possible actions you could take to make it work? Have you developed an action plan with short- and long-term goals? Have you planned alternative actions in case you run into obstacles or begin to self-sabotage? Have you set priorities?

- What are potential barriers that could interfere with success? What or who will motivate you? Whom can you call on to help you? Where can you go for support and advice?

- Have you set up a list of reinforcers and supports that will keep you motivated along the way? How will you reward yourself? What will you do if you do not meet the goals for a particular day? What alternative actions can you take? What will you use as motivation to stay on target?

- Have you established a set of guidelines for success? Will you have small goals to achieve at selected intervals or will you consider yourself successful only if you have met your ultimate goal?

DISCUSSION QUESTIONS

1. Define *health* and *wellness*. What components are included in the definitions of these terms?

2. In your opinion, are Canadians healthy today? Why or why not?

3. How are men and women treated differently in the health-care system? Why do you think these differences exist? What can be done to change this?

4. What are the leading causes of death in Canada? How do the current efforts at health promotion address these leading causes of death at both an individual and population level? Are these promotional efforts effective for you? Why or why not?

5. Briefly describe the health belief model, the theory of reasoned action, and the theory of planned behaviour. How well do they apply to university and college students and their health behaviours?

6. Explain the various factors (i.e., predisposing, reinforcing, and enabling) that influence college and university students to binge drink.

7. Describe the process you would follow to change a behaviour.

8. Why is it important that you are ready to change before attempting to change a behaviour?

APPLICATION EXERCISE

Reread the Consider This . . . scenario at the beginning of the chapter and answer the following questions.

1. Who do you think is healthier—Jonah or Camesha? Why?
2. From what you learned in this chapter, what steps should Jonah and Camesha take to change their behaviours?
3. As a friend, what can you do to be more supportive of the health of someone you know who is trying to make a change?
4. What health-risking behaviours are common on your campus? Do you think students are aware of the risks they are taking? Why or why not? Do you think they are ready for change? Why or why not?

MASTERINGHEALTH

Go to MasteringHealth for Assignments, the eText, and the Study Area with case studies, self quizzing, and videos.

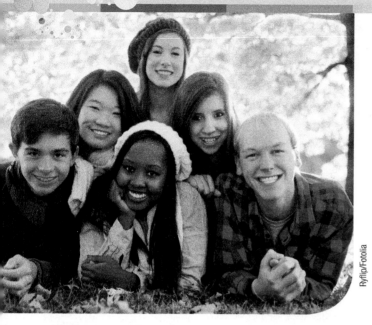

Ryflip/Fotolia

CHAPTER 2
PROMOTING AND PRESERVING YOUR PSYCHOSOCIAL HEALTH

◄◉ CONSIDER THIS . . .

Marisol is a 19-year-old first-year student majoring in liberal arts. She has become increasingly bored with her classes, finds little excitement in her days, and does not have the energy or desire to go out with friends. One weekend, she stayed in bed for two days "resting," and when she got up on Monday, she was still so tired that she could barely stay awake in class. She has difficulty concentrating, finds herself lounging on the couch playing with her iPad at every opportunity, and does not care whether her apartment is a mess. She has gone to the student health centre, and after several tests the doctor tells her that there is nothing physically wrong with her.

H ave you ever felt like Marisol? What do you think is wrong with her? What do you think contributes to her condition? Do you have friends showing similar signs? Why might a typical student health professional miss such obvious symptoms? What do you think Marisol should do to help herself get better? As a friend, what could you do to help her? What services and programs are available on your campus and in your community to help her?

LEARNING OUTCOMES

- Define psychosocial health and its components: intellectual, emotional, social, and spiritual health.

- Describe the external and internal factors influencing psychosocial health. Which of these factors can be changed?

- Identify common psychosocial problems, and explain their causes and available treatments.

- Describe the warning signs of suicide and the actions to take to help an individual contemplating suicide.

- Name the different types of mental health professionals and the most common types of therapy.

Most of us feel "down" occasionally; still, we get through the day in a reasonably productive, if not altogether exciting, way. We eventually sort through seemingly overwhelming problems, suppress our anxieties, and use our social support system (families, friends, and significant others) to help us through the low times. For some, though, these down times become persistent, nagging experiences that vary from small "downers" to "black holes" that they find increasingly difficult from which to emerge. Whether caused by temporary setbacks or major blows, these miserable moods sap our energy, reduce our physical reserves, waste our time, diminish our spirit, and take the joy out of our lives. They may even lead to a serious mental illness. Eventually, they may shorten our life span—reducing quantity as well as quality of life. How you feel and think about yourself, those around you, and your circumstances can tell you a lot about your psychosocial health. Like your physical health, your psychosocial or mental health has a profound impact on the quality and quantity of your life. You can enhance your psychosocial health just as you can your physical health, by becoming aware of relevant attitudes and behaviours and making changes where and when necessary.

DEFINING PSYCHOSOCIAL HEALTH

Psychosocial health or **mental health** encompasses the intellectual, emotional, social, and spiritual dimensions of health (see Figure 2.1). You are psychosocially or mentally healthy when you develop each of these dimensions to optimal levels. When you are psychosocially healthy, you have a reserve of energy for facing the normal ups and downs of life. You respond to challenges, disappointments, joys, frustrations, and pain by summoning up personal resources acquired through years of experience, and, when a needed resource is not available, you find ways to develop it. Your resiliency is strong, and you are motivated and actively involved in the process of living each day to the fullest.

Psychosocial health is the result of a complex interaction between your history and your conscious and unconscious thoughts about and interpretations of the past. Although definitions of psychosocial health vary, people who are psychosocially healthy share several basic characteristics (National Mental Health Association, 1988):

Psychosocial (or mental) health The intellectual, emotional, social, and spiritual dimensions of health.

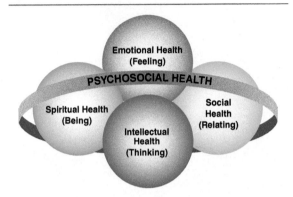

fear, love, anger, jealousy, guilt, or worry. They know who they are, have a realistic sense of their capabilities, and respect themselves even though they realize they are not perfect.

- **They feel comfortable with other people.** People who are psychosocially healthy have satisfying and lasting personal relationships and do not take advantage of others, nor do they allow others to take advantage of them. They give and receive love, consider others' interests, respect personal differences, and feel responsible for their fellow human beings.

- **They control tension and anxiety.** People who are psychosocially healthy recognize the underlying causes and symptoms of stress in their lives and consciously avoid illogical or irrational thoughts, unnecessary aggression, hostility, excessive excuse making, and blaming others for their problems. They use resources and learn skills to control reactions to stressful situations, including constructively expressing positive and negative feelings and learning to tolerate their frustrations.

- **They are able to meet the demands of life.** People who are psychosocially healthy try to solve problems as they arise, to accept responsibility for their thoughts and actions, and to plan ahead. They break down problems into manageable bits and work through them one piece or step at a time. They set realistic goals, think for themselves, and make independent decisions. Acknowledging that change is a normal part of life, they welcome new experiences.

- **They curb hate and guilt.** People who are psychosocially healthy acknowledge and combat their tendencies to respond with hate, anger, thoughtlessness, and selfishness. They do not take vengeance, nor do they allow feelings of inadequacy to build. They do not try to knock others

- **They feel good about themselves.** People who are psychosocially healthy are not overwhelmed by

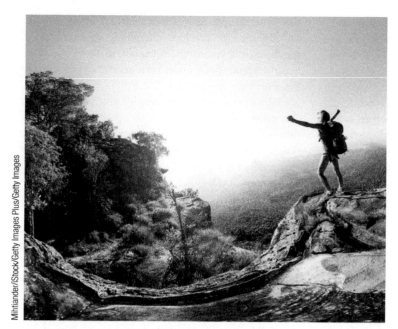
Mihtiander/iStock/Getty Images Plus/Getty Images

A joyful spirit and the resiliency to face life's ups and downs are measures of psychosocial health.

aside to get ahead but rather reach out to help others—even those they may not be fond of.

- **They choose a positive outlook.** People who are psychosocially healthy approach each day assuming it will go well. As Randy Pausch noted in *The Last Lecture*, " . . . there's a decision we all have to make and it seems perfectly captured in the Winnie-the-Pooh characters created by A.A. Milne. Each of us must decide: Am I a fun-loving Tigger or am I a sad-sack Eeyore?" (Pausch & Zaslow, 2008).

- **They enrich the lives of others.** People who are psychosocially healthy recognize that there are others whose needs may not be met. They try to help these people by doing simple things such as giving a ride to an elderly neighbour, bringing flowers to someone in pain, making dinner for someone who is hungry, volunteering at a community agency, and making charitable donations. They generally trust others and themselves.

- **They cherish the things that make them smile.** People who are psychosocially healthy make a special place in their lives for memories of the past. Family pictures, high-school mementos, souvenirs of past vacations, and other reminders of good experiences brighten their day. Fun is an integral part of their lives. Making time for themselves is also integral.

- **They value diversity.** People who are psychosocially healthy accept differences; they welcome into their lives people of a different sex, religion, sexual orientation, ethnicity, or political party. They often

go beyond accepting their differences and embrace and support them.

- **They appreciate and respect nature.** People who are psychosocially healthy enjoy and respect natural beauty and wonders. As mentioned in Chapter 1, the biophilia hypothesis refers to an instinctive bond between people and other living systems (Barbiero, Berto, & Pasini, 2011). People who are psychosocially healthy enjoy their surroundings (the environment and the living things within it), act responsibly, and are conscious of their place in the universe.

Of course, few of us ever achieve optimal levels in all these areas all the time. Attaining psychosocial health and wellness involves many complex processes and should be considered dynamic and rhythmical in nature, with ebbs and flows like the tide. This chapter will help you to understand not only what it means to be psychosocially healthy, but also the difficulties you may face in attaining and maintaining psychosocial health.

Intellectual Health: The Thinking You

As noted in Chapter 1, the term **intellectual health** is used to describe the "thinking" or "rational" part of psychosocial health. It describes your ability to perceive things happening around you in realistic ways, to use reasoning in problem solving, to interpret what is happening, and to evaluate your situation effectively and react appropriately. In short, you are able to sort through the clutter of events, variety of messages (conflicting and corroborating), and uncertainties of a situation and attach meaning (either positive or negative) to it based upon your experiences, attitudes, behaviours, and the environmental cues. Your values, attitudes, and beliefs about your health, your relationships with your family and others, and your life in general are usually—at least in part—a reflection of your intellectual health.

A person who is intellectually healthy enjoys life, the environment, and the people in it (Canadian Mental Health Association, 2009a). Such people tend to be creative, to learn, to try new things, and to take risks. They cope well in personal and professional situations of stress. They feel sad and angry when faced with the death of a loved one, a job loss or relationship problems, and

Intellectual health The "thinking" part of psychosocial health—includes values, attitudes, and beliefs.

other difficult events, but in time, with rational thinking and effective communication, they are able to move forward and enjoy life again. They also take responsibility for their actions. For example, if you choose to travel during 'reading week' knowing you have a major term paper and an exam when you return, you should not be disappointed with a "D" for your efforts when you quickly throw together a paper and study hurriedly for your exam. The intellectually healthy response is to take responsibility for your actions or lack of actions and plan differently next year or the next time by studying more before your holiday and/or spending some time writing the paper. You may even choose to travel at a different time.

When a person's intellectual health deteriorates, he or she may experience sharp declines in rational thinking and increasingly distorted perceptions. As a result, a person may become cynical and distrustful, experience volatile mood swings, or choose to be isolated from others. These negative reactions may threaten the quality and quantity of life of the person experiencing them, as well as the life and health of others. People showing such signs of extreme abnormal behaviours or mental health disorders are classified as having mental illnesses, discussed later in this chapter.

Emotional Health: The Feeling You

Emotional health refers to the "feeling," or subjective, side of psychosocial health and includes our "feeling" reactions to life. These "feeling" reactions are termed emotions. **Emotions** are intensified feelings or complex patterns of feelings that we experience on a minute-by-minute, day-to-day basis. Love, hate, hurt, despair, release, joy, anxiety, fear, frustration, and anger are some of the many emotions we experience. Typically, emotions are described as the interplay of four components: *physiological arousal, feelings, cognitive (thinking) processes,* and *behavioural reactions.*

There are four basic types of emotions: (1) emotions resulting from harm, loss, or threats; (2) emotions resulting from benefits or rewards; (3) borderline emotions, such as hope and compassion; and (4) more complex emotions, such as grief, disappointment, bewilderment, and curiosity (Lazarus, 1991). You may experience these emotions in combination at any time. You are also likely to experience a range in level of emotional responses from very intense to very little reaction. Further, your emotional responses to various settings and situations will vary on a day-to-day basis and may differ from how others experience

---

Emotional health The "feeling" part of psychosocial health; the "feeling" reactions to life.

Emotions Intensified feelings or complex patterns of feelings we experience.

---

the same setting or situation. Part of being psychosocially healthy involves evaluating your emotional responses, the environment leading to these responses, and the appropriateness of your actions or reactions to these emotional responses.

When you are emotionally healthy, you are usually able to respond appropriately to upsetting or uplifting events and are thus not likely to react in an extreme fashion, behave inconsistently, or adopt an offensive attack when you feel threatened. In other words, when you are emotionally healthy, you are less likely to let your feelings overpower you. How many times have you seen someone react with extreme anger by shouting, slamming a door, or punching a wall? Those are reactions of people who are not emotionally healthy. These people may be highly volatile and prone to unpredictable emotional outbursts and inappropriate, sometimes frightening, responses to events. An ex-boyfriend or girlfriend who becomes so angry that he or she hits and pushes you around or yells at you because he or she is jealous of you and/or your new relationship is demonstrating an unhealthy and dangerous emotional reaction.

Similarly, people going through a challenging break-up often have difficulty picking themselves up and moving on in healthy ways. Learning to acknowledge that it is okay to feel sad, unhappy, disappointed, or frustrated and getting help through counselling or talking with trusted friends is part of a healthy process of adapting and coping. Unfortunately many of us keep our emotions bottled up inside. Further, many of us, particularly men, think it shows weakness to seek help—whether professional or just from our friends (Canadian Mental Health Association, 2009b).

Poor emotional health often affects social health. Social isolation is one of the many potentially negative consequences of unstable emotional responses. Examples of poor emotional health include feeling and/or acting hostile, withdrawn, moody, grumpy, nasty, or irritable, as well as those who are overly quiet, cry easily, or demonstrate other disturbing emotional responses. Since people in a poor emotional state are not much fun to be around, their friends, family, and colleagues tend to avoid them at the very time they most need support.

For you and other students, a more immediate concern of poor emotional health may be the impact on your academic performance. Imagine studying for an exam or trying to write a paper after a fight with a close friend, partner, or family member, or when someone close to you has recently died. Emotional turmoil seriously affects your ability to concentrate, reason, or act in a rational way. Many otherwise rational people do things they would not normally do when they are going through a major emotional upset. As previously mentioned, those who show repeated and excessive abnormal behaviours are classified as having mental illnesses, which is discussed later in this chapter.

Social Health: Interactions with Others

As noted in Chapter 1, social health is the part of your psychosocial health dealing with your interactions with others on an individual and group basis, your ability to use—and to provide—social resources and support in times of need, and your ability to adapt to a variety of social situations. It is an integral component of psychosocial health. With the increased use of technology and social media, there have been significant changes in how we interact with others. However, many experts still suggest that face-to-face communication provides the most benefits for social well-being (Kraut et al., 1998).

When you are socially healthy, you have a wide range of social interactions with family, friends, and acquaintances, and are able to have healthy interactions with an intimate partner. You are able to listen, express yourself, form healthy relationships, act in socially acceptable and responsible ways, and find a fit for yourself in society. Numerous studies document the importance of social health in promoting physical and mental health, as well as enhancing longevity (Yang et al., 2016). Two factors, in particular, are important (Ritter, 1988):

- **Presence of strong social bonds. Social bonds**, or social linkages, reflect the general degree and nature of interpersonal contacts and interactions. Social bonds generally provide six major functions: (1) intimacy, (2) feelings of belonging to or integration with a group, (3) opportunities for giving or receiving nurturance, (4) reassurance of your worth, (5) assistance and guidance, and (6) advice. In general, when you are more "connected" to others, you manage your stress more effectively and are more resilient in response to life's crises.

- **Presence of key social supports. Social supports** refer to relationships that bring positive benefits to the individual. Social supports can be either expressive (emotional support, encouragement) or structural (housing, money). Social support can be provided informally by friends and family, or formally by professionals in various settings. People who are psychosocially healthy create a network of friends and family with whom they can give and receive informal support.

Social health also reflects the way you react to others around you. In its most extreme forms, a lack of social health is represented by acts of prejudice and bias toward other individuals or groups. **Prejudice** is defined as "a valenced affective or evaluative response (positive or negative) to a social category and its members" (Dovidio et al., 2010, p. 46). Further, Dovidio et al. (2010) go on to say that the most recognized definition of prejudice includes negative attitudes and behaviours towards a particular group and its members. In its most obvious manifestations, prejudice is reflected in acts of discrimination against others, in overt acts of hate and bias, and in purposeful intent to harm individuals or groups.

Spiritual Health: An Inner Quest for Well-Being

Although intellectual, emotional, and social health are key factors in your overall psychosocial functioning, it is possible to be intellectually, emotionally, and socially healthy and still not achieve your optimal levels of psychosocial well-being. What is missing? You may be missing that difficult-to-describe element that provides internal guidance and direction and gives zest to your life: the spiritual dimension. What does it mean to be spiritually healthy? As noted in Chapter 1, your spiritual health reflects your values, beliefs, and perceptions of the world and all living things. Spirituality is most often defined as a search for meaning, connectedness, energy, and transcendence, rather than simply a connection to a particular religion (Polzer, Casarez, & Engebretson, 2012). Spirituality refers to the deepest or innermost part of you, the part that helps you to make sense of the world and your part in it (Thompson Rivers University, 2013). It is at the core of where you gather your strength and hope. It is that from which you determine who you are and your purpose in life. Your spiritual health may involve a belief in a supreme being or a specified way of life as prescribed by a particular religion or it may relate to personal relationships or being at peace with nature and yourself.

Many of us live on a rather superficial material plane throughout our formative years. We have basic human needs that must be satisfied according to a set hierarchical order. We tend to be rather egocentric, or self-oriented, during these formative years and to seek immediate material and emotional gratification while denying or ignoring the spiritual aspect of our lives. When you worry about the clothes you wear, the car you drive, the appearance of your apartment, being seen with the 'right' people, and other material things, these are examples of this type of preoccupation. There comes a point, however, usually around midlife—or when a crisis occurs, such as a major illness or death of someone close to you—when you discover that the material

Social bonds Degree and nature of interpersonal contacts.

Social supports Structural and expressive aspects of social interactions.

Prejudice A negative evaluation of an entire group of people usually based on unfavourable and often mistaken ideas about the group.

FIGURE 2.2
Four Major Themes of Spirituality

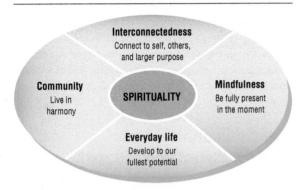

world cannot bring a sense of happiness or self-worth (O'Connell & O'Connell, 1992). You then recognize that things like prestige, money, power, and fame count for little in the larger scheme of life, and that if you were to die tomorrow these would not give meaning to your life—nor would you want your life to be defined by those material things. Whatever the reason, the realization that there is more to life brings new opportunities for understanding yourself and provides room for your spiritual growth. As you develop your spiritual health, you often come to recognize your uniqueness. You reach a better understanding of your strengths and weaknesses and your place in the world. Often, you find that your family, the environment, animals, friends, strangers who are suffering, and religion assume greater significance in your life. You then become more willing to give to others or attempt to improve the world around you. You do not have to wait until your middle years—or a crisis—to experience spiritual growth. You can choose to focus on your spiritual health now.

Attaining and maintaining your spiritual health take time and experience. The longer you live, the more you experience, the more you have to learn from. The more you ponder the meaning of your experiences, the greater your chances of achieving spiritual health. In its purest sense, as noted in Figure 2.2, spirituality addresses four main themes: interconnectedness, mindfulness, spirituality as a part of everyday life, and living in harmony with the community.

- **Interconnectedness. Interconnectedness** refers to your sense of belonging and connecting with yourself, with others, and with a larger meaning or purpose of life. Connecting with yourself involves exploring your feelings, assessing your reactions to people and experiences, and taking mental notes when your rhythm is disrupted by your reaction to

Interconnectedness A web of connections, including your relationship to yourself, to others, and to a larger meaning or purpose in life.

Mindfulness Awareness and acceptance of the reality of the present moment.

others or to situations. It also involves considering your values and achieving congruence between your goals and what you can do to achieve them without compromising your values.

- **Mindfulness. Mindfulness** refers to your ability to be fully present in the moment, to live in the now. It has been described as a way of nurturing greater awareness and clarity. It is a form of inner flow—a holistic sensation you feel when you are totally involved in the present (Astin et al., 2003; Bishop et al., 2004). You can achieve this inner flow or rhythm through an almost infinite range of opportunities for enjoyment and pleasure, either through the development and practice of physical and sensory skills in sport, music, dance, or yoga; or through the development of symbolic skills in areas such as poetry, philosophy, or mathematics.

- **Spirituality as a part of daily life.** Spirituality is embodied in the ability to discover and articulate your basic purpose in life; to learn how to experience love, joy, peace, and fulfillment; and to help yourself and others achieve their full potential (Bishop et al., 2004). This ongoing process of growth fosters three convictions: faith, hope, and love. *Faith* is the belief that helps you realize your unique purpose in life; *hope* is the belief that allows you to look confidently and courageously to the future; and *love* involves accepting, affirming, and respecting yourself and others regardless of who they are (Bishop et al., 2004).

- **Living in harmony with your community.** Your values are an extension of your beliefs about the world and your attitude toward life. These values are formed over time from your experiences, and are reflected in your hopes, dreams, desires, goals, ambitions, and personal and community-oriented actions (Bishop et al., 2004). Although you likely have some idea of what is important to you, you may not be aware of how your values impact upon you or those around you until a crisis forces you to reflect on your life. Volunteering to help others, doing charitable work, and donating resources to help people in need are ways to "give back" to the community and the people who support you. These kinds of altruistic actions—that is, the giving of yourself out of genuine concern for others—also play a significant role in your spiritual health (Karen et al., 2006).

Spirituality: A Key to Better Health

Although the specific impact of spirituality on your health remains elusive, many experts affirm the importance of this dimension in achieving health and wellness.

Studies of spirituality among post-secondary students from diverse universities and colleges indicated that spirituality played a role in their health, grades, and other aspects of their student life (Astin et al., 2004; Astin, Astin, & Lindholm, 2011). Astin et al. (2004) found a correlation between spirituality and health; more spiritually oriented students had better health, higher grades, more involvement in charitable organizations or volunteerism, and more interest in helping others. Other studies have also indicated a correlation between spirituality and positive health outcomes. For example, mindfulness therapies have been used effectively to treat depression, to reduce stress in outpatient therapy and in the nursing profession, with anxiety and heart disease treatments, and for other problems (Cohen-Katz et al., 2005; Segal, 2001; Tacon et al., 2003; Weiss, Nordlie, & Segal, 2005).

A Spiritual Resurgence

An increase in spiritual awareness does not necessarily equate with an increase in beliefs in a god or supreme being of some kind. You can find spiritual fulfillment in music, poetry, literature, art, nature, or intimate relationships (Elkins, 1998). Your spirituality might refer to a quest for self and selflessness—learning about yourself and how to willingly give of yourself to others. Understanding and appreciating yourself as a result of self-reflection can also help you deepen or appreciate your life experiences more fully than just living through them. This topic has received considerable scholarly and popular attention. The fact that self-help books focused on spirituality consistently top the bestseller lists demonstrates a strong interest in spirituality within contemporary society.

Putting Spirituality into Practice

How can you enhance the spiritual dimension of your psychosocial health? One of the most important things needed for developing your psychosocial health is to give yourself some time to pause and reflect upon your life. In these quiet moments, ask yourself the following: Am I doing what I most want to be doing? Do my actions reflect my values and beliefs? Do I treat others in ways similar to how I would want to be treated? As previously noted, some people focus on their spiritual development through a formal religion—for instance, by attending religious services, engaging in prayer, or taking part in the organized study or discussion of religious texts (such as the Bible or the Koran). Others will find meaningful volunteer experiences or spend more time in personal reflection. The World Giving Index noted that in 2013 44 percent of Canadians volunteered their time to a charity

or non governmental agencies (Charities Aid Foundation, 2014). Further, it was noted in the 2014 World Giving Index that Canada ranked third out of 146 countries for giving, with "helping a stranger," giving money, and volunteering time as the most common giving behaviours (Charities Aid Foundation, 2014). Regardless of what you choose to do, keep in mind that enhancing your spiritual health is as time-consuming, and requires as much effort as building your physical fitness or changing your dietary intake. The next section provides suggestions to help you find or develop your spiritual health.

Strategies for Finding Your Spiritual Side

Spirituality involves connectedness to others and to the broader community, so it is important that you take time for meaningful interactions with your friends, family, and people within the community with whom you may not interact regularly. What types of actions foster connectedness for you?

Volunteer. The ability to notice when others are in need, and reaching out to help them through volunteering, is an excellent way to feel connected with others and enhance your spiritual health. In the aftermath of world tragedies such as Hurricane Katrina and the earthquake in Haiti, thousands of people volunteered their time, money, and effort to help an entire population that was suffering. Recognizing that you are part of the greater system of humanity and that you have a role and responsibility to help others in need is a key part of your spirituality. Volunteering by helping your older neighbours clean their home or yard, working at an animal shelter, making food baskets at your school's food bank, or participating in a beach or highway cleanup are all a part of being responsible and finding a place to help in the greater scheme of things. Your college or university may provide some of you the opportunity for class-based or immersion service learning. Service learning refers to responding to a community need with service and then reflecting upon that experience in conjunction with what you are learning in class (Levesque-Bristol, Knapp, & Fisher, 2010). These opportunities—whether tutoring elementary school children, providing a physical activity program, assisting at a daycare, cleaning a local pond, assisting people with their income tax returns, teaching computer skills, or many other methods of helping with a community need—provide occasions to enhance your spiritual health through the positive feelings that often arise from giving of yourself. Volunteering can also be a huge boost for you when you are feeling down or wondering how you fit in.

Take Time to Reflect. Connecting with yourself is another method of finding your spiritual side. Commit to taking a few moments each day to think about who you are, what you value, what makes you feel good, or what things make you feel not so good. Setting aside some time to reflect can help you relieve tension, seek out answers to problems you are experiencing, or simply empty your mind and enjoy this time to yourself. Taking time to reflect may also help with managing your stress (see Chapter 3).

Get Involved in Service Learning.

As previously mentioned, service learning involves meaningful and productive contributions and relationships with the greater community. Community agencies and programs benefit from an enthusiastic, hardworking group of students who respond with service to their real needs. The students, in turn, have an opportunity to learn new or enhance previous skills and grow; they learn to look at the greater community and world around them and make links from that to what they are learning in the classroom. Some schools provide course-based and immersion service learning. Generally, students involved in course-based service learning volunteer their service over the term, whereas students involved in immersion service learning travel to provide a week or longer of in-depth service to another community. Regardless of the type of service learning, the intent is to reflect upon the experience and how it enhances your learning in the classroom.

FACTORS INFLUENCING PSYCHOSOCIAL HEALTH

Although it is relatively easy to define psychosocial health, it is much more difficult to explain why some people are psychosocially well almost all the time, others some of the time, and still others almost never. What factors influence your intellectual, emotional, social, and spiritual health? Are these factors changeable? What can you do to improve your psychosocial health? How can you enhance the positive qualities you already possess? See Table 2.1 for some general suggestions that may assist you in improving your psychosocial health.

Most of your intellectual, emotional, social, and spiritual reactions to life are a direct outcome of your experiences, along with social and cultural expectations. Each of you is born with the innate capacity to experience emotions. Some of you have a predisposition toward more emotionality than others. How you express your emotions has a lot to do with your interpretations of what you experience. These interpretations are often learned reactions to environmental and social stimuli.

External Influences

Your psychosocial health is based on how you perceive your experiences. While some experiences are under your control, others are not. External influences refer to those factors that you do not control, such as who raised you, the physical environment in which you live, and timelines imposed upon you by your professors.

Influences of the Family

Your families have a significant influence on your psychosocial development. As previously noted, children raised in healthy, nurturing, happy families where they learn about being responsible and accountable are more likely to become well-adjusted, productive adults. Children raised in dysfunctional families in which violence, abuse (sexual, physical, or emotional), negative behaviours, distrust, anger, dietary deprivation, drug use, parental discord, or other negative characteristics are present may have a harder time adapting to life. In dysfunctional families, security, unconditional love, and trust are lacking and the children are often confused and psychologically bruised. Yet not all people raised in dysfunctional families become psychosocially unhealthy. Conversely, not all people from healthy family environments are psychosocially healthy. Obviously more factors are involved in your "process of becoming" than just your family.

Influences of the Wider Environment

While isolated negative events may do little damage to psychosocial health, persistent stressors, uncertainties, and threats can cause significant problems. Children raised in environments where crime is rampant and daily safety is in question, for example, have an increased risk of psychosocial health issues among other things. Drugs, crime, violent acts, school failure, unemployment, and a host of other bad things can happen to individuals. That said, protective factors—such as having one or more positive role models in the midst of chaos, or a high level of self-esteem—can help children from even the worst environments grow up healthy and well adjusted.

Another important influence on psychosocial health is access to health services and programs designed to support the maintenance or enhancement of psychosocial health. Going to a support group or seeing a trained counsellor or therapist is often a crucial first step in prevention and intervention efforts. Unfortunately, individuals from a poor socioeconomic background (who often need the services most) may have more difficulty accessing such services.

TABLE 2.1

Psychosocial Health Tips

- **Daydream**—Close your eyes and imagine yourself in a dream location. Breathe slowly and deeply. Whether it is a beach, a mountaintop, a forest, or a favourite room from your past, let the comforting environment wrap you in a sensation of peace and tranquility.

- **"Collect" positive emotional moments**—Make it a point to recall times when you have experienced pleasure, comfort, tenderness, confidence, or other positive emotions. Display items that you like. You might have items that remind you of your achievements, your friends, or special times. Keep those special items close by.

- **Learn ways to cope with negative thoughts**—Negative thoughts can be insistent and loud. Learn to interrupt them. Do not try to block them (which seldom, if ever, works), and do not let them take over. Try distracting yourself or comforting yourself if you cannot solve the problem right away.

- **Do one thing at a time**—For example, when you are out for a walk or spending time with friends, turn off your cellphone and stop making that mental "to do" list. Be present; take in the sights, sounds, and smells you encounter.

- **Make your meals a special time**—Get rid of distractions such as the television, your cellphone, or other forms of technology and concentrate on enjoying your meal, whether you are by yourself or with others.

- **Be physically active**—Regular physical activity improves psychological well-being and can reduce depression and anxiety. Joining an exercise class or a gym can also reduce loneliness, since it connects you with a new set of people sharing a common goal.

- **Enjoy hobbies**—Taking up a hobby brings balance to your life by allowing you to do something you enjoy because you want to do it, free of the pressure of everyday tasks. It also keeps your brain active.

- **Set personal goals**—Goals do not have to be ambitious. You might decide to finish that book you started last year; to take a walk around the block every day; to learn to knit or play bridge; to call your friends instead of waiting for the phone to ring. Whatever goal you set, reaching it will build confidence and a sense of satisfaction.

- **Keep a journal (or even talk to the wall!)**—Expressing yourself after a stressful day can help you gain perspective, release tension, and even boost your body's resistance to illness.

- **Share humour**—Life often gets too serious, so when you hear or see something that makes you smile or laugh, share it with someone you know. A little humour can go a long way to keeping us mentally fit!

- **Volunteer**—The best way to feel better about yourself is to help someone in greater need. Check out local volunteer opportunities, widen your social network, experience new activities, and add another dimension to your life.

- **Treat yourself well**—Pay attention to your own needs and wants. Listen to what your body, your mind, and your heart are telling you. Trust your gut instinct. Eat healthy foods, limit junk foods, be physically active, and plan fun activities for yourself. Have a bubble bath. See a movie. Go for a walk. Call a friend or relative you have not talked to in ages. Sit on a park bench and breathe in the fragrance of flowers and grass. Whatever it is, do it just for you.

- **Do something that you have been putting off.** Cleaning out your closet or paying a bill that you have been putting off will make you feel like you have accomplished something.

- **Give yourself rewards.** Acknowledge that you are a great person by rewarding yourself occasionally. Reward yourself in a meaningful way, not in a way that contradicts living a healthy lifestyle.

- **Wear clothes that make you feel good about yourself.** You do not have to spend a lot to find clothes that make you feel good. Check out local thrift stores and consignment shops for great bargains.

- **Spend time with people.** People who make you feel better about yourself are great self-esteem boosters. Avoid people who treat you badly or make you feel bad about yourself.

- **Learn something new every day.** Take advantage of any opportunity to learn something new—you will feel better about yourself and be more productive.

Source: Courtesy of the Canadian Mental Health Association. Reprinted with permission.

Internal Influences

Although your life experiences influence you in fairly obvious ways, many internal factors also work subtly to shape who you are and who you become. Some of these factors include your traits, hormonal functioning, physical health status (including neurological or nervous system functioning), level of physical fitness, and selected elements of your mental and emotional health. If issues occur with any of these factors, overall psychosocial health can decline.

Self-Efficacy and Self-Esteem

During your formative years, your successes and failures in school, sports, friendships, family relationships, intimate relationships, jobs, and every other aspect of life subtly shape your perceptions and beliefs about

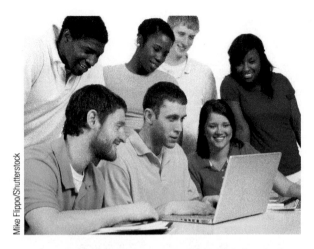

Past successes and happy experiences, often recalled through photos, mementos, and recollections, contribute to a person's psychosocial health.

your personal worth and ability to help yourself. These perceptions and beliefs in turn become internal influences on your psychosocial health.

Self-efficacy describes your belief about whether or not you can successfully engage in and execute a specific behaviour. If you experience success in academics, sports, or social life, you typically expect to be successful in these aspects in the future. If you fail an exam, were chosen last to be on a team, or have not been able to make friends easily, you may believe that failure is inevitable. In general, the more self-efficacious you are and the more your experiences have been positive, the more likely you are to keep trying to execute a specific behaviour successfully. When you have a high level of self-efficacy, you are also more likely to feel that you have **personal control** over situations or believe your internal resources allow you to control events. On the other hand, when you have low self-efficacy, you may give up easily or not even try to change your behaviours. Learning new skills and having successful experiences improves your confidence and leads to the expectation of future success.

Self-efficacy Belief in your ability to perform a task successfully.

Personal control Belief that your efforts can and do influence situations and interactions with others.

Self-esteem Your sense of self-respect or self-worth.

Learned helplessness An attitude of giving up and not trying because of past failures.

Learned optimism Pattern of responding that focuses on the positive, because you choose to view each situation positively and with a sense of hope.

Self-esteem refers to your sense of self-respect or self-worth. It can be defined as an evaluation of yourself and your personal worth. When you have high self-esteem, you tend to feel good about yourself and express a positive outlook on life. When you have low self-esteem, you tend not to be happy with yourself, to demean yourself, and to doubt your ability to succeed.

Your self-esteem forms as a result of the relationships you have with your parents and family during your formative years, with your friends as you grow older, with your significant others as you form intimate relationships, and with your teachers, coaches, co-workers, and others important to you throughout your lives. If you feel loved and valued in each of these relationships, you believe that you are inherently loveable and have a strong sense of self-esteem.

Learned Helplessness versus Learned Optimism

When you continually experience failure, you may develop a pattern of responding known as **learned helplessness**, in which you give up and do not take action to help yourself (Seligman, 1990). This attitude and resultant behaviour is due in part to society's tendency toward *victimology*, laying the blame for your problems on others or on the circumstances rather than accepting responsibility for your actions or lack of actions yourself. Although viewing yourself as a victim may help you to feel better temporarily, it does not address the underlying cause or causes of a problem. Ultimately, not taking responsibility for your actions erodes self-efficacy and fosters learned helplessness by developing an attitude that there is nothing you can do to improve the situation or the outcome, so you may as well give up.

Countering learned helplessness is the theory that you can also learn to be optimistic; this phenomenon is called, not surprisingly, **learned optimism** (Seligman, 1990). Scientists studying learned optimism have found that it is possible for you to make a conscious choice to take a more positive stance toward the world. For example, you can choose to see the glass as half full, instead of half empty. By changing your self-talk, examining your reactions and the way you assess what happens to you in life, and blocking negative thoughts and replacing them with positive thoughts, you can actually "learn" how to be optimistic or, perhaps more appropriately, you can choose to be optimistic.

Personality

Your personality is the unique mix of characteristics that distinguishes you from others. Hereditary, environmental, cultural, and experiential factors influence how you develop your personality. Your personality determines how you react to the challenges of life. It also determines how you interpret the feelings you experience and how you resolve the conflicts you feel about being denied the things you need or want.

You have the power not only to understand your behaviours but also to actively change them, and in this way shape your personality. Although much has been written about the importance of a healthy personality, there is little consensus about what exactly it is. In general, however, when you possess the following traits, you are likely to be psychologically healthy (Zimbardo, Weber, & Johnson, 2000):

- **Extroversion:** The ability to adapt to a social situation and demonstrate assertiveness as well as power or interpersonal involvement.
- **Agreeableness:** The ability to conform, be likeable, and demonstrate friendly compliance as well as love.
- **Openness to experience:** The willingness to demonstrate curiosity and independence (also referred to as *inquiring intellect*).
- **Emotional stability:** The ability to maintain control of your feelings.
- **Conscientiousness:** The qualities of being dependable and demonstrating self-control, discipline, and a need to achieve.

Resiliency and Developmental Assets

It has become well established that some people are much better prepared to meet the challenges of life than others. The combination of certain personality traits coupled with a supportive environment can equip you to deal effectively with life's many challenges. Individuals with this set of traits and circumstances are able to cope and even thrive in times of great stress or pressure. **Resiliency**, or *protective factors,* is a term used to describe those traits or characteristics that protect you or your community from threat or harm. In a sense, these traits may serve to inoculate you against potential ill health. When you have these assets, whether financial, emotional, spiritual, physical, intellectual, or social, and other positive forces in your life, you are likely to be resilient and bounce back when facing life's challenges.

ENHANCING PSYCHOSOCIAL HEALTH

You may believe that your psychosocial health is fairly well developed by the time you reach college or university. However, attaining self-fulfillment is a lifelong, conscious process that involves building your self-efficacy and self-esteem, understanding and controlling your emotions, maintaining support networks, and learning to solve problems and make decisions.

Developing and Maintaining Self-Esteem and Self-Efficacy

There are several ways to build your self-esteem and self-efficacy. These may include developing a support group, being a support for others, completing required tasks, forming realistic expectations, making and taking time for yourself, maintaining your physical health, and examining your problems and seeking help. Many of these suggestions overlap with suggestions previously made to enhance one or more components of your psychosocial health (see Table 2.1).

Developing a Support Group

One of the best ways to boost your self-esteem and self-efficacy is through contact within a group—peers who share your values. This kind of support network can help you to feel good about yourself. Although you might seek support in a wholly new group, remember that old ties are often the strongest. Keeping in contact with friends from your past and family members can provide a foundation of unconditional love that will help you through the many life transitions ahead.

Being a Support for Others

Feel better about yourself by helping others to feel good about themselves. Write more "thank you" cards, postcards, and "thinking of you" notes. Although personal, hand-written notes may seem a thing of the past, particularly with the various methods of electronic communication available today, they continue to provide meaningful messages to others that you care. Writing these notes—whether electronically or in 'hard' format—will build your self-esteem and that of your friends because of the good feelings they create. Become more interesting by being more interested (in people, current events, and so on). Send news clippings or forward interesting links and/or YouTube videos to family and friends. Join a discussion, political action, social justice, or recreational group.

Completing Required Tasks

Another way to boost your self-esteem or self-efficacy is to complete required tasks on time. You are not likely to succeed in your studies if you leave term papers until the night before they are due, or if you do not keep up with the reading for your courses or ask for clarification of points confusing you. Some university and college campuses provide study groups for various content areas. You can create a study group of your own too;

Resiliency Those traits or characteristics that protect you and your community from threat or harm.

point of view

SELF-HELP BOOKS: Beneficial or Baloney?

Self-help books abound! They cover everything from losing weight to having a better sex life to improving your golf swing to managing your finances. These books, and the programs, seminars, DVDs, and other products that support them, offer accessible, relatively inexpensive guidance to you when you are hoping to bring about positive change in your life. Are these books helpful, or are they a marketing scam, taking money from you without providing any real service?

ARGUMENTS IN FAVOUR OF SELF-HELP BOOKS

○ Self-help books can provide another perspective on a problem, helping you to become "unstuck."

○ Some books are directive and practical enough to help you positively change your life.

○ They provide useful information and point you to concrete and useful resources.

○ They provide a private way for you to find information about problems that you may find difficult to discuss.

○ Using a self-help book may help you to empathize more with another struggling person.

ARGUMENTS AGAINST SELF-HELP BOOKS

○ Books can't make you change—real change has to come from within.

○ These books often make claims of an outcome that seems too good to be true.

○ Merely reading the book may give you a false sense of solving a problem without actually dealing with it.

○ Self-help books encourage self-diagnosis, which can be risky if there are serious mental health issues.

○ Anyone can write a self-help book—and the book doesn't have to be based on scientific evidence.

○ When it comes to your health, it is worth it to find qualified health providers.

Where Do You Stand?

○ Do you think self-help books are helpful or harmful? In which situations do you think a self-help book is most likely to be valuable? Least valuable?

○ Would you use a self-help book? If so, how would you determine which one?

○ Do you know anyone who has used one? Did it help? How?

○ Suppose your younger cousin wanted to buy a self-help book. What advice would you give him or her?

you do not need to be an expert in a topic, instead what you need is a group of committed individuals willing to share their approach to a topic or problem. Your school's student services department may offer tips for managing time, understanding assignments, dealing with professors, and preparing for test taking. Poor grades, or grades that do not meet your expectations, are major contributors to diminished self-esteem and to emotional and intellectual distress among post-secondary students.

Forming Realistic Expectations

Developing or creating realistic expectations of yourself—and others—may also boost your self-esteem and self-efficacy. College or university is a time to explore your potential. If you expect perfect grades, many dates, a Hollywood-type romantic involvement, a high-paying job after graduation, and a beautiful home and car, you may be setting yourself up for failure. Assess your current resources and the direction in which you are heading. Set small, incremental goals that are possible for you to meet. Rather than suggesting, "I am going to get better grades," without some realistic actions or achievable, definable goals to support your intentions, decide that tomorrow you will spend two hours studying or go to the library to do research on a paper, or talk to your professor to see what he or she recommends to help you to better understand a particular topic.

Making and Taking Time for You

Taking time to enjoy the various components of your life is another way to boost your psychosocial health. Making that time available is critical. You may want to make time to participate in a sport as that often improves your self-esteem and self-efficacy. Alternatively, you may choose to meditate, volunteer your time to others in need, get a massage, or meet a new challenge, such as auditioning for a play, as a way to enhance your psychosocial health. Viewing each new activity as something to look forward to and an opportunity to grow is an important part of keeping excitement in your life.

Maintaining Physical Health

Maintaining physical health also contributes to self-esteem and to overall psychosocial health. Regular physical activity (see also Chapter 4) fosters a sense of well-being, improves mood, and can improve self-efficacy and self-esteem during all stages of life (Kilpatrick, 2008; Richardson et al., 2005; Schmalz et al., 2007). Nourishing meals that provide variety, balance, and moderation (see also Chapter 5) help you to feel good about yourself. Engaging in regular physical activity and eating well lead to weight maintenance (see also Chapter 6) rather than the usual weight gain, or "Frosh 15" (the 7 kilograms—or 15 pounds), experienced by many college or university students. Getting adequate sleep, managing your stress, and controlling your alcohol consumption are three other behaviours critical to maintaining your physical and mental health.

Eat More Vegetables and Fruit

The link between taking care of your physical body and psychosocial health seem to be well accepted and believed. Less well known is the importance of eating your vegetables and fruits. Research conducted by Blanchflower, Oswald, & Stewart-Brown (2012) relating vegetable and fruit consumption to seven measures of well-being found a strong positive correlation even when controlling for confounding factors such as income and education. This research notes dose-response in that those with the highest scores of well-being also ate more vegetables and fruit

(Blanchflower, Oswald, & Stewart-Brown, 2012). The highest correlation was found with individuals who consumed seven or eight vegetables and fruit.

Examining Problems and Seeking Help

Examining your problems and seeking help when needed will also boost your self-esteem and self-efficacy. Facing and solving problems can be one of life's most satisfying experiences. You do not necessarily have to deal with your problems alone. Help can come in the form of a friend, a group, or a mental health professional.

Getting Adequate Sleep

Getting adequate sleep is a key contributor to your physical and mental functioning. There are times when you may not get enough sleep and other times when you get too much sleep. Sleep serves at least two biological purposes: (1) conservation of energy, so that you are rested and ready to perform during high-performance daylight hours; and (2) restoration, so that neurotransmitters depleted during waking hours can be replenished. This process clears the brain of daily minutiae to prepare for a new day.

You likely can identify with that tired, listless feeling caused by sleep deprivation during periods of peak stress. There are times when you may not make enough time to sleep, have difficulty falling asleep, or do not stay asleep once you get there. Lack of sleep is especially common among post-secondary students given your relatively high workload and levels of anxiety and stress. Women, in particular, have problems with sleep (National Sleep Foundation, 2007).

How much sleep do you need? That depends on a number of factors. There is a genetically based need for sleep and it differs for each person and differs within each person depending upon where you are in your life cycle and what is happening in your life (National Sleep Foundation, 2011). That said, six to nine hours of sleep each night is generally recommended. Sleep duration is also controlled by *circadian rhythms*, which are linked to the hormone *melatonin*. You alter your sleep patterns by staying up late, drinking coffee, engaging in vigorous physical activities late at night, eating a heavy meal, or using an alarm or other wake-up device. *Sleep inertia* is a term used to describe the cognitive impairment, disorientation, and grogginess you experience when you first get up in the morning. This sleep inertia can impair your ability to think clearly and function effectively in tasks that occur shortly after you wake up. To wake up effectively and well rested, you should go to bed and get up regularly at the same time. Physical activity and a healthy breakfast (that is, three of the four food groups, low in fat, high in fibre) also help you to feel awake.

The characteristic stages of sleep range from wakefulness to drowsiness to light sleep, and then move to a deeper sleep. The most important period of sleep, a deeper sleep, is called "rapid eye movement" (REM) sleep and is essential to feeling rested and refreshed. You usually experience four to five periods of REM sleep where your heart rate increases, respiration speeds up, and dreaming tends to occur (Nordqvist, 2012). If you miss REM—which you do in an alcohol-induced sleep—you are left feeling groggy and sleep deprived. See also the "Focus on Sleep" section between Chapters 11 and 12.

Understanding the Mind–Body Connection

Can negative emotions and stress make you physically sick? Can positive emotions and happiness help you to feel well? Do positive emotions boost your immune system? Although considerable research has attempted to answer these questions, much remains unknown. The field of study is called psychoneuroimmunology: "the study of the interactions between psychological factors, the central nervous system, and immune function as modulated by the neuroendocrine system" (The Free Dictionary by Farlex, n.d.). Researchers in this field of study attempt to better understand the connections between the mind and the body. When you think about being in a good mood or feeling positive about things, you also tend to feel physically better—this research examines that more deeply. For decades, research focused primarily on negative emotions and disease; however, little is known about the role of positive emotions in preserving health and protecting against disease. Many believe that this end of the emotional continuum might hold the key to future advances in health, and that mind–body health science may expand into new areas and be accorded a higher level of importance as a result. One emotion that appears to have particularly positive benefits is *happiness*.

Happiness and Physical Health

Happiness refers to a number of positive states in which individuals actively embrace the world around them (Lemonick, 2005). As researchers examined characteristics of happy people, they found that this emotion had a profound impact on the body. Happiness, or related mood states such as hopefulness, optimism, and contentment, are believed to reduce the risk or limit the severity of cardiovascular disease, pulmonary disease, type 2 diabetes, hypertension, colds, and other infections (Lemonick,

Happiness Feeling of contentment created when expectations and physical, psychological, and spiritual needs are met and life is enjoyed.

Subjective well-being (SWB) An uplifting feeling of inner peace and/ or an overall feel-good state.

2005). Laughter increases heart and respiration rates, and reduces stress hormones in the same way as physical activity. For this reason, it has been promoted as a possible risk reducer for those with hypertension and other forms of cardiovascular disease (Kluger, 2005).

If happiness is good for your health, how do you "get happy?" **Subjective well-being (SWB)** refers to that uplifting feeling of inner peace or overall "feel-good state," which includes happiness. SWB is defined by three central components (Kluger, 2005):

1. **Satisfaction with present life.** When you are high in SWB, you tend to like your work (or stage of career development) and are satisfied with your current personal relationships. You are sociable, outgoing, and willing to open up to others. You also like yourself and enjoy good health and self-esteem.

2. **Relative presence of positive emotions.** When you are high in SWB, you more frequently feel pleasant emotions, mainly because you perceive the world around you in a generally positive way. You choose an optimistic outlook, and expect success in what you do.

3. **Relative absence of negative emotions.** When you have a strong sense of SWB, you experience fewer and less severe episodes of negative emotions, such as anxiety, depression, and anger.

Researchers also suggest that you may be biologically predisposed to happiness. In fact, happiness may be related to actual differences in brain physiology. *Neurotransmitters,* the chemicals that transfer messages between neurons, may function more efficiently when you are happy (Davidson, Maxwell, & Shackman, 2004). Others suggest that you can develop happiness by practising positive psychological actions (Diener & Seligman, 2004; Peterson & Seligman, 2004).

You do not have to be happy all the time to achieve overall subjective well-being. It is normal or usual to experience disappointment, unhappiness, and times when things do not go the way you expected or hoped. In these situations, if you have SWB, you are typically resilient, able to look on the positive side, able to get yourself back on track fairly quickly, and less likely to fall into despair over setbacks. Happiness does not depend on your age, sex, ethnicity, race, or socioeconomic status. Take the quiz at the end of the chapter on happiness and determine your satisfaction with life.

Humans are remarkably resourceful creatures. You will respond to great loss, such as the death of a loved one, or a traumatic event, with an initial period of grief, mourning, and sometimes anger. With time and the support of others, you will move forward and find satisfaction and peace with life once again. Typically, you learn from suffering and emerge stronger and more capable of dealing with the next crisis. You are likely to find some measure of happiness after the initial shock and pain of loss.

Does Laughter Enhance Psychosocial Health?

Remember the last time you laughed so hard that you cried or that your belly ached? Remember how relaxed you felt afterward? Humour is important for your daily life and current health, as noted in the following:

- Stressed people with a strong sense of humour become less depressed and anxious than those whose sense of humour is less well developed.

- Students who use humour as a coping mechanism report that it predisposes them to a positive mood.

- Telling a joke, particularly one that involves a shared experience, increases your sense of belonging and social cohesion.

Clearly, laughter enhances emotional and intellectual health. It also promotes social health: people like to be around others who are fun and who laugh easily. That is likely true for you too. Learning to laugh puts more joy into your everyday experiences and increases the likelihood that others will keep company with you.

Positive emotions such as joy, interest, and contentment serve valuable life functions. Joy is associated with playfulness and creativity. Interest encourages you to explore your world, which enhances your knowledge and cognitive ability. Contentment allows you to savour and integrate experiences, an important step in achieving mindfulness and insight. By building your physical, social, intellectual, and emotional resources, these positive feelings empower you to cope effectively with life's challenges. While the actual emotions may be transient, their effects can be permanent and provide lifelong enrichment (Fredrickson, 2000).

Psychosocial Health and Well-Being

In the 1970s and 1980s, a number of widely publicized studies of the health of widowed and divorced people indicated higher rates of illness and death than those of married people. Moreover, tests revealed below-normal immune-system functioning with follow-up studies indicating higher rates of cancer among people who were depressed (Igoumenou, 2010). Are these studies conclusive evidence of the mind–body connection? Probably not, because they did not take into account other factors relevant to health and disease. For example, some researchers suggest that people who are divorced, widowed, or depressed are more likely to

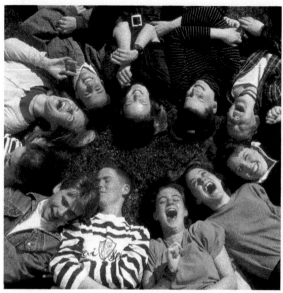

A powerful strategy for maintaining psychosocial health is to make time for friends and activities you enjoy and that bring laughter into your life.

drink and smoke, use drugs, eat and sleep poorly, and fail to engage in regular physical activity—all of which negatively affect the immune system. Another possibly relevant factor is that such people may be less tolerant of illness and more likely to report their problems (Gottman & Silver, 1999).

Keep in mind that the immune system changes measured in various studies of the mind–body connection are relatively small. They are nowhere near as large as what is found in people with HIV and AIDS, for example. The health consequences of such minute changes are difficult to gauge because the body can tolerate a certain amount of reduced immune function without illness developing. The exact amount the body is able to tolerate and under what circumstances are still unresolved questions (Grady, 1992). Thus, although there is a large body of evidence pointing to an association between physical and mental health, there is still much to learn about this relationship. In the meantime, maintaining an optimistic mindset continues to be sound advice as it relates to improved quality of life, regardless of whether or not it increases quantity of life.

UNDERSTANDING MOOD DISORDERS

In spite of your best efforts to remain psychosocially healthy, circumstances and events in your life are sometimes more than you can handle. Abusive relationships, stress, anxiety, loneliness, financial stress due to the high cost of post-secondary education, and other traumatic events can sap your spirits, causing you to turn inward or act in ways that are not so healthy. Chemical imbalances, drug interactions, trauma, neurological disruptions, and other physical problems can also contribute to these not-so-healthy behaviours. **Mental illnesses** are disorders that disrupt your thinking, feeling, moods, and behaviours, and cause a varying degree of impaired functioning in daily life.

Similar to a physical disease, mental illnesses can range from mild to severe and exact a heavy toll on the quality of life of the individual affected and those who come in contact with him or her. It is estimated that one in five Canadians will directly experience a mental illness at some point in his or her lifetime (Canadian Mental Health Association, 2013). In the most recent survey, 71.1 percent of Canadians (72.1 percent men; 70.1 percent women) reported very good or excellent mental health (Statistics Canada, 2014a) while 6.3 percent (5.6 percent men; and 7 percent of women) indicated fair or poor mental health (Statistics Canada, 2014b).

Depression

Depression is the most common emotional disorder in Canada; 11.2 percent of Canadians reported symptoms of depression in the recent 2012 Canadian Community Health Survey (Statistics Canada, 2013a). A major depressive episode is diagnosed when you are depressed and lose interest in most of your daily activities for at least two consecutive weeks (Langlois et al., 2011). Although depression can occur in any age group, onset is generally between 15 and 30 years (Langlois et al., 2011). According to the 2012 Canadian Community Health Survey, 4.7 percent of Canadians over the age of 15 were diagnosed with depression in the past 12 months. Over the course of their lives, females have a greater risk of depression than males: 14.1 versus 8.5 percent. Individuals between 45 and 64 years of age have the greatest possible and probable risk of depression (13.1 percent).

There are two acknowledged forms of depression: endogenous and exogenous depression. **Endogenous depression** is of biochemical origin. Neurotransmitters (chemicals that transmit nerve impulses across synapses) in the brain responsible for mood elevation become unbalanced for unknown reasons. A decrease in these neurotransmitters gives rise to outward expressions of depression. If not treated, endogenous depression may become chronic. **Exogenous depression**, on

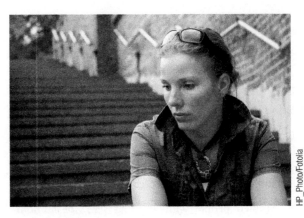

Without appropriate treatment, depression and anxiety can become overwhelming problems that affect psychosocial well-being and physical health.

the other hand, is usually caused by an external event such as the loss of something or someone of great value. People who experience exogenous depression can slide into chronic depression if unable to work through the grieving process necessary for overcoming event-related depression.

Similar symptoms appear in the two types of depression: lingering sadness; inability to find joy in pleasure-giving activities; loss of interest in work and reduced concentration; diminished or increased appetite; unexplainable fatigue; sleep disorders, including insomnia or early-morning awakenings; loss of sex drive; withdrawal from friends and family; feelings of hopelessness and worthlessness; and a desire to die. A person who is depressed may be unable to get out of bed in the morning or find it impossible to leave his or her house/room in residence.

A person who is depressed usually has low self-esteem. He or she may feel alone—separated from and unable to communicate with others. After a while, depression becomes a vicious circle. The person feels helpless and trapped, having no way out. He or she may feel that depression is a deserved punishment for real or imagined failings. Prolonged depression may cause a person to feel utterly worthless and to view suicide as the only way out.

Facts about Depression

Although depression appears to be one of the fastest-growing psychosocial health problems, contributing to 11 percent of all deaths (Langlois et al., 2011), the general public continues to be misinformed or ill-informed about many aspects of it. The following points may help you to better understand depression (Gertz, 1990).

- **Depression is not a natural reaction to crisis and loss.** Something has happened to the

---

Mental illnesses Conditions that result in abnormal thinking, feeling, moods, and behaviours, and cause a varying degree of impaired everyday functioning.

Endogenous depression A type of depression with a biochemical basis.

Exogenous depression A type of depression with an external cause, such as the death of a loved one or marital break-up.

mood and thinking of those who are depressed such that they experience pervasive pessimism, helplessness, despair, and lethargy, sometimes coupled with agitation. Individuals who are depressed may have difficulty at work or school and tend to have chronically negative interpersonal relationships. Symptoms may come and go, get worse, or stay stable, but they do not get better permanently without treatment. People who are depressed forget what it is like to feel normal.

- **People will not "snap out of" depression by using a little willpower.** Telling a depressed person to "snap out of it" is like telling a person with diabetes to produce more insulin. Treatment is needed. Initially, people who are depressed should examine their lifestyles and ensure they are making healthy choices regarding their physical activity, dietary intake, stress management, sleep, and so on. If changes in these behaviours do not help, then medical intervention in the form of antidepressant drugs and therapy may be necessary. Depression also tends to recur—more than half of those afflicted once will experience a recurrence. Understanding the seriousness of depression and supporting people in their attempts to recover is important.

- **Frequent crying is not a hallmark of depression.** Some depressed people do not cry at all. In fact, biochemists theorize that crying may actually ward off depression by releasing chemicals that the body produces as a positive response to distress.

- **Depression is not "all in the mind."** In fact, depressive illnesses originate with an inherited chemical imbalance in the brain. Depression-like symptoms can also be a side-effect of certain physiological conditions (or their treatment), such as thyroid disorders, Lyme disease, diabetes, multiple sclerosis, hepatitis, mononucleosis, rheumatoid arthritis, and pancreatic cancer.

- **No single psychotherapy method works for all cases of depression.** A variety of methods are available. What works best for each person is a treatment tailored to him or her that deals with his or her personal circumstances and experiences.

Treating Depression

Major depression is one of the most treatable of mental health problems (Langlois et al., 2011); various treatments available include lifestyle modification (engaging in regular moderate to vigorous physical activity, eating well, managing stress, getting adequate sleep, developing a strong social support system, and so on); talking to a physician, counsellor, psychologist, or psychiatrist; attending a support group; or taking

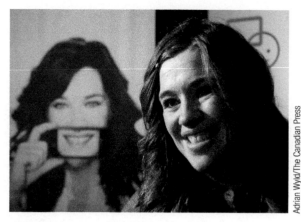

With the continued rise of public health campaigns, Canadians are becoming more familiar with depression.

a prescribed medication. Selecting the best treatment involves determining the type and degree of depression and its possible causes. Psychotherapeutic and pharmacologic modes of treatment are recommended for clinical (severe and prolonged) depression. Drugs often relieve the symptoms of depression, such as loss of sleep or appetite, while psychotherapy can improve the social and interpersonal functioning of the person who is depressed. Treatment may be weighted toward one or the other mode depending on the specific situation. In some cases, psychotherapy alone may be the most successful treatment. The two most common psychotherapeutic therapies for depression are cognitive and interpersonal therapy.

Cognitive therapy aims to help an individual look at life rationally and to address habitually pessimistic thought patterns. It focuses on the here and now rather than analyzing the past. It may take 6 to 18 months of weekly sessions comprising reasoning and behavioural exercises with a cognitive therapist to relieve a person of his or her depression. *Interpersonal therapy* is sometimes combined with cognitive therapy. It also addresses the present but differs from cognitive therapy in that its primary goal is to manage chronic issues with human relationships. Interpersonal therapists focus on individuals' relationships with their families and others.

Antidepressant drugs relieve symptoms in nearly 80 percent of people with chronic depression. In recent years, drug therapies have become so common that it is not unusual to know someone taking them. Despite their commonness, caution is warranted regarding the use of antidepressants. Many emergency-room visits occur when people misuse their antidepressants, in particular when they try to quit "cold turkey" or when they have drug interactions (see Chapter 9). Clinics have been established in large metropolitan areas to offer group support for people who are depressed. Some clinics treat all people who are depressed, while others restrict themselves to specific groups, such as widows, adolescents, or families and friends of people with depression.

Seasonal Affective Disorder

Seasonal affective disorder (SAD), a type of depression, affects approximately 2 to 3 percent of Canadians (Schlaepfer & Nemeroff, 2012). As much as 25 percent of the population in Canada experiences a milder form of the disorder known as the "winter blues." SAD strikes during the winter months and is associated with reduced exposure to sunlight. People with SAD experience irritability, apathy, carbohydrate craving and weight gain, increases in sleep time, and general sadness. It is believed that SAD is caused by a malfunction in the hypothalamus, the gland responsible for regulating responses to external stimuli. Stress may also play a role in SAD.

Certain factors seem to put people at risk for SAD. Women are four times more likely to suffer from SAD than men. Although SAD occurs in people of all ages, those between 20 and 40 years of age appear to be the most vulnerable (Whalen, n.d.). Certain families also appear to be at risk. People living in cities with cold, bright winters and with an active winter culture often have lower rates of SAD than expected. Vancouver has relatively high rates of SAD due to frequent overcast skies, while Saskatchewan has lower rates due to the frequency of sunshine in the winter. Some people experience a reduction in symptoms when they move south (Whalen, n.d.).

There are some simple but effective therapies for SAD (Whalen, n.d.). The most beneficial appears to be light therapy, in which an individual is exposed to lamps that mimic sunlight. In fact, following four days of daily light exposure, 80 percent of individuals experienced relief from their symptoms. Other forms of treatment include dietary modifications (eating more foods high in complex carbohydrates), increased physical activity, stress management, sleep restriction (limiting the number of hours slept in a 24-hour period), psychotherapy, and antidepressants.

Seasonal affective disorder (SAD) A type of depression that occurs in the winter months, when sunlight levels are low.

Anxiety disorders Disorders characterized by persistent feelings of threat and anxiety in coping with everyday problems.

Obsessive-compulsive disorder (OCD) A disorder characterized by obsessive thoughts or habitual behaviours.

Phobia A deep and persistent fear of a specific object, activity, or situation that results in a compelling desire to avoid the source of the fear.

Panic attack The sudden, rapid onset of disabling terror.

Anxiety Disorders

Anxiety disorders are the most common of mental health problems, occurring in about 1 in 10 people and more frequently in women than in men (Canadian Mental Health Association, 2009a). Anxiety disorders refer to a group of disorders that affect behaviour, thoughts, emotions, and physical health. These include obsessive-compulsive disorder, phobias, panic disorders, and post-traumatic stress disorder. People with anxiety disorders have intense, prolonged feelings of fright and distress for no apparent reason. It is believed that anxiety disorders are caused by a combination of genetics and personal circumstances. Anxiety disorders can be effectively treated with a combination of pharmaceutical intervention and cognitive-behavioural therapy (Canadian Mental Health Association, 2009a).

Obsessive-Compulsive Disorders

An **obsessive-compulsive disorder (OCD)** is an anxiety disorder that affects the thoughts, behaviours, emotions, and sensations of those who experience it (Canadian Mental Health Association, 2013). Obsessions—intrusive and illogical—are persistent ideas, thoughts, impulses, or images. Common OCDs revolve around contamination (therefore the need to wash the hands many times before eating), doubts (such as not being sure whether the lights were turned off), and disturbing sexual or religious thoughts. More harmful behaviours include pulling out the hair, eyebrows, or eyelashes, and other forms of self-mutilation.

It is believed that OCDs have a neurological and genetic basis. They occur equally in men and women of all ages, though usually before 40 years of age, and most often begin during adolescence or early childhood.

Phobias

A **phobia** is an anxiety disorder that involves a deep and persistent fear of a specific object, activity, or social situation, and results in a compelling desire to avoid the source of fear (Canadian Mental Health Association, 2009b). Phobias are thought to be more prevalent in women than in men. Simple phobias, such as fear of spiders, flying, or heights, can be treated successfully with behavioural therapy. Social phobias (fears related to interaction with others), such as fear of public speaking, inadequate sexual performance, and eating in public places, generally require more extensive therapy.

Panic Disorders

Another type of anxiety disorder is panic disorders which are expressed via a **panic attack**, the sudden onset of disabling terror (Langlois et al., 2011). These attacks can happen at any time: while sleeping, sitting in traffic, or just before you deliver your class presentation. Suddenly and unexpectedly, your heart starts to race, your face turns red, you cannot catch your breath, you feel nauseated, you start to perspire, and you may feel like you are going to pass out or are having a heart attack. Panic attacks may have no obvious link to environmental stimuli, or they may be learned responses to environmental stimuli. The exact causes of panic disorders remain unknown, although there appears to be a genetic component (Langlois et al., 2011). Stress and stimulant drugs, including caffeine, may also be related (Langlois et al., 2011).

Post-Traumatic Stress Disorder

Sometimes people experience something so unexpected and so shattering that it has a serious effect on them long after the danger has passed (Canadian Mental Health Association, 2009c). Examples of these experiences include traumas such as rape, abuse, assault, war, natural disasters (hurricanes, tornadoes, floods, forest fires), or airplane or car crashes. People who suffer serious after-effects of such experiences are afflicted by **post-traumatic stress disorder (PTSD)**. Common symptoms include flashbacks in which the terrifying experience is relived, nightmares, depression, detachment, and feelings of anger and irritability.

Schizophrenia

Perhaps the most frightening of all mental disorders is **schizophrenia**, a disease that affects about 1 percent of the Canadian population (Langlois et al., 2011). Schizophrenia is characterized by alterations of the senses (including auditory and visual hallucinations); the inability to sort out incoming stimuli and make appropriate responses; an altered sense of self; and radical changes in emotions, movements, and behaviours. Individuals with this disease often cannot function in society, unless treated pharmacologically (Langlois et al., 2011).

Schizophrenia is now recognized as a biological brain disease. It has become evident that the brain damage involved occurs very early in life, possibly as early as in the second trimester of fetal development. However, the disease most commonly has its onset in late adolescence.

Schizophrenia is treatable but not curable. Treatments usually include some combination of hospitalization, medication, and supportive psychotherapy. Supportive psychotherapy, as opposed to psychoanalysis, is used to help the individual acquire skills for living in society.

Despite its genetic roots, a stigma remains attached to schizophrenia. Families of individuals with schizophrenia often experience anger and guilt. They often need help in the form of information, family counselling, and advice on how to meet the needs for shelter, medical care, vocational training, and social interaction of their family member with schizophrenia.

SEX ISSUES IN PSYCHOSOCIAL HEALTH

Studies indicate that sex bias often gets in the way of correct diagnosis of psychosocial disorders. Doctors have arrived at different diagnoses even though symptoms were identical for males and females (Afifi, 2007). Further, women's illnesses were more likely to be diagnosed as psychiatric disorders with inappropriate medications prescribed (Afifi, 2007).

Depression and Sex

For reasons not well understood, women are twice as likely as men to develop depression (Statistics Canada, 2012b). Researchers have proposed biological, psychological, and social explanations. The biological explanation relates to women's hormone level changes observed during the menstrual cycle, pregnancy, miscarriage, postpartum period, pre-menopause, and menopause. Women also face various stressors related to their multiple roles and responsibilities—work, child-rearing, household work, relationships, and caring for older parents—at rates much greater than men. Although men's hormone levels appear to remain relatively stable throughout life, they too experience depression. For men, depression is often masked by alcohol or drug use or by the socially acceptable habit of working excessively long hours. Typically, men who are depressed present as irritable, angry, and discouraged rather than hopeless and helpless.

Not only are rates of depression different in men and women, they also have differences in coping strategies or response to certain events or stimuli, with women's coping strategies more likely to put them at greater risk of developing or maintaining depression. Men tend to distract themselves from a depressed mood, whereas women tend

---

Post-traumatic stress disorder A disorder characterized by terrifying flashbacks, detachment, and anxiety following a severe traumatic event.

Schizophrenia A mental illness characterized by irrational behaviours, severe alterations of the senses (hallucinations), and, often, an inability to function in society.

to focus on it. If focusing on depressed feelings intensifies these feelings, women's response style then may make them more likely than men to become clinically depressed.

PMS: Physical or Mental Disorder?

A major controversy regarding sex bias is the inclusion of a diagnosis for premenstrual syndrome (PMS) and premenstrual dysphoric disorder (PMDD) in the American Psychiatric Association's *Diagnostic and Statistical Manual of Mental Disorders*, fifth edition (known as *DSM-5*). Support for its inclusion was noted by Epperson et al. (2012). PMS is characterized by depression, irritability, and other symptoms of increased stress typically occurring just prior to menstruation and lasting for a day or two. Whereas PMS is somewhat disruptive and uncomfortable, it does not interfere with daily function; PMDD does. To be diagnosed with PMDD, a woman must have at least five symptoms of PMS for a week to ten days, at least one of which is serious enough to interfere with her ability to function at work or at home. In these more severe cases, antidepressants may be prescribed.

SUICIDE: GIVING UP ON LIFE

In its latest release Statistics Canada reported 3926 suicides in Canada for 2012, (equivalent to a rate of 17.2 and 5.4 per 100 000 for men and women, respectively) (Statistics Canada, 2012), lower than the worldwide rate of 16 per 100 000 people reported by the World Health Organization (2013). The pressures, joys, disappointments, challenges, and changes within the college or university environment are believed to contribute to these rates. However, young adults who choose not to go to post-secondary school and who search for directions in their career and relationship goals and other life aspirations are also at risk for suicide. Experts estimate that there may actually be more cases of suicide than reported due to the difficulty in determining the causes of suspicious deaths. Suicide is often a consequence of poor coping skills, lack of social support, lack of self-esteem, and the inability to see the way out of a bad or negative situation. Suicide can also be viewed as an extreme form of violence—anger, rage, and hopelessness turned inward rather than outward.

University or college students are more likely than the general population to attempt suicide; it is the second leading cause of death in people between the ages of 15 and 24. Although women attempt suicide at four times the rate of men, more than three times as many men as women actually succeed in ending their lives. Men may be more "successful" than women because they often choose more violent measures to kill themselves (that is, firearms versus an overdose of painkillers). The suicide rates are five to seven times higher among First Nations youth than for non-Aboriginal youth (Statistics Canada, 2013b).

People likely to commit suicide include those who are:

- experiencing a serious physical or mental illness,
- abusing alcohol or drugs,
- experiencing a major loss—such as the death of a loved one, unemployment, or divorce,
- experiencing major changes in life—for example, teenagers and seniors,
- have made previous suicide attempts, and
- have had a parent commit suicide (Canadian Mental Health Association, n.d.).

Many of us will be touched by a suicide at some time. In most cases, the suicide does not occur unpredictably. In fact, it is estimated that 8 out of 10 people who attempt suicide or die by suicide hint or talk openly about it beforehand (Canadian Mental Health Association, n.d.). Further, suicide is considered a process, not an event, with most contemplating their fate over a relatively long period of time.

Warning Signals of Suicide

Common warning signals of suicide include

- talk of suicide—for example, "no one cares if I live or die," or "I would be better off dead," or "it would be so much easier for everyone if I was dead"
- making a plan as to how a person might end his or her life
- increased risk taking
- writing or drawing about suicide (in a diary, for example)
- a preoccupation with death; giving away valued possessions
- a withdrawal from friends and family and from activities once found pleasurable
- hero worship of people who have died by suicide
- increased use of alcohol or drugs
- recent loss of a friend, family member, or parent, especially if they died by suicide
- conflicting feelings or sense of shame about being gay, straight, or transgendered

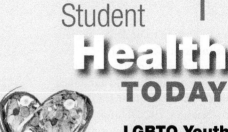

Student Health TODAY

LGBTQ Youth and Suicide Prevention

According to U.S. research among lesbian, gay, bisexual, transgender, and queer (LGBTQ) people, up to 40 percent of youth in grades 9 to 12 have considered suicide, compared with just over 10 percent of their heterosexual peers. Moreover, a study of 350 LGBTQ youth in Canada, the United States, and New Zealand found that over 4 out of 10 had considered suicide, and 1 in 3 had attempted suicide.

LGBTQ youth who come from highly rejecting families are more than eight times as likely to have attempted suicide as LGBTQ peers who reported no or low levels of family rejection. Furthermore, those that have experienced bullying in school and verbal or physical abuse by classmates are at greater risk for suicide. Other risk factors for suicide attempts include:

- A lack of social support
- A sense of isolation
- Stigma associated with seeking help

- Loss of a relationship
- Access to firearms and other lethal means

Protective factors to reduce suicide attempts include:

- Support through ongoing medical and mental health relationships
- Coping, problem-solving, and conflict-resolution skills
- Restricted access to highly lethal means of suicide
- Strong connections to family
- Family and parental acceptance of sexual orientation and/or gender identity
- School safety, support, connectedness and peer groups such as gay–straight alliances, LGBTQ groups, and so on
- Community support
- Positive role models and self-esteem
- Cultural and religious beliefs that discourage suicide and support self-preservation

Furthermore, there is growing awareness for the need to address LGBTQ suicide risk and possible interventions for reducing risk in national and provincial suicide prevention strategies and plans. Provide educational and resource materials on LGBTQ suicide and suicide risk to

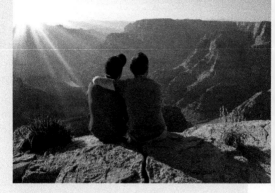

LGBTQ youth can experience unique challenges that may lead to depression or attempting suicide.

LGBTQ organizations, and encourage consideration of how suicide prevention can be advanced within the context of each organization's mission and activities.

Sources: Based on Rainbow Health Ontario, (2013). RHO Fact Sheet: LGBTQ Youth Suicide. Retrieved on October 11, 2016 from http://www.rainbowhealthontario.ca/resources/rho-fact-sheet-lgbt-youth-suicide/; Haas et al., "Suicide and Suicide Risk in Lesbian, Gay, Bisexual, and Transgender Populations: Review and Recommendations," *Journal of Homosexuality, 58,* no. 1 (2011), 10–51; The Trevor Project. Suicidal Signs and Facts. www.thetrevorproject.org/suicide-resources/suicidal-signs, (2010); M. Posner and L. Potter. "Suicide Risk and Prevention for Lesbian, Gay, Bisexual, and Transgender Youth," Suicide Prevention Resource Center, www.hhd.org/resources/publications/suicide-risk-and-prevention-lesbian-gay-bisexual-and-transgender-youth, 2008.

- mood swings, emotional outbursts, high level of irritability or aggression
- feelings of hopelessness (Canadian Mental Health Association, n.d.)

Taking Action to Prevent Suicide

Suicide is often seen as the only way out of an intolerable situation. People who commit suicide are often in such pain they cannot see any other way out. Crisis counsellors and help lines can help temporarily, but the only way to prevent suicide is to alleviate

conditions, situations, and substances that may precipitate attempts, including alcohol, drugs, loneliness, isolation, and access to guns. If someone you know threatens or displays warnings signs of suicide, take the following actions:

- **Monitor the warning signals.** Ensure that there is someone around the person as much as possible, 24/7 ideally.
- **Find a safe place to talk with the person.** Allow as much time as necessary. Talking about suicide will most likely decrease the chances that someone will act on his or her suicidal feelings.

- **Take any threat seriously.** Do not brush them off.
- **Do not belittle the person's feelings or say that he or she does not really mean it or could not succeed at suicide.** To some people, these comments offer the challenge of proving you wrong.
- **Let the person know how much you care about him or her.** State that you are there if he or she needs help.
- **Listen.** Try not to discredit or be shocked by what the person says to you. Empathize, and keep the person talking. Talk about stressors and listen to responses.
- **Ask the person directly, "Are you thinking of hurting or killing yourself?"**
- **Help the person think about alternatives.** Go with the person for help.
- **Make a plan with the person for the next few hours or days.** Help this person make contact with an appropriate health-care professional or make the contact yourself. Take this person to an appropriate health-care facility to meet with a counsellor.
- **If the person has a plan, remove any pills or guns; call 911 immediately for help.**
- **Tell your friend's spouse, partner, parents, brothers and sisters, or counsellor.** Do not keep your suspicions to yourself. Do not let a suicidal friend talk you into keeping your discussions confidential. Let your friend know you must share this information with a professional. If your friend is successful in a suicide attempt, you will have to live with the consequences of your inaction. Counselling services available on campus can help you talk with your friend and suggest options for you (Canadian Mental Health Association, n.d.).

WHEN MOOD DISORDERS AND SUBSTANCE USE DISORDERS MIX

Unfortunately, many Canadians suffering from mood disorders attempt to remedy or mask their pain by taking illegal substances. In fact studies show that over 50 percent of Canadians with mood disorders abuse alcohol and/or illegal drugs compared to 15 percent of the general population (Mood Disorder Society of Canada, 2009). It is a complex relationship, and health professionals are still trying to understand these connections. It has been described as the "chicken and egg syndrome." Mental health problems can be a risk factor for substance use problems, and substance abuse can be a risk factor for mood disorders (Canadian Mental Health Association, BC Division, 2005). If you are interested in learning more about substance abuse and responsible alcohol consumption please see Chapters 9 and 10.

SEEKING PROFESSIONAL HELP

Many Canadians feel that seeking professional help for psychosocial problems is an admission of personal failure. Typically, any physical health problem, such as an abscessed tooth or prolonged severe pain, sends us to the nearest dentist or physician. On the other hand, we tend to ignore psychosocial problems until they pose a serious threat to our well-being—and even then, we may refuse to ask for the help needed. Recently, however, an increasing number of Canadians are turning to mental health professionals for help. Researchers believe that more people want help today because "normal" living has become more difficult. Breakdown in support systems, high expectations of the individual by society, and dysfunctional families are cited as the three major reasons more people ask for help.

You should consider professional help under the following circumstances:

- you think you need help
- you experience wild mood swings
- your problem is interfering with your daily life
- your fears or feelings of guilt frequently distract you
- you begin to withdraw from others
- you hallucinate
- you feel that your life is not worth living
- you feel inadequate or worthless
- your emotional responses are inappropriate in various situations
- your daily life seems to be nothing but repeated crises
- you feel you cannot "get your act together"
- you are considering suicide
- you turn to drugs or alcohol to escape your problems
- you feel out of control

Types of Mental Health Professionals

Several types of mental health professionals, or providers, are available to help you. The most important criterion when choosing a provider is whether you feel you can work well with that person, not how many degrees he or she has.

Psychiatrist

A **psychiatrist** is a medical doctor. After obtaining a medical degree, a psychiatrist spends up to 12 years studying psychosocial health and disease. As a licensed physician, a psychiatrist can prescribe medications for various mental or emotional problems and may have admitting privileges at local hospitals. Some psychiatrists are affiliated with hospitals, while others are in private practice. Psychiatric fees are normally covered by provincial or territorial health insurance.

Psychoanalyst

A **psychoanalyst** is a psychiatrist or a psychologist with special training in psychoanalysis. Psychoanalysis is a type of therapy in which a person is helped to remember early traumas that block personal growth. Facing these traumas may help the individual to resolve his or her conflicts and begin to lead a more productive life.

Psychologist

A **psychologist** usually has a PhD or doctorate in counselling or clinical psychology. In addition, all provinces and territories require licensure for someone to use this title. Psychologists are trained in various types of 'talk' therapy. Most are trained to conduct individual and group counselling sessions. Psychologists may also be trained in certain specialties, such as family counselling, sexual counselling, or counselling related to compulsive behaviours. Psychologists may work in private practice or in publicly funded organizations. Some employee assistance programs cover a certain number of psychologist visits annually, and the extended health plan through your university or college may have some coverage for these fees.

Clinical/Certified/Psychiatric Social Worker

A **social worker** has at least a master's degree in social work (MSW) and two years of experience in a clinical setting. Some provinces and territories require an examination for accreditation in the College of Clinical Social Work. Some social workers work in clinical settings, whereas others have private practices. Certified clinical social workers (CSW) often work in private practices, and their clients are sometimes insured through employee assistance programs.

Counsellor

People with a variety of academic and experiential training call themselves counsellors. Most **counsellors** have a master's degree in counselling, psychology, educational psychology, or a related human service. Professional societies recommend at least two years of graduate coursework or supervised practice as a minimum requirement. Many counsellors are trained to do individual and group counselling. They often specialize in one type of counselling, such as family, marital, relationship, children, drug, divorce, behavioural, or personal counselling. Remember that in Canada anyone can use the title of therapist or counsellor. Before you begin treatment, you should consider the credentials of your counsellor, your desired outcomes, and your expectations, as well as those of your counsellor.

Psychiatric Nurse Specialist

Although all registered nurses can work in psychiatric settings, some have chosen to continue their education and specialize in psychiatric practice. The psychiatric nurse specialist can be certified by the Registered Psychiatric Nursing Association in some provinces.

Choosing a Therapist: Key Factors to Consider

When you are in emotional or psychological trouble, you are often in the most vulnerable of situations. The choices you make in times of desperation are often critical to your current and future health; yet, many people choose their therapists at random when they are at their lowest emotional point. Like auto mechanics, physicians, and professors, all therapists are not created equal, nor are they equally skilled at what they do. A degree or credential does not ensure compatibility with you, or even general competence. Take some time to check out the person you are going to see and evaluate that person during your first session; these are important first steps in taking care of yourself. While even the most thorough check does

Psychiatrist A licensed physician who specializes in treating mental and emotional disorders.

Psychoanalyst A psychiatrist or psychologist with special training in psychoanalysis.

Psychologist A person with a PhD and training in clinical or counselling psychology.

Social worker A person with a master's degree and at least two years' of clinical training.

Counsellor A person with a variety of academic and experiential training who deals with the treatment of emotional problems.

not guarantee satisfaction, assessing the following may help make your experience a positive and fulfilling one:

1. **Does the therapist have qualities you want in a close friend?** Early in your interaction with the therapist, you should find that the therapist is someone you like, admire, and respect—someone you relate to well and would be willing to trust with your most intimate thoughts. The therapist should convey a genuine interest in you and your problems, rather than watch the clock or check his or her book to schedule your next appointment. You should enjoy sitting in the room with this person and talking. In short, you need to "connect" with your therapist.

2. **Does the therapist act professionally?** Most therapists adhere to a very basic code of ethics. They set boundaries around their relationships with clients to ensure the clients' safety, foster a feeling of trust, and encourage confidence in their ability to help. There are exceptions, however. Signs of unprofessional behaviour include

   - suggestions of meetings or social interactions outside of your sessions, particularly if the therapist appears to be trying to be a personal friend or lover rather than maintaining a professional role
   - agreeing to counsel someone with whom there is a conflict of interest in the counselling situation. Former partners, business relationships, friends, and other clients should be off-limits
   - continually being late for sessions, seeming distracted in sessions, forgetting what you told them before and needing you to repeat things
   - spending too much time talking about him- or herself during the session rather than listening to you; identifying too much of what you are saying with him- or herself rather than your own situation
   - questionable billing practices, such as discrepancies in billing, billing errors to insurance companies, or seeming to want your business and the money rather than displaying a sincere desire to help
   - locking you into the therapist's own specialty; for example, a counsellor who specializes in alcoholism and adult children of alcoholics who continually tries to force you into the "adult child of alcoholic" box, even though this has little to do with your unique situation
   - continual interruptions of your session with phone calls, talking to the receptionist, or other diversions so that you do not get your full amount of time
   - never seeming to want to release you from therapy or encouraging an indefinite dependence on their help. Although the length of treatment varies with each client and his or her respective

problems, one of the goals of therapy should be to get out of therapy

3. **Does the therapist work with you to set your goals, thereby empowering you to get better at your own pace?** Good therapists will assess your general problem fairly early and set at least some provisional goals for you to work on. These usually take the form of small steps that you can tackle each week between sessions, or things that you can do to help you think about your issues and problems. If therapy takes place only in the office, the therapist is not moving you toward recovery. A good therapist is not a detective there to solve your problem per se; his or her role is to provide insight into the things you are doing or to help you understand how your situation and personal actions contribute to your problem(s). A good therapist should serve as a catalyst for you to help yourself, rather than serving as your saviour. Good therapists help you find your answers and build on your strengths, rather than just focusing on getting rid of your weaknesses.

4. **Is the therapist willing to let you conduct an interview before committing to his or her services?** Good therapists will allow you at least one meeting (often at a minimal or reduced charge) to check out the aforementioned information and to find out about their credentials, their counselling style, their personality, and the general "fit."

Most therapy should result in at least minor improvements in six to eight weeks. If you find that you are getting nowhere, if you are repeating the same things over and over, or if you find problems with any of the above, do not be afraid to find another therapist (*CBS This Morning*, 1996; Kalat, 1996).

What to Expect When You Begin Therapy

Before making an appointment, call for information and to briefly explain your needs. Ask about office hours, policies and procedures, fees, and insurance participation. Most of us have misconceptions about what therapy is and what it can do. The first visit serves as a sizing-up between you and the therapist. The therapist will record your history and details about the problem that has brought you to therapy. Answer honestly and do not be embarrassed to acknowledge your feelings. It is critical to the success of your treatment that you trust the therapist enough to be open and honest. Do not expect the therapist to tell you what to do or how to behave. The responsibility for improved behaviour lies with you. If, after your first visit (or even after several visits), you feel you cannot work with this person, say so. You have the right to find a therapist with whom you feel comfortable.

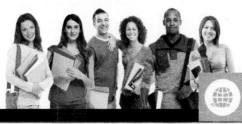
TAKING CHARGE: Managing Your Psychosocial Health

Psychosocial health involves many intricately woven components. Finding the best way to achieve optimal psychosocial health requires careful introspection and planned action. The following questions and questionnaire may provide depth to your understanding of your psychosocial health.

- Why is being psychosocially healthy important to you? To the people close to you?
- What steps can you take to improve your intellectual health? What actions can you take today that will improve your emotional health? What steps can you take to improve your social health? What can you do to improve your spiritual health?
- If you thought you had a psychosocial problem, would you seek help? Why or why not? Who could you seek help from?

Remember that achieving optimal mental health is influenced by many factors. Keep in mind the following points and act upon them whenever possible

- Consider life an opportunity for discovery and learning.
- Accept yourself as the best that you are able to be right now.
- Remember that nobody is perfect.
- Remember that the most difficult times in life occur during transitions and can be opportunities for growth even though they may be painful.
- Remember that there are other perspectives than your own.
- Recognize the sources of your anxiety and act to reduce them.
- Ask for help when you need it; discuss your problems with others.
- Become sensitive to and aware of your body's physical and mental signals—take care of yourself.
- Find a meaning for your life and work toward achieving your goals.
- Develop strategies to get through problem situations.
- Remain open to emotional experiences—give yourself to today rather than waiting for tomorrow.
- Even when you fail, be proud of yourself for trying.
- Keep your sense of humour—learn to laugh at yourself.
- Never quit trying to grow, to experience, to love, and to live life to its fullest.

FIGURE 2.3
Satisfaction with Life Scale

How happy are you?
Read the following statements, and then rate your level of agreement with each one using the 1–7 scale.

1	2	3	4	5	6	7
Strongly disagree	Disagree	Slightly disagree	Neither agree nor disagree	Slightly agree	Agree	Strongly agree

1. In most ways, my life is close to my ideal. _____
2. The conditions of my life are excellent. _____
3. I am satisfied with my life. _____
4. So far I have gotten the important things I want in life. _____
5. If I could live my life over, I would change almost nothing. _____

Total score: _____

Scoring:
31–35: You are very satisfied with your life 26–30: Satisfied 21–25: Slightly satisfied
20: You are neither satisfied nor dissatisfied 15–19: Slightly dissatisfied 10–14: Dissatisfied 5–9: Very dissatisfied

Source: Based on W. Pavot and E. Diener, "Review of the Satisfaction with Life Scale," *Psychological Assessment 5* (1993): 164–172.

DISCUSSION QUESTIONS

1. What is psychosocial health? What are the indicators of psychosocial health?

2. Discuss the factors that influence your overall level of psychosocial health. Why do you think the university or college environment may provide a challenge to your psychosocial health? What factors can you change? Which ones may be more difficult to change? How do you cope with factors you cannot change?

3. What steps could you take today to improve your psychosocial health? Which steps require long-term effort?

4. What factors contribute to psychosocial difficulties and illnesses? Which of the more common psychosocial illnesses are likely to affect people in your age group? What can you do to prevent these happening in you?

5. What are the warning signs of suicide? What would you do if you heard a stranger in the cafeteria say to no one in particular that he was going to "do the world a favour and end it all?" What if this person was a friend; how would you react then?

6. Describe the different types of health professionals and therapies. What services are provided by your student health centre? Which service/professional would you recommend for which service?

APPLICATION EXERCISE

Reread the "Consider This . . ." scenario at the beginning of the chapter and answer the following questions.

1. How psychosocially healthy is Marisol?

2. What factors contribute to Marisol's current health status?

3. What services on your campus would be available to help Marisol improve her psychosocial health?

4. As a friend, what could you do to help Marisol?

MASTERINGHEALTH

Go to MasteringHealth for Assignments, the eText, and the Study Area with case studies, self quizzing, and videos.

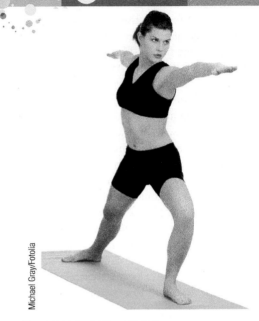

Michael Gray/Fotolia

CHAPTER 3

UNDERSTANDING AND COPING WITH LIFE'S STRESSORS

◄●) CONSIDER THIS . . .

Rhett is taking a full load of classes in his first year of post-secondary studies. He is living with his best friend from high school in a residence on campus and goes home one weekend each month. He is involved in several student organizations and plays intramural sports. He is doing well in his science courses but struggling in his arts classes. Although he tries to study in his room, he finds residence life too distracting and had to find somewhere else to study. The library is often overcrowded and he has difficulty finding a spot. He feels he wastes precious studying time trying to find a place to set up his books and things. Rhett tries to get to bed by midnight; however, the noise level in the residence often keeps him awake until 1 or 2 a.m. Since being on campus, he eats fewer vegetables and fruit and more pasta, pizza, burgers, and fries. Unlike many of his friends who say they know what they are planning to do when they graduate, Rhett is still searching for his career path.

Are Rhett's experiences common for first-year university or college students? What components of first-year post-secondary studies might cause him to feel stressed? What advice would you give him as a first-year student?

LEARNING OUTCOMES

- Define stress, stressors, and stress reaction.

- Explain the three phases of the general adaptation syndrome and describe what happens physiologically and psychologically when under stress.

- Discuss psychosocial, environmental, and self-imposed sources of stress. Describe the stressors particularly relevant to university and college students.

- Identify stress management techniques.

- Clarify the immune system's response to acute and chronic stress.

Stress: hard to live with and almost impossible to live without. You are likely bombarded by a host of subtle and not-so-subtle internal and external factors that may lead you to feel stressed from the moment you wake until you fall asleep. Even as you sleep, noise, temperature changes, and other activities can lead to a stress response. Rarely does a day go by without someone you know talking about being under stress—from homework, part-time or full-time job responsibilities, financial pressures, relationships, volunteer-related responsibilities, technology, or other problems. Despite your best efforts to ignore it, You cannot run from, hide from, or wish away stress-inducing factors. You may be one of those people for whom 'stress' is the stimulus for growth and higher levels of achievement. Or you may be one of those people for whom 'stress' increases the likelihood of dysfunctional or abnormal behaviours or illness.

Stress in itself is neither positive nor negative. Rather, it is our reactions to it that can be described as positive or negative (Tavakolia, 2010). Whether you are aware of it or not, your reactions to stress can become the habits that lead you either to health-enhancing personal growth or to debilitation in the form of migraines, substance misuse and abuse, circulatory disorders, asthma, gastrointestinal problems, and hypertension (high blood pressure). In addition, your responses to stress can lead to psychological and social problems, including dysfunctional relationships. In this chapter, we explore why and how these reactions take place and how you may be able to control them and channel your efforts more effectively so that your health and wellness is not compromised.

WHAT IS STRESS?

Many things that contributed to making you who you are also influence how you respond to potentially stress-inducing events in your life. Stress responses—such as breaking out in a cold sweat before asking someone to go out on a date, becoming anxious or irritated around people who speak too slowly or drive too cautiously, feeling nervous when meeting new people, a racing heart rate when you are called upon to make a response in class, feeling edgy or pumped when it is time to play a game—are all unique by-products of past experiences. Your family, friends, environmental conditions, general health status, drug use, personality, and support systems influence how you respond to a given event.

Stress means different things to different people (Koolhaas et al., 2011). Often, we think of **stress** as an externally imposed factor that threatens or makes a demand on our minds and bodies (Canadian Mental Health Association, 2009). If your professor tells you that you have a 10-page paper due next week, that is an external stressor. Most stress is actually self-imposed and is usually the result of an internal state of emotional tension that occurs in response to the various demands of living. Stress can be defined by the physiological and psychological responses to the demands placed upon us (Selye, 1974). In other words, stress refers to the mental and physical response of our bodies to the various demands or expectations placed upon us in our daily lives. It is your thoughts about the situation you are in that are the critical factors; if you decide the demands of the situation outweigh the skills you have, then you are likely to judge the situation as stressful and react with a stress response (Canadian Mental Health Association, 2009).

A **stressor** is any physical, social, or mental event or condition that forces your mind and body to react or adjust (Tavakolia, 2010). Stressors can be tangible, such as an angry parent or a disgruntled roommate, or intangible, such as the mixed emotions associated with meeting your significant other's parents for the first time. Adjustment is your attempt to cope with a given situation (Koolhaas et al., 2011). As you try to adjust to the various stressors in your life, strain can develop. Strain is the wear and tear your body and mind sustains during the process of adjusting to or resisting a stressor.

Most of your daily activities involve situations or events that might elicit a stress response. Positive stress, or stress that results from generally positive situations, is called **eustress**. Getting married, starting school, beginning a career, developing new friendships, and learning a new physical skill can lead to eustress. **Distress**, or negative stress, is caused by things such as financial problems, injury or illness, the death of a loved one, trouble at work, academic difficulties, the unexpected ending of a relationship, and not being sure of your purpose in life. Both types of stress provide you with an opportunity for personal growth and can lead to personal satisfaction.

Although the mind and body each react to eustress and distress, it is most often the reactions to distress that cause concern. Most often, you cannot prevent distress; like eustress, it is simply a part of your life. However, you can learn to recognize the events likely to cause stress and to anticipate your reactions to them by learning to practise prestress coping skills and develop post-stress management techniques. Developing these skills depends on your understanding of the major components of stress. It is also important to recognize which of your stressors are under your control and can be

---

Stress Our mental and physical responses to the demands placed upon us.

Stressor A physical, social, or mental event or condition that forces us to adjust to it.

Eustress Stress perceived as "good" because it potentially results in positive change.

Distress Stress perceived as "bad" because it potentially results in negative change.

managed using a problem-solving focus versus those that are not within your control and may be better managed using an emotion-focus.

The Mind–Body Connection: Physical Responses

The mind–body connection was briefly discussed in Chapter 2 and is related to the field of **psychoneuroimmunology (PNI)**, which involves research regarding the complex interactions between the psychological and physiological systems of the body (The Free Dictionary by Farlex, n.d.). When stress is experienced, the complex intricacies of physical and emotional reactions to it cause the body to wear down over time. As a result, stress is often described generically as a "disease of prolonged arousal" that often leads to other negative health effects.

Much of the initial impetus for studying the health effects of stress came from prospective observations. Specifically, researchers in the Framingham Study noted that highly stressed individuals were significantly more likely to experience cardiovascular diseases (Bressert, 2006). Monkeys exposed to high levels of unpredictable stressors in studies also showed significantly increased levels of disease and mortality (Bressert, 2006). In a study of susceptibility to cold viruses, subjects who reported recent high levels of stressors were much more likely to catch a cold after inhaling large doses of a cold virus through their nose than their counterparts who reported fewer stressors (Bressert, 2006). While the battle over the legitimacy of these observations continues to be waged in research labs, the correlation of too much stress over long periods of time to selected ailments has gained credibility. What do repeated experiences of the stress response actually do to the body? Why are health and wellness experts concerned about repeated responses or reactions to stress? What are the short- and long-term health implications of the stress response? Why is so much emphasis placed on learning how to manage the stress response?

Stress and Impaired Immunity

Although the health effects of prolonged stress responses provide solid evidence of the direct and indirect impact of stress on body organs, researchers continue to seek more answers regarding the physiological and psychological mechanisms that lead to specific diseases. The science of PNI, as previously mentioned, analyzes the relationship between the mind's response to stress and the functioning of the immune system. Further, the field of PNI also examines the beneficial role of

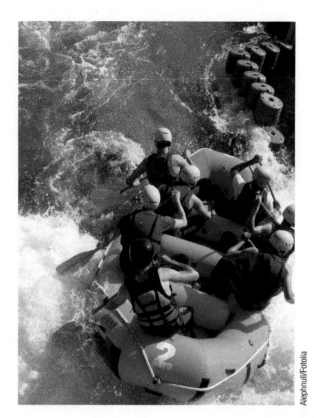

Stress is a positive factor in life when it creates opportunities for personal growth and satisfaction rather than psychological or physiological wear and tear.

enhancing physiological functioning (e.g., engaging in regular physical activity) and better management of stress and the stress response.

Much of the preliminary PNI data on stress and immune functioning focused on the hypothesis that during periods of prolonged stress, elevated levels of adrenal hormones, including cortisol, destroy or reduce the ability of the white blood cells known as "natural killer T cells." Killer T cells aid in the immune response and, when they are suppressed, the body is less effective at combatting illnesses. In addition to killer T suppression, many other body processes are disrupted and overall disease-fighting capacity is reduced. Considerable research supports the hypothesis of a relationship between increased stress levels and greater risk of disease in times of grief, social disruption, poor mood, and so forth, but there is still much to be learned about possible mediating factors (Trueba & Ritz, 2013). Although not enough is yet known about the mechanisms behind this relationship, various potential avenues have been investigated involving various components and processes of the immune system, including the impact of stress on the T helper (Th) cell immune process (Trueba & Ritz, 2013).

Psychoneuroimmunology (PNI) Science that focuses on the intricate relationship between the mind and body and its relationship to health.

Student
Health
TODAY

The Look of Stress

We have seen that look: dark circles under the eyes, pained expression, furrowed brow, and deep lines along a downturned mouth. Usually these relate to too little sleep, too much worry, and "too much to do and no end in sight." Prolonged stress that is not managed poses real threats to your appearance that will not be erased with a good night's sleep.

STRESS AND HAIR LOSS

Too much stress can lead to hair loss, even baldness, in men and women. The most common type of stress-induced hair loss is *telogen effluvium*. Often seen in individuals who have experienced a death in the family or a difficult pregnancy, or lost a dramatic amount of weight, this condition pushes colonies of hair into a resting phase. Over time (usually a few months), simply washing or combing the hair may cause clumps of it to fall out.

A similar stress-related condition known as *alopecia areata* occurs when stress triggers white blood cells to attack and destroy hair follicles, usually in patches. If stress is prolonged, varying degrees of baldness can occur. The good news is that you can reverse the hair loss process in both conditions with sleep, stress management, and sound nutrition.

STRESS AND WEIGHT GAIN

Prolonged stress can result in weight gain. In fact, stress is linked to belly fat. One of the most important strategies for weight maintenance may be to reduce and manage your stress. Exactly how this works is not clear; however, most theories point to prolonged increases in stress hormones.

Stress increases levels of hormones, such as *cortisol*, that stimulates release of glucose into the bloodstream. When blood sugar levels rise, the body secretes insulin to bring these levels down. When stress is chronic, insulin levels can remain elevated, causing fat cells to enlarge and fat to be more readily stored in the body. Prolonged rises in blood sugar and insulin also increase risk for pre-diabetes and diabetes. There also is evidence that prolonged elevations of cortisol may slow your metabolism, thereby making it even more difficult to maintain weight.

As cortisol levels increase, you may find that you actually crave foods, particularly sweet foods made from refined carbohydrates. In addition, cortisol may cause you to feel hungry and eat more than you normally would. Rather than settling down and cooking a healthier meal with plenty of vegetables, whole grains, and lean meat, people who are frustrated, keyed up, angry, or depressed are more likely to choose

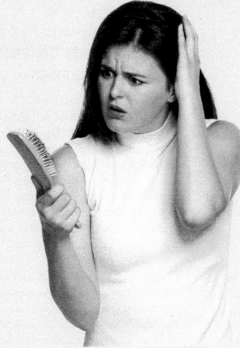

Lubava/Shutterstock

Losing hair? Maybe you need to de-stress?

fast foods and mindlessly munch on chips, candy, or other 'junk' food for comfort.

Sources: Based on D. K. Hall-Flavin, "Stress and Hair Loss: Are They Related?" Mayo Clinic, October 4, 2008, www.mayoclinic.com/health/stress-and-hair -loss/AN01442; S. George, S. Khan, H. Briggs, and J. Abelson, "CRH-stimulated Cortisol Release and Food Intake in Healthy, Non-obese Adults," *Psychoneuroendrocrinology 35*, no. 4 (2010): 607–12; M. Berset, N. Semmer, A. Elfering, N. Jacobshagen, and L. Meier, "Does Stress at Work Make You Gain Weight? A Two-year Longitudinal Study," *Scandinavian Journal of Work, Environment, & Health 37*, no. 1 (2011): 45–53; L. Bacon and L. Aphramor, "Weight Science: Evaluating the Evidence for a Paradigm Shift," *Nutrition Journal 10*, no. 9 (2011). DOI:10.1186/1475-2891-10-9. www .nutritionj.com/content/10/1/9; J. Tomiyama, T. Mann, D. Vinas, J. M. Hunger, J. Dejager, and S. E. Taylor, "Low Calorie Dieting Increases Cortisol," *Psychosomatic Medicine 72*, no. 4 (2010): 357–64.

THE GENERAL ADAPTATION SYNDROME

Every living organism attempts to achieve a state of balance known as **homeostasis**. In homeostasis, all physiological and psychological systems function smoothly, maintaining equilibrium. When a stress is perceived, the mind and body adjust with an **adaptive response**, or an attempt to restore homeostasis. This adaptive response varies in intensity and physical manifestation from person to person and from stressor to stressor. Further, this response varies within an individual from time to time, even in reaction to the same stressor.

The physiological and psychological responses to stress follow a pattern first recognized in 1936 by Selye (1974). The three-stage response to stress is called the **general adaptation syndrome (GAS)**. The phases of the GAS are alarm, resistance, and exhaustion (see Figure 3.1).

Alarm Phase

During the alarm phase, the body detects a stressor that disturbs homeostasis. The brain subconsciously perceives the stressor and prepares the body either to fight or to run away, a response sometimes called the "fight or flight response." The subconscious perceptions and consideration of the stressor stimulate the areas in the

brain responsible for emotions. Emotional stimulation, in turn, starts the physical reactions associated with stress (see Figure 3.2). This entire process usually takes only a few seconds.

When the mind perceives a stressor (either real or imaginary), such as a potential attacker, the cerebral cortex, the region of the brain that interprets the nature of an event, is called to attention. If the cerebral cortex consciously or unconsciously perceives a threat, it triggers an instantaneous **autonomic nervous system (ANS)** response that prepares the body for action (that is, fight or flight). This is an innate response to stress that was developed when our ancestors had to flee or protect themselves from life-threatening predators or even while hunting for their food. The ANS is the portion of the central nervous system that regulates bodily functions that are not normally under conscious control, such as heart rate, breathing, and glandular function. When we are stressed, the rate of these bodily functions increases to give us the physical strength to protect ourselves against an attack, or to mobilize internal forces. The ANS has two branches. One branch, the **sympathetic nervous system (SNS)**, energizes the body for either fight or flight by signalling the release of several stress hormones that increase heart and breathing rates, as well as many other responses. The other branch, the **parasympathetic nervous system (PNS)**, slows all the systems stimulated by the stress response. In other words, the PNS works in opposition to the SNS and attempts to restore homeostasis. In a healthy person, these two systems work together to maintain balance or homeostasis. The problem is, our innate reaction to stress is not very practical as most of the stressors we encounter in modern life do not require a fight or flight response (e.g., lossing your keys or being stuck in traffic). As a result our bodies have pent up energy that is not expended through fleeing or physically defending ourselves. Moreover, long-term stress can cause this balance to become strained, resulting in chronic physical and mental problems. In fact our bodies may make adjustments to our state of balance and attempt to reach homeostasis while still under stress.

Homeostasis A balanced or rhythmic physical and mental state in which the body's systems function smoothly.

Adaptive response Form of adjustment in which the mind and body work to restore homeostasis.

General adaptation syndrome (GAS) The pattern followed in our physiological and psychological responses to stress, consisting of the alarm, resistance, and exhaustion phases.

Autonomic nervous system (ANS) The portion of the central nervous system that regulates bodily functions and is not normally consciously controlled.

Sympathetic nervous system (SNS) Branch of the ANS responsible for stimulating the stress response.

Parasympathetic nervous system (PNS) Part of the ANS responsible for slowing systems stimulated by the SNS.

FIGURE 3.1

The General Adaptation Syndrome

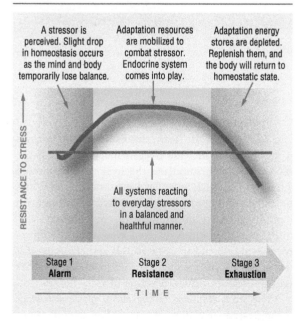

A stressor is perceived. Slight drop in homeostasis occurs as the mind and body temporarily lose balance.

Adaptation resources are mobilized to combat stressor. Endocrine system comes into play.

Adaptation energy stores are depleted. Replenish them, and the body will return to homeostatic state.

RESISTANCE TO STRESS

All systems reacting to everyday stressors in a balanced and healthful manner.

Stage 1
Alarm

Stage 2
Resistance

Stage 3
Exhaustion

TIME

FIGURE 3.2
The Body's Physiological Response to Stress

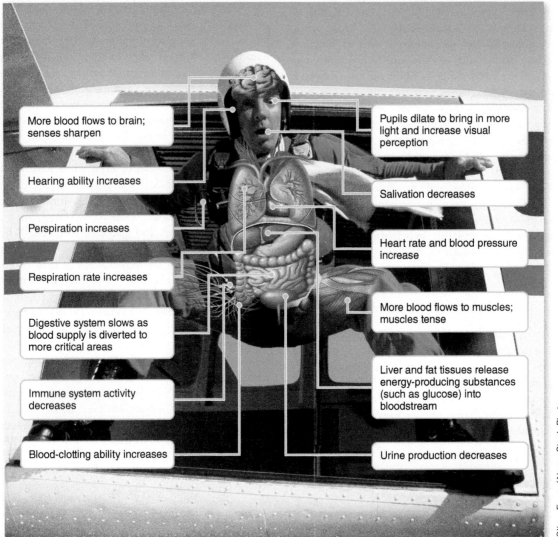

More blood flows to brain; senses sharpen

Hearing ability increases

Perspiration increases

Respiration rate increases

Digestive system slows as blood supply is diverted to more critical areas

Immune system activity decreases

Blood-clotting ability increases

Pupils dilate to bring in more light and increase visual perception

Salivation decreases

Heart rate and blood pressure increase

More blood flows to muscles; muscles tense

Liver and fat tissues release energy-producing substances (such as glucose) into bloodstream

Urine production decreases

Oliver Furrer/Alamy Stock Photo

The response of the SNS to various stressors involves a complex series of biochemical exchanges between different parts of the body. The **hypothalamus**, a section of the brain, functions as the control centre and determines the overall reaction to stressors. When the hypothalamus perceives that extra energy is needed to fight or flee a stressor, it stimulates the adrenal glands, located near the top of the kidneys, to release the hormone **epinephrine**, also called adrenaline.

Hypothalamus A section of the brain that controls the SNS and directs the stress response.

Epinephrine Also called adrenaline, a hormone that stimulates body systems.

Epinephrine causes more blood to be pumped with each beat of the heart, dilates the alveoli (air sacs in the lungs) to increase oxygen intake, increases the rate of breathing, stimulates the liver to release more glucose (which fuels muscular contractions), and dilates the pupils to improve visual sensitivity. The body is then poised to act immediately. As epinephrine secretion increases, blood is diverted away from the digestive system, which can cause nausea and cramping if it occurs shortly after eating. Further, epinephrine dries nasal and salivary tissues, resulting in a dry mouth.

The stress response of the alarm phase also leads to longer-term reactions to stress. The hypothalamus triggers the pituitary gland, which, in turn, releases another powerful hormone, **adrenocorticotrophic hormone (ACTH)**. ACTH signals the adrenal glands to release **cortisol**, a hormone that facilitates the release of stored nutrients to meet energy demands. Finally, other parts of the brain and body release endorphins, the body's naturally occurring opiates, that relieve pain that might be caused by a stressor or the body's response to the stressor.

Resistance Phase

The resistance phase of the GAS begins almost immediately after the alarm phase has started. In the resistance phase, the body adjusts in a way that allows the system to begin the various processes required to return to homeostasis. As the sympathetic nervous system works to energize the body via the hormonal actions of epinephrine, norepinephrine, cortisol, and other hormones, the parasympathetic nervous system counters this by working to keep these energy levels under control and to return the body to a normal level of functioning.

Exhaustion Phase

In the exhaustion phase of the GAS, the physiological and psychological energy used to respond to a stressor (that is, the fight or flight response) has been depleted. Short-term responses to stress would not deplete all a person's energy reserves, but chronic stressors or repeated bouts with the stress response often result in recurring states of alarm and resistance. When a person no longer has the adaptation energy stores to respond to a distressor, burnout and serious illness may result.

SOURCES OF STRESS

Eustress and distress have many sources, including psychosocial factors, such as change, pressure, inconsistent goals and behaviours, conflict, overload, and burnout; environmental stressors, such as natural and human-made disasters; and self-imposed stressors, including factors related to self-concept (Koolhaas et al., 2011).

Psychosocial Sources of Stress

As you learned in Chapter 2, psychosocial health refers to the intellectual, social, emotional, and spiritual dimensions of your health. A combination of these components defines how you perceive your life, relate to others, and react to stress. Many psychosocial factors in your daily life may lead you to feel stressed. Your interactions with others, the subtle and not-so-subtle expectations you have of yourself and others; the expectations others have of you; and the social conditions where you work, play, and live force you to adjust and readjust continually. Some of these stressors present real threats to your mental or physical well-being; others might lead you to worry about things that may never happen. Still other stressors result from otherwise good psychosocial events—being around someone you are attracted to, meeting new friends, moving to a new place, celebrating a win or successful paper or exam, and travelling.

Change

There is the potential to experience stress any time there is change, whether good or bad, in your normal daily routine. The more changes you experience and the more adjustments you must make as a result, the greater your stress response may be. Holmes and Rahe (1967) analyzed the social readjustments experienced by more than 5000 patients, noting which events seemed to occur just before the onset of disease. They determined that certain events (positive and negative) were predictive of increased risk for illness (Holmes & Rahe, 1967). Holmes and Rahe (1967) called their scale for predicting stress overload and the likelihood of illness the Social Readjustment Rating Scale (SRRS). The SRRS has since been modified for certain groups, including university or college-aged students. Although many other factors should also be considered, it is generally believed that the more stressors you have, the more likely you are to experience negative effects on your health and wellness and the more important it is to address your behaviours or situations before health problems occur. See the Rate Yourself box at the end of this chapter to assess your personal levels of stress.

While the SRRS focused on major sources of stress such as a death in the family, Lazarus (1985) focused on petty annoyances, irritations, and frustrations—collectively referred to as hassles—as sources of stress. Minor hassles—losing your keys, having the grocery bag rip on the way to the door, slipping and falling in front of others as you walk to your seat in class, finding that you went through a whole afternoon with a big chunk of spinach stuck in your front teeth—may seem unimportant in the long term, but in the short term, they cause distress, and Lazarus' research suggested

Adrenocorticotrophic hormone (ACTH) A pituitary hormone that stimulates the adrenal glands to secrete cortisol.

Cortisol Hormone released by the adrenal glands that facilitates the release of stored nutrients to meet energy demands.

that the cumulative effects of these minor hassles may be harmful in the long term (Lazarus, 1985).

Pressure

Pressure occurs when you feel forced to speed up, slow down, intensify, or shift the direction of your behaviours to meet a higher standard of performance (Geukes et al., 2013). Pressures can be based on your personal goals and expectations or on a concern about what others might think of you. Pressure can also come from outside influences. Among the most significant and consistent of these are seemingly relentless demands from society or the media to look a certain way, compete in all that you do, and be all that you can be. The forces that push you to attempt to shape your body into an image that may not even be physiologically realistic for you (see also Chapter 6 and the Focus on Body Image feature later in this text) or to compete for the best grades, the nicest cars, the most attractive partners, and the highest paying jobs create a lot of pressure to be the personification of success (Geukes et al., 2013). Being pressured into doing something you do not want to do (for example, to go to a movie or party because everyone else is going, when you really want to study or read) can also be a source of frustration or stress.

Inconsistent Goals and Behaviours

You might find that the negative stress effects are magnified when you experience a conflict between your goals (what you hope to obtain in life) and your behaviours. For instance, you want good grades and your family expects them, yet you party and procrastinate throughout the term, spending very little time studying. Thus, your behaviours are inconsistent with your goals. On the other hand, if you choose to use your time well, study hard, and are committed to your school work, your goals and behaviours are congruent and you will not experience this kind of negative stress. Alternatively, your goal for your post-secondary experience may be to experience as much 'life' as possible, and, in that regard, the time you spend partying and not studying is congruent with your goals and less likely to cause you stress. Thwarted goals may lead to frustration, and frustration has been shown to be a significant disrupter of homeostasis (see Figure 3.3).

Determining whether your behaviours are consistent with your goals is an essential component of your efforts to maintain rhythm in your life. If you consciously strive to attain your goals in a very direct manner, your chances of success are greatly improved. If you deviate from the plan, or if you act in a manner that is inconsistent with

Conflict Simultaneous existence of incompatible demands, opportunities, needs, or goals.

Overload A condition in which we feel pressured by constant and overwhelming demands made upon us.

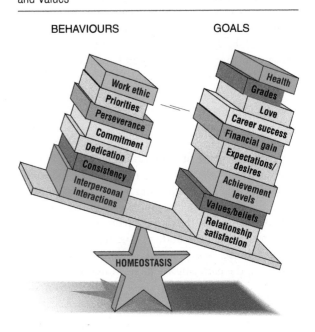

FIGURE 3.3

Homeostatic Balance Requires Actions Related to Goals and Values

BEHAVIOURS   GOALS

Work ethic
Priorities
Perseverance
Commitment
Dedication
Consistency
Interpersonal interactions

Health
Grades
Love
Career success
Financial gain
Expectations/ desires
Achievement levels
Values/beliefs
Relationship satisfaction

HOMEOSTASIS

your goals, significant stress can result that makes achieving your goals impossible and they may then become negative sources of stress.

Conflict

Of all life's difficulties, **conflict** is probably the most common. In fact, conflicts are ubiquitous, they occur between people, between people and the environment, between organizations, and even between countries (Ware & Young, 2010). Conflict occurs when you are forced to make challenging decisions concerning two or more competing motives, behaviours, or impulses; or when you are forced to face two incompatible demands, opportunities, needs, or goals (Yan & Zeng, 2011). What if your best friend chooses to smoke marijuana and you do not want to, yet you fear rejection? Or what if your friends are making fun of a classmate, encouraging you to join in, but you recognize that behaviour as hurtful? Such conflicts occur every day. Worrying about the alternatives, fretting, stewing, and becoming overly anxious are common responses when conflict occurs.

Overload

Overload occurs when you experience excessive time pressures, excessive responsibility, lack of support, or excessive expectations of yourself and those around you. Have you ever felt that you had so many responsibilities that you could not do them all? Have you longed for a weekend when you could just curl up and read a good book or take time out with friends and not feel guilty about all the work you have to do or the responsibilities you have toward others? These feelings typically occur when you have been under continuous pressure for some time and are experiencing overload. You may feel overloaded if you experience anxiety about tests and assignments, do not feel very good about yourself and what you have done, and think about dropping classes or dropping out of school, and other problems. In severe cases, you may be unable to see any solutions, and may experience depression or other forms of mental illness (see Chapter 2) or resort to overeating or consuming alcohol or drugs as a method of coping.

Burnout

If you regularly feel overload, frustration, and disappointment, you may eventually experience **burnout**, a state of physical and mental exhaustion caused by an excessive and continuous response to stress. People involved in the helping professions, such as teaching, social work, drug counselling, nursing, and psychology, appear to experience high levels of burnout, as do police officers, firefighters, and air-traffic controllers, who work in high-pressure, dangerous jobs.

Other Forms of Psychosocial Stress

Other forms of psychosocial stress include problems with adaptation (difficulty in adapting to life's changes), frustration (thwarting or inhibiting of natural or desired behaviours or goals), overcrowding (the presence of too many people in your space), discrimination (unfavourable actions taken against people based on prejudices concerning race, ethnicity, religion, social status, gender, sex, sexual orientation, lifestyle, national origin, or physical characteristics), and socioeconomic events (inflation, unemployment, or poverty). People of different ethnic backgrounds and individuals who are part of the LGBTQ community may face disproportionately heavy impacts from these sources of stress. You should not underestimate the effect of these other sources of stress, particularly those related to discrimination. If you believe you are being discriminated against, or feel impoverished, these realities are lived every day and do not go away, and as a result are a continuous stress that you experience.

Environmental Stress

Environmental stress results from events occurring in our physical environment. Environmental stressors include natural disasters, such as floods, earthquakes, hurricanes, tornadoes, hail storms, blizzards, ice storms, forest fires, and industrial disasters, such as chemical spills, accidents at nuclear power plants, and explosions. Often as damaging as one-time disasters are **background distressors**, such as noise, air, and water pollution or heat, humidity, cold, and wind-chills—although you may not be aware of them, and their effects may not become apparent for decades. As with other distressors, your body responds to environmental distressors with the GAS. If you cannot escape background distressors, you may exist in a constant resistance phase, which can also contribute to your development of stress-related disorders.

Self-Imposed Stress

Self-Concept and Stress

How you feel about yourself, your attitudes toward others, and your perceptions and interpretations of the stressors in your life are part of the psychological component of stress. Also included are the coping mechanisms you learned to use in various situations in response to stress.

The psychological system that governs your stress responses is called the **cognitive stress system** (Morris, 1993). It recognizes stressors; evaluates them on the basis of self-concept, past experiences, and emotions; and makes decisions about how to best cope with them. Your sensory organs serve as input channels for information reaching your brain. From that point on, attention to the problem, memory, reasoning, and problem-solving processes are organized in various parts of the brain before you respond to the stressor. Because learning and memory involve the changing of various proteins in brain neurons, the emotions you experience during the stress response also "tickle" the memory-storage neurons and contribute to your responses. Behaviourally, you respond to the stressor in ways consistent with your memories of similar situations.

Your self-esteem has the potential to also significantly affect various disease processes. If your self-esteem is low, that in and of itself is a self-imposed distressor that can impair your immune system's ability to combat disease. Some researchers believe that chronic distress can depress the immune system and thus increase the symptoms of such diseases as acquired immune deficiency syndrome (AIDS), herpes, multiple sclerosis, and Epstein-Barr syndrome.

Burnout Physical and mental exhaustion as a result of the continuous experience of overload.

Background distressors Environmental stressors, such as heat, humidity, noise, and so on that result in the GAS even though you may be unaware of them.

Cognitive stress system The psychological system that governs your emotional responses to stress.

Self-esteem is closely related to the emotions engendered by past experiences. If you have low self-esteem, you are more likely to feel helpless anger, an emotion experienced when you have not learned to express your anger in appropriate ways. Often when you experience helpless anger, you feel you are wrong to feel angry and instead of expressing your anger in a healthier way, you turn it inward. You may "swallow" your anger in food, alcohol, or other drugs, or act in other self-destructive ways. In the next section, you can ask yourself a series of questions to better understand how you express your anger.

Expressing your anger constructively is an important skill involved in learning to cope with intimate relationships, family interactions, and other stressful situations. Consider the following suggestions:

Determine the reason behind your anger. Is it due to a real event (for example, someone you trusted is spreading gossip about you) or to a perception you have about a situation (friends are avoiding you, so you think they have heard something in the grapevine that resulted in them ignoring you)?

Do not let your anger build. When you become angry, take control, and decide what actions you need to take. Try not to act rashly, nor should you stew for too long. Employ the 24–48 hour rule. Allow 24 hours to pass; if you are still angry, take action to manage the situation. If more than 48 hours pass and you do not do anything, let it go; it was not that important after all.

If you decide to confront a person, select an appropriate time and place for the meeting. Do not attack your target unexpectedly or in the presence of others—the person may become defensive. Give the person a general idea of what you want to discuss ahead of time and choose the appropriate time and location together.

Stick to the main reason for your anger. Bringing up a whole list of things that have made you angry over the last year will complicate the issue and make the other person want to create his or her own list of wrongs that you have committed. Plan in advance which issue you want to discuss. Be careful of using all inclusive statements such as "You always . . ." or "You never. . . ."

Attack the problem rather than the person. ("It made me angry that we had to leave early" instead of "You made me angry because you made us leave early.") Do not get into a battle over personal characteristics. Use "I" statements to communicate resentment or disappointment ("I feel angry that we had to leave the party so early"). "You" statements often put people on the defensive.

Listen carefully to what the other person has to say. Do not interrupt; give the other person a chance to speak. Listen rather than planning what you are going to say next. If the other person starts wandering from the issue, gently bring him or her back to the point. If the

other person attacks you personally, stay in control and do not allow yourself to fight back.

Treat the other person with respect. Even though you may say the right things, your gestures and body language can reveal that you do not value what the other person has to say, that you are hostile, or that you are losing patience. Drumming your fingers, sighing, or rolling your eyes while the other person is talking will likely add tension. Remember, communication is 90 percent nonverbal. In other words, your body's language must match your verbal language to be believed.

Recognize when to quit. Sometimes even the best-laid plans go awry. No matter what you do, the problem may appear impossible to resolve. In such situations, knowing when to quit, either temporarily or permanently, is a key factor in controlling anger and the stress that results from it. Agree to disagree. Nobody has to "win" the argument.

When it is over, let it be over. After you have done all that you can do, let go of your anger. Do not dwell in the past. Acknowledge your right to be angry, recognize it for what it was, and move on.

Personality Types and Hardiness

Your personality type may also contribute to the kind and degree of self-imposed stress you experience. The coronary-disease-prone personality was first described by Friedman and Rosenman (1974) in *Type A Behavior and Your Heart*. Although this work is now considered controversial, it is the basis for much current research.

Friedman and Rosenman (1974) identified two stress-related personality types: Type A and Type B. Type A personalities were described as hard-driving, competitive, anxious, time-driven, impatient, angry, and perfectionistic. Type B personalities were described as relaxed and noncompetitive. According to Rosenman and Friedman (1974), people with Type A characteristics were more prone to heart attacks than their Type B counterparts.

Researchers today believe that more needs to be discovered about Type A and Type B personalities before we can say that all people with a Type A personality will have greater risks for heart disease than those with a predominantly Type B personality. First, most people are not one personality type or the other all the time. Second, there are many other unexplained variables that must be explored, such as why some Type A personalities seem to thrive in stress-filled environments. Now labelled Type C personalities, these individuals appear to succeed more often than Type B personalities and have good health even while displaying Type A patterns of behaviour.

Critics of the supposed links between these personality types and risk of disease argue that attempts to explain ill health by means of personal behavioural patterns have been crude. For example, Ragland and Brand (1989) contend that the Type A personality may be more complex than previously described. These researchers identified a "toxic core" in some Type A personalities. People with this toxic core are angry, distrustful of others, and have above-average levels of cynicism. Generally, people who are angry and hostile also have below-average levels of social support and other increased risks for ill health. It may be this toxic core rather than the hard-driving nature of the Type A personality that makes people more prone to self-imposed stress and its consequences (Ragland & Brand, 1989).

Modification of the Type A personality is possible when particular "learned" behaviours are adjusted. For example, if you have a Type A personality, it is possible to reduce your hurried behaviours and become more tolerant, patient, and better-humoured. Unfortunately, many do not decide to modify their Type A habits until after becoming ill or suffering a heart attack or other circulatory system distress. Prevention of heart and circulatory disorders resulting from stress entails recognizing and changing dangerous behaviours before damage is done.

Psychological hardiness has been identified as a characteristic that may relate to your ability to cope with stress (Akhshabi et al., 2013). When you are psychologically hardy, you are characterized by control, commitment, challenge, choices, and connectedness (sometimes called the Type C personality) (Hystad, Eid, & Laberg, 2011). When you have this Type C personality, you take control of the actions under your control and accept responsibility for your behaviours (Hystad et al., 2009). You also have a sense of commitment, good self-esteem, and understand your purpose in life (Hystad et al., 2009). When you are psychologically hardy, you choose to commit yourself to the things that matter to you and say no when the situation is not of personal importance (Hystad et al., 2009). You will see challenges, change, or struggles in life as stimulating opportunities for personal growth (Hystad et al., 2009). When you are psychologically hardy, you also make lifestyle choices that enhance your health, such as eating well, being physically active regularly, getting adequate sleep, developing meaningful relationships, making time for yourself, and so on. Finally, you connect to others in meaningful ways. This connectedness provides a level of social support that is also health enhancing. Another C that fits this psychologically hardy profile refers to courage—when you are psychologically hardy, you have the courage to take actions that match your values and beliefs, even if they are not the culturally accepted norm (Dungy, 2010).

Self-Efficacy and Control

Whether you are able to cope successfully with stressful situations often depends on your level of self-efficacy, or belief in your skills and performance abilities (Hystad et al., 2009). If you have been successful in mastering similar problems in the past, you are more likely to believe in your effectiveness in future situations. Similarly, if you have repeatedly tried and failed, you may lack the confidence in your abilities to deal with your problems. In some cases, this insecurity may prevent you from even trying to cope, which is also known as **learned helplessness**. this is the sense of learned helplessness also discussed in Chapter 2.

In addition, if you believe you lack control in a situation, you may become easily frustrated and give up quickly. If you think you have little to no personal control over your life and what happens to you, then you might have an external locus of control (a belief that an outside power—fate or destiny—controls your life) and a low level of self-efficacy. When you are confident that your behaviours will influence the ultimate outcome of the events in your life, you likely have an internal locus of control (the belief that you are in control of your life). When you feel limited control over your life and the outcome of various situations, you tend to have higher levels of stress.

STRESS AND THE POST-SECONDARY STUDENT

Stress related to university or college life is more far-reaching than simply the pressure to excel academically. As a post-secondary student, you experience numerous distressors, including changes related to being away from home for the first time; climatic differences between home and school; pressure to make friends in a new and sometimes intimidating setting; the feeling of anonymity imposed by larger classes; test-taking anxiety; and pressures related to time management, social pressures, and a desire to conform. Some of you are stressed by athletic team requirements, on-campus food selection, roommates' habits, peers' expectations, new questions about personal values and beliefs, relationship problems, fraternity or sorority demands, financial worries, changed sleeping habits (including reduced sleep), and the need to be technologically savvy. Older students can also experience distressors from competing with 18- to 21-year-olds, in addition to the pressure of determining future career path and managing responsibilities regarding their family and home.

Technological advances have created new pressures for you with the expectation that you will be constantly connected through various forms of social media (see also the

Psychological hardiness A personality characteristic characterized by control, commitment, challenge, choices, connectedness, and courage.

point of view

WHAT CAUSES YOU MORE STRESS?
Life Stressors or Daily Hassles?

As mentioned in this chapter, you respond to stress in your own way. You also respond to various challenges and not to others. Learning about what you respond to and how you typically respond to it is part of stress management. It is also important to learn what types of situations are more stressful for you. Which are you less effective in managing? Consider the following two lists and determine which requires more effort on your part in learning to manage your stress. Consider other life stressors and daily hassles too.

LIFE STRESSORS

- Moving
- Starting or ending a relationship
- Someone in your family or close circle of friends becoming seriously ill
- Someone in your family or close circle of friends dying
- Staring a new job
- Changing programs or direction of study
- Travelling
- Managing your finances
- Being different than others
- Being bullied

DAILY HASSLES

- Your roommate leaving dishes in the sink
- Someone butting ahead of you in line at meal hall
- Running out of deodorant
- Someone whispering in front of you in class
- Waiting in the slow line to pay for your textbooks (or groceries, or any other item)
- Losing your student card
- Forgetting your lunch at home
- Arriving at class and finding it cancelled
- Your lab experiment not working
- Your roommate borrowing something without asking

section Taming Technostress in this chapter). Further, computer-related tasks potentially take longer than expected (such as sifting through the abundance of materials to find credible and relevant information), in addition to repetitive strain injuries related to overuse and poor body mechanics while on a computer. Most colleges and universities offer stress management workshops through their health centres or student counselling departments.

You should not ignore the following symptoms of stress overload. If you experience one or more of these symptoms, act promptly to reduce their impact:

- difficulty keeping up with classes or difficulty concentrating on and finishing tasks
- frequent clashes with close friends, family, or intimate partners about trivial issues such as housekeeping

- frequent mood changes or overreaction to minor problems
- lethargy caused by lack of sleep or excessive frustration
- lack of interest in social activities or tendency to avoid others
- avoidance of stressors through use of drugs or alcohol or through other extreme behaviours
- sleep disturbances, TV or computer/technology-related addiction, free-floating anxiety, or an exaggerated sense of self
- difficulty in maintaining an intimate relationship
- lack of interest in sexual relationships or inability to participate in satisfactory sexual relationships
- tendency to be intolerant of minor differences of opinion

- hunger and cravings or tendency to overeat or to eat while thinking of other things
- lack of awareness of sensory cues
- inability to listen or tendency to jump from subject to subject in conversation
- stuttering or other speech difficulties
- accident-proneness
- difficulty finding the right words to say or misspeaking quite frequently

STRESS MANAGEMENT

Stress can be challenging or defeating depending upon how we learn to view it. The most effective way to not allow stress to take over our lives is to develop relevant skills and attitudes known collectively as stress management. Stress management consists primarily of finding balance or rhythm in your life. As previously mentioned, we have chosen to use the term *rhythm* rather than *balance* because it is not likely that you will achieve balance or an equal amount of time for your work and play, family and personal time. Rather, you need to find a rhythm that allows you to rest/sleep; relax; be physically active; eat well; and have the personal and social time so you can meet your work, school, family, community, social, and financial responsibilities. As you find this rhythm in your life, you need to make choices to react constructively to your stressors. Eliot (1984) offers two rules for trying to cope with life's challenges: "Don't sweat the small stuff," and remember that "it's all small stuff."

Dealing with Stress

The first step of stress management is to thoroughly examine any problem involving stress. Figure 3.4 shows a decision-making model for managing your response to stress. As the model shows, dealing with stress involves assessing all aspects of a stressor, examining how you currently respond to it and how you may be able to change your response, and evaluating various methods of coping with stress. Some stressors you cannot change, such as professors' assignments or unexpected distressors like car accidents or storm damage. Inevitably, you will take classes that bore you and for which you find no application to real life. And, of course, you will feel powerless when a loved one has died. These facts themselves cannot be changed; only your reactions or responses to these situations can be altered. As mentioned previously, when you have control over the

FIGURE 3.4

A Decision-Making Model for Stress Management

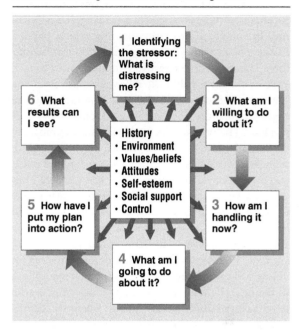

Source: Lefton, Lester A., *Psychology*, 5th Ed., © 1994, p. 485. Reprinted and electronically reproduced by permission of Pearson Education, Inc., Upper Saddle River, New Jersey.

stressor, you should engage in problem-focused stress management; that is, you should find a way to handle the problem. Alternatively, if you have no control over the stressor, you should engage in emotion-focused stress management; that is, you should manage your response to the stressor. More details are provided in the following text.

Assessing Your Stressors

After recognizing a stressor, you need to assess it. Can you alter the circumstances in any way to reduce the amount of distress you are experiencing, or must you change your behaviours and reactions? For example, if you have five term papers for five courses due during the semester, you will probably quickly assess that you cannot alter the circumstances: your professors are unlikely to change their requirements. You can, however, alter your behaviours by working on one or two of the papers well before their due dates and space the work you need to do for the others over time to avoid last-minute stress from trying to write them all in the week before they are due. Another example is your boss being vague about directions for job-related tasks. You cannot change your boss; you can, however, ask your boss to clarify what is expected of you—in writing, if an oral response is insufficient.

Recognizing and Changing Your Responses

Recognizing and changing your responses to stressors requires self-reflection, practice, and emotional control. It is important to recognize your typical physical and mental responses to stress so that you can manage these responses more effectively in future situations. If your roommate is habitually messy and this causes you stress, you can choose from several responses. You can express your anger by yelling, you can pick up the mess and leave a nasty note, you could ask your roommate to pick up after him- or herself, explaining your need for tidiness to work effectively (or whatever reason it is that you prefer a tidy living situation), or you can defuse the situation with humour. The first response that comes to mind is not always the best response. Try to stop before you react, to gain the time you need to find an appropriate response—one that you will not regret. Ask yourself, "What is to be gained from my response?" or "How will my response mediate this type of behaviour in the future?" Many people change their responses to potentially stressful events through cognitive coping strategies. These strategies help them prepare for stressors through gradual exposure to increasingly higher stress levels.

Learning to Cope

Everyone copes with stress and their stress responses in different ways (Canadian Mental Health Association, 2009). Some methods are positive and effective, while others have the potential to be negative and infective. Some people choose to drink or take drugs in the effort to cope. Others speak to counsellors or other trained personnel. Still others try to get their minds off their stress by engaging in physical activity, exercise, or other relaxation techniques. Regardless of how you cope with a given situation, conscious efforts to deal with it are an important step in stress management. Using drugs or alcohol may only provide temporary relief. Similarly, though physically and mentally beneficial, exercise and other relaxation techniques do not solve the issue or issues resulting in the stress response; you may still have to take action to deal with the situation.

Downshifting

Today's lifestyles are hectic and pressure-packed, with self-imposed stress often a result of trying to keep up. You may wonder if "having it all" is worth it, and may take a step back and simplify your life. This simplification is known as "downshifting." Moving from a big city to a small town or moving from a big house to a smaller home and a host of other changes typify downshifting.

Downshifting involves a fundamental alteration in values and honest introspection about what is important in your life. When you consider any form of downshift or perhaps even start your career this way, it is important to move slowly and consider the following:

- **Determine your ultimate goal.** What is most important to you, and what will you need to reach that goal? What can you do without? Where do you want to live? Where do you want to work?

- **Make a short- and long-term plan for simplifying your life.** Set up your plan in doable steps, and work toward each step with realistic short- and long-term goals. Determine the people and organizations to whom it is important to give your time and say no to those requests from people and organizations that do not share your values.

- **Complete a financial inventory.** How much money will you need to do the things you want to do? Will you live alone or share costs with roommates? Do you need a car, or can you rely on active transportation, such as walking, cycling, skating, or scootering, or use public transportation? Pay off credit cards and eliminate existing debt, or consider debt consolidation. Get used to paying with cash or your debit card. If you do not have the cash or money available in your account, do not buy. Remember, your lifestyle may be different as a student compared to when you were working or living at home.

- **Select the right career.** Look for work that you enjoy; salary should not be the deciding factor. Can you be happy in a lower-paying job that is less stressful and provides you with sufficient challenge and the opportunities for the personal and professional growth that you consider important? What do you need to make your work fulfilling?

- **Consider options for saving money.** Downshifting does not mean you renounce money; it means you choose not to let money dictate your life. It's still important to save. If you are just getting started, you need to prepare for emergencies and future plans.

- **Clear out/clean out.** A cluttered life can be distressing. Take an inventory of material items, and get rid of things you have not worn or used in the last year or so. Donate these items to appropriate charities.

Taming Technostress

Another potential cause of stress today is related to the burgeoning technology available. Interestingly a report by Canadian Internet Business (McKinnon, 2014) found that Canadians are online using a desktop or laptop computer for approximately 4.53 hours per day. In addition, they are connected to mobile devices (smartphone, iPad, or tablet) for an average of 1.51 hours per day. With societies ongoing dependence on mobile devices, it is expected that daily use will continue to rise.

We now seem to have cellphones or smartphones that ring or vibrate constantly with incoming calls, text, or email messages; an email inbox that seems to never be empty no matter how often you attempt to address what is in it; laptop computers or iPads that somehow end up in your luggage when you go on vacation; voice message systems that do not allow you to talk to a live person; and slower downloads than we now expect (Zielinski, 2004). Can you feel your heart rate speeding up just thinking about these situations?

On campuses across the country, students, faculty, staff, and administrators are using electronic organizers, the internet, and other forms of technology. Email, inter/intranet, and smartphones are no longer flashy new tools, but as commonplace as the backpack. Unfortunately, many people feel frustrated and distressed in their struggle to adapt to increasingly complex technology. You may find that technology has the potential to be a daily terrorizer that raises your blood pressure, frustrates you, and prevents you from ever really getting away from it all. In short, you may be a victim of stressors that previous generations only dreamed (or had nightmares) about. Known as "technostress," this problem is defined as "personal stress generated by reliance on technological devices . . . a panicky feeling when they fail, and a state of near-constant stimulation, or being perpetually 'plugged in'." When technostress grabs you, it may interact with other forms of stress to create a synergistic, never-ending form of stimulation that keeps your stress response reverberating all day (Zielinski, 2004).

Part of the problem, ironically, is that technology enables you to be productive. Because it encourages polyphasic activity, or "multitasking," you are forced to juggle multiple thoughts and actions at the same time, such as walking and talking on cellphones or walking and texting. You may even find it difficult to concentrate in class because of the incessant buzzing from your own device compelling you to check and respond to your latest text message! Ironically, you are actually less efficient when you multitask than when you focus on one project at a time (Shellenbarger, 2003). Moreover, there is clear evidence that multitasking contributes to auto accidents and other harmful consequences, including short-term memory loss. What is less clear is what happens to you when you are always plugged in. What are the symptoms of technology overload? It evokes typical stress responses by increasing heart rate and blood pressure and causing irritability and memory disturbances. It is possible that over time, if you are continually over-stressed, you may lose the ability to

relax and find that you feel nervous, anxious, and have trouble concentrating. Weil and Rosen (2004) describe *technosis,* a syndrome in which people get so immersed in technology that they risk losing their own identity. Ask yourself the following questions—if you answer yes, you may be too dependent on technology. Do you rely on preprogrammed systems to contact others? Do you feel stressed if you have not checked your email within the last couple of hours? Are you lost without your smartphone?

Suggestions for Fighting Technostress.

- **Enjoy the natural environment.** Take some time away from all forms of technology. Try to find a place that has few people and little noise—that usually means outdoors. Do NOT bring your technology with you, or at the very least turn it off and keep it in your pocket.

- **Become aware of what you are doing.** Log the time you spend texting, searching the net, and writing or responding to email, and so on. Set up a schedule to limit your use of technology. For example, spend no more than one to two hours per day answering texts and emails, or on Facebook.

- **Give yourself more time for everything you do.** If you are surfing the web for resources for a term paper, start earlier rather than the night before the paper is due.

- **Manage the telephone—do not let it manage you.** Rather than interrupting what you are doing to answer, screen calls with an answering machine or caller ID. Get rid of call waiting, which forces you to juggle multiple calls, and subscribe to a voice mail service that takes messages when you are on the phone. Manage the time you spend texting, particularly when you are studying. Turn the sound off. Check and reply to your messages during your breaks from studying.

- **Take regular breaks from your technology (and studying).** Even when working, take a short break every hour: get up, walk around, stretch, do deep breathing, get a glass of water, use the washroom, and so on.

- **If you are working on the computer, look away from the screen and focus on something far away every 20–30 minutes.** Stretch your shoulders and neck hourly as you work. In fact, you should get up and move (as mentioned previously). Play soft background music to help you relax.

- **When working on the computer, focus on one task at a time.** If you are working on a paper, close your email and instant messaging so that you can focus on your paper and not feel pressured to respond because you've got mail or someone has logged on to instant messaging.

- **Resist the urge to buy the newest and fastest technology.** Such purchases not only cause financial stress but also add to stress levels with the typical glitches that occur when installing and adjusting to new technology.
- **Do not take laptops, hand-held devices, or other technological gadgets on vacation.** Use your cellphone for emergencies; turn it and your voice messaging system off.
- **Back up materials on your computer at regular intervals.** Writing a term paper only to lose it during a power outage will likely lead to undue duress.
- **Expect technological change.** The only constant with technology is improvement and change. No matter how at ease you are with your current computer or smartphone at some point you will need to move on to a new one.

Managing Emotional Responses

Have you ever gotten all worked up about something you thought was happening only to find that your perceptions were totally wrong or that poor communication resulted in a misinterpretation of events? This happens a lot of the time. You may get upset by your faulty perceptions rather than reality. For example, imagine you find out that your friends were invited to a party but you were not. You are likely to become angry as well as hurt or disappointed. Self-doubt will likely follow, and you will wonder if anybody likes you. Yet the reality may be that you were invited, but your invitation was lost or misplaced.

Stress management requires that you examine your emotional responses, including your self-talk and explanatory style. With any emotional response to a distressor, you are responsible for your emotions and resulting behaviours. Learning to tell the difference between normal emotions and those based on irrational beliefs can help you to express them in a healthy and more appropriate way. Admitting your feelings and allowing them to be expressed either through communication or action is a stress management technique that can help you get through many difficult situations. Talking yourself through the situation—in a positive way—and explaining yourself to others, accepting responsibility when appropriate, and avoiding blaming others for your mistakes or setbacks are also part of managing your emotional responses and behaviours. It is also important in this regard to develop appropriate expectations for yourself and others.

Learning to Laugh and Cry

Learning to express your emotions freely may be a difficult task for you. However, it is a task worth learning. Have you ever noticed that you feel better after a good laugh or cry? It was not your imagination. Laughing and crying stimulate the heart and temporarily invigorate many body systems. Heart rate and blood pressure then decrease significantly, allowing your body to relax.

Managing Social Interactions

The importance of social interaction should not be underestimated in your stress management plans. Consider the nature and extent of your friendships. Do you have a friend or several friends with whom you can share intimate thoughts and feelings? Is there someone you can call for help or in case of an emergency? Do you trust your friends to be supportive? Do you think your friends will be honest and tell you if you are doing something risky or inappropriate? Having someone to listen to you when needed and give helpful advice is an invaluable stress management tool. It is less important to have a wide circle of acquaintances than it is to have a few really good friends. Different friends often serve different needs, so having more than one friend is beneficial. During your university and college years, your friends often fulfill roles that family members held in the past. As you continue to develop and cultivate friendships, look for individuals who:

- have values similar to your own
- have similar interests that you can enjoy together
- have different interests that force you to grow and explore new ideas
- are good listeners, give and share freely, are tolerant, and do not rush to judgment
- are trustworthy
- consider your needs in addition to their own
- are not unusually critical, negative, selfish, or pessimistic
- are responsible and value doing well in school (assuming you value and are responsible for your education)
- know when and how to have fun
- are willing to be physical-activity buddies or study partners with a mutual interest in a healthy lifestyle
- know how to laugh, cry, engage in meaningful conversation, and feel comfortable with silence

Just as it is important to find these characteristics in your friends, it is also important for you to bring these qualities to your friendships. Sometimes, focusing on others can help you get your problems into perspective and control.

Making the Most of Support Groups

Support groups can also be an important part of your stress management. Friends, family members, and co-workers can provide you with emotional and physical support. Although the ideal support group differs for each of you, you should have one or two close friends in whom you can confide and neighbours with whom you can trade favours. You should participate in community activities at least once a week. Part of your support group may also involve a significant other; a healthy, committed relationship can provide vital support.

If you do not have a close support group, you should know where to turn when the pressures of life seem overwhelming. Family members are often a steady base of support on which you can rely. Most colleges and universities have counselling services available at no cost for short-term crises. Members of the clergy or others involved in chaplaincy, instructors, and residence supervisors can also be supportive resources. You should also be able to find counselling services in the local community. All services are confidential.

Taking Mental Action

Stress management calls for mental action in two areas. First, positive self-efficacy, or the belief in your abilities or capacity to manage your stress, comes from learned habits. If you believe you have what it takes to handle the challenges that come your way, you will be less likely to feel overwhelmed. Successful stress management also involves developing and practising self-efficacy skills. For example, when things seem overwhelming, remind yourself of situations you handled well in the past and challenges you have already overcome; do not assume the situation is beyond your control. Second, because you cannot always anticipate what the next distressor will be, you need to develop the mental skills necessary to manage your reaction to stresses when they happen. The ability to think about and react quickly to stress comes with time, practice, experience with a variety of stressful situations and coping methods, and patience. Most of all, you must strive to become more aware of situations that potentially induce stress and act quickly to deal with them. Rather than seeing stressors as adversaries, learn to view them as exercises in life, challenges to be overcome, or obstacles to be cleared.

Changing the Way You Think

Once you realize that some of your thoughts or self-talk may be negative, irrational, or overreactive, making a conscious effort to reframe or change the way you have been thinking and focus on more positive ways of thinking is a key element of stress management. Here are some specific actions you can take to develop these mental skills.

- **Worry constructively.** Do not waste time and energy worrying about things you cannot change or things that may never happen. For example, do not fret over the weather forecast even if rain or a storm is predicted for when you want to travel on the weekend. Wait until the weekend comes to adjust your plans accordingly.

- **Look at life as fluid and rhythmical.** Accept change as a natural part of living and growing rather than resisting it. For example, if your roommate decides to move out, see that as an opportunity to live with someone different, to experience a new friendship.

- **Consider alternatives.** Remember that there is seldom only one appropriate action. Anticipating options will help you plan for change and adjust more rapidly. For example, when faced with several assignments or mid-term exams scheduled for the same day, there are a variety of approaches you can take. You might speak to each professor and outline your situation, hoping for some rescheduling, or you might simply start each assignment right away and plan your time accordingly.

- **Have moderate expectations.** Aim high, but be realistic about your circumstances and capabilities. Be realistic about your grades—90s are rare in college and university! Aiming to maintain honours status may be more appropriate for you.

- **Weed out trivia.** Do not sweat the small stuff, and remember that most of it is small stuff. So, if someone took the last bit of salad ahead of you in the food line, do not fret about it; move onto your next option or wait until more salad is brought out.

- **Do not rush into action.** Think before you act. Use the 24–48 hour rule. If something happens that angers or disappoints you, leave it for 24 hours. If you are still disturbed, address the situation. If you leave it for 48 hours, it must not be important enough for you to follow up.

- **Keep things in perspective.** Try not to exaggerate the importance of what has happened. Yes, failing an exam or a paper is not a good thing. Still, consider how much it is actually worth and, in the whole scheme of life, how significant is it?

- **Focus on the positive.** Become selectively aware of the positive aspects of negative or unplanned situations. For example, if you get caught in traffic or have to wait in line to pay for your groceries, plan your day ahead or think about how you might form your argument for your upcoming paper. If your partner ends your relationship, think about the extra time you will have to yourself or for your friends and family.

- **See stumbling blocks as challenges rather than barriers.** Expect challenges and difficulties rather than resisting them. So, when your schedule becomes full with many papers to write, exams to prepare for, and classes to attend, see that as the opportunity to organize your time well and to follow a planned agenda versus just seeing it as "stressful."

- **When you think "I cannot do it," break the task into smaller pieces and work on one small part at a time.** For example, if you have a paper and a laboratory report due on the same day, break each down into logical pieces and work on one piece at a time.

- **Reframe.** Rather than seeing the situation as a stumbling block, see it as a challenge and an opportunity. For example, if your date is no longer available to go out, see the unexpected evening alone as an opportunity to unwind with a workout or a warm bubble bath, rather than getting angry or frustrated.

Taking Physical Action

Learning to use physical activity to prevent, alleviate, and manage stress will complement the emotional strategies you employ in stress management.

Physical Activity

Moderate and vigorous intensity physical activities play a critical role in stress management. When engaged in moderate or vigorous intensity physical activity, your body releases endorphins (mood-enhancing, pain-killing hormones) into the bloodstream. Being physically active also increases your energy, reduces hostility, and improves mental alertness. Vigorous physical activity is particularly effective as an immediate response to stress because it can immediately alleviate or reduce your stress symptoms/response. Engaging in vigorous physical activity helps reduce the effects of the fight or flight response and brings your body back to homeostasis. Try to get at least 20 to 30 minutes of aerobic exercise three

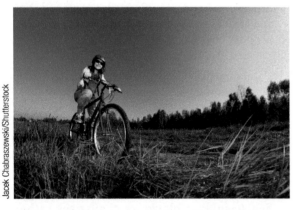

Moderate and vigorous intensity aerobic exercise is an effective stress management tool.

Jacek Chabraszewski/Shutterstock

or four times a week for added benefits in the hormonal regulation of stress. A quiet walk can also refresh your mind, calm your stress response, and replenish your adaptation energy stores. Plan walking breaks alone or with friends. In fact, walking and talking is often an effective way to manage stress—physically and mentally. Stand up and stretch after prolonged periods of study at your desk. This short period of physical activity may provide the break you really need. For more information about physical activity, see Chapter 4.

Relaxation

Similar to regular physical activity, relaxation can help you to cope with stressful feelings, preserve energy stores, and dissipate the excess hormones associated with the GAS. Relaxation may involve a warm bath, or some time sitting quietly and listening to music, or it may involve sitting comfortably repeating a mantra (a word to help you relax). There are various forms of relaxation that you can use. Generally, relaxation helps you refocus your energies and you should practise it daily. When you begin to feel your body respond to stress—eustress or distress—make time to relax to give yourself added strength and to alleviate the negative physical effects of the GAS. As your body relaxes, your heart rate lowers, your blood pressure and metabolic rate decrease, and many other body-calming effects occur, allowing you to channel energy more effectively. Diaphragmatic breathing and progressive muscle relaxation can be effectively used for relaxation.

Diaphragmatic or deep breathing: Typically, we breathe only using the upper chest and thoracic region rather than involving the abdominal region. Diaphragmatic breathing refers to deep breathing that maximally expands the chest by including the lower abdomen. This technique is commonly used in yoga exercises (Dold, 2004). The diaphragmatic breathing process occurs in three stages:

- **Stage 1:** Assume a comfortable position. Whether sitting or lying down on your back, find the most natural position to be in. Close your eyes, unbutton your shirt or binding clothes, remove your belt, or unbutton your pants. Often it works best to hold your hands over your abdomen and get used to feeling the rise and fall of your stomach.

- **Stage 2:** Concentrate on the act of breathing. Shut out external noise. Focus on inhaling, exhaling, and the route the air is following. Try saying to yourself, "Feel the warm air coming into your nose, warming your windpipe, and flowing into your lungs, expanding first your chest and then your belly."

- **Stage 3:** Visualize. The above stages seem to work best when combined with visualization. A common example is to visualize clean, fresh, invigorating air slowly entering the nose and then being exhaled as grey, stale air. Such processes, particularly when they involve the whole body, seem to help individuals become refreshed from their experience.

Progressive muscle relaxation: Progressive muscle relaxation involves systematically contracting and relaxing each of several muscle groups; breathing deeply and concentrating on the muscles being contracted and relaxed are part of this process. Again, find a comfortable position and begin a deep-breathing cycle. The difference from diaphragmatic breathing is that, as you concentrate on inhaling, you will also contract a particular muscle group (for example, the hand and fingers). Hold that position for a short period and then, as you exhale, slowly release the muscles that you have been contracting. Repeat and add more muscle groups. You might start with the hands, then move to the forearms, the entire arms, the neck, then move to the shoulders, back, buttocks, thighs, lower legs, and finish with the feet. You can add components of other relaxation techniques to this experience by saying, "My hands are getting warmer, my arm is getting warmer," and so on as you work to gain maximum control of blood flow and muscle tension in a region.

Eating Well

Is food a destressor? Do Mom's chocolate chip cookies or Grandma's apple pie really make you feel better? Whether foods can calm us and nourish our psyches is a controversial question. However, what is clear is that having a balanced, healthy dietary intake will provide you with the stamina needed to get through problems and may stress-proof you in ways not fully understood. It is also known that undereating, overeating, emotional eating, and a dietary intake that is insufficient in variety, balance, and moderation can create distress in your body. For more information about the benefits of healthy eating for overall health and wellness, see Chapter 5.

Learning Time Management

Time—everybody needs more of it, especially when you are trying to meet the demands of classes, social life, part-time jobs, family obligations, and needed relaxation and physical activity. The following tips regarding time management should become a part of your stress management program:

- **Clean off your desk.** According to Jeffrey Mayer, author of *Winning the Fight between You and Your Desk,* most of us lose time looking for things that are lost on our desks, on our computers, or in our homes. Go through the things on your desk, recycle the unnecessary papers, and organize the remaining papers in "to do" piles.

- **Never handle papers more than once.** When bills and other papers come in, take care of them immediately. Write out a cheque and hold it for mailing or arrange for payment through electronic banking. Get rid of the envelopes. Read your mail and file it or toss it. If you have not looked at something in over a year, recycle it. The same can be said for your email. Read it, handle it, and then delete it.

- **Prioritize your tasks.** Make a daily "to do" list and stick to it. Categorize the things you must do today, the things that you have to do but not immediately, and the things that it would be nice to do. Prioritize the 'must do now' and 'have to do later' items and put deadlines next to each. Only consider the 'nice to do' items if you finish the others or if this list includes something fun for you.

- **Avoid interruptions.** When you have a project that requires your total concentration, schedule uninterrupted time. Turn off your phone and email. Close your door and post a Do Not Disturb sign. Go to a quiet room in the library or student union where no one will find you. Protect your time so you can use it well.

- **Do not be afraid to say "no."** Too often, we overcommit ourselves. It is okay to say "No, I am too busy," "No, I am not really interested," or "I would like to help out; however, I am already committed to too many projects at this time."

- **Reward yourself for being efficient.** If you planned to take a certain amount of time to finish a task and you finish early, take some time for yourself. Go for a walk. Read for pleasure. Spend some time with your friends. Take some time to cook or try out a new recipe. Differentiate between rest breaks and work breaks. Work breaks simply mean that you switch tasks for a while. Rest breaks get you away from work and let you spend time for yourself.

- **Use time to your advantage.** If you are a morning person, plan your work to take advantage of that time. If you know that by Friday afternoon you will be tired and worn out, plan to work then on tasks that require minimal concentration. Take breaks when needed. Use physical activity as an energizer.

- **Remember that time is precious.** Many people learn to value their time only when they face a terminal illness. Value each day. Time spent not enjoying life is a tremendous waste of potential.

- **Become aware of your own time patterns.** For many of us, minutes and hours drift by without us even noticing them. Chart your daily schedule, hour by hour, for one week as shown in Table 3.1. Note the time that was wasted, when it was wasted, and think of the reasons that may have led to that. Note also the time spent in productive work or restorative pleasure. Determine how you could be more productive and make more time for yourself.

TABLE 3.1

A Time Management Chart

Time	What Did You Do?	Was This a Good Use of Your Time?	Why or Why Not?
7:00 a.m.			
8:00 a.m.			
Etc.			

Using Alternative Stress Management Techniques

The popularity of stress management has increased the amount of advertising for various "stress fighters" such as hypnosis, massage therapies, and meditation. Some universities and colleges may provide these services through extended health coverage. Most should be available in your local community.

Massage Therapy

If you have ever had someone massage your stiff neck or aching feet, you know that massage is an excellent means of relaxation and thus a potential form of stress management. Massage therapists use techniques that vary from the aggressive methods typical of Swedish massage to gentler methods such as acupressure and Esalen massage. Before selecting a massage therapist, check his or her credentials carefully. He or she should have training from a reputable program that teaches scientific principles for anatomical manipulation. Each province and territory has different requirements to become a registered massage therapist—check out the Canadian Massage Therapy Alliance website at www .cmta.ca for specific information.

Meditation

Another way to relax and manage stress is through meditation. **Meditation** generally focuses on visualization and deep breathing, allowing tension to leave the body with each exhalation. There is no "right" way to meditate. Although there are several common forms of meditation, most involve sitting quietly and comfortably for 15 to 20 minutes, focusing on a particular word or symbol, controlling your breathing, and getting in touch with your inner self. The deep breathing typically used is described on page 70 in the Relaxation section titled "Diaphragmatic or Deep Breathing." Visualization can be added to this deep breathing. Visualization, or the creation of mental scenes,

Meditation A relaxation technique that involves deep breathing and potentially visualization.

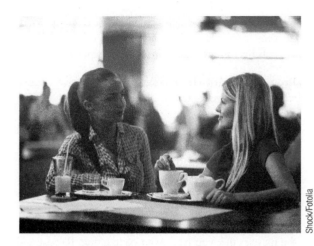

Being able to talk comfortably to someone close to you is part of stress management.

Shock/Fotolia

works by engaging your imagination of the physical senses of sight, sound, smell, taste, and feel to replace stressful stimuli with peaceful or pleasurable thoughts. Your choice of mental images is unlimited and should reflect a scene that brings you peace; this might be a beach or mountain lake, a mountain range, or a field of flax or grain blowing in the wind.

The following simple guidelines may also help you manage the amount of stress you experience as well as your stress response.

- **Plan life, not time.** Determining what you want from life rather than what you can get done may help change the way you use time. Evaluate all your activities, even the most trivial, to determine whether they add to your life. If they don't, get rid of them.

- **Decelerate.** Rushing is part of the Canadian work ethic and mindset that says "Busy is better." It can be addictive. When rushed, ask yourself if you really need to be. What is the worst that could happen if you slow down? Tell yourself at least once a day that failure seldom results from doing a job slowly or too well. Failures happen when rushing causes a lack of attention to detail.

- **Learn to delegate and share.** The need to feel in control is powerful. If you are unusually busy, leave details to someone else. Do not be afraid to ask others to help or share the workload and responsibilities.

- **Learn to prioritize.** Give priority to what is most critical to your life, your job, or your current situation. Decide what things you can do, what things you must do, and what things you want to do, and delegate the rest to someone else either permanently or until you complete some of your priority tasks. Before you take on a new responsibility, finish or drop an old one.

- **Schedule time alone.** Find time each day for quiet thinking, reading, physical activity, or other enjoyable activities.

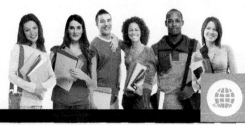

assess
YOURSELF

Go to MasteringHealth to complete this questionnaire with automatic scoring

How Stressed Are You?

Let's face it: Some periods in life, including your college years, can be especially stressful! Learning to "chill" starts with an honest examination of your life experiences and your reactions to stressful situations. Respond to each section, assigning points as directed. Total the points from each section, then add them and compare them to the life-stressor scale.

1 Recent History

In the last year, how many of the following major life events have you experienced? (Give yourself **five points** for each event you experienced; if you experienced an event more than once, give yourself **ten points**, etc.)

1. Death of a close family member or friend _____
2. Ending a relationship (whether by choice or not) _____
3. Major financial upset jeopardizing your ability to stay in college or university _____
4. Major move, leaving friends, family, and/or your past life behind _____
5. Serious illness (you) _____
6. Serious illness (of someone you're close with) _____
7. Marriage or entering a new relationship _____
8. Loss of a beloved pet _____
9. Involved in a legal dispute or issue _____
10. Involved in a hostile, violent, or threatening relationship _____

Total _____

2 Self-Reflection

For each of the following, indicate where you are on the scale of 0 to 5.

	Strongly Disagree					Strongly Agree
1. I have a lot of worries at home and at school.	0	1	2	3	4	5
2. My friends and/or family put too much pressure on me.	0	1	2	3	4	5
3. I am often distracted and have trouble focusing on schoolwork.	0	1	2	3	4	5
4. I am highly disorganized and tend to do my schoolwork at the last minute.	0	1	2	3	4	5
5. My life seems to have far too many crisis situations.	0	1	2	3	4	5
6. Most of my time is spent sitting; I don't get much exercise.	0	1	2	3	4	5
7. I don't have enough control in decisions that affect my life.	0	1	2	3	4	5
8. I wake up most days feeling tired/like I need a lot more sleep.	0	1	2	3	4	5
9. I often have feelings that I am alone and that I don't fit in very well.	0	1	2	3	4	5
10. I don't have many friends or people I can share my feelings or thoughts with.	0	1	2	3	4	5
11. I am uncomfortable in my body, and I wish I could change how I look.	0	1	2	3	4	5

(continued)

	Strongly Disagree					Strongly Agree
12. I am very anxious about my major and whether I will get a good job after I graduate.	0	1	2	3	4	5
13. If I have to wait in a restaurant or in lines, I quickly become irritated and upset.	0	1	2	3	4	5
14. I have to win or be the best in activities or in classes or I get upset with myself.	0	1	2	3	4	5
15. I am bothered by world events and am cynical and angry about how people behave.	0	1	2	3	4	5
16. I have too much to do, and there are never enough hours in the day.	0	1	2	3	4	5
17. I feel uneasy when I am caught up on my work and am relaxing or doing nothing.	0	1	2	3	4	5
18. I sleep with my cell phone near my bed and often check messages/tweets/texts during the night.	0	1	2	3	4	5
19. I enjoy time alone but find that I seldom get enough alone time each day.	0	1	2	3	4	5
20. I worry about whether or not others like me.	0	1	2	3	4	5
21. I am struggling in my classes and worry about failing.	0	1	2	3	4	5
22. My relationship with my family is not very loving and supportive.	0	1	2	3	4	5
23. When I watch people, I tend to be critical and think negatively about them.	0	1	2	3	4	5
24. I believe that people are inherently selfish and untrustworthy, and I am careful around them.	0	1	2	3	4	5
25. Life is basically unfair, and most of the time there is little I can do to change it.	0	1	2	3	4	5
26. I give more than I get in relationships with people.	0	1	2	3	4	5
27. I tend to believe that what I do is often not good enough or that I should do better.	0	1	2	3	4	5
28. My friends would describe me as highly stressed and quick to react with anger and/or frustration.	0	1	2	3	4	5
29. My friends are always telling me I "need a vacation to relax."	0	1	2	3	4	5
30. Overall, the quality of my life right now isn't all that great.	0	1	2	3	4	5

Total _____

Scoring

Total your points from sections 1 and 2.

Although the following scores are not meant to be diagnostic, they do serve as an indicator of potential problem areas. If your scores are:

0–50, your stress levels are low, but it is worth examining areas where you did score points and taking action to reduce your stress levels.

51–100, you may need to reduce certain stresses in your life. Long-term stress and pressure from your stresses can be counterproductive. Consider what you can do to change your perceptions of things, your behaviors, or your environment.

101–150, you are probably pretty stressed. Examine what your major stressors are and come up with a plan for reducing your stress levels right now. Don't delay or blow this off because it could lead to significant stress-related problems, affecting your grades, your social life, and your future!

151–200, you are carrying high stress, and if you don't make changes, you could be heading for some serious difficulties. Find a counselor on campus to talk with about some of the major issues you identified above as causing stress. Try to get more sleep and exercise, and find time to relax. Surround yourself with people who are supportive of you and make you feel safe and competent.

DISCUSSION QUESTIONS

1. Compare and contrast distress and eustress. In what way are both types of stress harmful? Why do both have to be managed?

2. Describe the alarm, resistance, and exhaustion phases of the general adaptation syndrome. Discuss the physiological and psychological responses that take place during the stress response. At what point should you intervene with some form of stress management?

3. What are the major factors that seem to influence the nature and extent of a person's stress susceptibility? Explain how social support, self-esteem, and personality type may make you more or less susceptible to stress.

4. Why are university and college students particularly susceptible to overload and burnout? What services are available on your campus and in your community to help you deal with excessive stress?

5. What can university and college students do to build resilience against negative stress effects? What actions can you take to manage your stressors? How can you help others to manage their stressors more effectively?

6. Identify the stress management techniques described in this chapter. Of these, which do you think would be most useful for you? Why?

APPLICATION EXERCISE

Reread the "Consider This . . ." scenario at the beginning of the chapter and answer the following questions.

1. How common is it for first-year students like Rhett to experience stress? Why?

2. If you were Rhett, what would you do to do better academically in your arts classes? What kind of help is available on your campus if you had a similar problem? How do you access these services?

3. Are Rhett's experiences with residence life similar to what you might experience on your campus? What suggestions could you make to him so that he enjoys this part of campus life and still does well academically?

4. Is it important for Rhett to know precisely what career he is headed for? Why or why not?

MASTERINGHEALTH

Go to MasteringHealth for Assignments, the eText, and the Study Area with case studies, self quizzing, and videos.

focus on

Spiritual Health

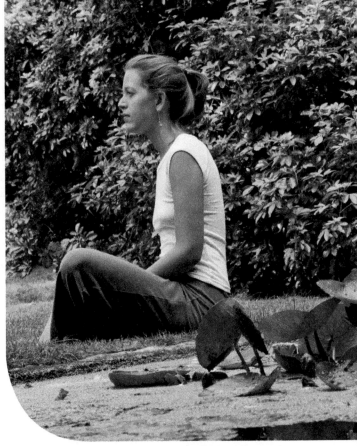

Igor S. Srdanovic/Shutterstock

Isla's favourite spot on campus is the Art Gallery. Whether she is feeling stressed about exams or is mulling over an important decision, a few minutes alone in the gallery seems to help. Sometimes she sits quietly and looks at just one piece of art. Sometimes she walks through the gallery, barely pausing at each piece. When she sits or stands looking at a piece of art, she breathes deeply and lets her thoughts turn to gratitude for her health, her family, and the opportunity to study. However she spends her time, Isla leaves feeling refreshed and refocused, with greater confidence in her ability to tackle the challenges of her day.

Isla's desire to find a sense of purpose, meaning, and harmony in her life is shared by a majority of college and university students (Franke et al., 2010). A large study of post-secondary students measured in their frosh and again in their senior years found that interest in the following goals increased:

- Integrating spirituality into my life
- Developing a meaningful philosophy of life
- Helping others who are in difficulty
- Influencing social values

Further, juniors and seniors wanted to participate in community action programs and expressed more desire to understand other countries and cultures than first year students (Franke et al., 2010). Lastly, students also reported high levels of satisfaction with, and the importance of, expressing diverse beliefs on their campus.

In Chapter 1, spiritual health was identified as one of the key dimensions of health. Isla's sense of wonder and respect for art, her gratitude for the good things in her life, and her belief in a "universal spirit" suggest that spiritual health is an important focus of her daily life, bringing her greater awareness and serenity. This 'focus on' section will explore ways to enhance your spiritual health.

WHAT IS SPIRITUALITY?

From one day to the next, you might attempt to satisfy your needs for belonging and self-esteem by acquiring material possessions. But at some point, you will likely come to realize that new gadgets, clothes, or concert tickets do not necessarily make you happy or improve your sense of self-worth. That is when you begin to contemplate another side of yourself: your spirituality.

Spirituality is not easy to define. Although part of the universal human experience, it is highly personal and involves feelings and senses that are often intangible. In this way, spirituality defies the boundaries a strict definition would impose. The root, *spirit,* in many cultures refers to *breath,* or the force that animates life. When you are "inspired," your energy flows. You are not held back by doubts about the purpose or meaning of your work and life. Indeed, many definitions of spirituality incorporate this sense of transcendence. For example, the National Cancer Institute (2011)

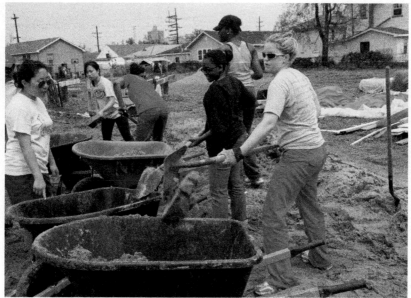

One of the ways you might express your spirituality is by working to reduce suffering in the world; you might contribute your time and skills to volunteer organizations, as these students are doing by working to build homes for Habitat for Humanity.

defines **spirituality** as your sense of peace, purpose, and connection to others, and beliefs about the meaning of life. Similarly, Koenig (2008), defines *spirituality* as your quest for understanding answers to ultimate questions about life, meaning, and your relationship with the sacred or transcendent. The sacred or transcendent could be a higher power or it could relate to your relationship with nature or forces we cannot explain.

Religion and Spirituality: Distinct Concepts

Spirituality may or may not lead to participation in organized **religion**; that is, a system of beliefs, practices, rituals, and symbols designed to facilitate

closeness to the sacred or transcendent (Koenig, 2008). In other words, although spirituality and religion share common elements, they are not the same thing. You may consider spirituality important in your life, but not necessarily in the form of religion (Pew Research Center, retrieved 2008). Table 1 identifies some characteristics that distinguish between religion and spirituality.

Most people (70 percent) affiliated with a religious tradition agreed that other religions are also valid (Pew Research Center, retrieved 2008). Perhaps this is because the major religions express a belief in a unifying spiritual concept, a oneness with a greater power. It seems that a majority of people recognize and respect this underlying unity of spiritual ideas, expressed in different religious and spiritual practices.

TABLE 1

Characteristics Distinguishing Religion and Spirituality

Religion	Spirituality
Community focused	Individualistic
Observable, measurable, objective	Less measurable, more subjective
Formal, orthodox, organized	Less formal, less orthodox, less systematic
Behaviour oriented, outward practices	Emotionally oriented, inwardly directed
Authoritarian in terms of behaviours	Not authoritarian, little accountability
Doctrine separating good from evil	Unifying, not doctrine oriented

Source: National Center for Complementary and Alternative Medicine (NCCAM), "Prayer and Spirituality in Health: Ancient Practices, Modern Science," *CAM at the NIH 12,* no. 1 (2005): 1–4.

Spirituality Your sense of peace, purpose, and connection to others and beliefs about the meaning of life.

Religion A system of beliefs, practices, rituals, and symbols designed to facilitate closeness to the sacred or transcendent.

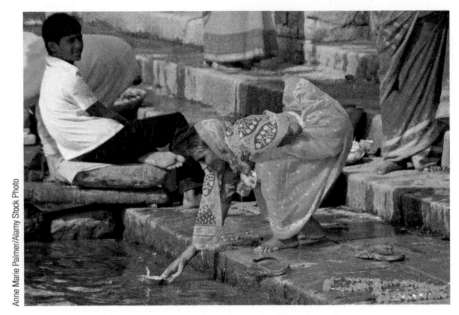

Many people find that religious practices, such as attending services or making offerings—such as the small lamp this Hindu woman is placing in the sacred Ganges River—help them to focus on their spirituality. However, religion does not have to be part of your spiritual life.

Spirituality Integrates Three Facets

Three facets of human existence as presented in Figure 1 are believed to constitute the core of human spirituality: relationships, values, and purpose in life (Seaward, 2012). In other words, your spiritual well-being is characterized by healthy relationships, strong personal values, and a sense that you have a meaningful purpose in life.

- **Relationships.** Have you ever wondered if someone you were attracted to is really right for you? Or if you should break off a long-term relationship? Have you ever wished you had more friends, or that you were a better friend to others and to yourself? Have you ever tried to make a connection with some sort of Presence or Higher Self? These sorts of questions are natural triggers for spiritual growth: As you contemplate who you choose as a life partner or how to mend a quarrel with a friend, you foster your inner wisdom. At the same time, healthy relationships are a sign of spiritual well-being. When you treat yourself and others with respect, honesty, integrity, and love, you manifest your spiritual health.

- **Values.** Your personal **values** are your principles—not only the things you say you care about, but also the things that cause you to behave the way you do. For instance, if you value honesty, then you are not likely to tell a professor that you were sick all weekend and unable to complete your paper, when you really were partying. In other words, your value system is the set of fundamental rules by which you conduct your life. When you attempt to clarify your values and live according to them, you engage in spiritual work. Spiritual health is characterized by a strong personal value system.

FIGURE 1

Three Facets of Spirituality

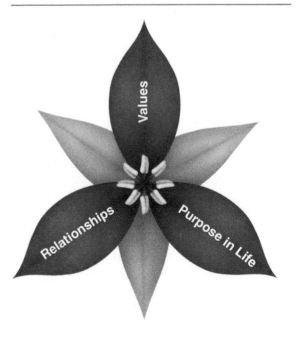

Values Principles that influence your thoughts and emotions and guide the choices you make in your life.

- **Meaningful Purpose in Life.** What career do you plan to pursue after you graduate? Do you hope to marry? Do you plan to have or adopt children? What things will make you happy and feel "complete?" How do these choices reflect what you hold as your purpose in life? At the end of your days, what things would you want people to say about how you lived your life and what your life meant? Contemplating these questions fosters spiritual growth. When you are spiritually healthy, you are able to articulate your purpose, and to make choices that reflect this purpose. In thinking about your purpose, avoid the temptation to get too ambitious, as in, "I am here to eradicate world hunger!" Instead, try to articulate what you see as your unique contribution to the world—something you can actually do, starting now.

Spiritual Intelligence Is an Inner Wisdom

Your relationships, values, and sense of purpose together contribute to your overall **spiritual intelligence (SI)**. Zohar (1997) defined SI as "an ability to access higher meanings, values, abiding purposes and unconscious aspects of the self." Included in SI are qualities such as the ability to think outside of the box, humility, and access to energies that come from a source beyond the ego (Zohar, 1997). SI helps you use meanings, values, and purposes to live a richer and more creative life (Zohar, 1997). SI also helps you find a moral and ethical path to help guide you through life. Further, SI helps you in the search for your meaning and purpose in life.

WHY IS IT BENEFICIAL TO FOCUS ON YOUR SPIRITUAL HEALTH?

Spiritual Health Contributes to Physical Health

An area of particular interest is the association between spiritual health and general health. It is believed that the positive influence spirituality has on health may be due to improved immune function, cardiovascular function, and/or other physiological changes (U.S. Department of Health and Human Services, 2011). Further, some believe that certain spiritual practices can affect the mind, brain, body, and behaviour in ways that have potential to treat many health problems

and to promote healthy behaviour. Ongoing research is investigating the role of spirituality in treating specific pain conditions, irritable bowel syndrome, insomnia, and other chronic medical conditions.

The improved health and longer life in spiritually healthy people may be a result of their greater self-control and mindfulness training. That is, people who are more spiritually healthy and incorporate mind–body practices may have an increased capacity to practise healthy behaviours and reduce the likelihood of overeating, smoking, excessive alcohol consumption, and the use of other drugs. They may also be more likely to cope better with stress on a daily basis (U.S. Department of Health and Human Services, 2011). Further, when you do get sick, your spiritual or religious well-being may help restore health and improve quality of life by (National Cancer Institute, 2010):

- decreasing anxiety, depression, anger, discomfort, and feelings of isolation
- decreasing alcohol and drug use
- decreasing blood pressure and the risk of heart disease
- increasing the person's ability to cope with the effects of illness and with medical treatments
- increasing feelings of hope and optimism, freedom from regret, satisfaction with life, and inner peace

Several studies show an association between spiritual health and your ability to cope with any of a variety of physical illnesses in addition to cancer (University of Maryland Medical Center, 2009). For example, a study of people living with chronic pain and neurological conditions showed a benefit from spiritual health and mind–body techniques (Wells et al., 2010). Other studies looking at individuals with diabetes and other chronic conditions also identified benefits for those who incorporated spiritual practices on a regular basis, including adherence to medications and decreased muscle tension (Cotton et al., 2006).

Spiritual Health Contributes to Psychological Health

Current research also suggests that spiritual health contributes to psychological health. For instance, high levels of spirituality relate to lower levels of anxiety and depression (Peterson, Johnson, & Tenzek, 2010). Further, activities such as yoga, deep meditation, and prayer positively affect brain chemistry. When such activities are practised along with taking antidepressant medications, this can be a very effective treatment for psychological conditions.

Spiritual intelligence (SI) The ability to access higher meanings, values, abiding purposes, and unconscious aspects of the self, a characteristic that helps you to find a moral and ethical path to guide you through life.

People who belong to a spiritual community also benefit from increased social support. For instance, participation in religious services, charitable organizations, and social gatherings can help avoid isolation. At such gatherings, clerics and other members may offer spiritual support for challenges that participants may be facing. Or a community may have retired members who offer child care or meals for members with disabilities or transportation or those needing to get to medical appointments. All such measures can contribute to members' overall feelings of security and belonging.

Spiritual Health Contributes to Reduced Stress

Managing stress is the likely mechanism among spiritually healthy people for improved health and longevity and for better coping with illness (National Cancer Institute, 2010). Further, positive religious coping supports effective stress management (Winter et al., 2009). Finally, increasing mindfulness through meditation reduces stress levels not only in people with physical and mental disorders, but in healthy people as well (Chiesa & Serretti, 2009).

WHAT CAN YOU DO TO FOCUS ON YOUR SPIRITUAL HEALTH?

Cultivating your spiritual side requires as much time and effort as becoming physically fit or improving your diet. The following might help you to develop your spiritual health by training your body, expanding your mind, tuning in, and reaching out.

Train Your Body

For thousands of years, in regions throughout the world, seekers have cultivated transcendence through physical means. One example is the practice of various forms of **yoga**. Although in the West we think of yoga as controlled breathing and physical postures, traditional forms emphasize meditation, chanting, and other practices believed to cultivate unity with the *Atman,* or Absolute.

Yoga A physical and mental process involving controlled breathing, physical postures *(asanas)*, meditation, chanting, and other practices believed to cultivate unity with the *Atman,* or Absolute.

Try yoga on your campus or in your community. Choose a form that feels right to you: *hatha yoga* focuses on flexibility, deep breathing, and tranquility; *ashtanga yoga* is fast-paced and demanding, and appropriate for developing physical fitness. Dress comfortably in relaxed fabrics that are somewhat close fitting so that, when you bend at the waist or lift your leg, you do not feel constricted or exposed. At the beginning of the class, the instructor will likely lead you through some gentle warm-up poses, and then add more challenging poses with coordinated inhalations and exhalations to align, stretch, and invigorate each region of your body. Bring a yoga mat to create your space and to cushion your joints as you work through the postures.

Training your body to improve your spiritual health does not necessarily require formal practices such as yoga. By energizing your body and sharpening your mental focus, jogging, biking, aerobics, or any other exercise you do every day can contribute to your spiritual health. The ancient Eastern meditative movement techniques of tai chi or qigong can also increase physical activity, mental focus, and deep breathing. Both have been shown to have beneficial effects on bone health, cardiopulmonary fitness, balance, and quality of life (Jahnke et al., 2010). To transform your exercise session into a spiritual workout, begin by acknowledging gratitude for your body's strength and speed, then, throughout the session, be mindful of your breathing. Mindful breathing is discussed more below.

You can also cultivate spirituality through fully engaging your body's senses. Think of vision, hearing, taste, smell, and touch as five portals to spiritual health. Viewing an engaging piece of artwork or listening to beautiful music can calm the mind and soothe the spirit. A key reason that Isla, in our opening story, finds sustenance in art is that she engages her senses—gazing at the art, listening to the quiet, and feeling the calm surround her.

The flip side of cultivating your senses is depriving them! Closing your eyes and sitting in silence removes the distraction of visual and auditory stimuli, helping you to focus within. To take advantage of silence, turn off your cellphone and take a long, solitary walk preferably away from traffic and other distracting noises.

Expand Your Mind

Psychological counselling may also be used to improve your spiritual health. Therapy helps you let go of the hurts of the past, accept your limitations, manage stress and anger, reduce anxiety and depression, and take control of your life—all steps toward spiritual growth.

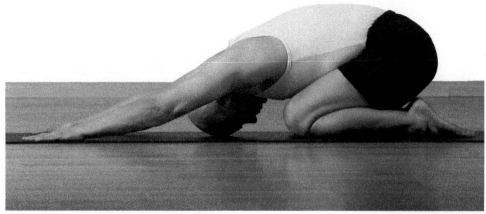

Erik Isakson/Blend Images/Alamy Stock photo

Yoga incorporates a variety of poses (called asanas), from energetic to restful. This yoga student is performing a restful asana known as the child's pose.

Another practical way to expand your mind is to study the sacred texts of the world's major religions and spiritual practices. Many seekers find guidance in the writings of great spiritual teachers. Libraries and bookstores are filled with volumes that explore the diverse approaches humans take to achieve spiritual fulfillment.

Finally, you can expand your awareness of different spiritual practices by exploring meditation groups, taking classes in spirituality or comparative religions, attending meetings of student organizations where different religious tenets are explored, going to different houses of worship in your community, attending public lectures and critically evaluating whether the speakers demonstrate a spiritual bent or reflect bias or exclusion in their lectures, and checking out the official websites of various spiritual and religious organizations.

Tune in to Yourself and Your Surroundings

Focusing on your spiritual health has been likened to tuning in on a radio—inner wisdom is perpetually available, but if you fail to tune your "receiver," you will not be able to hear it for all the "static" of daily life. Fortunately, four ancient practices still used throughout the world can help you tune in. These are contemplation, mindfulness, meditation, and prayer, which you can think of as studying, observing, emptying, and communing with the divine.

- **Contemplation.** If you were to look up the word *contemplation* in a dictionary, you would find that it means a study of something—whether a candle flame or a theory of quantum mechanics. With spirituality, **contemplation** usually refers to concentrating the mind on a spiritual or ethical question or subject, a view of the natural world, or an icon or other image representative of divinity. For instance, a Zen Buddhist might contemplate a riddle, called a *koan,* such as, what is the sound of one hand clapping? A Sufi might contemplate the 99 names of God. A Roman Catholic might contemplate an image of the Virgin Mary. If you do not have a religious affiliation, you might contemplate the natural world, a favourite poem, or an ethical question such as, what is the origin of evil?

When practising contemplation, it can be helpful to keep a journal to record any insights that arise. In addition, journaling itself can be a form of contemplation. For example, you might want to make a list of 20 things in your life that you are grateful for or write a poem of forgiveness to yourself or a loved one. You might also use your journal to record inspirational quotations that you encounter in your readings.

- **Mindfulness.** A practice of focused, non-judgmental observation, **mindfulness** is the ability to be fully present in the moment (Figure 2). If you have ever been immersed in a moment, experiencing it completely using all your senses—sight, hearing, taste, smell, touch—this is mindfulness. Examples include watching the sun set over a mountain, watching the sun rise along the ocean, listening to a pianist playing Bach, and performing a challenging calculation in math. In other words, mindfulness is an awareness of present-moment reality—a holistic sensation of being totally involved in the moment (Brantley, 2011).

Contemplation A practice of concentrating the mind on a spiritual or ethical question or subject, a view of the natural world, or an icon or other image representative of divinity.

Mindfulness A practice of purposeful, non-judgmental observation in which we are fully present in the moment.

FIGURE 2
Qualities of Mindfulness

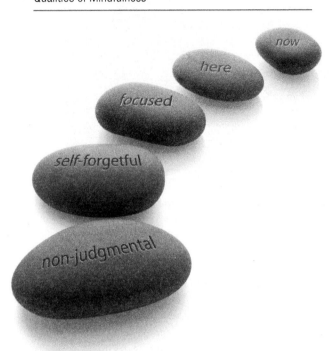

Michael Valdez/iStock/Getty Images Plus/Getty Images

So, how do you practise mindfulness? Living mindfully means allowing yourself to become more deeply and completely aware of what it is you sense in each moment (Brantley, 2011). So the next time you eat an orange, pay attention! What does it feel like to pierce the skin with your thumbnail? Do you smell the orange as you peel it? What does the rind really look like? What does the rind feel like on your skin, under your nails? How does the orange splatter as you separate it into segments? What does it taste like? How does the taste change from the first bite to the last?

Think of physical and mental challenges, such as a competitive diver leaping from the board, a physician attempting a difficult diagnosis, the creative and performing arts such as sculpting, painting, writing, dancing, or playing a musical instrument. Even household activities such as cooking or cleaning can foster mindfulness—as long as you pay attention while you do them!

In this era of global environmental concerns, you can also cultivate mindfulness by paying attention to how your choices affect the world. This means more than simply reduce, reuse, recycle. Mindfulness of our environment calls on you to examine your values and behaviours as you share the Earth every moment of each day.

Meditation A practice of emptying the mind of thought.

• **Meditation. Meditation** is a practice of emptying the mind, of cultivating stillness. Although the precise details vary, the fundamental task is the same: to quiet the mind, to stop the "chatter," "static," or "monkey mind." For thousands of years, humans of different cultures and traditions found that achieving periods of meditative stillness each day enhances their spiritual health. Today, researchers are beginning to discover why. Using brain-scanning techniques, researchers have found that experienced meditators show significantly increased levels of *empathy*, the ability to understand and share another person's experience (National Center for Complementary and Alternative Medicine, 2009). Meditation also increased the capacity for forgiveness among college students (Oman et al., 2008) and improves the brain's ability to process information; reduces stress, anxiety, and depression; improves concentration; and decreases blood pressure (National Center for Complementary and Alternative Medicine, 2009).

So, how do you meditate? Briefly, begin by sitting in a quiet place with low lighting where you will not be interrupted. You might choose a "full lotus" position, with both legs bent fully at the knees, each ankle over the opposite knee. If a full lotus position is not possible, try a modified lotus position, in which your legs are simply crossed in front of you. Lying down is not recommended because you might fall asleep. Rest your hands palm upward on your knees. This position uncrosses the two bones of the forearm. Your eyes can be open, half-open, or closed. Once in a position conducive to meditation, start to empty your mind. There are different ways to clear your mind:

• **Mantra meditation.** Focus on a *mantra*, a single word such as *Om, Amen, Love,* or *God*. Keep repeating this word silently to yourself. When a distracting thought arises, set it aside. It may help to imagine the thought as a leaf, and mentally place it on a gently flowing stream that carries it away. Do not fault yourself for becoming distracted. Simply notice the thought, release it, and return to your mantra.

• **Breath meditation.** Count each breath. Pay attention to each inhalation, the brief pause that follows, and the exhalation. Together, these equal one breath. When you have counted ten breaths, return to one. As with mantra meditation, as distractions arise, release them and return to the breath.

• **Colour meditation.** When your eyes are closed, you may perceive a field of colour, such as a deep blue "pearl." Focus on this colour. Treat distractions as for other forms of meditation.

• **Candle meditation.** With your eyes open, focus on the flame of a candle. Allow your eyes to soften as you meditate on this object. Treat distractions as for other forms of meditation (Reese, 2011).

After several minutes of meditation, and with practice, you may come to experience a sensation sometimes described as "dropping down," in which you feel yourself release into the meditation. In this state, which can be likened to a wakeful sleep, distracting thoughts are far less likely to arise, and you may receive surprising insights.

In the beginning, try meditating for 10 to 20 minutes a session, once or twice a day. In time, increase your sessions to 30 minutes or more. As you meditate for longer periods, you will likely find yourself feeling more rested and less stressed throughout your day, and you may experience the increased levels of empathy recorded among expert meditators.

- **Prayer.** In **prayer**, rather than emptying the mind, an individual focuses the mind in communication with a transcendent Presence. Spiritual traditions throughout the world distinguish several forms for this type of communication. Prayer offers a sense of comfort; a sense that you are not alone; and an avenue for expressing concern for others, for admission of transgressions, for seeking forgiveness, and for renewing hope and purpose. Focusing on the things you are grateful for in life can help you to look to the future with hope and give you the strength to get through the most challenging times.

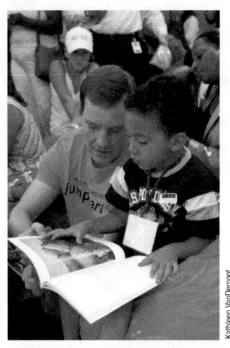

Volunteering can be a fun and fulfilling way to broaden your experience, connect with your community, and focus on your spiritual health.

Reach Out to Others

Altruism, the giving of yourself out of genuine concern for others, is a key aspect of a spiritually healthy lifestyle. Volunteering, choosing to work for a not-for-profit organization, donating money or other resources to a food bank or other program, or even spending an afternoon picking up litter in your neighborhood are all ways to serve others and simultaneously enhance your spiritual health. Most colleges and universities offer opportunities for community practicums and service that can also facilitate future career opportunities.

Community service can also take the form of **environmental stewardship**, which is defined as the responsibility for environmental quality shared by all those whose actions affect the environment (Environmental Protection Agency, 2010). Responsibility manifests in action; simple actions such as reducing and recycling, turning off the lights, turning the heat down when going to bed or when not at home, replacing old light bulbs with energy-efficient varieties, and taking shorter showers are part of environmental stewardship.

Prayer Communication with a transcendent Presence.

Altruism The giving of yourself out of genuine concern for others.

Environmental stewardship Making responsible decisions for the long-term health of the environment.

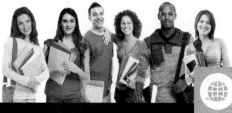
What Is Your Spiritual IQ?

Answer each question as follows:

0 = not at all true for me
1 = somewhat true for me
2 = very true for me

_____ **1.** I frequently feel gratitude for the many blessings of my life.

_____ **2.** I am often moved by the beauty of Earth, music, poetry, or other aspects of my daily life.

_____ **3.** I readily express forgiveness toward those whose missteps have affected me.

_____ **4.** I recognize in others qualities more important than their appearance and behaviours.

_____ **5.** When I do poorly on an exam, lose an important game, or am rejected in a relationship, I am able to know that the experience does not define who I am.

_____ **6.** When fear arises, I am able to know that I am eternally safe and loved.

_____ **7.** I meditate or pray daily.

_____ **8.** I frequently and fearlessly ponder the possibility of an afterlife.

_____ **9.** I accept total responsibility for the choices that I have made in my life.

_____ **10.** I feel that I am on Earth for a unique and sacred reason.

Scoring

The higher your score on this quiz means the higher your spiritual intelligence. To improve your score, consider the suggestions for spiritual practices from this chapter.

Developing Your Spiritual Health

The Assess Yourself activity gave you the chance to evaluate your spiritual intelligence, and the chapter introduced you to some practices used by others to enhance their spiritual health. Consider taking some of the small but significant steps listed below to further the development of your spiritual health.

Today, You Can:

- Find a quiet spot; turn off your cellphone; close your eyes; and contemplate, meditate, pray, or be mindful of your surroundings for 10 minutes.

- In a journal or on your computer, compile a list of things you are grateful for. Include at least 10 things: people, pets, talents and abilities, achievements, favourite places, foods . . . whatever comes to mind!

Within the Next Two Weeks, You Can:

- Explore the options on campus for psychotherapy, join a spiritual or religious student group, or volunteer with a student organization working for positive change.

- Think of a person in your life with whom you have experienced conflict. Spend a few minutes contemplating forgiveness toward this person and then write him or her an email or letter apologizing for any offense you may have given and offering your forgiveness in return. Wait for a day or two before deciding whether you are ready to send the message.

By the End of the Semester, You Can:

- Develop a list of spiritual texts that you would like to read during your break.

- Explore options for volunteer work when you have more time in the summer.

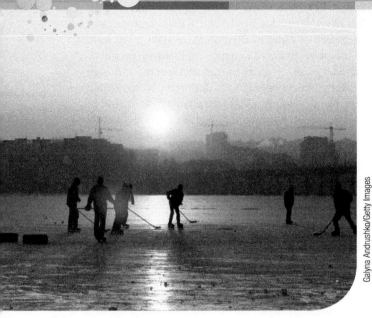

Galyna Andrushko/Getty Images

CHAPTER 4

ENGAGING IN PHYSICAL ACTIVITY FOR HEALTH, FITNESS, AND PERFORMANCE

CONSIDER THIS . . .

While in high school, Laura participated in many physical activities, including organized sports such as volleyball, soccer, swimming, and track. Among the many lifestyle changes she encountered during her first year of post-secondary studies was the need to spend time alone in sedentary scenarios such as reading, writing, and studying. Laura had seen some of her friends struggle to include any physical activity or exercise in their student lives. Despite the academic demands of her first semester at school, Laura was determined to make time for exercise and worked out daily, alternating physical activities focused on cardiorespiratory endurance and muscular strength and endurance each day. She studied for long solitary hours and got high grades, though she averaged less than six hours of sleep a night. By the end of each week, Laura usually felt lonely and tired and was not sure she could continue this routine.

Is Laura overdoing it? What potential problems can you foresee if she continues her first-semester schedule? What changes should Laura make in her lifestyle to feel less lonely and tired?

LEARNING OUTCOMES

- Discuss physical activity and exercise for health, physical fitness, and performance.

- Define the components of a health-related physical fitness program and describe the exercise frequency, intensity, time, and type to build and/or maintain fitness in each component.

- Identify and discuss the recommendations for physical activity promoted in Canada's Physical Activity Guide for Healthy Active Living.

- Discuss common barriers to students' physical activity participation and methods to overcome them.

- Describe common physical fitness-related injuries as well as methods to reduce your risk of these injuries.

Participation in regular physical activity provides a wide range of physical, social, and mental health benefits for children and adults of all ages (CSEP, 2012a; World Health Organization, 2003) These health benefits are a result of an increased energy expenditure and improved physical literacy, which contribute to overall improvement in the quality and quantity of life (Bouchard et al., 1988; Cardoso et al., 2010; International Physical Literacy Association [IPLA], 2015). **Physical literacy** is described as the motivation, confidence, physical competence, knowledge, and understanding to value and take responsibility for engagement in physical activities for life (IPLA, 2015). Physical activity and physical literacy go hand-in-hand. Regular physical activity helps to protect against developing many chronic diseases (Bauer et al., 2014; Bouchard et al., 1988). Furthermore, engaging in weekly physical activity helps to control stress, increases self-esteem, and contributes to an overall "feel-good" feeling. It is no wonder that physical activity is often viewed as the key to health and considered a tool for disease prevention (Warburton, Whitney, & Bredin, 2006a; 2006b). Despite the numerous multi-media campaigns to raise awareness about the benefits and importance of physical activity, only 15 percent of Canadian adults meet the current physical activity recommendations (Colley et al., 2011) of 150 minutes of moderate to vigorous physical activity (MVPA) each week (Tremblay et al., 2011). **MVPA** refers to physical activities that cause adults to sweat a little and breathe harder (CSEP, 2012a). Even more disturbing is that only 9 percent of Canadian children and adolescents ages 5-17 years old meet the minimal recommendation of 60 minutes of daily MVPA (Government of Canada, 2016). From six years of age and older males tend to be more physically active than females. Further, children are more active than adolescents (Colley et al., 2011; Thompson, 2005; Thompson et al., 2009), and adolescents are more active than adults. Research also indicates that your physical activity level as a child and adolescent influences your attitudes and behaviours toward your physical activity as an adult (Thompson, Humbert, & Mirwald, 2003; Froehlich Chow & Humbert, 2013). Moreover, if you were not provided opportunities to engage in physical activity and develop your physical literacy during your early years, which includes learning **fundamental movement skills** such as how to kick a ball or hop on one foot, you would be far less likely to engage in physical activity and sports in later years. Failing to develop these skills often leads to negative physical activity experiences in physical education or sport during elementary and high school years. However, it is important to remember that you develop physical literacy over the course of your lifetime and staying physically active is important for all ages. Therefore, if you have had negative experiences or are currently inactive, you should not give up, as your university or college years provide an excellent opportunity to break from the past and develop positive physical activity attitudes and behaviours that will increase the quality and quantity of your life. Keep in mind that changes in physical activity level are common, with most people regularly cycling through more and less physically active times. For example, over a 10-year span, 26.8 percent of Canadians over the age of 12 became more physically active while 21.5 percent became less active (Statistics Canada, 2008). What is more important is reducing the length of time you are inactive and remembering that every minute counts.

PHYSICAL ACTIVITY FOR HEALTH, FITNESS, AND PERFORMANCE

Physical activity refers to all body movements produced by skeletal muscles resulting in energy expenditure (Health Canada, 2004). Walking, swimming, gardening, and housework are examples of physical activity. Physical activities can vary by intensity. For example, walking to class typically requires little effort, while walking up hill and carrying a backpack is more intense. There are three general categories of physical activity defined by the purpose for which they are done: physical activity for health, physical activity for fitness, and physical activity for performance.

Research shows us that participating in regular moderate-to-vigorous intensity physical activity, including walking, gardening, participation in gym classes, and sports is associated with significantly lower all-cause mortality and increased overall health and wellness (Hallal & Lee, 2013). In fact, doctors in the province of Quebec have recently received new prescription pads that allows them to not only prescribe physical activity, but also indicate how much and what type of activities their patients should be engaging in (CBC, 2015).

Physical literacy The motivation, confidence, physical competence, knowledge, and understanding to value and take responsibility for engagement in physical activities for life.

MVPA Moderate to vigorous physical activity (MVPA) are physical activities that cause adults to sweat a little and breathe harder.

Fundamental movement skills Fundamental movement skills (FMS) are the movement patterns that involve different body parts. They are the foundation movements or precursor patterns to the more specialized, complex skills used in play, games, sports, dance, gymnastics, outdoor education, and physical recreation.

Physical activity Body movements produced by skeletal muscles resulting in energy expenditure.

Physical Activity for Health

Canadian researchers Warburton et al. (2006b) concluded from their review of research on physical activity and health that "there is irrefutable evidence of the effectiveness of regular physical activity in the primary and secondary prevention of several chronic diseases (for example, cardiovascular disease, diabetes, cancer, hypertension, obesity, depression and osteoporosis and premature death)" (p. 801). It is becoming quite common for medical doctors to prescribe exercise to patients suffering chronic diseases and/or mental illness (Sallis 2015). Moreover, a position stand from the American College of Sports Medicine indicates the evidence for positive health benefits from engaging in a physically active lifestyle is irrefutable and the benefits outweigh the risk (Garber et al., 2011). Just adding more physical activity to your day can benefit your health. In fact, if *all* Canadians followed the physical activity recommendations in Canada's Physical Activity Guidelines (CPAG), about one-third of deaths related to coronary heart disease; one-quarter of deaths related to stroke and osteoporosis; one-fifth of deaths related to colon cancer, high blood pressure, and type 2 diabetes; and one-seventh of deaths related to breast cancer could be prevented (Warburton et al., 2007).

The recommendations in the CPAG, designed for Canadian adults between the ages of 18 and 64 years are to obtain at least 150 minutes of moderate or more intense physical activity each week and flexibility activities should be engaged in three to five days per week (Tremblay et al., 2011). Examples of moderate-intensity physical activities include brisk walking, cycling, dancing, and so on. Vigorous-intensity physical activities make you quite warm and breathe quite quickly, as you would while jogging or playing a game of basketball. Further, this physical activity should be accumulated in 10-minute or longer time periods (Tremblay et al., 2011). It is also recommended that activities that are bone and muscle strengthening should be engaged in at least two times per week (Tremblay et al., 2011).

A physically active lifestyle might include choices such as walking or cycling to school, parking further away from your destination, taking movement breaks while studying, or taking the stairs instead of the elevator (CSEP, 2012a). You can also choose to be more physically active in your leisure or "down" time by dancing, playing Frisbee, or walking your dog. Every little bit helps, so get out of your seat and move more, more often. In fact, research indicates that there are health risks for individuals who meet the minimal physical activity requirements but spend the rest of their time in sedentary pursuits (Patel et al., 2010). As a result, sedentary behaviour guidelines have been developed for children and youth, and similar guidelines will be developed for adults. Recent research has shown that

TABLE 4.1

The Health and Performance-Related Components of Physical Fitness

Health-Related Components
Cardiorespiratory endurance
Muscular strength
Muscular endurance
Flexibility
Body composition
Performance-Related Components
Power
Speed
Balance
Agility
Reaction time
Coordination

Source: Based on T. Baranowski, et al., "Assessment, Prevalence, and Cardiovascular Benefits of Physical Activity and Fitness in Youth," *Medicine and Science in Sports and Exercise 24* (June 1992): supplement, S238.

if you have to be sedentary for more than an hour at a time you should take a break and move around for a few minutes each hour. Another way to reduce sedentary time is to consider working at a standing desk or replace your desk chair with a stability ball. For more information regarding your need for physical activity and to reduce your sedentary time or to obtain a copy of Canada's Physical Activity Guidelines, go to www.csep.ca.

Physical Activity for Fitness

Exercise refers to a particular kind of physical activity. Although all exercise is physical activity, not all physical activity would be considered exercise. For example, walking from your car to class is physical activity, whereas regularly going for a brisk, 30-minute walk is exercise. **Exercise** is defined as planned, structured, and repetitive bodily movements done to improve or maintain one or more components of physical fitness, such as cardiorespiratory endurance, muscular strength and endurance, or flexibility (Health Canada, 2004). **Physical fitness** refers to a set of attributes that are either health- or performance-related (see Table 4.1). The health-related attributes—cardiorespiratory endurance, muscular strength and endurance, and flexibility—allow you to perform moderate- to vigorous-intensity physical activity on a

Exercise Planned, structured, and repetitive physical activity done to improve or maintain one or more components of physical fitness.

Physical fitness A set of attributes that are either health- or performance-related.

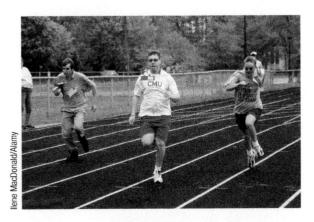
It is important for all people, including those with disabilities, to develop optimal levels of physical fitness to participate in physical activities they enjoy—including competitive sports.

regular basis without undue fatigue and with energy left over to handle physical or mental emergencies (Health Canada, 2004).

To become physically fit, you need to do more than make physically active lifestyle choices. You also need to do particular exercises for a particular length of time, at a specific intensity, and for a certain number of times each week. More details regarding building and maintaining your physical fitness are presented later in this chapter.

Some people have physical limitations that might be viewed as preventing them from being able to get the exercise recommended to achieve and/or maintain physical fitness. These individuals can and should be physically active and, in particular, should exercise to obtain their personal optimal level of physical fitness, as well as the health-related benefits to improve their overall wellness. CSEP (2012b) has developed physical activity guidelines for individuals with special needs. For example, a woman with arthritis in her knee and hip joints might not be able to run or even walk long distances, but she can participate in water exercises, since these would not add to the stress on her joints. Similarly, a man who uses a wheelchair may not be able to jog, but he can meet the physical activity recommendations and work on his physical fitness by swimming or playing wheelchair basketball or rugby and performing resistance training exercises with his upper body.

Physical Activity for Performance

People who participate in athletics use physical activity, or more specifically, specific exercises or training, to improve their performance. In this regard, specific exercises are undertaken to increase not only the relevant health-related components of physical fitness, such as cardiorespiratory endurance, muscular strength

and endurance, and flexibility, but also power, agility, speed, coordination, and the other performance-related attributes of physical fitness. Plyometrics are an example of a training technique often used to improve performance. Plyometrics are exercises that contract muscles in a certain order to increase power. An example is doing push-ups with a hand-clap between each one. In addition to developing power, plyometrics can be used to improve body control and the speed at which you change directions (a component of agility).

Although many recreational exercisers use interval training to improve their speed as well as their cardiorespiratory fitness, performance training is safest for individuals who already have a higher level of physical fitness. Generally, those who engage in performance training will achieve or attempt to achieve a level of physical fitness close to or at their genetic potential. In order to continue to obtain fitness improvements it is important to incorporate changes and increase the challenge of an exercise plan over time. Key components of an exercise plan, such as how to create and adapt an effective plan, are discussed later in this chapter.

In this regard, careful monitoring of the training plan is essential, since there is an increased risk of injury and overtraining, which are also discussed later in this chapter.

BENEFITS OF REGULAR PHYSICAL ACTIVITY

Improved Cardiorespiratory Endurance

A regular program of moderate or more intense aerobic physical activity improves the efficiency of your cardiovascular and respiratory systems. It enables the heart to pump more blood with each beat, thus lowering resting heart rate; it improves the body's capacity to take in and distribute oxygen to working muscles; and it strengthens the muscles responsible for respiration. See also Chapter 12 for more details regarding exercise and the heart.

Reduced Risk of Heart Disease

Your heart is a muscle (called cardiac muscle) made up of highly specialized tissue. Because muscles become stronger and more efficient with use, regular physical activity of sufficient intensity strengthens the heart, enabling it to pump more blood with each beat. This increased efficiency means that your heart requires fewer beats per minute to circulate blood throughout your body to maintain function. In this way, a stronger, more efficient heart is better able to meet the demands of life.

Prevention of Hypertension

Hypertension is the medical term for chronic high blood pressure. It is a cardiovascular disease itself and increases the risk of coronary heart disease and stroke. Hypertension causes the heart to work harder with each beat because of increased resistance due to less pliable arterial walls. Hypertension may also occur when blood flow is restricted as it may be in an artery that is partially clogged with fatty stores (see Chapter 12 for more details).

Regular moderate-intensity physical activity lowers systolic and diastolic blood pressure by about 10 mmHg in people with mild to moderate hypertension (Cardoso et al., 2010). Regular physical activity can also reduce systolic and diastolic blood pressure in people with normal blood pressure (Cardoso et al., 2010).

Improved Blood Lipid and Lipoprotein Profile

Lipids are fats that circulate in the bloodstream and are stored in various places in your body. A high level of blood lipids (cholesterol and triglycerides) increases risk of coronary heart disease (Third Report of the National Cholesterol Education Program Expert Panel on Detection, Evaluation, and Treatment of High Blood Cholesterol in Adults, 2001). Risk increases for heart disease because the heart has to work harder with each beat as a result of the reduced blood flow caused by the narrowing of the arteries that occurs with high blood fats as they "build up" on the artery walls. Regular aerobic exercise reduces low-density lipoproteins (LDLs—"bad cholesterol"), total cholesterol, and triglycerides (a blood fat), thus reducing plaque build-up in the arteries, while increasing high-density lipoproteins (HDLs—"good cholesterol") (Herzberg, 2004). Higher HDL levels are associated with lower risk for coronary artery disease because they remove some of the "bad cholesterol," thus reducing fatty plaque accumulation from coronary artery walls and easing the work effort of the heart. Again, this is discussed in more detail in Chapter 12.

Improved Bone Health

Osteoarthritis is a nonfatal but incurable disease characterized by degeneration of joint cartilage and irritation of surrounding bone and soft tissues. Affecting 1 in 10 Canadians, osteoarthritis is the most prevalent chronic joint condition in Canada. Women are afflicted more frequently than men (Stupar et al., 2010). Supervised walking and weight-loss programs can improve physical capacity while reducing knee-joint osteoarthritis symptoms (Felson et al., 1992; Messier et al., 2013).

A common affliction in the older population is osteoporosis, a disease characterized by low bone mass and deterioration of bone tissue, which increases fracture risk. Although men and women are both negatively affected by osteoporosis, the prevalence is greater in women. Weight-bearing and strength-building physical activities are recommended to maintain bone health and to prevent osteoporotic fractures (Spence & Humphries, 2001). Bone, like other human tissues, responds to the demands placed upon it (the overload principle), and unless the mechanical stresses placed on bone by a particular physical activity exceed the level of stress the bone has adapted to, bone mass and structure will not adapt (Dunlop et al., 2009). Women (and men) have much to gain by remaining physically active as they age—bone mass levels have been found to be significantly higher among physically active women than among those who are sedentary (Andreoli et al., 2012). However, it appears that the full bone-related benefits of physical activity can be achieved only with sufficient hormone levels (estrogen in women, testosterone in men) and adequate calcium, vitamin D, and total calorie intake.

Improved Weight Management

Although there are many physical and mental health benefits from participating regularly in physical activity, for many people, the desire to lose or maintain weight is their primary reason. The role physical activity plays in your weight maintenance and weight loss is important, but it is equally, if not more, important to also consider your sedentary behaviours—particularly when they are uninterrupted—as well as your dietary intake (see Chapter 6 for more details). Physical activity of all kinds has a direct positive effect on metabolic rate in that more calories are required to supply the energy needed to perform that physical activity. As well, your metabolic rate remains elevated for several hours following vigorous physical activities. Resistance training exercises also have a small direct and more impactful long-term effect on metabolic rate. Specifically, resistance training itself does not require substantive energy to be completed, however, when you increase your muscle mass, your overall metabolic demands increase because muscle mass is a metabolically active tissue.

Improved Quantity and Quality of Life

Prevention of Type 2 Diabetes

Diabetes is a complex metabolic disorder that affects many Canadians. It is believed that a healthy dietary intake combined with sufficient physical activity could prevent many of the current cases of type 2 diabetes (Pelletier et al., 2012; Tudor-Locke, Bell, & Meyers, 2000). A large epidemiological study found that for every 2000 calories of energy expended during leisure-time physical activities, the incidence of diabetes was reduced by 24 percent (Helmrich, Ragland, & Paffenbarger, 1994). Perhaps the most encouraging finding was that the protective effect of physical activity was greatest among individuals at the highest risk (Helmrich, Ragland, & Paffenbarger, 1994).

Increased Longevity

Experts have long debated the relationship between physical activity and longevity. For decades, most research failed to show an increase in life expectancy through physical activity alone. Then, a classic prospective study of Harvard alumni over more than 30 years reported that inactive men were at a greater risk of premature death from all causes than men who engaged in regular physical activity (Paffenbarger et al., 1986). How much physical activity was required to produce this effect? Inactive men who included a brisk 30- to 60-minute walk each day experienced the most significant increases in their life expectancies (Blair et al., 1989).

Improved Immunity to Disease

Will regular physical activity improve your immunity? Research suggests that regular moderate-intensity physical activity makes people less susceptible to disease, but that this potential benefit depends upon whether the physical activity was perceived as pleasurable or stressful (Eichner, 1993; Right to Play, n.d.). Often, the relationship of physical activity to immunity or, more specifically, to disease susceptibility is described as a J-shaped curve (Gleeson, 2007). In other words, susceptibility to disease decreases as you move from sedentary to moderately active, then increases again as you engage in more extreme levels of physical activity or exercise such as the training required of world-class or Olympic athletes (Gleeson, 2007). Further, athletes engaging in marathon-type events or very intense physical training programs have been shown to be at a greater risk for upper respiratory tract infections such as colds and the flu (Moreira et al., 2009). In fact, research shows that marathon runners experienced twice as many upper respiratory tract infections as non-runners

(Robson-Ansley et al., 2012). The reason for this difference relates to the intensive, rather than moderate, intensity exercise, resulting in a nonspecific depression of the immune system that results in increased susceptibility to infections for these individuals (Lewicki et al., 1987).

Just how physical activity alters immunity is not well understood. We do know that moderate-intensity physical activity temporarily increases our white blood cells (WBCs), the blood cells responsible for fighting infection. How long does one have increased immunity? It is suggested that after 30 minutes or more of physical activity, WBCs may be elevated for 24 hours or more before returning to normal levels (Eichner, 1993).

Improved Mental Health and Stress Management

Although most people who engage in regular physical activity are not aware of the beneficial physiological changes of their activity apart from those that are most noticeable, such as weight loss or weight maintenance, most experience the psychological benefits. While these psychological benefits are difficult to quantify and describe, they are the reasons for continuing to be physically active.

Regular vigorous physical activity has been shown to "burn off" the chemical by-products released by our nervous system during its normal response to stress. Elimination of these biochemicals reduces our stress response by accelerating the neurological system's return to homeostasis. For this reason, regular physical activity of moderate to vigorous intensity should be an integral component of your stress management plan (see also Chapter 3).

Regular physical activity can improve physical appearance by toning and developing muscles and, combined with a healthy dietary intake, reducing (or maintaining) body fat. Feeling good about your appearance is an integral component of your self-esteem. Other improvements to your physical self-esteem result from learning new skills, developing increased ability and capacity in recreational activities, and "sticking with" a physical activity plan.

Quite simply, you are likely to feel good about yourself overall when you engage in physical activity regardless of whether it is a workout, a walk, a game of tag, raking the lawn, or some other physical activity inside or outside. This overall feeling or a sense of general satisfaction, though difficult to quantify or measure, provides immediate feedback from your participation and therefore has the potential to be more motivational than things like reduced risk of chronic disease—which you cannot feel.

IMPROVING CARDIORESPIRATORY ENDURANCE

Cardiorespiratory endurance, or cardiovascular fitness, refers to the ability of the heart, lungs, and blood vessels to function efficiently. Our lives depend on our cardiorespiratory system's ability to deliver oxygenated blood and nutrients to our body tissues and to remove carbon dioxide and other metabolic waste products. The primary category of physical activity known to improve cardiorespiratory fitness is aerobic exercise. The term *aerobic* means "with oxygen" and describes any type of exercise, typically performed at moderate to vigorous intensity, for extended periods of time. Aerobic activities such as brisk walking, jogging, bicycling, skating, and swimming are among the best exercises for improving or maintaining cardiorespiratory fitness.

Aerobic power is the term used to describe the current functional status of the cardiovascular system (that is, the heart, lungs, blood vessels) and refers specifically to the volume of oxygen consumed by the muscles during exercise, maximal aerobic power (often referred to as VO_{2max}) (Thompson, 2005). Maximal aerobic power refers to the maximal capacity of the cardiorespiratory system. The most common measure of maximal aerobic capacity is determined from a walk or run on a treadmill. In this test, you will walk or run at an easy pace, and then, at set time intervals, gradually increase the workload (that is, a **graded exercise test** in which a combination of running speed and the angle of incline is used to make the exercise more physically demanding) to arrive at your point of maximal exertion. It may be more correct to say your peak exertion rather than maximal exertion, or the greatest value that can be measured in an exercise test. The higher your cardiorespiratory endurance, the more oxygen you can transport to exercising muscles and the longer you can maintain a high intensity of exercise before exhaustion. Other less valid, but reliable methods of measuring aerobic capacity can be used to estimate VO_{2max}. These submaximal tests use stationary bicycles, walk/run tests, shuttle runs, step tests, or walk tests to quantify the aerobic fitness levels in people of all ages and of all abilities. You may have performed one or more of these aerobic capacity tests in your physical education classes.

It is important for you to complete the Physical Activity Readiness Questionnaire (PAR-Q; available at www.csep.ca) prior to engaging in physical activity or any tests to measure your physical fitness (Canadian Society for Exercise Physiology, 2003). If you answer yes to any of the questions on the PAR-Q or if you have certain medical conditions, such as asthma, diabetes, heart disease, or obesity, you should consult a physician to ensure that physical activity is safe for you. Further, you should engage in a walking/jogging program at low intensity before you attempt to measure your maximal or peak aerobic capacity.

CARDIORESPIRATORY FITNESS PROGRAMS

When creating a cardiorespiratory fitness program, there are many variables to consider. Generally, what is needed is an aerobic physical activity you enjoy that works your heart at a moderate or greater intensity, approximately 70 to 90 percent of your maximum heart rate, which corresponds to a workload of 55 to 85 percent of your VO_{2max} (Fox, Bowers, & Foss, 1989) for a continuous length of time (20 to 30 minutes) at least three days per week.

The most effective aerobic exercises for building cardiorespiratory endurance are total body activities involving large muscle groups of your body.

Determining Exercise Frequency

If you have been physically inactive for the past few months or longer, the frequency of your aerobic exercise should begin at three times per week. If you exercise less frequently (that is, once or twice per week), you will achieve fewer health benefits and are not likely to improve your cardiorespiratory fitness. Exercising three to five times per week is the general recommendation for improving cardiorespiratory endurance. Your ultimate goal should be to exercise five times a week. Exercising your cardiovascular system more than five days a week will not lead to higher levels of cardiorespiratory fitness and may increase your risk of injury. To avoid overuse injuries and monotony, vary your aerobic exercises and take a day off when needed.

Determining Exercise Intensity

An aerobic exercise program must employ sustained, moderate or greater intensity physical activity to improve cardiorespiratory endurance.

Cardiorespiratory endurance The ability of the heart, lungs, and blood vessels to function effectively and efficiently.

Aerobic power The current functional status of a person's cardiorespiratory system; measured as VO_{2max} and referring specifically to the volume of oxygen consumed by the muscles during exercise.

Graded exercise test A test of aerobic capacity administered by a physician, exercise physiologist, or other trained person.

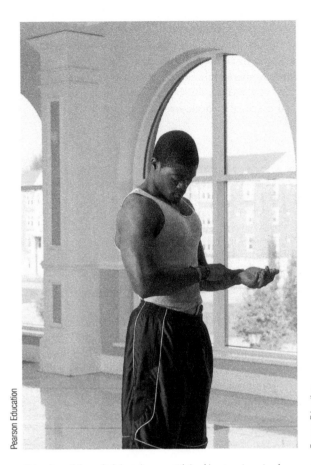
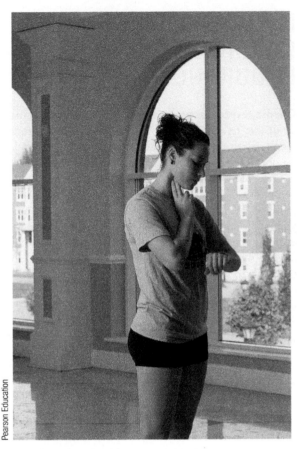

Palpation of the radial (wrist) or carotid (neck) artery is a simple means of determining heart rate.

A common measure of exercise intensity is your heart rate. As previously mentioned, the exercise intensity required to improve cardiorespiratory endurance is a heart rate between 70 and 90 percent of your maximum heart rate (Warburton, Whitney Nicol, & Bredin, 2006a). To calculate your **target heart rate**, subtract your age from 220 (for males) or 226 (for females) (Warburton, Whitney Nicol, & Bredin, 2006a). The result is your maximum heart rate (HR_{max}). You then determine your target heart rate by calculating the desired percentage of maximum heart rate—that is, 70–90 percent. Thus, if you are a 20-year-old male, your estimated maximum heart rate is 200 (220 − 20 = 200). Your target exercising heart rate would be somewhere between 140 (200 × 0.70 = 140) and 180 (200 × 0.90 = 180) beats per minute. If you have been sedentary for a long time, set a lower target heart rate, somewhere between 50 and 60 percent of your maximum. As your cardiorespiratory fitness improves, you can gradually increase your target heart rate using small increments—for example, from 50 to 55 percent, then from 55 to 60 percent, and then from 60 to 65 percent, and so on. It is not recommended to engage in aerobic exercise for health benefits to exceed 90 percent of maximum heart rate.

Once you know your target heart rate, you can determine how close you are to this value during your workout. You will need to stop exercising briefly to measure your heart rate. To take your pulse, lightly place your index and middle fingers (not your thumb) over one of the major (carotid) arteries in your neck, along either side of your Adam's apple, or on the radial artery on the inside of your wrist. Be sure to start counting your pulse immediately—the first count is "0"—after you stop exercising, as your heart rate decreases quickly. Using a watch or clock, take your pulse for six seconds and multiply this number by 10 (just add a zero to your count) to get the number of beats per minute. If necessary, increase or decrease the pace or intensity of your workout to achieve your target heart rate. Alternatively, you can take your pulse for 10 seconds and multiply the result by 6 to get the number of beats per minute.

A target heart rate of 70 percent of maximum is sometimes called the "conversational level of exercise" because you are able to talk with a partner while exercising (Stamford, 1993). If you are breathing so hard that talking is difficult, the intensity of your exercise is

Target heart rate The desired intensity of aerobic exercise for improving or maintaining cardiorespiratory fitness; calculated as a percentage of maximum heart rate (220 [for males] or 226 [for females] minus age).

too high. Conversely, if you are able to sing or laugh heartily while exercising, the intensity of your exercise is insufficient for improving or maintaining cardiorespiratory endurance.

Determining Exercise Time

Time refers to the number of minutes of exercise performed at the specified intensity during any one session. When the intensity of the exercise is 70 to 90 percent HR_{max}, only 20 to 30 minutes are needed to induce a training effect. Although many individuals engage in exercise sessions lasting longer than 30 minutes, greater improvements to cardiorespiratory fitness are not realized.

Determining Exercise Type

Type or specificity, refers to the specific physical activity you chose to improve a component of your health related fitness. For example, if you want to increase cardiorespiratory endurance you might plan to jog, run, swim or engage in some other aerobically challenging activity.

The Recovery

It is recommended that you take at least 18 to 24 hours between workouts aimed at improving cardiorespiratory fitness to allow the body sufficient time to recover and, more importantly, to adapt to the overload applied, so that the body can become more cardiorespiratory fit (Garber et al., 2011; Warburton, Whitney Nicol, & Bredin, 2006a).

Although not a specific principle, remember that any physical activity, even if it does not meet all the exercise characteristics mentioned in this chapter, will benefit your overall health and help you to feel better about yourself almost immediately.

IMPROVING MUSCULAR STRENGTH AND ENDURANCE

Musculoskeletal health (that is, strength, endurance, and flexibility) also significantly impacts health and overall wellness. Specifically, musculoskeletal health is associated with a reduced risk for coronary heart disease and osteoporosis, as well as improved glucose tolerance and ease of completing the tasks of daily living (Kell, Bell, & Quinney, 2001). **Muscular strength** refers to the maximal amount of force a muscle or group of muscles is capable of exerting in one contraction. The most common way to measure strength is to determine the maximum amount of weight you can lift once. This value is called **one repetition maximum (1RM)**. Your 1RM can also be predicted from a 10RM test (Powers et al., 2006). **Muscular endurance** is defined as a muscle's or group of muscles' ability to exert force repeatedly without fatiguing or the ability to sustain a muscular contraction. The more repetitions you can perform successfully (for example, push-ups) or the longer you can hold a certain position (for example, flexed arm hang), the greater your muscular endurance. Muscular endurance is often measured from the number of curl-ups or push-ups an individual can do. Push ups may be a measure of strength for some people when they are only able to complete a few (less than 6) in the correct form.

Principles of Strength Development

There are three key principles—tension, overload, and specificity—to follow to increase your muscular strength and endurance (Mackenzie, 2000).

The Tension Principle

The key to developing strength is to create sufficient tension within a muscle or group of muscles. The most common way to create tension in a muscle is the use of external resistance such as that found in weightlifting. While weightlifting is one method of producing tension in a muscle, many other types of physical activity have the same effect—for example, lifting your own body weight (push-ups or pull-ups) or riding a bicycle up a steep hill. It really does not matter what type of resistance you choose to develop tension in your muscles; what matters is that you use sufficient and appropriate resistance to improve muscular strength and/or endurance dependent upon your physical fitness goals.

The Overload Principle

The overload principle is the most important of the three key principles for improving muscular strength. Everyone begins a resistance training

Musculoskeletal health The combination of strength, endurance, and flexibility and their influence on various components of health.

Muscular strength The maximal amount of force that a muscle or group of muscles is capable of exerting.

One repetition maximum (1RM) The maximum amount of weight/resistance that can be lifted/moved only once.

Muscular endurance A muscle's or group of muscles' ability to exert force repeatedly or to sustain a contraction without fatiguing.

FIGURE 4.1

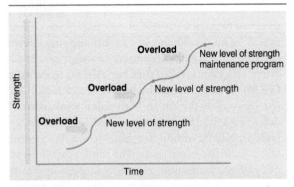

The overload principle must be followed to increase strength or endurance. Notice that once the muscle has adapted to the original overload, a new overload must be placed on the muscle for subsequent gains in strength or endurance to occur.

Source: Data from Philip A. Sienna, *One Rep Max: A Guide to Beginning Weight Training*, Fig. 2.1, 8. © 1989. Wm. C. Brown Communications, Inc., Dubuque, Iowa.

program with an initial level of strength. To increase strength, you must then regularly create tension in your muscles greater than you are accustomed to. This overload forces your muscles to adapt by getting larger (**hypertrophy**), stronger, and thus capable of generating more tension. Figure 4.1 illustrates a continual process of overload and adaptation resulting in improved strength. If you do not create an overload—if you "underload" your muscles—you will not increase strength. Conversely, if you create too great an overload, you may experience muscle injury, muscle fatigue, and even a loss of strength. Once you reach your strength goal, no further overloading is necessary. Your next challenge is to maintain that level of strength by continuing to engage in a regular (once or twice per week) total-body resistance exercise program.

Hypertrophy Increased size (girth) of a muscle.

Isometric muscle contraction Force produced without muscle movement.

The Specificity of Training Principle

This principle refers to the manner in which a specific body system responds to the physiological demands placed upon it. According to the specificity principle, you get a specific response or adaptation to the exercises you do. If the specific overload you impose is designed to improve strength in the muscles of your chest and back, the response to that demand (overload) will be improved strength in the chest and back, not in the overall body. Therefore, to improve overall or total body strength, you must include exercises for all the major muscle groups. You must also ensure that your overload is sufficient to increase strength and not only endurance.

The Recovery Principle

Allow 48 hours for the body to "recover" from and adapt to the resistance training undertaken (that is, to become stronger) (Hitchcock, 2011). This does not mean that you cannot resistance train daily, but rather that you need to design your workout so that you alternate which muscles you concentrate on when resistance training. Keep in mind that your core body is always involved in your training and you may need to take a day off to ensure that it too has sufficient time to heal and adapt to the overloads undertaken. Again, it is recommended that you learn to listen to your body and adapt accordingly.

Types of Muscle Contractions

When your skeletal muscles receive a stimulus from your nervous system to contract, they respond by developing tension and producing a measurable force. Your skeletal muscles contract in three different modes—isometric, concentric, and eccentric—to produce this force (Knuttgen & Kraemer, 1987). In an **isometric muscle contraction**, force is produced by the muscle without movement. Isometric

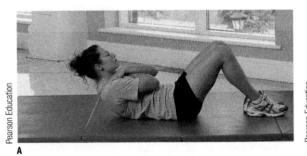

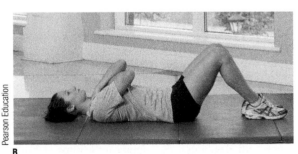

These photographs illustrate concentric and eccentric muscle actions. In A, the abdominal muscles shorten, a concentric muscle action, while producing tension in the lifting phase of a curl-up. In B, the abdominal muscles lengthen, an eccentric muscle action, while producing tension as the body returns to its starting position.

muscle contractions do not create joint motion. Muscles act isometrically to stabilize a particular body part while another body part is moving, or when a maximal resistance is met and the force produced cannot overcome the resistance. One example is the unsuccessful attempt to push a car out of a snow bank. Although you push with all your might, the car does not move (and neither do your joints). The muscles involved are producing force in an isometric way. Another example related to resistance training is trying to lift a barbell that is too heavy for you. The more you try, the more tired your muscles become, but the barbell never leaves the floor. Isometric muscle contractions are important because they are involved in maintaining body stability. Not all isometric contractions require maximal efforts as maintaining your balance and body alignment while holding a push-up (e.g., in the plank position or in downward dog) is another example of isometric muscle contractions.

A **concentric muscle contraction** is one in which force is produced while the muscle shortens. Joint movement is always produced during concentric muscle actions. Raising the body in a curl-up is an example of a concentric action of the abdominal muscles. Usually, but not always, concentric muscle contractions produce movement in a direction opposite to the downward pull of gravity.

Eccentric muscle contraction describes a muscle's ability to produce force while lengthening. Typically, eccentric muscle actions occur when movement is in the same direction as the pull of gravity. If you want to be sure that a given resistance exercise has an eccentric phase, you must use the type of resistance that requires you to achieve the starting position before your next repetition. For example, in a curl-up, you lower your upper body slowly to the starting point of the exercise in an eccentric contraction of the abdominal muscles.

All factors being equal, the greatest amount of force is produced during eccentric muscle contractions, followed by isometric and then concentric muscle contractions. Changes in muscle size and strength are affected by the type of resistance exercise and by the type of muscle contraction(s) you use during your workout. When using free weights (barbells, dumbbells), the typical sequential pattern of concentric–eccentric muscle contractions during resistance training contributes to improved muscle strength and muscle fibre size. If your resistance training program uses only concentric muscle contractions, you will need to perform at least twice as many repetitions to achieve the same results as you would attain by using concentric–eccentric combinations (Hilliard-Robertson et al., 2003; Roig et al., 2008).

Methods of Providing Resistance

There are four commonly used methods of applying resistance for muscular strength and endurance training: body weight resistance; and fixed, variable, and accommodating resistance devices.

Body Weight Resistance

Muscular strength and endurance can be improved without exercise equipment, using your body weight as the resistance. For many individuals, using their body weight as resistance in a variety of exercises can be as effective as external resistance in developing and maintaining muscular strength and endurance. Exercises such as curl-ups, push-ups, and pull-ups require your muscles to lift and return your body weight off and back down to the floor, involving concentric and eccentric muscle contractions. Other effective exercises include isometric contractions found in yoga and Pilates such as the downward dog and forward, back, and side planks.

Fixed Resistance

Fixed resistance exercises provide a constant resistance throughout a full range of movement. Barbells and dumbbells provide fixed resistance because their weight or the amount of resistance applied does not change as you exercise. However, due to the biomechanics of human motion, the muscle forces that must be exerted to move the weight are lower at some joint angles and higher at others. Any given muscle generates the least amount of force at the beginning and ending positions of a resistance exercise, and the most force when the joint involved in the exercise approximates a right angle (90 degrees). As a result, the disadvantage of fixed resistance exercises is that the extent to which a muscle is overloaded varies throughout the exercise, and the exercise may not fully develop the muscle.

Variable Resistance

Whether found at a health club or in your home workout area, variable resistance equipment alters the resistance encountered by a muscle at each joint angle so that the effort by the muscle is consistent throughout the full range of motion. Variable resistance machines are typically single-station devices (for example, Nautilus), but some have multiple stations at which muscles of the upper and lower extremities can be exercised (for example, Soloflex).

Concentric muscle contraction Force produced while shortening the muscle.

Eccentric muscle contraction Force produced while lengthening the muscle.

Accommodating Resistance

Accommodating resistance devices (isokinetic machines) maintain a constant speed through the range of motion. The exerciser performs at a maximal level of effort, while the exercise machine controls the speed of the exercise and does not allow any faster motion. The body segment being exercised must move at a rate faster than or equal to the set speed to encounter resistance.

Getting Started

You will find some general principles useful whatever your strength training goals. If sufficient tension is generated within a muscle, it will respond by becoming stronger regardless of the type of muscle action or resistance used. To design your program, first determine your 1RM for each muscle or muscle group you plan to exercise. Then, develop specific training goals as well as the strategies to achieve those goals.

Strength Training

There are almost as many ways to develop muscular strength as there are participants in strength training programs. Given the specificity principle, it is important to select at least one resistance exercise for each major muscle group in the body to develop total body strength. Generally, strength training exercises are done in a set, or series, of multiple repetitions using the same resistance. For increases in muscular strength, the amount of resistance should be at least 60 percent or greater of your 1RM for a given exercise, with two to six repetitions of the exercise performed per set (Garber et al., 2011). Generally, a resistance that you can move or lift only two or three times is a good place to start. It is further recommended that one to three sets be performed. It is also recommended that you first complete a number of repetitions, then sets, before increasing the amount of resistance (Garber et al., 2011).

Since resistance training exercises cause microscopic damage (tears) to muscle fibres, and the rebuilding process takes about 24 to 48 hours, resistance training programs should incorporate at least one day of rest (and recovery) between workouts to allow the muscle or muscle groups to adapt. Thus, the recommended frequency of programs to build muscular strength is two to four days per week (Kraemer & Ratamess, 2004).

To summarize, if your exercise efforts are intended to build muscular strength, you should perform each strength building exercise at an intensity greater than 60 percent of your 1RM for one to three sets of two to six repetitions, two to four days per week. See also Table 4.2.

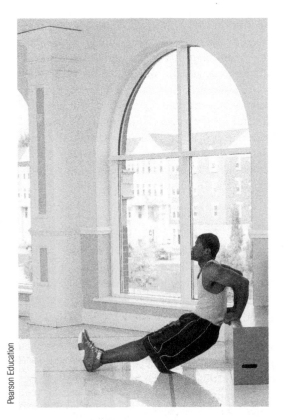
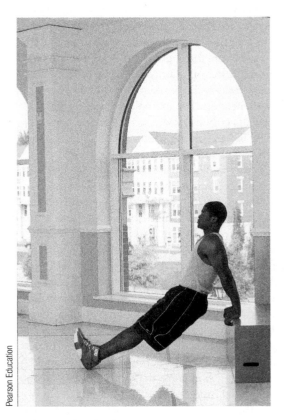

Using your body weight can be an effective way to build or maintain muscular strength and endurance.

TABLE 4.2

Guide to Manipulating Training Variables to Achieve Muscular Strength and Endurance Training Goals

	Endurance	Strength
Sets	2–6	1–3
Repetitions	10–15	2–6
Resistance (% of maximum)	< 60	> 60
Rest between sets (seconds)	30–60	120
Frequency per week (days)	2–4	2–4
Rest between workouts (days)	1–2	1–2

Muscular Endurance Training

In contrast to the exercise requirements to result in enhanced muscular strength, muscular endurance is improved by performing a relatively high number of repetitions with a relatively low resistance. To increase your muscular endurance, add variety to your training program with exercise devices equipped with an ergometer, such as a stationary bicycle, rowing machine, elliptical, or stair-climbing machine. With these and other devices, you can control the cadence of the activity and/or adjust the amount of resistance you encounter. Performing thousands of repetitions during a 20-minute (or longer) workout using a relatively low resistance will quickly develop muscular endurance in the muscles exercised. Other activities that build muscular endurance include hiking, wall climbing, jogging, and cycling. These latter types of exercises also provide cardiorespiratory benefits if you select an intensity that allows you to reach your target heart rate. You can also build muscular endurance through resistance training by performing two to six sets of 10 to 15 repetitions at a resistance of less than 60 percent of your 1RM, two to four days per week (Garber et al., 2011; Warburton, Whitney Nicol, & Bredin, 2006a). See also Table 4.2.

IMPROVING YOUR FLEXIBILITY

Flexibility refers to the range of motion, or the amount of movement possible, at a particular joint or series of joints. Although this component of physical fitness is often overshadowed by muscular strength and cardiorespiratory endurance, it should not be overlooked because inflexible muscles are susceptible to injury. Improving your range of motion through stretching exercises will enhance the efficiency and fluidity of your movements as well as your posture.

A regular stretching program may also enhance psychological well-being in that the exercises used often involve deep breathing and a focus on relaxation.

Types of Stretching Exercises

Flexibility is most often enhanced by controlled stretching of muscles (Quinn, 2013). The primary strategy is to decrease the resistance to stretch (tension) within a tight muscle targeted for increased range of motion (Quinn, 2013). To do this, you repeatedly stretch the muscle to its point of tension and its two tendons of attachment to elongate them.

The safest exercises for improving flexibility involve **static stretching**. Static stretching techniques slowly and gradually lengthen a muscle or group of muscles. For this type of stretching, various positions and postures are used with the "stretch" held to a point where tension (mild discomfort) is felt within the muscle (Quinn, 2013). This end position is then held for 10 to 60 seconds, and is repeated two or three times in close succession (Quinn, 2013). With each repetition of a static stretch, your range of motion improves temporarily and, when done regularly, range of motion increases for longer periods of time. Stretching regularly (at least four, and preferably seven, days a week) will effectively result in a more permanent elongation of the targeted muscle or muscle group and thus permit a greater range of motion at a given joint.

In regard to athletic performance, static stretching immediately prior to dynamic or all-out performances such as sprinting may have a negative effect on the athlete's performance (Behm & Kibele, 2007). Thus, to minimize the risk of reduced performance and potentially injuries, it is recommended that the warm-up should include light to moderate intensity physical activity followed by large size dynamic stretching and completed with sport-specific dynamic activities on increasing intensity (Behm & Chaouchi, 2011).

YOGA, TAI CHI, AND PILATES

Three popular styles of exercise that include stretching are yoga, tai chi, and Pilates. In addition to improving flexibility, these types of exercise may increase muscular strength and endurance as well as focus on the mind–body connection through concentration on breathing and

Flexibility The range of motion, or the amount of movement possible, at a particular joint or series of joints.

Static stretching Assuming a "stretching" position—at the point of tension—for 10 to 30 seconds in which there is a gradual lengthening of a muscle.

point of view

TO SUPPLEMENT OR NOT TO SUPPLEMENT?

Enter a varsity athlete's gym, your campus fitness centre, or your community wellness centre and you are bound to see one or more individuals who are "jacked" or "ripped" proudly showing off their six-pack abs readily. You might wonder what and how much exercise it takes to look like that. You may also wonder if those individuals have done it all on their own or have they used performance-enhancing supplements? Would performance-enhancing substances make it easier?

ARGUMENTS IN SUPPORT OF USING PERFORMANCE-ENHANCING SUBSTANCES

- muscle size increases rapidly
- rapid increase in muscular power and strength
- less time and effort required to get the body shape desired
- others are doing it, so why not you?

ARGUMENTS AGAINST USING PERFORMANCE-ENHANCING SUBSTANCES

- in addition to the well-known effects of feminization in males and masculinization in females who take anabolic steroids, there is considerable risk of serious liver injury, stroke, kidney failure, and pulmonary embolism (blockage of an artery in the lung) with anabolic steroid use
- use of nonanabolic substances carries risk of allergies and the possibility that the product you bought is not what you paid for
- supplements are costly
- these are unnatural products that do not belong in the body
- it is cheating to use some sort of performance-enhancing substance

Where Do You Stand?

○ Do you think performance-enhancing substances are safe? See Table 4.3 for more details. Why or why not?

○ Would you use performance-enhancing substances to look more muscular? Why or why not?

○ If your younger brother or sister wanted to use a performing-enhancing substance, what would you say? What training advice might you give?

---

body position. Some people see these three activities as strongly connected to the development of their spiritual health, particularly when time is spent relaxing, breathing deeply, and trying to clear the mind.

Yoga

Although yoga originated in India about 5000 years ago, it is currently one of the most popular physical activities that involves static stretching. Yoga blends the mental and physical aspects of exercise, a union of mind and body that provides a relaxing and satisfying experience that many find enhances their spiritual health. If done regularly, the combination of mental focus and physical effort improves flexibility, vitality, posture, agility, and coordination.

The practice of yoga focuses on controlled breathing as well as purely physical exercise. In addition to its mental dimensions, yoga incorporates a complex array of static stretching exercises expressed as postures—or asanas. Over 200 postures/asanas exist and about 50 are commonly practised. During a session, participants move to different asanas and hold them for 30 seconds or more. Asanas, singly or in combination, can be changed and adapted for

TABLE 4.3

Performance-Enhancing Dietary Supplements and Drugs—Their Uses and Effects

	Primary Uses	Side Effects
Creatine Naturally occurring compound that helps supply energy to muscle	• To improve postworkout recovery • To increase muscle mass • To increase strength • To increase power	• Weight gain, nausea, muscle cramps • Large doses have a negative effect on the kidneys
Ephedra and Ephedrine Stimulant that constricts blood vessels and increases blood pressure and heart rate	• Weight loss • Increased performance	• Nausea, vomiting • Anxiety and mood changes • Hyperactivity • In rare cases, seizures, heart attack, stroke, psychotic episodes
Anabolic Steroids Synthetic versions of the hormone testosterone	• To improve strength, power, and speed • To increase muscle mass	• In adolescents, stops bone growth; therefore reduced adult height • Masculinization of females; feminization of males • Mood swings • Severe acne, particularly on the back • Sexual dysfunction • Aggressive behaviour • Potential heart and liver damage
Steroid Precursors Substances that the body converts into anabolic steroids, e.g., androstenedione (andro), dehydroepiandrosterone (DHEA)	• Converted in the body to anabolic steroids to increase muscle mass	• In addition to side effects noted with anabolic steroids, body hair growth, increased risk of pancreatic cancer
Human Growth Hormone Naturally occurring hormone secreted by the pituitary gland that is essential for body growth	• Anti-aging agent • To improve performance • To increase muscle mass	• Structural changes to the face • Increased risk of high blood pressure • Potential for congestive heart failure

Sources: Based on "The Risks and Dangers Involved in Bodybuilding Supplements," retrieved April 20, 2013 from securitynews.hubpages.com/hub/The-Risks-and-Dangers-Involved-in-Bodybuilding-Supplements; Mayo Clinic Staff, "Performance-Enhancing Drugs and Your Teen Athlete," MayoClinic.com, January 2009, www.mayoclinic.com/health/performance-enhancing-drugs/SM00045; Office of Diversion Control, Drug and Chemical Evaluation Section, "Drugs and Chemicals of Concern: Human Growth Hormone," August 2009, www.deadiversion.usdoj.gov/drugs_concern/hgh.htm; Office of Dietary Supplements, National Institutes of Health, "Ephedra and Ephedrine Alkaloids for Weight Loss and Athletic Performance," Updated July 2004, http://ods.od.nih.gov/factsheets/EphedraandEphedrine.

young and old or to accommodate physical limitations or disabilities. Asanas can also be combined to provide well-conditioned athletes with a challenging workout!

A typical yoga session will move the spine and joints through their full range of motion. Yoga postures lengthen, strengthen, and balance musculature; leading to increased flexibility, stamina, and strength—and many people report a psychological sense of general well-being too. Table 4.4 details three popular types of yoga.

Tai Chi

Tai chi is an ancient form of exercise that combines stretching, balance, coordination, and meditation. It is designed to increase range of motion and flexibility while reducing muscular tension. Based on Chi Kung, a Taoist philosophy dedicated to spiritual growth and good health, tai chi was developed about 1000 CE by monks to defend themselves against bandits and warlords. It involves a series of positions called "forms," based on Chinese martial arts, that are performed continuously.

TABLE 4.4

Popular Yoga Styles

- *Iyengar yoga* focuses on precision and alignment in the poses. Standing poses are basic to this style and are often held longer than in other styles.
- *Ashtanga yoga* in its pure form is based on a specific flow of poses with an emphasis on strength and agility that creates internal heat. *Power yoga,* a style growing in popularity, is a derivative of ashtanga yoga.
- *Bikram yoga*, or hot yoga, is similar to power yoga but does not incorporate a specific flow of poses. Literally the hottest yoga going, it is performed in temperatures of 38°C, or even a bit higher. Proponents say that the heat increases the body's ability to move and stretch without injury.

Further, tai chi is often described as "meditation in motion" because it promotes serenity through gentle movements—connecting the mind and body.

Pilates

Pilates was developed by Joseph Pilates in 1926. It teaches body awareness, good posture, and easy, graceful body movements. Pilates improves flexibility, agility, coordination, strength, tone, and economy of motion. It might alleviate back pain. Pilates combines stretching with movement against resistance aided by devices such as tension springs or heavy rubber bands. Pilates differs from yoga and tai chi in that it includes a component specifically designed to increase strength. The method consists of a sequence of carefully performed movements. Some are carried out on specially designed equipment, while others are performed on mats. Each exercise strengthens the muscles involved and has a specific breathing pattern associated with it.

BODY COMPOSITION

Body composition is the final component of health-related physical fitness and is unique in that you do not exercise or train specifically to improve it, but rather changes often happen to it as a result of the exercises done to improve the various components of physical fitness. As will be noted in Chapter 6, body composition describes the relative portions of fat and lean tissues in the body. Body composition parameters are influenced by regular physical activity and exercise in terms of total body mass, fat mass, fat-free mass, and regional fat distribution. Generally, aerobic physical activities improve body composition because they expend calories and contribute to weight maintenance and/or loss. Similarly, strength training activities may improve body composition directly and indirectly. Direct improvements may be noted by increases in lean body mass. Indirect improvements may be noted as a result of a higher metabolism because of the increased

lean body mass. For more details on body composition, including its measurement, refer to Chapter 6.

PLANNING YOUR PHYSICAL FITNESS TRAINING PROGRAM

Identifying Your Physical Fitness Goals and Designing Your Program

Before you start a physical fitness training program, determine your personal health and physical fitness needs, limitations, exercise likes and dislikes, daily schedule, and goals. Regardless of your reason for starting an exercise or training program, your most important goal should be to commit to it regularly.

When creating a plan, it is important that your goals represent your present fitness level, age, health, skills, interest, and availability. A great way to develop your exercise program is to follow the FITT principle (AAHPERD, 1999). This principle helps you to develop a physical activity plan that outlines how often (Frequency), how hard (Intensity) how long (Time) a person exercises, and what kinds (Type) of exercises are selected. It also emphasizes that every plan should have a schedule that progresses over time. The body adapts quickly to an overload and unless you continue to overload your body your progress will quickly plateau. For example, if jogging is the physical activity you choose, you might start first with walking. Once you can comfortably walk briskly for 20 to 30 minutes at a time, you can safely start to jog. Still, you want to start slowly, alternating jogging and walking (1 minute of jogging, 1 minute of walking; progress to 2 minutes of jogging, 1 minute of walking, and so on) until you develop a cardiorespiratory fitness level that enables you to jog continuously for 20 to 30 minutes.

To optimize your physical fitness training, develop a workout schedule that is challenging and realistic. An important step in adopting a new behaviour is

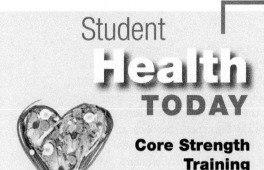

Student Health TODAY

Core Strength Training

The body's core muscles are the foundation for all movement. These muscles include the deep back and abdominal muscles that attach to the spine and pelvis. The contraction of these muscles provides the basis of support for movements of the upper and lower body and powerful movements of the extremities.

A weak core generally results in poor posture, lower back pain, and muscle injuries. A strong core provides a more stable platform for movements, thus reducing the chance of injury.

You can develop core strength by doing various exercises including calisthenics, yoga, or Pilates. Holding yourself in a front or reverse plank ("up" and reverse of a push-up position) and holding or doing abdominal curl-ups are examples of exercises that increase core strength. Increasing core strength does not happen from one single exercise, but rather from a structured regime of postures and exercises. Although exercises using instability devices (stability ball, wobble boards, etc.) are effective for increasing strength of the core, they should be used in conjunction with, not instead of, a physical fitness program that follows the FITT prescription.

Sources: Based on V. Baltzpoulos, "Isokinetic Dynamometry," in *Biomechanical Evaluation of Movement in Sport and Exercise: The British Association of Sport and Exercise Sciences Guidelines,* eds. C. Payton and R. Bartlett (New York: Routledge, 2008), 105; J. R. Fowles, "What I Always Wanted to Know about Instability Training," *Applied Physiology, Nutrition, and Metabolism 35,* no. 1 (2010): 89–90; D. G. Behm et al., "The Use of Instability to Train the Core Musculature," *Applied Physiology, Nutrition, and Metabolism 35,* no. 1 (2010): 91–108; D. G. Behm et al., "Canadian Society for Exercise Physiology Position Stand: The Use of Instability to Train the Core in Athletic and Nonathletic Conditioning," *Applied Physiology, Nutrition, and Metabolism 35,* no. 1 (2010): 109–12.

developing a new routine (as described in Chapter 1). Care must be taken to ensure that you do not set yourself up for failure before you begin by choosing an overly ambitious schedule. If you decide to walk six times per week, but are able to complete only four sessions, you might feel you failed to achieve your goal. It is very important to set yourself up for success by making your goals realistic and achievable—success in meeting and exceeding your short-term goals will give you the positive energy and confidence to move forward with your program and reach your long-term goals. For many people, it is also important to keep a record of their workouts as well as the progress made in each. Something as simple as checkmarks on the calendar for the days you exercised can provide the visual signs of success to help to keep you motivated. More detailed records provide positive feedback and motivation by allowing you to look back to see where you started and how much you have progressed over time. It is also important to regularly evaluate your progress because, as mentioned previously, progress over time is key to improving your health related fitness. The FITT principle also states that an effective physical activity plan should include activities that will improve *all* of the following health-related fitness components: cardiorespiratory endurance, muscular strength, muscular endurance, and flexibility.

Warm-Up and Cool-Down

Every exercise session should begin with a warm-up and finish with a cool-down. Your warm-up should include 5 to 15 minutes of large body movements that increase your body temperature, potentially followed by light stretching for the muscle groups you are about to use. Warm-up is not the time to improve flexibility. The length of your warm-up is dependent upon how psychologically prepared you are to move; if you are geared up and ready to go, the warm-up may not take as long (approximately five minutes), whereas if you are not quite in the mood to exercise, the warm-up may take longer (approximately 15 minutes). A warm-up should gradually increase heart rate and core body temperature, improve joint lubrication, increase muscles' and tendons' elasticity and flexibility, and enhance your performance during the workout that follows.

The cool-down should be similar to the warm-up, with 5 to 10 minutes of moderate- to low-intensity cardiorespiratory activity, followed by 5 to 10 minutes of stretching exercises. The purpose of the cool-down is to gradually reduce your heart rate, blood pressure, and body temperature to pre-exercising levels. In addition, a cool-down reduces the risk of blood pooling in the extremities, and facilitates quicker recovery between exercise sessions. Because of the body's increased temperature, the cool-down is an excellent time to stretch and increase flexibility.

Cardiorespiratory Endurance

It is important to spend a significant portion of your exercise time developing your aerobic fitness. Choose physical activities that you like. Many people find cross training—alternating participation in two or more activities (such as jogging and swimming)—more enjoyable than long-term participation in only one activity. Cross training is also beneficial in that it strengthens a variety of muscles and reduces your risk of overuse injuries. It may potentially lead to higher levels of physical fitness as well. Jogging, brisk walking, swimming, cycling, rowing, step aerobics, and cross country skiing are excellent activities for developing cardiovascular fitness.

Resistance Training

It is important to include strengthening exercises in your training plans as well. Although regular aerobic exercise will contribute to building and maintaining muscular endurance, it will not build or maintain muscular strength. Different exercises using free weights, your own body weight, a resistance band, or machines can be combined in many ways to create an effective resistance-training workout. As previously mentioned, physical activities such as yoga, tai chi, and Pilates can also be effective at building strength depending upon what is done.

Flexibility

For optimal flexibility, static stretching exercises should be performed every day following a general warm-up to raise the core body temperature and increase the elasticity of muscles and tendons. Many people find that stretching between sets during their resistance training sessions is quite effective. The target muscles are already warm, and since the stretches are performed during the rest time between sets, no additional time for stretching is required at the beginning or end of the workout.

FITNESS-RELATED INJURIES

There are two basic types of injuries stemming from participation in fitness training-related activities: overuse and traumatic.

Causes of Fitness-Related Injuries

Overuse injuries Injuries that result from the cumulative effects of day-after-day stresses placed on tendons, muscles, and joints.

Traumatic injuries Injuries that are usually accidental in nature and occur suddenly and violently (for example, fractured bones, ruptured tendons, and sprained ligaments).

Overtraining is the most frequent cause of injuries associated with physical fitness training. **Overuse injuries** occur because of cumulative, day-after-day stresses placed on body parts (tendons, bones, and ligaments). The forces that occur normally during physical activity are not enough to result in an injury, but when applied on a daily basis for weeks or months, they can result in an injury. That is why people who sustain this type of injury typically cannot pinpoint a particular time or day when they were injured. Common sites of overuse injuries are the leg, knee, shoulder, and elbow joints. While participating in your personal fitness program, listen to your body's warning signs. Muscle stiffness and soreness, bone and joint pains, and whole-body fatigue are common warning signs of an overuse injury. To minimize your risk of an overuse injury, vary your physical activities and exercises throughout the week. Further, set appropriate and realistic short- and long-term training goals.

Traumatic injuries, which occur suddenly and violently, typically by accident, are the second major type of fitness training–related injuries. Typical traumatic injuries are broken bones, torn ligaments and muscles, contusions, and lacerations. Most traumatic injuries are unavoidable—for example, spraining your ankle by landing on another person's foot after jumping up for a rebound in basketball. If your traumatic injury causes a noticeable loss of function and immediate pain or pain that does not go away after 30 minutes, you should have a physician examine it.

Prevention

To minimize your risk of injuries, it is important to examine the equipment you use—the actual exercise equipment you use and the shoes you wear.

Appropriate Footwear

When you purchase running shoes or sneakers, look for several key components. Proper footwear can decrease the likelihood of foot, knee, or back injuries. Biomechanics research suggests that running is a "collision" sport—that is, the runner's foot collides with the ground with a force three to five times the runner's body weight with each stride (Brody, 1987). The force not absorbed by the running shoe is transmitted upward into the foot, leg, thigh, and back. Our bodies are able to absorb forces such as these, but may be injured by the cumulative effects of repetitive impacts (for example, running 65 kilometres per week). Therefore, the ability of running shoes to absorb shock is a critical factor to consider when you purchase footwear for your physical activities. Proper fit is also important. In addition, it is crucial to replace footwear regularly (some suggest after running approximately 1000 kilometres) to ensure that the shock absorbency is still effective. You will notice when it is time to replace your shoes as they will feel less cushiony and you might experience some knee, ankle, or foot pain (Vonhof, 2011). Other physical activities or sports (basketball, soccer, cycling, mountain climbing) require different footwear performance, and the requirements of the physical activity or sport should be considered when you prepare yourself to engage in those activities or sports.

Appropriate Protective Equipment

It is essential to use well-fitted, appropriate equipment for your physical activities. For some activities, there is specialized protective equipment to reduce your chances of injury. In tennis, for example, the use of the "right" racquet with the "right" tension helps prevent the general inflammatory condition known as "tennis elbow."

Eye injuries can occur in virtually all physical activities, though the risk of injury is much greater in some activities than others. As many as 90 percent of eye injuries resulting from racquetball and squash are preventable with appropriate eye protection—for example, goggles with polycarbonate lenses (Erie, 1991).

According to the Canadian Cycling Association, cycling is one of the most popular recreational activities in Canada and continues to grow every year. The selection of the right-sized bicycle frame and correct seat height, coupled with the use of a bicycle helmet, padded grips/handlebars, and padded cycling gloves, can significantly reduce injuries. In the past, head injuries accounted for 85 percent of all deaths attributable to bicycle accidents; however, the wearing of bicycle helmets has significantly reduced the number of skull fractures and facial injuries among recreational cyclists (Wasserman & Buccini, 1990). Cyclists should wear bicycle helmets that meet the criteria established by the Canadian Standards Association (see www.bhsi.org/stdcomp.htm).

Common Overuse Injuries

The three most common overuse injuries are plantar fasciitis, "shin splints," and "runner's knee."

Plantar Fasciitis

Plantar fasciitis is an inflammation of the plantar fascia, a broad band of dense, inelastic tissue (fascia) that runs from the heel to the toe on the bottom of your foot (Molloy, 2012). The main function of the plantar fascia is to protect the nerves, blood vessels, and muscles of the foot from injury. In repetitive, weight-bearing activities such as walking and running, the plantar fascia may become inflamed. Common symptoms include pain and tenderness under the ball of the foot, at the heel, or at both locations (Molloy, 2012). The pain of plantar fasciitis is particularly noticeable during your first steps out of bed in the morning. If not treated properly, this injury may progress in severity to the point that

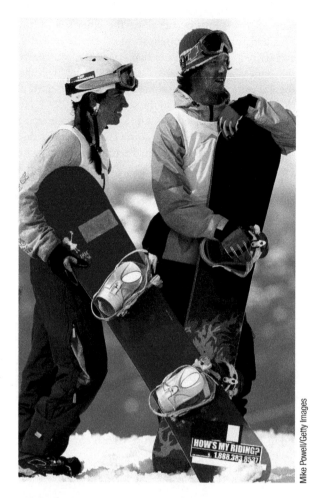

Mike Powell/Getty Images

While appropriate clothing and equipment help prevent injuries in any physical activity, a workout partner is also an important safeguard.

weight-bearing exercise is too painful to endure. Uphill running is not advised since each uphill stride severely stretches (and thus irritates) the already inflamed plantar fascia. Plantar fasciitis can be prevented by regular stretching of the plantar fascia prior to exercise and by wearing footwear with good arch support and shock absorbency. Stretching the plantar fascia involves slowly pulling all five toes upward toward your head, holding for 10 to 15 seconds, and repeating this three to five times on each foot before exercising.

Shin Splints

Shin splints is a general term for any pain that occurs on the front part of the lower legs affecting 4 to 35 percent of the athletic and military populations (Batt, 2011). More than 20 medical conditions have been identified within the broad description of shin splints. Problems range from stress fractures of the tibia (shinbone) to severe inflammation in the muscular compartments of the lower leg, which can interrupt the flow of blood and nerve conduction to the foot. The most common type of shin splints occurs along the inner side of the tibia and is usually a combination of muscle irritation and irritation of the tissues that attach the muscles to the bone (Biber Brewer & Gregory, 2012). Typically, there is pain and swelling along the middle one-third of the postero-medial tibia in the soft tissues.

Sedentary people who start a new weight-bearing physical activity program are at the greatest risk for shin splints, though well-conditioned aerobic exercisers who rapidly increase their distance or pace may also be at risk. Running and exercise classes are the most frequent cause of shin splints, but those who do a great deal of walking (for example, postal carriers or restaurant staff) may also develop shin splints.

To minimize your risk, wear shoes with good arch support and shock absorbency (Batt, 2011). Many athletic retail stores can help you choose appropriate footwear based upon pronation and comfort. If the severity of your shin splints increases to the point that you cannot comfortably complete your desired physical activity, see your physician. Specific pain on the tibia or on the fibula (the adjacent, smaller bone) should be examined for possible stress fracture. Reducing the frequency, intensity, and time of weight-bearing exercises may be required. You may also be advised to substitute a non-weight bearing exercise such as swimming, cycling, or rowing during your recovery period.

Runner's Knee

Runner's knee describes a series of problems involving the muscles, tendons, and ligaments of the knee. The most common problem is abnormal movement of the patella or kneecap (Brody, 1987). Women are more commonly affected than men because of their anatomical structure. Specifically, their wider pelvis results in a lateral pull on the patella by the muscles that act on the knee. In women (and some men), the lateral pull on the patella causes irritation of the cartilage on the back of the patella as well as to the nearby tendons and ligaments. The main symptom is the pain experienced when downward pressure is applied to the patella after the knee is straightened fully. Additional symptoms include swelling, redness, and tenderness around the patella, and a dull, aching pain in the centre of the knee (American Academy of Orthopedic Surgeons, 1991). With these symptoms, your physician will probably recommend that you stop running for a few weeks and reduce daily physical activities that put compressive forces on the patella (for example, exercise on a stair-climbing machine or doing squats with heavy resistance) until you no longer feel any pain around your kneecap.

Treatment

RICE Acronym for the standard first-aid treatment for injuries: rest, ice, compression, and elevation.

Treatment for virtually all fitness training-related injuries involves **RICE:** rest, ice, compression, and elevate. Rest is required to eliminate the risk of further irritating the injured body part. Immobilization of the injured body part can be accomplished with a 10- or 15-centimetre wide elastic bandage which applies indirect pressure to damaged blood vessels to help stop bleeding. Be careful that the wrap is not on so tightly that it interferes with normal blood flow. A throbbing hand or foot indicates that the immobilization is too tight and it should be loosened. Cold is applied to relieve pain and to constrict the blood vessels to reduce internal or external bleeding associated with the injury. To prevent frostbite or other irritation to the skin, do not apply ice directly to your skin; instead, place a layer of wet towelling between the ice and your skin. Ice should be applied to a new injury for approximately 20 minutes every hour for the first 24 to 72 hours. Elevation of the injured extremity above the level of the heart also helps to control internal or external bleeding by making the blood flow uphill to reach the injured area.

Exercising in the Heat

For physical activities outside, the function of your exercise clothing is far more important than how you look in them. For some physical activities, you will need clothing that allows maximal body heat dissipation—for example, light-coloured nylon shorts and a mesh tank top while running in hot weather. For other physical activities, you will need clothing that permits significant heat retention without allowing you to become sweat-soaked—for example, layers of polypropylene and/or wool clothing while cross-country or downhill skiing.

Exercising in hot or humid temperatures increases your risk of a heat-related injury. However, if you are in good physical condition, wear appropriate clothing, and drink plenty of fluids, you can safely withstand a wide range of temperatures and humidity when engaged in physical activity. Heat stress, which includes several potentially fatal illnesses resulting from an elevated core body temperature, should be a concern when exercising in warm, humid weather. In these conditions, your body's rate of heat production often exceeds its ability to cool. You can prevent heat stress by following certain precautions. First, acclimatize yourself properly to hot and/or humid climates. The process of heat acclimatization, which increases your body's cooling efficiency, requires about 10 to 14 days of gradually increased exercise in a hot environment. Second, reduce your risk of dehydration by replacing fluids before, during, and after exercise. Third, wear clothing appropriate for the activity and the environment. Finally, use common sense—for example, when the temperature is 30°C and the humidity is 90 percent, postpone your usual lunchtime run until the evening or re-schedule for the early morning. You may even choose a different physical activity or exercise, one that is indoors in an air-conditioned facility or one that is in water.

The three heat stress illnesses, progressive in their level of severity, are heat cramps, heat exhaustion, and heat stroke. The least serious problem, **heat cramps**, is easily prevented by adequate fluid replacement and a dietary intake that includes the electrolytes lost during sweating (sodium and potassium). Sport drinks may be effective in this regard (more on these in Chapter 5). **Heat exhaustion** is most often caused by excessive water loss because of intense or prolonged exercise or physical work in a hot and/or humid environment. Symptoms of heat exhaustion include nausea, headache, fatigue, dizziness and faintness, and, paradoxically, "goosebumps" and chills. When suffering from heat exhaustion, your skin will be cool and moist. Heat exhaustion is actually a mild form of shock, in which the blood pools in the arms and legs away from the brain and major organs of the body. **Heat stroke**, often called sunstroke, is a life-threatening emergency condition with a 20- to 70-percent death rate (Hafen & Karren, 1992). Heat stroke occurs during vigorous exercise when the body's heat production significantly exceeds its cooling capacity. Core body temperature can rise from normal (37°C) to 40.5°C to 43°C within minutes after the body's cooling mechanism shuts down. A rapid increase in core body temperature can cause brain damage, permanent disability, and death. Common signs of heat stroke are dry, hot, and usually red skin, very high body temperature, and a very rapid heart rate.

Heat stress illnesses can occur in situations in which the danger is not obvious. Serious or fatal heat stroke may result from prolonged sauna or steam baths, prolonged total immersion in a hot tub or spa, or by exercising in a plastic or rubber head-to-toe "sauna suit." If you experience any of the symptoms mentioned here while exercising, stop immediately, move to the shade or a cool spot to rest, and drink plenty of cool fluids. To prevent overhydration or hypernatremia, be careful to also replace lost electrolytes.

Exercising in the Cold

When you are physically active in cool or cold weather, especially in windy conditions, your body's heat loss is frequently greater than its heat production. Under these conditions, **hypothermia**—a potentially fatal condition resulting from abnormally low body core temperature—can result. Hypothermia can occur as a result of prolonged, vigorous exercise (for example, snowboarding or rugby) in 4°C to 10°C temperatures, particularly if there is rain, snow, or a strong wind.

As your body core temperature drops from the normal 37°C to 34°C, you will begin to shiver. Shivering—the involuntary contraction of nearly every muscle in your body—is designed to increase your body temperature by generating heat through muscle activity. During this first stage of hypothermia, you may also experience cold hands and feet, poor judgment, apathy, and amnesia (Thornton, 1990). Shivering ceases in most hypothermia victims as their core body temperature drops to between 32°C and 30°C, a sign that the body has lost its ability to generate heat. Death from hypothermia usually occurs at core body temperatures between 26.5°C and 24°C.

To prevent hypothermia, follow these guidelines: analyze weather conditions and your risk of hypothermia before engaging in your planned outdoor physical activity, remembering that wind and humidity are as significant as temperature; use the "buddy system"—that is, have a friend join you for your cold-weather outdoor activities; wear layers of appropriate clothing to prevent excessive heat loss (for example, polypropylene or woolen undergarments, a Gore-Tex windbreaker, and wool hat and gloves); and, finally, don't allow yourself to become dehydrated.

Your Movement Journey

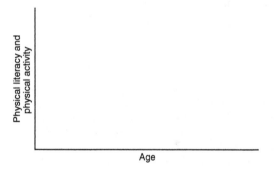

Before completing the "Assess Yourself" exercise you might take a minute to consider your movement journey over the course of your life. Create a simple line graph depicting how your physical activity levels and physical literacy has changed from preschool (age three to five years) to your current age. Your physical activity and physical literacy levels will make up the vertical axis and your age will make up the horizontal axis. Physical activity and physical literacy levels can be depicted with different coloured lines. Consider how your physical activity and physical literacy levels have changed and fluctuated over the course of your lifetime. The goal of this activity to help you understand how your life journey has contributed to your current physical activity levels and physical literacy. This will also help you to set new physical activity goals.

Heat cramps Muscle cramps that occur during or following exercise in warm/hot conditions.

Heat exhaustion A heat stress illness caused by significant dehydration resulting from exercise in hot and/or humid conditions; frequent precursor to heat stroke.

Heat stroke A deadly heat stress illness resulting from dehydration and overexertion in hot conditions; can result in body core temperature rising rapidly from normal to 43°C in just a few minutes.

Hypothermia A potentially fatal condition resulting from abnormally low body core temperature.

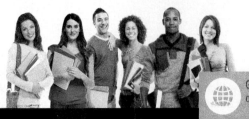

TAKING CHARGE: Managing Your Physical Activity Behaviours

The decision to become physically active is easy to make but not always easy to put into action. Physical activity should be enjoyable so, in addition to considering the health benefits, you should choose activities that you enjoy and that help you to feel good about yourself.

Begin by making a list of your favourite physical activities. Which of these increases or helps to maintain cardiorespiratory efficiency, muscular strength and endurance, and flexibility? Your list may include walking, dancing, playing intramural sports, as well as exercises such as weight lifting, jogging, cycling, and swimming. Which would you like to make part of your program? Next, you need to find time to exercise and be physically active. Do you have extra time you could set aside? Can you use your time more effectively so that you do have time for physical activity and/or exercise? If not, how could physical activity become part of your daily activities? Could you walk to and from your classes? Rather than watch TV or have a coffee for a study break, could you do some physical activities? Could your social time include physical activities?

The following suggestions might assist you in becoming regularly physically active:

- **Start slowly.** For the first-time exerciser or for someone who has been inactive for a considerable period of time, any type and amount of physical activity is a step in the right direction. If you have been inactive for a long time or are overweight or obese, 5 minutes of walking may be all that you can do when you start. Do not be discouraged; start there and progress as your fitness improves.
- **Make only one lifestyle change at a time.** Attempting too many changes at once invites failure. Success with one behaviour change encourages you to make other positive lifestyle changes.
- **Have reasonable expectations of yourself and your training program.** Many people become exercise dropouts because their expectations are too high. Be patient with yourself and your body. Give it sufficient time to reach your physical fitness goals.
- **Choose a specific time to be physically active and stick with it.** Learning to establish priorities and keeping to a schedule are vital steps toward improved physical fitness. In fact, it is beneficial to schedule your physical activity as you would your classes and meetings so that the time is protected for you. Experiment by exercising at different times of the day to learn what time works and feels best for you.
- **Prepare yourself to be physically active; plan ahead.** If you plan to exercise first thing in the morning, put out your exercise clothes the night before. Similarly, if you plan to be physically active over your lunch break, pack your workout clothes and put them by the door so you do not forget them when you leave for the day.
- **Be physically active with a friend.** Reneging on an exercise or physical activity commitment is more difficult if your plans include a friend. Enjoy the social aspects of exercising with a friend. Partners can motivate and encourage one another, provided they remember that progress will not be the same for each of them.
- **Make physical activity a positive habit.** Usually, if you are able to do a physical activity for three weeks, you will be able to incorporate it into your lifestyle. Be aware that for some individuals exercise can become a negative habit (addiction).
- **Keep a record of your progress.** A personal journal can be a good motivator. Your journal could include various facts about your physical activities (frequency, intensity, time, type) and chronicle your emotions and personal achievements as you progress in your training.
- **Take lapses in stride.** Physical deconditioning—a decline in fitness level—occurs at about the same rate as physical conditioning. If you have not exercised for three or more weeks after regular training, you will notice lower levels of cardiorespiratory and muscular fitness. First, renew your commitment, and then restart your exercise program.

Before you start your physical activity or exercise program, it may be useful to learn what is available to you:

- Does your campus have facilities for physical activity and physical fitness training? Where are these facilities? Are they conveniently located? Is the use of facilities included in your student fees? What hours are those facilities available?
- What intramural and exercise programs are available on campus? How can you sign up for these?

- What community facilities are available for physical activity? Where are these facilities? Are they conveniently located? Have you considered using these facilities? Why or why not? What is the cost of a membership? Hours of usage?
- Does your community have walking and/or bicycling trails? Are the places you need to go regularly (for example, the grocery store) within walking distance? Is the scenery pleasant when you walk? These factors are associated with a higher level of walking (Spence et al., 2006). Do they matter to you as well? Why or why not?
- What opportunities are available for you to volunteer at a local physical fitness or wellness facility? Have you considered volunteering to help low-income individuals or individuals with a physical or mental disability in physical activity or physical fitness programs? Why or why not?
- Are there opportunities within your college or university for you to be involved in providing physical activity programs to children or adolescents? How can you get involved in them?

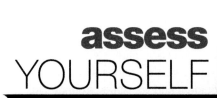

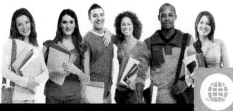

Go to MasteringHealth to complete this questionnaire with automatic scoring

How Physically Fit Are You?

Before you start your new physical fitness program, consider establishing your baseline or start values so that every so often you can test yourself again and monitor your improvement.

Evaluating Your Cardiorespiratory Endurance

Find a local track, typically 400 metres, to perform your test. You want to walk around this track four times (1.6 km or 1 mile) as fast as you can. Choose a speed that you can walk at for the entire duration of the test. Use the chart below to estimate your cardiorespiratory fitness level based upon your age and sex. Aim for at least the 'good' zone.

Fitness Category	Age (years)			
	13–19	20–29	30–39	40+
Men				
Very poor	>17:30	>18:00	>19:00	>21:30
Poor	16:01–17:30	16:31–18:00	17:31–19:00	18:31–21:30
Average	14:01–16:00	14:31–16:30	15:31–17:30	16:01–18:30
Good	12:30–14:00	13:00–14:30	13:30–15:30	14:00–16:00
Excellent	<12:30	<13:00	<13:30	<14:00
Women				
Very poor	>18:01	>18:31	>19:31	>20:01
Poor	16:31–18:00	17:01–18:30	18:01–19:30	19:31–20:00
Average	14:31–16:30	15:01–17:00	16:01–18:00	18:01–19:30
Good	13:30–14:30	13:30–15:00	14:00–16:00	14:30–18:00
Excellent	<13:30	<13:30	<14:00	<14:30

Because the one-mile walk test is designed primarily for older or less conditioned individuals, the fitness categories listed here do not include a "superior" category.

Source: Modified from *Rockport Fitness Walking Test.* Copyright © 1993. The Rockport Company, LLC. Reprinted with permission.

(continued)

Evaluating Your Muscular Strength and Endurance

A number of tests are proposed by the Canadian Society for Exercise Physiology (CSEP) for determining muscular strength and endurance. The most commonly used tests are partial curl-ups and push-ups. Other tests include grip strength and vertical jump.

The partial curl-up measures the muscular endurance of the abdominal musculature. In the partial curl-up, the trunk is raised no more than 30 to 40 degrees above the mat so that the shoulders are raised about 15 to 25 cm. A full sit-up is not used because of the stress placed on the lower back when performed and because they also require hip flexor action when performed. Curl-ups are timed and performed at a slow and controlled cadence of 25 curl-ups per minute to a maximum of 25. Knees are bent at a 90 degree angle and feet remain flat on the floor. Please refer to Table 4.5 to determine your 'health benefit zone'.

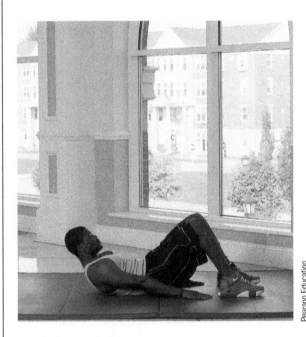

Partial curl-up.

Push-ups provide a measure of the muscular endurance of the upper body, including the shoulders, arms, and chest. There is no time or ceiling limit for the measurement of push-ups. Start by positioning yourself on the ground (see figures to the left) on your toes if you are male, on your knees if you are female. Your hands should be below your shoulders and your body extended in a straight line. Push your body up by straightening your elbows using your toes/knees as a pivot. Lower your body until your chin is close to the mat. Neither your stomach nor your thighs should contact the ground. Keep your back straight and lower your entire body as a unit. Please refer to Table 4.5 to determine your 'health benefit zone'.

Evaluating Your Flexibility

The most commonly used test to measure flexibility is the sit and reach test or trunk forward flexion. Another test endorsed by CSEP is back extension. The sit and reach test measures the ability of the back to flex, which involves the muscles of the lower back and of the back of the legs (that is, hamstrings). It is recommended that you warm-up prior to performing this test. Sit upright, shoes removed, feet flat against the box. With your feet in place, knees straight, extend your hands palms down as far as possible forward in a smooth, fluid movement. Lowering your head may help you to reach further. Please refer to Table 4.5 to determine your 'health benefit zone'.

Evaluating Your Body Composition

Your body composition can be measured in a number of ways. One method involves determining your body mass index (BMI) from your height and weight. Although widely used in population studies as an indicator of overweight and obesity, BMI does not actually provide a measure of fatness and so

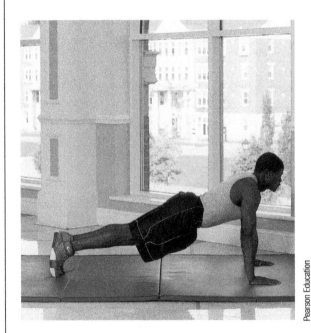

Push-up from toes.

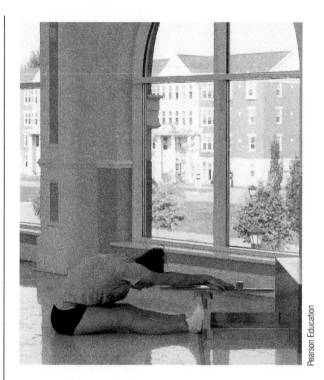

Trunk flexibility is usually evaluated using the sit and reach test.

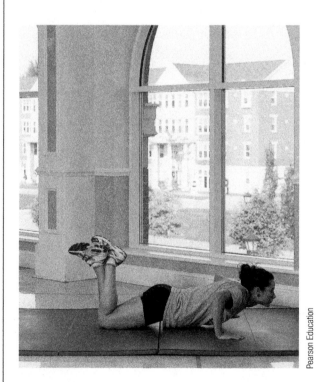

Push-up from knees.

is not really a measure of body composition. Waist circumference is a simple measure that provides a relatively valid measure of abdominal fatness; however, it too does not actually provide a measure of body composition. When measuring your waist circumference, you should use a nonelastic measuring tape and place it snugly around your waist- at the level of your umbilicus (i.e., belly button) or at the obvious waist narrowing. Record to the nearest 0.5 cm. Please refer to Tables 4.6, 4.7, and 4.8 to determine your 'health benefit zone'.

Sum of five skinfolds is a measurement of body composition advocated by the CSEP. Skinfold measurements provide an indication of subcutaneous fat (that is, fat that lies directly below the skin) and since half the fat in a normal-fat individual lies below his or her skin, an estimate of body composition can be made. Five measurements (triceps, biceps, subscapular, iliac crest, and medial calf) are taken, totalled, and compared to the health benefit zones. Alternatively the subscapular and iliac crest can be made for an indication of trunk fatness. Please refer to Tables 4.6, 4.7, and 4.8 to determine your 'health benefit zone'.

Critical Thinking

Your friend Silke catches everyone's eye: five years of intense bodybuilding have created a sleek, "jacked," hard body. She plans to enter bodybuilding contests within the next year. Silke started working out in high school after her father had a heart attack at age 38. Her family doctor pointed out that her family had a history of cardiovascular disease and that she should take steps to lower her own risk.

Although aerobic exercise was the doctor's suggestion, Silke works out two to three hours a day in the weight room, usually powerlifting to build bigger muscles for competition. When she had a higher-than-normal blood pressure reading last week, she was convinced that she had to train harder. From what you have learned, you want to suggest that she add aerobic exercise and flexibility training to her workout. However, because you do little more than walk 30 minutes a day, you are afraid she will not take your suggestion seriously.

Using the DECIDE model described in Chapter 1, decide how you could approach Silke to urge her to take a more balanced and perhaps more realistic approach to her workout regime.

(continued)

TABLE 4.5

Healthy Musculoskeletal Fitness: Norms and Health Benefit Zones by Age Groups and Gender

	Age (yrs) 15–19					
	*Push-Ups (#)		#Trunk Fwd Flexion (cm)		$Partial Curl-Up (#)	
Gender	M	F	M	F	M	F
ZONE Excellent	≥ 39	≥ 33	≥ 39	≥ 43	≥ 25	≥ 25
Very good	29–38	25–32	34–38	38–42	23–24	23–24
Good	23–28	18–24	29–33	34–37	21–22	21–22
Fair	18–22	12–17	24–28	29–33	16–20	16–20
Needs improvement	≤ 17	≤ 11	≤ 23	≤ 28	≤ 15	≤ 15
	Age (yrs) 20–29					
	Push-Ups (#)		Trunk Fwd Flexion (cm)		Partial Curl-Up (#)	
Gender	M	F	M	F	M	F
ZONE Excellent	≥ 36	≥ 30	≥ 40	≥ 41	≥ 25	≥ 25
Very good	28–35	21–29	34–39	37–40	23–24	23–24
Good	22–27	15–20	30–33	33–36	21–22	19–22
Fair	17–21	10–14	25–29	28–32	13–20	13–18
Needs improvement	≤ 16	≤ 9	≤ 24	≤ 27	≤ 12	≤ 12
	Age (yrs) 30–39					
	Push-Ups (#)		Trunk Fwd Flexion (cm)		Partial Curl-Up (#)	
Gender	M	F	M	F	M	F
ZONE Excellent	≥ 30	≥ 27	≥ 38	≥ 41	≥ 25	≥ 25
Very good	22–29	20–26	33–37	36–40	23–24	22–24
Good	17–21	13–19	28–32	32–35	21–22	16–21
Fair	12–16	8–12	23–27	27–31	13–20	11–15
Needs improvement	≤ 11	≤ 7	≤ 22	≤ 26	≤ 12	≤ 10
	Age (yrs) 40–49					
	Push-Ups (#)		Trunk Fwd Flexion (cm)		Partial Curl-Up (#)	
Gender	M	F	M	F	M	F
ZONE Excellent	≥ 22	≥ 24	≥ 35	≥ 38	≥ 25	≥ 25
Very good	17–21	15–23	29–34	34–37	22–24	21–24
Good	13–16	11–14	24–28	30–33	16–21	13–20
Fair	10–12	5–10	18–23	25–29	11–15	6–12
Needs improvement	≤ 9	≤ 4	≤ 17	≤ 24	≤ 10	≤ 5
	Age (yrs) 50–59					
	Push-Ups (#)		Trunk Fwd Flexion (cm)		Partial Curl-Up (#)	
Gender	M	F	M	F	M	F
ZONE Excellent	≥ 21	≥ 21	≥ 35	≥ 39	≥ 25	≥ 25
Very good	13–20	11–20	28–34	33–38	20–24	16–24
Good	10–12	7–10	24–27	30–32	14–19	9–15
Fair	7–9	2–6	16–23	25–29	9–13	4–8
Needs improvement	≤ 6	≤ 1	≤ 15	≤ 24	≤ 8	≤ 3

	Gender	Push-Ups (#) M	Push-Ups (#) F	Trunk Fwd Flexion (cm) M	Trunk Fwd Flexion (cm) F	Partial Curl-Up (#) M	Partial Curl-Up (#) F
ZONE	Excellent	≥ 18	≥ 17	≥ 33	≥ 35	≥ 25	≥ 18
	Very good	11–17	12–16	25–32	31–34	16–24	11–17
	Good	8–10	5–11	20–24	27–30	10–15	6–10
	Fair	5–7	1–4	15–19	23–26	4–9	2–5
	Needs improvement	≤ 4	≤ 1	≤ 14	≤ 23	≤ 3	≤ 1

* Push-Ups: The Canadian Physical Activity, Fitness & Lifestyle Approach: CSE-Health & Fitness Program's Health-Related Appraisal and Counseling Strategy, 3rd Edition, © 2003. Reprinted with permission from the Canadian Society for Exercise Physiology.

Trunk Fwd Flexion: From "The Canadian Physical Activity, Fitness & Lifestyle Approach: CSEP'S-Health & Fitness Program's Health-Related Appraisal and Counseling Strategy", © 2003. Used with permission.

$ Partial Curl-Up: From "The Canadian Physical Activity, Fitness & Lifestyle Approach: CSEP'S-Health & Fitness Program's Health-Related Appraisal and Counseling Strategy", © 2003. Used with permission.

TABLE 4.6

Health Benefit Zones by Age and Sex: Body Weight, Adiposity, and Fat Distribution*

		Age (yrs) 15–19						
**Measures		BMI		SO5S		WG		SO2S	
Sex	M	F	M	F	M	F	M	F
	18	17	25	36	67	61	11	13
	19	18	27	40	68	63	12	14
	19	19	28	43	64	64	13	16
	20	19	29	46	70	65	13	17
	20	19	31	49	72	65	14	18
	20	20	32	51	72	66	15	19
	21	20	33	54	73	67	15	20
	21	20	35	56	74	67	16	21
	21	21	36	58	75	68	17	22
	22	21	38	61	76	68	17	23
	22	22	40	63	77	69	18	24
	22	22	42	66	78	70	19	26
	22	22	44	69	79	70	21	27
	23	23	47	72	80	71	22	29
	23	23	51	77	81	72	24	31
	24	24	54	83	82	72	27	33
	25	25	61	89	84	74	28	37
	26	26	69	97	88	77	32	42
	28	28	82	116	95	81	42	49

		Age (yrs) 20–29						
**Measures		BMI		SO5S		WG		SO2S	
Sex	M	F	M	F	M	F	M	F
	19	18	26	37	71	61	13	13
	20	18	29	40	73	63	14	14
	21	19	30	43	75	64	16	16
	21	19	32	46	76	65	17	17
	22	20	34	49	77	65	18	18
	22	20	36	51	78	66	19	19
	22	20	38	53	79	66	20	20
	23	21	40	56	81	67	21	21
	23	21	43	58	81	68	23	22
	23	21	46	60	82	69	25	23
	24	22	49	63	83	70	27	24

(continued)

TABLE 4.6 (continued)

Age (yrs) 20–29

**Measures	BMI		SO5S		WG		SO2S	
Sex	M	F	M	F	M	F	M	F
	24	22	52	65	84	71	28	26
	25	22	55	69	85	72	30	27
	25	23	58	72	86	73	32	29
	26	23	62	76	87	75	35	31
	27	24	68	81	89	77	38	33
	27	25	74	86	91	78	41	36
	28	26	82	95	93	81	46	42
	30	28	94	111	97	86	54	48

Age (yrs) 30–39

**Measures	BMI		SO5S		WG		SO2S	
Sex	M	F	M	F	M	F	M	F
	20	19	28	40	75	63	14	14
	21	19	32	45	77	64	17	15
	22	20	35	48	79	65	19	17
	22	20	38	52	80	66	20	18
	23	21	41	55	81	68	22	20
	23	21	44	58	82	69	24	21
	24	22	46	61	83	70	26	23
	24	22	49	63	83	71	27	24
	24	22	52	66	85	72	29	25
	25	23	55	69	86	73	31	27
	25	23	58	72	87	74	33	28
	26	23	60	76	88	75	35	30
	26	24	63	79	89	76	37	32
	27	24	67	83	90	77	39	34
	28	25	71	88	92	79	42	36
	28	26	76	93	94	81	45	39
	29	27	82	99	96	83	48	43
	30	29	89	109	99	86	53	48
	32	31	101	128	106	91	59	59

Age (yrs) 40–49

**Measures	BMI		SO5S		WG		SO2S	
Sex	M	F	M	F	M	F	M	F
	21	19	28	42	78	65	15	14
	22	20	37	48	80	67	20	16
	23	20	40	51	82	68	22	18
	23	21	44	56	84	69	24	20
	24	21	46	59	85	70	26	21
	24	22	48	62	86	72	27	23
	25	22	51	66	87	73	29	25
	25	23	53	69	88	74	31	26
	25	23	56	73	89	75	32	28
	26	24	58	77	91	76	34	29
	26	24	60	81	92	77	35	32
	27	25	63	86	93	78	36	34
	27	25	66	90	94	80	38	37
	28	26	69	94	96	81	40	40
	28	27	72	98	98	83	42	43
	29	28	75	105	100	85	44	46
	30	29	79	113	102	88	47	50
	31	31	86	125	105	92	50	56
	32	34	97	150	114	99	56	65

DISCUSSION QUESTIONS

1. Consider the Canadian Guidelines for Physical Activity and the percentage of adult Canadians who achieve them; identify the practical, economic, and environmental roadblocks that make it difficult to attain and maintain a physically active lifestyle in Canada.

2. Suggest ways that Canadians of all ages—children, adolescents, adults, and older adults—could incorporate more physical activity into their lives. When answering this question, consider each demographic group in a rural, urban, and suburban environment. What could the various levels of government (federal, provincial/territorial, municipal) do to enhance the physical activity level of Canadians? Should the private sector also get involved? How? What is the role of education in promoting physical activity? How can this role be better played?

3. What is the difference between physical activity and physical fitness? How do each relate to health? What are the physiological and psychological benefits of engaging in regular physical activity and/or achieving a higher level of physical fitness?

4. When exercising to improve your cardiorespiratory endurance, how can you monitor the intensity of your exercise? How frequently do you need to exercise? For how long? What kind of physical activities would you do? Why should you consider cross training?

5. Compare and contrast strength training using your body as resistance versus weight training machines or free weights. Which would you prefer? Why?

6. How can you improve your flexibility? When is the most effective time to improve flexibility? Why?

7. Create and populate a table with columns for the FITT prescription (Frequency, Intensity, Time, and Type) and rows for cardiorespiratory endurance, muscular strength, muscular endurance, and flexibility.

8. How can you prevent fitness training-related injuries? How does footwear play a role in preventing injuries?

APPLICATION EXERCISE

Reread the "Consider This . . ." scenario at the beginning of the chapter and answer the following questions.

1. Assuming that Laura's workouts were 45 to 60 minutes long and alternated each day between cardiorespiratory and muscular strength training, was she exercising appropriately? What amount of exercise is too much? Too little? Just right? How can you tell?

2. Given that Laura is still tired and lonely even though she works out regularly, what advice would you give her? Is fatigue simply a part of university or college life, or can it be managed? How could you suggest she manage her loneliness?

MASTERINGHEALTH

Go to MasteringHealth for Assignments, the eText, and the Study Area with case studies, self quizzing, and videos.

CHAPTER 5
EATING FOR OPTIMAL HEALTH AND PERFORMANCE

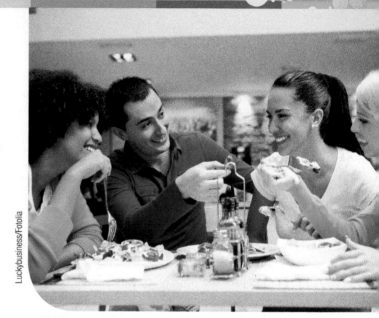

Luckybusiness/Fotolia

LEARNING OUTCOMES

- Summarize the history of Eating Well with Canada's Food Guide and the objectives that guided each stage of its development.

- Describe how to obtain a healthy dietary intake using the Food Guide and the Food Guide for First Nations, Inuit and Métis.

- Review each major essential nutrient and the purpose each serves in maintaining overall health.

- Identify typical problems university or college students experience when trying to eat well.

- Identify current food safety concerns and what students can do to ensure their food is safe for consumption.

◄◉ CONSIDER THIS . . .

Ahmed is a first-year student living in residence and using the food services provided. At "food hall," the same sorts of choices are available to Ahmed each day (burgers and fries, pizza, stir fry, pasta and sauce, soup, sandwiches, and tossed salads), foods are often overcooked, there are few fresh vegetables or fruits, and beverages offered include soft drinks, iced tea, milk, and various watered-down juices. Although Ahmed eats daily at "food hall," he supplements his food intake with fast food, ice cream, and other salty and/or sweet snacks. Ahmed is gaining weight and not feeling very good about himself physically or emotionally. Ahmed wants to eat better, but when he goes to "food hall" or out to eat, he is not sure what to do differently.

What factors contribute to students' attitudes and behaviours toward their food choices? Why do some students find it difficult to eat well? Do you think Ahmed should change his eating habits? Why or why not? What would you suggest he do differently? Do you or your friends have similar problems? Where on your campus could you go for help?

You face dietary choices and nutritional challenges that your grandparents never dreamed of—exotic foods; dietary supplements; artificial sweeteners; no-fat, low-fat, and artificial-fat alternatives; cholesterol-free, trans fat-free, sugar-free, low sodium, high-protein, high-carbohydrate, gluten-free, and low-calorie products. Thousands of alternatives bombard us daily. Caught in the crossfire of claims advertised by the food industry and advice provided by health and nutrition experts, most find it challenging to make wise dietary choices. The ability to sift through the untruths, half-truths, and scientific realities to select a dietary plan that satisfies individual preferences and needs is an essential health-promoting skill—particularly when you are living away from home for the first time. Past patterns of eating influence current dietary attitudes and behaviours. Understanding the reasons behind your dietary attitudes and behaviours might help you make more positive dietary choices.

HEALTHY EATING

We often take our ability to eat what we want, when we want, where we want, and how we want for granted. We assume we will have sufficient food to get us through the day, and rarely are forced to eat foods we do not like for survival. Although we have undoubtedly experienced **hunger**, few of us have suffered the type of hunger that continues for days and threatens survival. We often eat because of **appetite**, a learned psychological desire to eat whether or not we are hungry. Our appetite can be triggered by smell, taste, time of day, special occasions, or proximity to favourite foods such as freshly baked bread, pizza, or chocolate chip cookies. Other factors also stimulate our desire to eat, including cultural and social meanings attached to food, convenience and advertising, habit or custom, emotional comfort, nutritional value, social interaction, and regional/seasonal trends. Finding the right balance between eating to maintain body functions (eating to live) and eating to satisfy our appetite and/or cultural needs (living to eat) is a problem for many, as evidenced by the increased prevalence of overweight and obesity in our population.

Many factors influence what you eat, when you eat, why you eat, where you eat, and how much you eat. Although your great-grandparents typically sat down to eat at least three big meals per day, they also laboured heavily in the fields or at other physical work, effectively using the calories consumed. Today, eating three large meals each day combined with a sedentary lifestyle—at work and at play—will likely result in weight and fat gain. Social pressures, including family traditions, social events that involve food, and busy work schedules, also influence the quality and quantity of your dietary intake. Another factor that influences your eating is culture. In fact, culture permeates all aspects of life, including food preparation, food selection, and attitudes and behaviours toward eating. Some of the attitudes and behaviours relate to what, how much, where, why, and when food is consumed as well as who with (or without). Food may also be consumed to sooth the spirit. The next few paragraphs describe the cultural influence of three traditions and the potential relationships to health: Mediterranean, Asian, and Western (World Cancer Research Fund/American Institute for Cancer Research, 2007). Each of these traditions is influenced by ethnic and religious beliefs in addition to culture, climate, terrain, material resources, and technology. In regard to your dietary intake and overall health, you can learn from other cultural eating practices and potentially adapt your eating attitudes and behaviours.

Dietary Patterns Around the Globe

The traditional Mediterranean diet found in Spain, southern France and Italy, former Yugoslavia, Greece, Turkey, Cyprus, Crete, Lebanon, Israel, Palestine, Egypt, Libya, Algeria, Tunisia, and Morocco typically includes a lot of bread and other cereal products (usually made of wheat), vegetables and fruits, fish, cheese, olive oil, tree nuts such as walnuts and almonds, and wine (in non-Islamic countries) (World Cancer Research Fund/American Institute for Cancer Research, 2007). Food is flavoured extensively with herbs and spices. Little meat is consumed, and when it is, it is most often included in everyday dishes.

Although Asian cuisines (including those of India, Sri Lanka, Thailand, Cambodia, Vietnam, China, Japan, and Korea) can be very diverse, the traditional Asian diet typically includes rice as its staple cereal and main source of energy (World Cancer Research Fund/American Institute for Cancer Research, 2007). The consumption of vegetables, fruits, and fish varies based upon prosperity. Similar to the Mediterranean dietary intake, herbs and spices are used extensively to flavour food. Tea is the traditional hot drink. Both the Mediterranean and traditional Asian diets are linked to lower risks of coronary heart disease, lower rates of obesity, type 2 diabetes, and some types of cancers (see Chapter 12).

In Canada

"Traditional" dietary patterns considered Western are a result of an industrialized food system (World Cancer Research Fund/American Institute for Cancer Research, 2007). The traditional Western diet is energy

Hunger The feeling associated with the physiological need to eat.

Appetite The desire to eat; often more psychological than physiological.

dense and includes increasingly more processed foods. Specifically, the traditional Western diet includes large amounts of meat, milk and milk products, fatty and/or sugary foods (that is, processed meats, pastries, baked goods, confectionery, and so on), and alcoholic drinks. Further, relatively low intakes of vegetables and fruits are common in traditional Western cuisine. As a result, the typical Western dietary intake tends to be high in calories, fat, and sugar and low in fibre. This diet is associated with overweight and obesity, as well as a greater risk for type 2 diabetes, cardiovascular disease, stroke, some cancers, and other chronic diseases.

Nutrition is the science that investigates the relationship between physiological function and the elements of the foods we eat. With the abundance of food available in our society, the options available, and easy access to almost every **nutrient** (water, proteins, carbohydrates, fats, vitamins, and minerals) 24 hours a day, Canadians should have few nutritional problems. However, our "diet of affluence" may be responsible for many diseases and disabilities. This country's history as a land of agricultural abundance accounts for the traditional Canadian diet: high in fats and calories with typically large servings of red meats, potatoes, and rich desserts. More recent trends indicate that Canadians are changing to a white-meat diet (that is, poultry and fish) with fewer fats and more vegetables and fruits. Still, many of us do not eat well. Much of our preoccupation with food and our tendency to eat too much of certain foods and too little of others stems from our eating habits in early childhood (to age five).

EATING WELL WITH CANADA'S FOOD GUIDE

In July 1942, the Official Food Rules, Canada's first food guide, was introduced (Health Canada, n.d.a). The main objectives of the Official Food Rules were to promote healthy eating, prevent nutritional deficiencies, and improve the health of Canadians while recognizing the impact of wartime food rationing. Although the Food Guide has been transformed many times, it has never wavered from its original purpose of guiding food selection and promoting the health of Canadians. In addition to new looks and formats, the title of Canada's Food Guide has changed over time: from Canada's Official Food Rules (1942), to Canada's Food Rules (1944, 1949), to Canada's Food Guide (1961, 1977, 1982), to Canada's Food Guide to Healthy Eating (1992), and most recently to Eating Well with Canada's

Nutrition The science that investigates the relationship between physiological function and the essential elements of foods we eat.

Nutrients The constituents of food that sustain us physiologically: water, proteins, carbohydrates, fats, vitamins, and minerals.

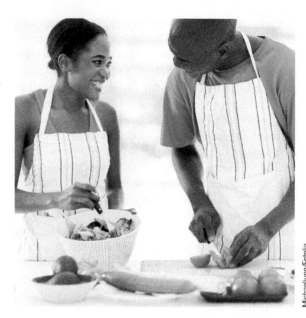

It takes knowledge, resources, and planning to make healthy food choices, whether eating out, choosing food in the dining hall, or cooking meals at home.

Food Guide (2011). In addition, Health Canada also created Eating Well with Canada's Food Guide-First Nations, Inuit and Metis, which is available in several Indigenous languages (Figure 5.1).

The newest version of the Food Guide is intended to help a broader age range of Canadians, since it can be applied to anyone two years of age and older. Specifically, the objectives of the new Food Guide are to:

- describe a pattern of eating sufficient to meet nutrient needs,
- describe a pattern of eating that reduces risk of nutrition-related health problems,
- describe a pattern of eating that supports the achievement and maintenance of a healthy body weight,
- describe a pattern of eating that reflects the diversity of foods available to Canadians,
- support Canadians' awareness and understanding of what constitutes a pattern of healthy eating, and
- emphasize that healthy eating and regular physical activity are important for health (Health Canada, n.d.b).

Figure 5.1 shows Eating Well with Canada's Food Guide (2011). Examples of one serving from each of the major food groups are also depicted.

Daily recommended serving sizes from each food group are depicted by sex in Figure 5.2. The Food Guide is a specific recommendation to include a small amount of unsaturated fat each day (that is, 30 to 45 millilitres or 2 to 3 tablespoons.). The Food Guide continues to advocate for variety, balance, and moderation in your food intake. It is recommended that you eat as many different foods

FIGURE 5.1

Eating Well with Canada's Food Guide

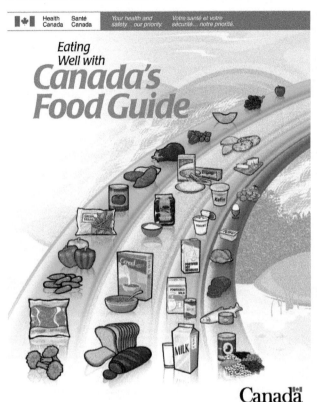

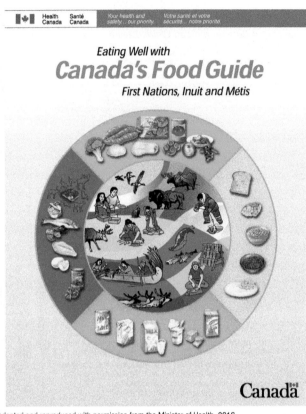

from each food group as possible to obtain variety. Generally, focusing on lots of "colour" on your plate helps to achieve variety in your food consumption. In terms of balance, it is recommended that you obtain the minimum number of servings from each food group *before* eating "extras" or "others" (that is, foods that do not fit into a specific food group, such as chips, soft drinks, chocolate bars, cookies, candies, and so on). Finally, moderation refers to total calorie consumption as well as consumption of individual foods. In other words, moderate consumption meets your caloric needs and does not involve excessive consumption, nor does it involve an excessive consumption of one particular food (that is, a whole box of crackers or pint of ice cream). It also should be emphasized that in eating healthily, all foods fit. In other words, all foods can be part of healthy eating; some, like "extras" or "others," we simply need to eat less of.

THE DIGESTIVE PROCESS

Food provides the chemicals we need for physical activity and body maintenance. Because our bodies cannot synthesize or produce certain essential nutrients, we must get them from the foods we eat. Nutrients are the elements of food that physiologically sustain us, and, as mentioned, these include water, protein, carbohydrates, fats, vitamins, and minerals. Before foods can be utilized, the digestive system must break them down into smaller, more usable forms. The process by which foods are broken down and absorbed or excreted by the body is known as the **digestive process**.

Even before you take your first bite, your body has already begun a series of complex digestive responses. Your mouth prepares for the food by increasing saliva production. **Saliva** contains mostly water, which aids in chewing and swallowing, but it also contains important enzymes that begin the process of food breakdown. One such enzyme, amylase, initiates the digestive process for carbohydrates. From your mouth, food passes down your **esophagus**, a 23- to 25-centimetre tube that connects the mouth to the stomach. A series of contractions and relaxations by the muscles lining your esophagus gently moves food to the next

Digestive process The process by which foods are broken down and absorbed or excreted by the body.

Saliva Fluid secreted by the salivary glands that contains enzymes that assist in the digestion of some foods.

Esophagus Tube that transports food from the mouth to the stomach.

FIGURE 5.2
Daily Recommended Food Guide Servings

Recommended Number of Food Guide Servings per Day

Age in Years	Children			Teens		Adults			
	2-3	4-8	9-13	14-18		19-50		51+	
Sex	Girls and Boys			Females	Males	Females	Males	Females	Males
Vegetables and Fruit	4	5	6	7	8	7-8	8-10	7	7
Grain Products	3	4	6	6	7	6-7	8	6	7
Milk and Alternatives	2	2	3-4	3-4	3-4	2	2	3	3
Meat and Alternatives	1	1	1-2	2	3	2	3	2	3

The chart above shows how many Food Guide Servings you need from each of the four food groups every day.

Having the amount and type of food recommended and following the tips in *Canada's Food Guide* will help:

- Meet your needs for vitamins, minerals and other nutrients.
- Reduce your risk of obesity, type 2 diabetes, heart disease, certain types of cancer and osteoporosis.
- Contribute to your overall health and vitality.

Make each Food Guide Serving count...
Wherever you are – at home, at school, at work or when eating out!

▶ **Eat at least one dark green and one orange vegetable each day.**
Go for dark green vegetables such as broccoli, romaine lettuce and spinach.
Go for orange vegetables such as carrots, sweet potatoes and winter squash.
▶ **Choose vegetables and fruit prepared with little or no added fat, sugar or salt.**
Enjoy vegetables steamed, baked or stir-fried instead of deep-fried.
▶ **Have vegetables and fruit more often than juice.**

▶ **Make at least half of your grain products whole grain each day.**
Eat a variety of whole grains such as barley, brown rice, oats, quinoa and wild rice.
Enjoy whole grain breads, oatmeal or whole wheat pasta.
▶ **Choose grain products that are lower in fat, sugar or salt.**
Compare the Nutrition Facts table on labels to make wise choices.
Enjoy the true taste of grain products. When adding sauces or spreads, use small amounts.

▶ **Drink skim, 1%, or 2% milk each day.**
Have 500 mL (2 cups) of milk every day for adequate vitamin D.
Drink fortified soy beverages if you do not drink milk.
▶ **Select lower fat milk alternatives.**
Compare the Nutrition Facts table on yogurts or cheeses to make wise choices.

▶ **Have meat alternatives such as beans, lentils and tofu often.**
▶ **Eat at least two Food Guide Servings of fish each week.***
Choose fish such as char, herring, mackerel, salmon, sardines and trout.
▶ **Select lean meat and alternatives prepared with little or no added fat or salt.**
Trim the visible fat from meats. Remove the skin on poultry.
Use cooking methods such as roasting, baking or poaching that require little or no added fat.
If you eat luncheon meats, sausages or prepackaged meats, choose those lower in salt (sodium) and fat.

Enjoy a variety of foods from the four food groups.

Satisfy your thirst with water!
Drink water regularly. It's a calorie-free way to quench your thirst. Drink more water in hot weather or when you are very active.

*Health Canada provides advice for limiting exposure to mercury from certain types of fish. Refer to www.healthcanada.gc.ca for the latest information.

What is One Food Guide Serving?
Look at the examples below.

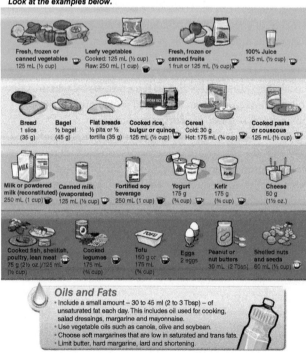

digestive organ, the **stomach**. Here, food mixes with enzymes and stomach acids. Hydrochloric acid works in combination with pepsin, another enzyme, to break down proteins. In most people, the stomach secretes enough mucus to protect the stomach lining from these harsh digestive juices. In others, there are problems with the lining that result in ulcers or other gastric problems.

Further digestive activity takes place in your **small intestine**, an 8-metre-long coiled tube containing three sections: the duodenum, the jejunum, and the ileum. Each section secretes digestive enzymes that, when combined with enzymes from the liver and the pancreas, contribute to the breakdown of proteins, fats, and carbohydrates. Once broken down, these nutrients are absorbed into the bloodstream and supply body cells with energy. The liver is the major organ that determines whether nutrients are stored, sent to cells or organs, or excreted. Solid wastes consisting of fibre, water, and salts are dumped into the large intestine, where most of the water and salts are reabsorbed into the system and the fibre is passed out through the anus. The entire digestive process takes approximately 24 hours (see Figure 5.3).

Stomach Large muscular organ that temporarily stores, mixes, and digests foods.

Small intestine Muscular, coiled digestive organ; 8 metres in length, consists of the duodenum, jejunum, and ileum.

FIGURE 5.3
The Digestive Process

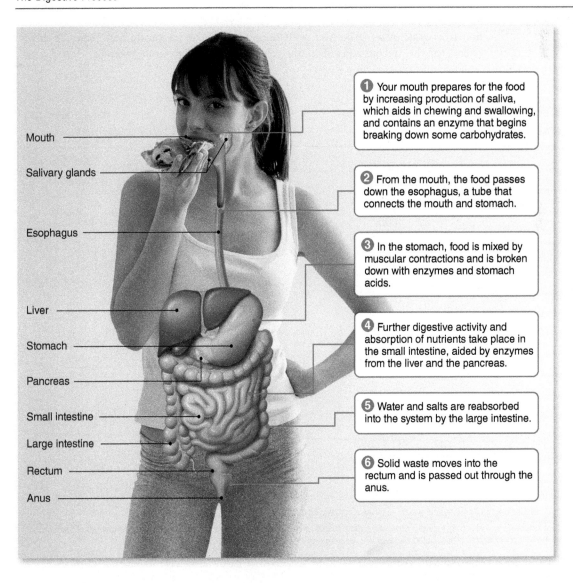

Mouth

Salivary glands

Esophagus

Liver

Stomach

Pancreas

Small intestine

Large intestine

Rectum

Anus

1 Your mouth prepares for the food by increasing production of saliva, which aids in chewing and swallowing, and contains an enzyme that begins breaking down some carbohydrates.

2 From the mouth, the food passes down the esophagus, a tube that connects the mouth and stomach.

3 In the stomach, food is mixed by muscular contractions and is broken down with enzymes and stomach acids.

4 Further digestive activity and absorption of nutrients take place in the small intestine, aided by enzymes from the liver and the pancreas.

5 Water and salts are reabsorbed into the system by the large intestine.

6 Solid waste moves into the rectum and is passed out through the anus.

Dietary Reference Intake vs. Recommended Nutrient Intake

Scientists in Canada and the United States collaborated to develop new, common recommendations for nutrient intake. Canada previously used Recommended Nutrient Intake (RNI) while the United States utilized the Recommended Dietary Allowance (RDA), with slight variations between the two. These new recommendations, called Dietary Reference Intakes (DRIs), are based on the amount of water, proteins, carbohydrates, fats, vitamins, and minerals we need to avoid deficiencies and reduce risk for chronic diseases while attempting to avoid overconsumption (Thompson, Manore, & Sheeska, 2007). The RDA is now a reference standard within the DRIs and represents the average nutrient intake that meets the requirements of 97 to 98 percent of healthy males and females at a particular age (Thompson, Manore, & Sheeska, 2007). Another term to become familiar with in regard to nutrient consumption is *adequate intake* (AI). AI refers to the recommended average daily nutrient intake based on observed or experimentally determined estimates of nutrient intake for a group of healthy people (Thompson, Manore, & Sheeska, 2007). These estimates are used when an RDA cannot be established and are assumed to be adequate.

Calorie A unit of measure that indicates the amount of energy obtained from a particular food.

OBTAINING ESSENTIAL NUTRIENTS

Calorie

A kilocalorie is a unit of measure used to quantify the amount of energy in food. On nutrition labels and in consumer publications, the term is shortened to **calorie**. Energy is defined as the capacity to do work. We derive energy from the energy-containing nutrients in the foods we eat. These energy-containing nutrients— proteins, carbohydrates, and fats—provide calories. Vitamins, minerals, and water do not. Table 5.1 shows the caloric needs for various individuals.

TABLE 5.1

Estimated Daily Calorie Needs

	Calorie Range	
	Sedentary*	Active†
Children		
2–3 years old	1000	1400
Females		
4–8 years old	1200	1800
9–16	1400	2200
14–18	1800	2400
19–30	1800	2400
31–50	1800	2200
51+	1600	2200
Males		
4–8 years old	1200	2000
9–16	1600	2600
14–18	2000	3200
19–30	2400	3000
31–50	2200	3000
51+	2000	2800

*A lifestyle that includes only the light physical activity associated with typical day-to-day life.

†A lifestyle that includes physical activity equivalent to walking more than 5 kilometres (3 miles) per day at 5 to 6 kilometres (3 to 4 miles) per hour, in addition to the light physical activity associated with typical day-to-day life.

Source: U.S. Department of Agriculture and U.S. Department of Health and Human Services, *Dietary Guidelines for Americans, 2010*, 7th ed. (Washington, DC: U.S. Government Printing Office).

Water

Most of us are aware that we could survive much longer without food than without water. Even in severe conditions, the average person can go for weeks without certain vitamins and minerals before experiencing serious deficiency symptoms. However, **dehydration** (abnormal depletion of body fluids) can cause serious health-related issues within hours, and death after a few days.

Between 50 and 60 percent of our total body weight is water. The water in our system bathes cells, aids in fluid and electrolyte balance, maintains pH balance, and transports molecules and cells throughout the body. Water is the major component of blood, which carries oxygen and nutrients to the tissues and is responsible for maintaining cells in working order.

The Dietitians of Canada (2013) suggest approximately 12 cups of beverages for men and 9 for women each day. More specifically, the DRI for men between the ages of 19 and 50 years is 3.7 litres of total water per day (includes 3.0 litres of beverages), while the recommendation for women (ages 19 to 50 years) is 2.7 litres (includes 2.2 litres of beverages). Individual needs vary according to dietary factors, age, size, environmental temperature and humidity levels, physical activity, and the effectiveness of the individual's system. It is not unusual for athletes to lose one to two litres of fluid per hour in hot, humid weather when exercising. To maintain hydration levels, athletes should weigh themselves before and after their workouts and drink one litre of fluid for every kilogram of weight lost. There is considerable variation between and within athletes regarding water and salt losses and thus, individual prescription is required and athletes should take personal responsibility for their hydration needs (Maughan & Shirreffs, 2010). Thirst is not a good indicator of your need for fluids. In fact, if you wait until you are thirsty to replenish your fluids, you have waited too long. The best method of ensuring that your body is adequately hydrated is to monitor the colour of your urine. If it is a pale yellow, your body is sufficiently hydrated; if it is a darker yellow, your body needs fluids.

Are sports drinks necessary? Not likely as often as they are consumed. Most sport drinks are absorbed as effectively as water, and some are absorbed better than juice. In terms of hydration, it is important to note that people are likely to drink more fluid when it is flavoured. The intent of sport drinks is to replenish electrolytes lost through perspiration. They are also used to replenish glycogen or energy stores. Thus, when your perspiration is profuse for 60 minutes or longer, a sports drink may be necessary. However, for physical activity of shorter duration or that is not accompanied by heavy sweating, a sports drink is not needed; water can adequately meet your needs.

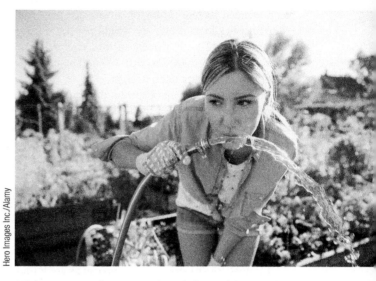

Hero Images Inc./Alamy

While you may not be conscious of your body's need for water, it is actually the most necessary nutrient.

Milk also has the potential to hydrate the body and replenish nutrients following exercise or sport training (Laidlaw, 2007). Milk is a liquid that not only hydrates but also is a rich source of carbohydrates for energy as well as a rich source of protein, which is vital for muscle repair. Milk also contains the electrolytes sodium and potassium, which are involved in the body's hydration process—and with which sports drinks are often fortified.

Proteins

Next to water, proteins are the most abundant substances in the human body. **Proteins** are major components of nearly every cell and are often referred to as "building blocks" because of their role in the development and repair of bone, muscle, skin, and blood cells. Proteins are also the key elements of the antibodies that protect us from disease, of enzymes that control chemical activities in the body, and of hormones that regulate bodily functions. Moreover, proteins aid in the transport of iron, oxygen, and nutrients to the body's cells. Finally, proteins are also involved in fluid, electrolyte, and acid–base balance (pH). Normally, proteins are not a source of energy, but can be broken down to supply energy if carbohydrates and fat are not available. Proteins provide 4 calories of energy per gram of intake.

Most Canadians consume more protein than needed. In particular, they consume too much protein in the form of meat and high-fat dairy products, which are associated with higher blood cholesterol levels (Thompson, Manore, & Sheeska, 2007). The

Dehydration Abnormal depletion of body fluids.

Proteins An essential constituent of nearly all body cells, necessary for the development and repair of bone, muscle, skin, and blood, and key elements of antibodies, enzymes, and hormones.

recommended protein intake for the average person is 0.8 gram per kilogram of body weight per day, equivalent to about 12 to 20 percent of total energy intake (Thompson, Manore, & Sheeska, 2007). The excess is stored, like other extra calories, as fat.

Proteins are made up of smaller molecules known as **amino acids**. Amino acids are composed of chains that link together like beads on a necklace in differing combinations. More than 22 amino acids are found in animal tissue, and humans cannot synthesize all of them. The nine amino acids that the adult body cannot make adequately are referred to as **essential amino acids** (Aristoy & Toldra, 2012). These are histidine, isoleucine, lysine, methionine, phenylalanine, threonine, tryptophan, leucine, and valine (Aristoy & Toldra, 2012). They must be obtained from the foods we eat.

Complete (high-quality) proteins are found in foods that naturally contain the nine essential amino acids together. If we consume a food deficient in an essential amino acid, the total amount of protein that can be synthesized by the other amino acids is limited by the missing amino acid(s). It is important to remember that the fact that essential amino acids are present in a food does not guarantee that they will be synthesized. The quality of protein depends on the presence of amino acids in digestible form and in amounts proportional to body requirements.

The most common sources of dietary protein in Canada are meats, poultry, seafood, dairy products, eggs, soy products, legumes, whole grains, and nuts. In addition to providing high-quality proteins, some of these foods (that is, meats, poultry, high-fat dairy products, and eggs) also contain high levels of saturated fat. Selecting leaner cuts of meat, removing the fat and skin from poultry, and choosing low-fat dairy products will enable you to get high-quality proteins with less fat.

Proteins from most plant sources are **incomplete proteins** in that they are missing one or two essential amino acids. It is relatively easy for the non–meat eater to combine plant foods effectively and eat complementary sources of plant protein. An excellent example is eating peanut butter on whole-grain bread. Although separately peanut butter and whole wheat bread are deficient in essential amino acids, eating them together provides high-quality protein because all amino acids are eaten at the same time.

As illustrated in Figure 5.4, plant sources of protein fall into four general categories: legumes (beans, peas, peanuts, and soy products), grains (whole grains,

---

Amino acids The building blocks of protein.

Essential amino acids Nine of the basic nitrogen-containing building blocks of protein that the body cannot produce.

Complete (high-quality) proteins Proteins that contain all nine essential amino acids.

Incomplete proteins Proteins lacking in one or more essential amino acids.

Carbohydrates Basic nutrients that supply the body with energy (4 kcal/gram).

FIGURE 5.4
Complementary Proteins

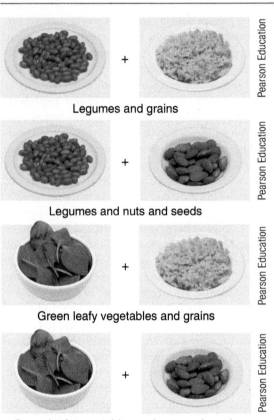

Legumes and grains

Legumes and nuts and seeds

Green leafy vegetables and grains

Green leafy vegetables and nuts and seeds

Pearson Education

corn, and pasta products), nuts and seeds, and other vegetables, such as leafy greens and broccoli. Mixing two or more foods from each of these categories at the same meal provides all the essential amino acids necessary to ensure adequate protein absorption. People not interested in obtaining all their protein from plants can combine incomplete plant proteins with complete low-fat animal proteins such as poultry, seafood, and lean cuts of pork or beef. Further, low-fat cottage cheese, skim milk, egg whites, and nonfat dry milk provide high-quality proteins, few calories, and little dietary fat.

CARBOHYDRATES

Carbohydrates upply us with the energy we need to sustain normal daily activity. In comparison to proteins or fats, carbohydrates are broken down more quickly and efficiently, yielding a fuel called glucose. All body cells can burn glucose for fuel; moreover, glucose is the only fuel that red blood cells can use and is the primary fuel for the brain. Carbohydrates are the best fuel for moderate to intense exercise because they can be readily broken down to glucose even when we're breathing hard and our muscle cells are getting less oxygen.

Like proteins, carbohydrates provide 4 calories per gram. The RDA for adults is 130 grams of carbohydrate per day (Institute of Medicine of the National Academies, 2005). There are two major types: simple and complex.

Simple Carbohydrates

Simple carbohydrates or simple sugars are found naturally in fruits, many vegetables, and dairy. The most common form of simple carbohydrates is glucose. Fruits and berries contain fructose (commonly called fruit sugar). Glucose and fructose are **monosaccharides**. Eventually, the human body converts all types of simple sugars to glucose to provide energy to cells.

Disaccharides are combinations of two monosaccharides. Perhaps the best known example is sucrose (granulated table sugar). Lactose (milk sugar), found in milk and milk products, and maltose (malt sugar) are other examples of common disaccharides. Disaccharides must be broken down into monosaccharides before the body can use them. Sugar is found in high amounts in a wide range of processed food products. A classic example is the amount of sugar in one can of pop: more than 49 millilitres (10 teaspoons) per can! Moreover, such diverse items as ketchup, barbecue sauce, and flavoured coffee creamers derive 30 to 65 percent of their calories from sugar. Read food labels carefully before purchasing. If sugar or one of its aliases (including high fructose corn syrup and cornstarch) appears near the top of the ingredients list, then that product contains a lot of sugar and is probably not your best nutritional bet. Also, most labels list the amount of sugar as a percentage of total calories.

Complex Carbohydrates: Starches and Glycogen

Complex carbohydrates are found in grains, cereals, legumes, and other vegetables. Also called **polysaccharides**, they are formed by long chains of monosaccharides. Like disaccharides, they must be broken down into simple sugars before the body can use them. **Starches**, glycogen, and fibre are the main types of complex carbohydrates. Starches make up the majority of the complex carbohydrate group and come from flours, breads, pasta, rice, corn, oats, barley, potatoes, and related foods. The body breaks down these complex carbohydrates into glucose, which can be easily absorbed by cells and used as energy or stored in the muscles and the liver as **glycogen**. When the body requires a sudden burst of energy, it breaks down glycogen into glucose.

Complex Carbohydrates: Fibre

Fibre, sometimes referred to as "bulk" or "roughage," is the indigestible portion of plant foods that helps move foods through the digestive system, delays absorption of cholesterol and other nutrients, and softens stools by absorbing water. Dietary fibre is found only in plant foods, such as fruits, vegetables, nuts, and grains (Institute of Medicine of the National Academies, 2005).

Fibre is either *soluble* or *insoluble*. Soluble fibres, such as pectins, gums, and mucilages, dissolve in water, form gel-like substances, and can be digested easily by bacteria in the colon. Major food sources of soluble fibre include citrus fruits, berries, oat bran, dried beans, and some vegetables. Insoluble fibres, such as lignins and cellulose, typically do not dissolve in water and cannot be fermented by bacteria in the colon. They are found in most fruits and vegetables and in **whole grains**, such as brown rice, wheat, bran, and whole-grain breads and cereals. The AMDR (Acceptable Macronutrient Distribution Range: these come from Health Canada and are related to the Dietary Reference Intakes) for carbohydrates is 45 to 60 percent of total calories, and health experts recommend that the majority of this intake be fibre-rich carbohydrates.

The best way to increase your intake of dietary fibre is to eat more complex carbohydrates, such as whole grains, fruits, vegetables, dried peas and beans, nuts, and seeds. A few years ago, fibre was thought to be the remedy for just about everything. It is believed that a dietary intake high in fibre provides the following:

- protection against colorectal cancer
- protection against breast cancer
- protection against constipation
- protection against diverticulosis
- protection against heart disease
- protection against diabetes
- enhanced weight control

The AI for fibre is 25 grams per day for women and 38 grams per day for men—or

---

Simple carbohydrates Found primarily in fruits; are quickly digested.

Monosaccharide A simple carbohydrate that contains only one molecule of sugar.

Disaccharide A combination of two monosaccharides.

Complex carbohydrates Found in grains, cereals, and vegetables; require more time to be digested.

Polysaccharide A complex carbohydrate formed by the combination of long chains of saccharides.

Starches are a carbohydrate that provides your body with energy and is found in foods such as grain, rice, and potatoes.

Glycogen The polysaccharide form in which glucose is stored in the liver.

Fibre Refers to the nondigestible part of plants.

Whole grains Unprocessed and contain all three parts of a grain, including the germ, endosperm, and bran.

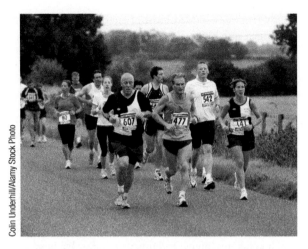

Carbo-loading before an endurance event is a strategy used by many athletes to build energy reserves for the last few kilometres.

an amount equivalent to 14 grams of fibre for every 1000 calories consumed (Thompson, Manore, & Sheeska, 2007). Most Canadians do not eat sufficient fibre; thus, to increase your dietary intake of fibre, the following steps are recommended:

- Select breads and cereals made with whole grains such as wheat, oats, barley, and rye.

- Choose foods with at least two to three grams of fibre per serving.

- Choose fresh fruits and vegetables whenever possible. When appropriate, eat the peel or skin of fresh fruits and vegetables (potatoes, pears, apples, mangoes, kiwi fruit, and so on).

- Eat legumes frequently—every day, if possible.

- Drink plenty of fluids.

Fats

Fats (or lipids), another basic nutrient, are perhaps the most misunderstood of the body's required energy sources. Fat is a source of essential fatty acids (omega-3 and omega-6) and plays a vital role in the maintenance of healthy skin and hair, insulation of the body organs against shock, maintenance of body temperature, and the proper functioning of the cells themselves. Fats help our food taste better, provide texture to food, and carry the fat-soluble vitamins A, D, E, and K to the cells. They also provide a concentrated form of energy at nine calories per gram. Despite all the essential roles fat has in our bodies, we are still recommended to limit our dietary intake to less than 30 percent of our total calories.

Although a moderate consumption of fats is essential to health, overconsumption can be dangerous. The most common form of fat circulating in the blood is **triglyceride**, which makes up about 95 percent of total body fat. When we consume too many calories, the excess is converted into triglycerides in the liver, which are stored in obvious places on our bodies. The remaining 5 percent of body fat is composed of substances such as **cholesterol**, which can accumulate on the inner walls of arteries, causing a narrowing of the channel through which blood flows. This buildup, "plaque," is a major cause of arteriosclerosis (discussed in detail in Chapter 12).

Fat cells consist of chains of carbon and hydrogen atoms. Those not able to hold any more hydrogen in their chemical structure are labelled **saturated fats**. These generally come from animal sources, such as meats and dairy products, and are solid at room temperature. **Unsaturated fats**, which come from plants and most vegetable oils, are generally liquid at room temperature and have room for additional hydrogen atoms in their chemical structure. The terms *monounsaturated fat* and *polyunsaturated fat* refer to the relative number of hydrogen atoms missing. Peanut and olive oils are high in monounsaturated fats, whereas corn, sunflower, and safflower oils are high in polyunsaturated fats.

Healthier fats contain polyunsaturated and monounsaturated fatty acids (found in vegetable oils—canola, soybean, olive—soft non-hydrogenated margarines, nuts, seeds, avocados, olives, and fatty fish (Conrad, n.b.); we should include approximately 45 millilitres (2–3 tablespoons) of these fats in our daily dietary intake (Health Canada, n.d.b). Part of our fat intake should include omega-3 and omega-6, which are polyunsaturated fatty acids. Canadians typically ingest sufficient omega-6 fats in the form of polyunsaturated margarines and sunflower, corn, and sesame oil. However, our intake of omega-3 fatty acids tends to be low. As such, we need to increase our intake of fish, flaxseed, walnuts, canola, and soybean oil (Conrad, n.d.). It should be pointed out that the omega-3 fatty acids found in fish are more readily used by the body than those found in plants.

Another group of fats we need to be aware of are **trans fatty acids** or trans fats. Trans fats are fatty acids produced by adding hydrogen molecules to liquid oil to make the oil solid. Unlike regular fats and oils, these "partially hydrogenated" fats stay solid or semisolid at room temperature. They change into irregular shapes at the molecular level, priming them to clog arteries.

Fats Basic nutrients that provide taste and texture to food, absorb vitamins A, D, E, and K, and are needed for the proper functioning of cells, insulation of body organs against shock, maintenance of body temperature, and healthy skin and hair.

Triglyceride The most common form of fat in the body.

Cholesterol A form of fat circulating in the blood that can accumulate on the inner walls of arteries.

Saturated fats Fats that are unable to hold any more hydrogen in their chemical structure; derived mostly from animal sources; solid at room temperature.

Unsaturated fats Fats that have room for more hydrogen in their chemical structure; derived mostly from plants; liquid at room temperature.

Trans fatty acids Fatty acids produced when polyunsaturated oils are hydrogenated to make them more solid.

Colin Underhill/Alamy Stock Photo

Trans fats are used in margarines, commercially baked goods, and many restaurant deep fryers. Trans fats are more harmful than saturated fats because they increase LDL levels and decrease HDL levels in the bloodstream (Mah, n.d.). In other words, they increase our "bad" cholesterol and decrease our "good" cholesterol. Canada was the first country in the world to include trans fat on food labels; starting in December 2005, all prepackaged food sold in Canada had to include the trans fat content. In regard to food labelling, "trans fat free" or "0 trans fat" can be used only if the stated serving amount contains less than 0.2 grams of trans fats or if the total amount of saturated and trans fat in a stated serving is 2 grams or less (Mah, n.d.). In 2007, the Canadian Federal Government established two key recommendations in regards to the use of trans fats: (1) limit the trans fat content of vegetable oils and soft, spreadable margarines to 2% of the total fat content; and (2) limit the trans fat content for all other foods to 5% of the total fat content, including ingredients sold to restaurants (Health Canada, 2015). On November 7, 2013, the Food and Drug Administration of the United States announced that they were phasing out the use of artificially created trans fats (RT Question More, 2013).

Reducing Fat in Your Diet

Finding the best ways to reduce fat in your dietary intake is largely dependent on you determining what does and does not work for you and your lifestyle. The following basic guidelines are a place to start:

- Know what you are putting in your mouth. Read food labels. No more than 10 percent of your total calories should come from saturated and/or trans fat, and no more than 30 percent should come from all forms of fat combined.

- Choose fat-free or low-fat versions of foods whenever possible. Do not eat more of these because they are fat-free or low-fat than you would the full-fat versions.

- Use olive oil for baking, stir frying, and sautéing.

- Whenever possible, use liquid, diet, or whipped margarine: these forms have less trans fat than solid fat.

- Choose lean meats, seafood, or poultry. Remove skin and visible fat. Broil or bake whenever possible. In general, the more well-done the meat, the fewer the calories from fat. Drain fat after cooking.

- Limit intake of cold cuts, bacon, sausage, hot dogs, and organ meats.

- Select nonfat or low-fat dairy products whenever possible.

- When cooking, substitute chicken broth, wine, vinegar, low-fat/no-fat dressings and low-fat/no-fat sour cream for butter, margarine, oils, regular fat sour cream, mayonnaise, and salad dressings.

- Remember to think of your food intake as an average over a day or several days. If you have a high-fat breakfast or lunch, have a low-fat dinner to balance it out.

- The small choices you make daily add up to make a tremendous difference in the amount of fat you eat over time. Trimming just 5 millilitres (1 teaspoon) of fat each day can cut more than 2 kilogram from your dietary intake in one year—without removing great-tasting foods or causing noticeable changes. Consider the following:

1. "Butter" your toast, muffins, or bagels with "fruit-only" jams instead of butter, margarine, cream cheese, or other high-fat spreads.
   - 15 mL butter or margarine — 108 calories — 12 g fat
   - 15 mL sugarless jam — 8 calories — 0 g fat

2. Sauté or stir fry meat and vegetables in chicken broth or wine (most of which burns off during cooking) rather than oil.
   - 15 mL oil — 240 calories — 27 g fat
   - wine or broth — 0 calories — 0 g fat

3. Remove the skin from chicken before cooking.
   - 100 g breast — 193 calories — 8 g fat
   - 100 g skinless breast — 142 calories — 3 g fat

4. Use low-fat or no-fat salad dressings on your sandwiches and salads.
   - 15 mL mayonnaise — 100 calories — 11 g fat
   - 15 mL low-fat dressing — 7 calories — 0 g fat

5. Choose nonfat frozen yogurt instead of ice cream.
   - 125 mL ice cream — 400 calories — 25 g fat
   - 125 mL nonfat yogurt — 120 calories — 0 g fat

6. Mix in a blender three parts low-fat cottage cheese with one part nonfat yogurt and use as a 'mock' cream cheese dip, spread, or topping.
   - 30 mL cream cheese — 99 calories — 10 g fat
   - 30 mL mock cream cheese — 20 calories — 0 g fat

7. Eat broth-based rather than cream-based soups.

- 250 mL cream of chicken soup   191 calories   15 g fat
- 250 mL chicken noodle soup   75 calories   2 g fat

8. Eat seafood at least twice per week.

- 85 g top round beef   162 calories   5 g fat
- 100 g skinless chicken breast   142 calories   3 g fat
- 85 g cod   70 calories   0.5 g fat

9. Substitute two egg whites for one whole egg in recipes or omelettes.

- 1 whole egg   79 calories   6 g fat
- 2 egg whites   32 calories   0 g fat

10. Choose meatless entrées such as lentil soup or vegetarian chili.

- 270 g beef chili   256 calories   6 g fat
- 270 g lentil soup   164 calories   1 g fat

(*Healthy Homestyle Cookings* by Evelyn Tribole, MS, RD Rodale Press, 1994. Reprinted with permission.)

Vitamins

Although they do not provide energy (that is, calories), **vitamins** are potent, essential, organic compounds that promote growth and help maintain life and health. Every minute of every day, vitamins help maintain your nerves and skin, produce blood cells, build bones and teeth, heal wounds, and convert food energy to body energy.

Age, heat, and other environmental conditions can destroy vitamins in food. Vitamins are classified as either fat-soluble, meaning that they are absorbed through the intestinal tract with the help of fats, or water-soluble, meaning that they are easily dissolved in water. Vitamins A, D, E, and K are fat-soluble; B-complex vitamins and vitamin C are water-soluble. Fat-soluble vitamins tend to be stored in the body, and toxicity can occur if too much is consumed. Water-soluble vitamins are generally excreted and cause few toxicity problems. Tables 5.2 and 5.3 provide a list of water-soluble and fat-soluble vitamins, the recommended dietary intake, best sources, and major functions in the body, as well as the symptoms of deficiency and toxicity.

Vitamins Essential organic compounds that promote growth and reproduction and maintain life and health.

Functional foods Foods believed to have specific health benefits and/or to prevent disease.

Antioxidants Substances believed to protect against tissue damage at the cellular level.

Few Canadians suffer from vitamin deficiencies, particularly if they consume the recommended number of servings from each of the food groups most days of the week. Further, you can assume you are obtaining the DRIs for each vitamin (and mineral) if your dietary intake follows the principles of variety (lots of colour too), balance, and moderation.

Nevertheless, Canadians continue to purchase and consume large quantities of vitamin supplements. For the most part, vitamin supplements are unnecessary and in certain instances may even be harmful.

Antioxidants

Beneficial foods termed **functional foods** are based on the ancient belief that eating the right foods may not only prevent disease, but also cure some diseases. Some of the most popular functional foods today are items containing **antioxidants** or other *phytochemicals* (from the Greek word meaning *plant*). Among the more commonly cited nutrients touted as providing a protective antioxidant effect are vitamin C, vitamin E, and beta-carotene, a precursor to vitamin A. It is believed these substances may protect people from damage caused by *free radicals*. Free radicals are unstable molecules formed during metabolism that can damage or kill healthy cells, cell proteins, or DNA. Free radical formation is a natural process that cannot be avoided; antioxidants can neutralize free radicals, slow their formation, and may even repair the damage.

Many claims about the benefits of antioxidants in reducing the risk of heart disease, improving vision, and slowing the aging process require more research to provide conclusive recommendations. Two relatively large, longitudinal epidemiological studies provided promising results suggesting that antioxidants in foods, mostly those found in vegetables and fruits, protect against cognitive decline and risk of Parkinson's disease (Bjelakovic et al., 2007; Kang & Grodstein, 2008). Other studies indicate that these vitamins, particularly when taken as supplements, have no effect on atherosclerosis (Clarke et al., 2010; Cook et al., 2007; Siekmeier, Steffen, & Marz, 2007). Controversy exists regarding the benefits of vitamin C as some people who consume diets rich in vitamin C develop fewer cancers, but other studies detect no effect (Albanes, 2009). Other studies report that high-dose vitamin C given intravenously, rather than orally, may be effective in treating cancer and protecting from diseases affecting the central nervous system (Lin et al., 2009).

Possible effects of vitamin E intake are even more controversial. Researchers have theorized that because many cancers result from DNA damage, and because vitamin E appears to protect against DNA damage, vitamin E should reduce cancer risk. The majority of

TABLE 5.2

A Guide to Water-Soluble Vitamins

Vitamin Name and Recommended Intake	Reliable Food Sources	Primary Functions	Toxicity/Deficiency Symptoms
Thiamin (vitamin B_1) RDA: Men = 1.2 mg/day Women = 1.1 mg/day	Pork, fortified cereals, enriched rice and pasta, peas, tuna, legumes	Required as enzyme cofactor for carbohydrate and amino acid metabolism	**Toxicity:** none known **Deficiency:** beriberi, fatigue, apathy, decreased memory, confusion, irritability, muscle weakness
Riboflavin (vitamin B_2) RDA: Men = 1.3 mg/day Women = 1.1 mg/day	Beef liver, shrimp, milk and dairy foods, fortified cereals, enriched breads and grains	Required as enzyme cofactor for carbohydrate and fat metabolism	**Toxicity:** none known **Deficiency:** ariboflavinosis, swollen mouth and throat, seborrheic dermatitis, anemia
Niacin, nicotinamide, nicotinic acid RDA: Men = 16 mg/day Women = 14 mg/day UL = 35 mg/day	Beef liver, most cuts of meat/fish/poultry, fortified cereals, enriched breads and grains, canned tomato products	Required for carbohydrate and fat metabolism; plays role in DNA replication and repair and cell differentiation	**Toxicity:** flushing, liver damage, glucose intolerance, blurred vision differentiation **Deficiency:** pellagra; vomiting, constipation, or diarrhea; apathy
Vitamin B_6 (pyridoxine, pyridoxal, pyridoxamine) RDA: Men and women 19–50 = 1.3 mg/day Men > 50 = 1.7 mg/day Women > 50 = 1.5 mg/day UL = 100 mg/day	Chickpeas (garbanzo beans), most cuts of meat/fish/poultry, fortified cereals, white potatoes	Required as enzyme cofactor for carbohydrate and amino acid metabolism; assists synthesis of blood cells	**Toxicity:** nerve damage, skin lesions **Deficiency:** anemia; seborrheic dermatitis; depression, confusion, and convulsions
Folate (folic acid) RDA: Men = 400 µg/day Women = 400 µg/day UL = 1000 µg/day	Fortified cereals, enriched breads and grains, spinach, legumes (lentils, chickpeas, pinto beans), greens (spinach, romaine lettuce), liver	Required as enzyme cofactor for amino acid metabolism; required for DNA synthesis; involved in metabolism of homocysteine	**Toxicity:** masks symptoms of vitamin B_{12} deficiency, specifically signs of nerve damage **Deficiency:** macrocytic anemia; neural tube defects in a developing fetus; elevated homocysteine levels
Vitamin B_{12} (cobalamin) RDA: Men = 2.4 µg/day Women = 2.4 µg/day	Shellfish, all cuts of meat/fish/poultry, milk and dairy foods, fortified cereals	Assists with formation of blood; required for healthy nervous system function; involved as enzyme cofactor in metabolism of homocysteine	**Toxicity:** none known **Deficiency:** pernicious anemia; tingling and numbness of extremities; nerve damage; memory loss, disorientation, and dementia
Pantothenic acid AI: Men = 5 mg/day Women = 5 mg/day	Meat/fish/poultry, shiitake mushrooms, fortified cereals, egg yolks	Assists with fat metabolism	**Toxicity:** none known **Deficiency:** rare
Biotin RDA: Men = 30 µg/day Women = 30 µg/day	Nuts, egg yolks	Involved as enzyme cofactor in carbohydrate, fat, and protein metabolism	**Toxicity:** none known **Deficiency:** rare
Vitamin C (ascorbic acid) RDA: Men = 90 mg/day Women = 75 mg/day Smokers = 35 mg more per day than RDA UL = 2000 mg	Sweet peppers, citrus fruits and juices, broccoli, strawberries, kiwi	Antioxidant in extracellular fluid and lungs; regenerates oxidized vitamin E; assists with collagen synthesis; enhances immune function; assists in synthesis of hormones, neurotransmitters, and DNA; enhances iron absorption	**Toxicity:** nausea and diarrhea, nosebleeds, increased oxidative damage, increased formation of kidney stones in people with kidney disease **Deficiency:** scurvy, bone pain and fractures, depression, and anemia

Note: RDA = Recommended Dietary Allowance; AI = Adequate Intakes; UL = Tolerable Upper Level Intakes. Values are for all adults aged 19 and older, except as noted. Values increase among women who are pregnant or lactating.

Source: Thompson, Janice J.; Manore, Melinda, *Nutrition: An Applied Approach*, 2nd ed., © 2009. Reprinted and electronically reproduced by permission of Pearson Education, Inc., New York, NY.

TABLE 5.3
A Guide to Fat-Soluble Vitamins

Vitamin Name and Recommended Intake	Reliable Food Sources	Primary Functions	Toxicity/Deficiency Symptoms
Vitamin A (retinol, retinal, retinoic acid) RDA: Men = 900 µg Women = 700 µg UL = 3000 µg/day	Preformed retinol: beef and chicken liver, egg yolks, milk Carotenoid precursors: spinach, carrots, mango, apricots, cantaloupe, pumpkin, yams	Required for ability of eyes to adjust to changes in light; protects colour vision; assists cell differentiation; required for sperm production in men and fertilization in women; contributes to healthy bone and healthy immune system	**Toxicity:** fatigue; bone and joint pain; spontaneous abortion and birth defects of fetuses in pregnant women; nausea and diarrhea; liver damage; nervous system damage; blurred vision; hair loss; skin disorders **Deficiency:** night blindness, xerophthalmia; impaired growth, immunity, and reproductive function
Vitamin D (cholecalciferol) AI (assumes that person does not get adequate sun exposure): Adult 19–70 = 15 µg/day 600 IU/day Adult > 70 = 20 µg/day 800 IU/day UL = 50 µg/day 4000 IU/day	Canned salmon and mackerel, milk, fortified cereals	Regulates blood calcium levels; maintains bone health; assists cell differentiation	**Toxicity:** hypercalcemia **Deficiency:** rickets in children; osteomalacia and/or osteoporosis in adults
Vitamin E (tocopherol) RDA: Men = 15 mg/day Women = 15 mg/day UL = 1000 mg/day	Sunflower seeds, almonds, vegetable oils, fortified cereals	As a powerful antioxidant, protects cell membranes, polyunsaturated fatty acids, and vitamin A from oxidation; protects white blood cells; enhances immune function; improves absorption of vitamin A	**Toxicity:** rare **Deficiency:** hemolytic anemia; impairment of nerve, muscle, and immune function
Vitamin K (phylloquinone, menaquinone, menadione) AI: Men = 120 µg/day Women = 90 µg/day	Kale, spinach, turnip greens, brussels sprouts	Serves as a coenzyme during production of specific proteins that assist in blood coagulation and bone metabolism	**Toxicity:** none known **Deficiency:** impaired blood clotting; possible effect on bone health

Note: RDA = Recommended Dietary Allowance; AI = Adequate Intakes; UL = Tolerable Upper Level Intakes. Values are for all adults aged 19 and older, except as noted. Values increase among women who are pregnant or lactating.

Source: Thompson, Janice J.; Manore, Melinda, *Nutrition: An Applied Approach,* 2nd ed., © 2009. Reprinted and electronically reproduced by permission of Pearson Education, Inc., New York, NY.

studies have demonstrated no effect or, in some cases, a negative effect (Slatore et al., 2008).

Carotenoids are part of the red, orange, and yellow pigments found in vegetables and fruits. Beta-carotene, the most researched carotenoid, is a precursor of vitamin A. This means that vitamin A can be produced in the body from beta-carotene; like vitamin A, beta-carotene has antioxidant properties. Although there are over 600 carotenoids in nature, two that have received a great

deal of attention are *lycopene* (found in tomatoes, papaya, pink grapefruit, and guava) and *lutein* (found in green leafy vegetables such as spinach, broccoli, kale, and brussels sprouts). As such, lycopene may be effective in reducing the risk of cancer. A landmark study assessing the effects of tomato-based foods reported that men who ate 10 or more servings of lycopene-rich foods per week had a 45 percent lower risk of prostate cancer (Haseen et al., 2009). However, subsequent research has questioned the benefits of lycopene, and some professional groups are modifying their endorsements of

Carotenoids Fat-soluble plant pigments with antioxidant properties.

tomato-based products (Boffetta et al., 2010; Jatoi et al., 2007). Lutein is most often touted as a means of protecting the eyes, particularly from age-related macular degeneration, a leading cause of blindness for people aged 65 and older.

Vitamin D

In addition to playing a vital role in bone health for people of all ages, vitamin D may have a positive effect on reducing risk for some types of cancers, in particular colorectal cancer, and other immune-related diseases (Dietitians of Canada News Releases, 2006).

The dietary reference intakes (DRIs) recommend that adults up to the age of 50 obtain 200 IU each day, those between the ages of 51 and 70 require 400 IU per day, and individuals over the age of 71 need 600 IU per day. Further, the Osteoporosis Society of Canada recommends that adults over the age of 50 and at risk for osteoporosis obtain 800 IU of vitamin D or the equivalent of 750 mL of milk (around three glasses) per day.

You normally obtain vitamin D in one of two ways: from the sun via UVB radiation absorbed through your skin, and through your dietary intake, most often from fortified cows' milk. Other dietary sources include fatty fish, such as salmon and sardines, infant formulas, meal replacements, and nutritional supplements.

All Canadians—and anyone else who lives above 37° latitude—may be at risk in the winter months of obtaining insufficient vitamin D when there is insufficient UVB radiation from the sun, partly because of the reduced daylight hours and partly because of the level of the solstice. Other groups particularly at risk include:

- The elderly—because they produce less vitamin D in their bodies as a result of aging. Other contributing factors include an inadequate dietary intake, and limited exposure to the sunlight because the elderly are more likely to be housebound.

- Individuals with dark skin—because the darker one's skin, the lower the production of vitamin D.

- Exclusively breast-fed infants—because the vitamin D content of breast milk is not sufficient.

- Individuals who wear clothing covering the majority of their body when outside—because there is no exposed skin to absorb vitamin D from the sun and its UVB radiation.

- Individuals with low dietary intakes of vitamin D.

Minerals

Minerals are the inorganic, indestructible elements that aid physiological processes in the body. Without minerals, vitamins could not be absorbed. Minerals are readily excreted and usually not toxic. Macrominerals are minerals that the body needs in fairly large amounts: sodium, calcium, phosphorus, magnesium, potassium, sulphur, and chloride. Trace minerals include iron, zinc, manganese, copper, iodine, and cobalt, so-called because only trace amounts of these minerals are needed. Serious problems may result if excesses or deficiencies occur. Specific types of minerals, the recommended dietary intake, best sources, and their major functions in the body, as well as symptoms of deficiency and toxicity, are listed in Tables 5.4 and 5.5. Although minerals are necessary for body function, there are limits to how much of them we should consume.

Sodium

Sodium is necessary for the regulation of blood and body fluids, for the transmission of nerve impulses, for heart activity, for muscle contraction, and for other metabolic functions. Sodium also enhances flavour, balances the bitterness of some foods, acts as a preservative, and tenderizes meat. Although vital to our survival—and to the good taste of food—we tend to consume much more sodium than we need. The AI for sodium is 1500 mg per day for the average adult (Thompson, Manore, & Sheeska, 2007), yet most Canadians consume two to three times this amount with most of their sodium coming from pre-salted processed and restaurant foods (CSPI, 2012). Health Canada (2010) reports that the average Canadian consumes 3400 mg of sodium per day. Further, over 85 percent of men and between 63 and 83 percent of women had sodium intakes exceeding the upper limit (set at 2300 mg/day) (Health Canada, 2010). The most common source of sodium for Canadians is table salt (that is, sodium chloride, which is about 40 percent sodium and 60 percent chloride by weight) (Thompson, Manore, & Sheeska, 2007). The remainder of dietary sodium comes from the water we drink and highly processed foods such as pickles, salty snack foods, processed cheeses, many breads and bakery products, smoked meats and sausages, many fast-food entrées, and soft drinks.

Many experts believe there is a link between excessive sodium intake and hypertension (high pressure). As a result, many organizations recommend that Canadians cut back on sodium consumption to reduce their risk for cardiovascular diseases, debilitating bone fractures, and other health problems (Mah, n.d.).

Calcium

The issue of calcium consumption has gained national attention with the rising incidence

Minerals Inorganic, indestructible elements that aid physiological processes.

TABLE 5.4

A Guide to Major Minerals

Mineral Name and Recommended Intake	Reliable Food Sources	Primary Functions	Toxicity/Deficiency Symptoms
Sodium AI: Adults = 1.5 g/day (1500 mg/day)	Table salt, pickles, most canned soups, snack foods, cured luncheon meats, canned tomato products	Fluid balance; acid–base balance; transmission of nerve impulses; muscle contraction	**Toxicity:** water retention, high blood pressure, loss of calcium **Deficiency:** muscle cramps, dizziness, fatigue, nausea, vomiting, mental confusion
Potassium AI: Adults = 4.7 g/day (4700 mg/day)	Most fresh fruits and vegetables: potato, banana, tomato juice, orange juice, melon	Fluid balance; transmission of nerve impulses; muscle contraction	**Toxicity:** muscle weakness, vomiting, irregular heartbeat **Deficiency:** muscle weakness, paralysis, mental confusion, irregular heartbeat
Phosphorus RDA: Adults = 700 mg/day	Milk/cheese/yogurt, soymilk and tofu, legumes (lentils, black beans, peanuts), nuts (almonds, pecans), poultry	Fluid balance; bone formation; component of ATP, which provides energy for our bodies	**Toxicity:** muscle spasms, convulsions, low blood calcium **Deficiency:** muscle weakness, muscle damage, bone pain, dizziness
Chloride AI: Adults = 2.3 g/day (2300 mg/day)	Table salt	Fluid balance; transmission of nerve impulses; component of stomach acid (HCL); antibacterial	**Toxicity:** none known **Deficiency:** dangerous blood acid–base imbalances, irregular heartbeat
Calcium RDA: Adult males 19–70 = 1000 mg/day Adult females 19–50 = 1000 mg/day Adult females 51–70 = 1200 mg/day Adults > 70 = 1200 mg/day UL = 2500 mg/day for adults 19–50; adults > 50 = 2000 mg/day	Milk/yogurt/cheese (best absorbed form of calcium), sardines, collard greens and spinach, calcium-fortified juices	Primary component of bone; acid–base balance; transmission of nerve impulses; muscle contraction	**Toxicity:** mineral imbalances, shock, kidney failure, fatigue, mental confusion **Deficiency:** osteoporosis, convulsions, heart failure
Magnesium RDA: Men 19–30 = 400 mg/day Men > 30 = 420 mg/day Women 19–30 = 310 mg/day Women > 30 = 320 mg/day UL = 350 mg/day	Greens (spinach, kale, collards), whole grains, seeds, nuts, legumes (navy and black beans)	Component of bone; muscle contraction; assists more than 300 enzyme systems	**Toxicity:** none known **Deficiency:** low blood calcium; muscle spasms or seizures; nausea; weakness; increased risk of chronic diseases such as heart disease, hypertension, osteoporosis, and type 2 diabetes
Sulfur No DRI	Protein-rich foods	Component of certain B vitamins and amino acids; acid–base balance; detoxification in liver	**Toxicity:** none known **Deficiency:** none known

Note: RDA = Recommended Dietary Allowance; AI = Adequate Intakes; UL = Tolerable Upper Level Intake. Values are for all adults aged 19 and older, except as noted.

Source: Thompson, Janice J.; Manore, Melinda, *Nutrition: An Applied Approach*, 2nd ed., © 2009. Reprinted and electronically reproduced by permission of Pearson Education, Inc., New York, NY.

TABLE 5.5

A Guide to Trace Minerals

Mineral Name and Recommended Intake	Reliable Food Sources	Primary Functions	Toxicity/Deficiency Symptoms
Selenium RDA: Adults = 55 µg/day UL = 400 µg/day	Nuts, shellfish, meat/fish/poultry, whole grains	Required for carbohydrate and fat metabolism	**Toxicity:** brittle hair and nails, skin rashes, nausea and vomiting, weakness, liver disease **Deficiency:** specific forms of heart disease and arthritis, impaired immune function, muscle pain and wasting, depression, hostility
Fluoride AI: Men = 4 mg/day Women = 3 mg/day UL = 2.2 mg/day for children 4–8 years; children > 8 years = 10 mg/day	Fluoridated water and other beverages made with this water	Development and maintenance of healthy teeth and bones	**Toxicity:** fluorosis of teeth and bones **Deficiency:** dental caries, low bone density
Iodine RDA: Adults = 150 µg/day UL = 1100 µg/day	Iodized salt and foods processed with iodized salt	Synthesis of thyroid hormones; temperature regulation; reproduction and growth	**Toxicity:** goiter **Deficiency:** goiter, hypothyroidism, cretinism in infant of mother who is iodine deficient
Chromium AI: Men 19–50 = 35 µg/day Men > 50 = 30 µg/day Women 19–50 = 25 µg/day Women > 50 = 20 µg/day	Grains, meat/fish/poultry, some fruits and vegetables	Glucose transport; metabolism of DNA and RNA; immune function and growth	**Toxicity:** none known **Deficiency:** elevated blood glucose and blood lipids, damage to brain and nervous system
Manganese AI: Men = 2.3 mg/day Women = 1.8 mg/day UL = 11 mg/day for adults	Whole grains, nuts, legumes, some fruits and vegetables	Assists many enzyme systems; synthesis of protein found in bone and cartilage	**Toxicity:** impairment of neuromuscular system **Deficiency:** impaired growth and reproductive function, reduced bone density, impaired glucose and lipid metabolism, skin rash
Iron RDA: Men = 8 mg/day Women 19–50 = 18 mg/day Women > 50 = 8 mg/day	Meat/fish/poultry (best absorbed form of iron), fortified cereals, legumes, spinach	Component of hemoglobin in blood cells; component of myoglobin in muscle cells; assists many enzyme systems	**Toxicity:** nausea, vomiting, and diarrhea; dizziness, confusion; rapid heartbeat; organ damage; death **Deficiency:** iron-deficiency microcytic anemia, hypochromic anemia
Zinc RDA: Men 11 mg/day Women = 8 mg/day UL = 40 mg/day	Meat/fish/poultry (best absorbed form of zinc), fortified cereals, legumes	Assists more than 100 enzyme systems; immune system function; growth and sexual maturation; gene regulation	**Toxicity:** nausea, vomiting, and diarrhea; headaches; depressed immune function; reduced absorption of copper **Deficiency:** growth delays, delayed sexual maturation, eye and skin lesions, hair loss, increased incidence of illness and infection
Copper RDA: Adults = 900 µg/day UL = 10 mg/day	Shellfish, organ meats, nuts, legumes	Assists many enzyme systems; iron transport	**Toxicity:** nausea, vomiting, and diarrhea; liver damage **Deficiency:** anemia, reduced levels of white blood cells, osteoporosis in infants and growing children

Note: RDA = Recommended Dietary Allowance; AI = Adequate Intakes; UL = Tolerable Upper Intake Level. Values are for all adults aged 19 and older, except as noted.

Source: Thompson, Janice J.; Manore, Melinda, *Nutrition: An Applied Approach,* 2nd ed., © 2009. Reprinted and electronically reproduced by permission of Pearson Education, Inc., New York, NY.

of osteoporosis (see Chapter 17) among the elderly, particularly among older women. Calcium plays a vital role in building strong bones and teeth, contracting muscles, clotting blood, transmitting nerve impulses, regulating heartbeat, and balancing fluid within cells. Most Canadian adults between ages 19 and 50 years do not consume the recommended 1000 milligrams of calcium per day, with particularly inadequate intakes in older Canadians (50+ years), who are advised to consume 1200 milligrams of calcium per day (Vatanparast, Dolega-Cieszkowski, & Whiting, 2009). Another reason to ensure adequate calcium intake relates to obesity prevention. Research suggests a positive relationship between calcium intake and healthy weight maintenance in that people who consume sufficient calcium are more likely to not be overweight or obese (Tremblay & Chaput, 2008). Another potential related negative trend is the replacement of milk with soft drinks as a choice beverage with or without meals. Soft drinks not only contain a high percentage of free sugars but also do not provide the nutrients found in milk.

Increasing Your Dietary Calcium Intake

Because calcium intake is so important throughout your life, it is critical that you consume the minimum required each day. In most cases, more than half our calcium intake comes from milk, one of the best sources of dietary calcium. Although many green, leafy vegetables are sources of calcium, some contain oxalic acid, which makes their calcium harder to absorb. Broccoli, cauliflower, and many peas (black eyed peas, chick peas, etc.) and beans (pinto beans and soybeans) are good sources of calcium. Many nuts, particularly almonds, Brazil nuts, and hazelnuts, and seeds, such as sunflower and sesame, contain calcium as well. Molasses is a source of calcium, as are canned salmon (if you eat the bones) and sardines. Some fruits—such as citrus, figs, raisins, and dried apricots—have moderate amounts of calcium too.

Of interest to those who drink carbonated soft drinks is that the added phosphoric acid (phosphate) in these drinks can cause you to excrete calcium. Calcium and phosphorus imbalances can lead to kidney stones, hypertension, diabetes, and other calcification problems (Parasuraman & Venkat, 2010).

Vitamin D improves absorption of calcium; thus, exposure to sunlight is like having an extra calcium source. Stress, on the other hand, contributes to calcium depletion. Although calcium supplements are available, the best way to meet your needs is to consume calcium as part of a balanced, varied dietary intake throughout the day in foods containing protein, vitamin D, and vitamin C for optimum absorption.

Anemia Iron-deficiency disease that results from the body's inability to produce hemoglobin.

Iron

Iron deficiency is the most common nutrient deficiency worldwide, affecting more than 2 billion people or about one-third of the population. Although less prevalent an issue in Canada, it is still the most common nutrient deficiency. Females aged 19 to 50 require 18 milligrams of iron per day, and males of all ages about 8 milligrams per day; both should stay below 45 milligrams per day (Dietitians of Canada, 2010). After the age of 50 (postmenopausal for women), women's requirements drop to 8 milligrams of iron per day, and they should continue to not get more than 45 milligrams per day (Dietitians of Canada, 2010). Pregnant women should aim for at least 27 milligrams of iron per day, but, as always, remain below 45 milligrams per day (Dietitians of Canada, 2010). Iron deficiencies can lead to **anemia**, a problem resulting from the body's inability to produce hemoglobin, the bright red, oxygen-carrying component of the blood. When this occurs, body cells receive less oxygen, and carbon dioxide wastes are removed less efficiently, resulting in a person feeling tired and run down. Another problem with iron deficiency is that the immune system becomes less effective, which can lead to increased risk of illness. A less common problem, iron toxicity, is caused by too much iron in the blood. Women are more likely than men to suffer from iron deficiency problems, partly because they typically eat less than men and because of blood loss from menstrual flows.

Sex Differences in Nutritional Needs

Men and women differ in body size, body composition, and overall metabolic rates. These differences result in slightly different requirements for most nutrients throughout the life cycle. It also means that men and women face some unique challenges in meeting their dietary goals. Some of these differences have already been discussed. However, there are some dietary factors that need further consideration. One factor is that women have a lower ratio of lean body mass to adipose (fatty) tissue at all ages. These differences are minute prior to puberty and then become considerably different (Malina, Bouchard, & Bar-Or, 2004). As a result of this difference and the fact that men have more fat-free mass and, in particular, lean body mass after puberty, their metabolism is higher, meaning that they require more calories than women to do the same things.

Different Cycles, Different Needs

Women also have many more "landmark" times in their lives when their nutritional needs vary significantly. From menarche to menopause, women undergo cyclical physiological changes that can have dramatic effects on metabolism, nutrition needs, and efforts to maintain a nutrition plan. For example, during pregnancy and lactation, nutrition requirements increase substantially. Those unable to follow the dietary recommendations may gain more weight during pregnancy and retain it afterward. During the menstrual cycle, many women report significant food cravings that result in overeating. At menopause, nutrition needs change again rather dramatically. With the hormone estrogen reduced, the body needs more calcium to combat losses in bone mineral density.

Eating Too Much Meat!

Although men do not have the same cyclical patterns, they often have dietary excesses or habits resistant to change. Consider the following:

- Men who eat red meat as a main dish five or more times a week are at a four times higher risk of colorectal cancer than men who eat red meat less than once a month.

- Men who eat a lot of red meat are more than twice as likely to get prostate cancer.

- For every three servings of vegetables or fruits consumed per day, men can expect a 22 percent lower risk of stroke.

- High vegetable and fruit dietary intakes may lower the risk of lung cancer in smokers from 20 times the risk of nonsmokers to "only" 10 times the risk. They may also protect against oral, throat, pancreas, and bladder cancers, all of which are more common in smokers.

- While obesity seems to be a factor in cancer of the esophagus, an increasingly common malignancy among men, consumption of vegetables and fruits can reduce this risk.

- Other research supporting a greater vegetable and fruit intake (for men and women) suggests that well-being and happiness are positively associated with intake with the highest levels of well-being noted with seven or eight daily servings of vegetables and fruit (see Chapter 2 for more details) (Blanchflower, Oswald, & Stewart-Brown, 2012).

VEGETARIANISM

For a variety of reasons, some people choose not to eat meat; approximately 4 percent of Canadians are identified as **vegetarian** (Thompson, Manore, & Sheeska, 2007). Vegetarianism can provide a positive alternative to the typical high-fat, high-calorie, meat-based cuisine

of most Canadians. However, without knowledge and careful food selection, people who follow one or more of the vegetarian diets can experience deficiencies.

The term *vegetarian* means different things to different people. Strict vegetarians, or vegans, avoid all foods of animal origin, including dairy products and eggs. The people who fall into this category must carefully plan their dietary intake to ensure they obtain the necessary nutrients. Far more common are people who are lacto-vegetarians. These people eat dairy products but avoid flesh foods; as a result, their diet is often low in fat and cholesterol, but only if they consume skim milk and other low-fat or nonfat dairy products. Ovo-vegetarians add eggs to their diet, while lacto-ovo-vegetarians eat dairy products and eggs. Pesco-vegetarians eat seafood, dairy products, and eggs, while semi-vegetarians eat poultry, seafood, dairy products, and eggs. Some people in the semi-vegetarian category prefer to call themselves non–red meat eaters.

Generally, people who follow a vegetarian dietary intake weigh less and have better cholesterol levels, fewer problems with irregular bowel movements (constipation and

> **Vegetarian** A term with a variety of meanings: vegans avoid all foods of animal origin; lacto-vegetarians avoid flesh foods and eat dairy products; ovo-vegetarians avoid flesh foods and eat eggs; lacto-ovo-vegetarians avoid flesh foods and eat dairy products and eggs; pesco-vegetarians avoid meat but eat seafood, dairy products, and eggs; semi-vegetarians eat chicken, seafood, dairy products, and eggs.

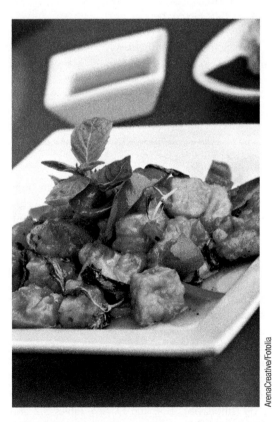

Meals like this provide variety, moderation, and balance. Adding brown rice, whole wheat pasta, or quinoa, as well as a small glass of milk, further provides essential nutrients.

ArenaCreative/Fotolia

Student
Health
TODAY

Sports Drinks or Chocolate Milk: Which to Use after a Workout?

You know it is important to replenish fluids following a workout, but you may not be sure what the best choice is for you. Generally, water is the best fluid to choose before, during, and after a workout. However, there are situations in which you might need to choose something different.

The rationale for drinking fluids other than water ranges from preference to the physiological need to replenish lost nutrients. Most sports drinks are absorbed as effectively as water, and some are absorbed better than juice, another popular thirst-quencher. Some people are likely to consume more when their drink is flavoured, a point that may be significant in ensuring proper hydration. Keep in mind, however, that the intent of sports drinks is to replenish electrolytes lost through

perspiration, as well as to quickly replenish glycogen or energy stores. When perspiration is profuse (that is, 60 minutes or more of sweating), sports drinks may be helpful in replacing these lost electrolytes. However, if you have been physically active for a shorter duration or your exercise is not accompanied by heavy sweating, a sports drink is not needed and may add unnecessary calories and electrolytes to your diet. For a shorter, easier workout, water can probably meet your needs.

Recently, research has been given to milk and its potential to hydrate the body and replenish nutrients. Milk is a liquid that not only hydrates but also is a source of electrolytes (sodium and potassium), as well as nutrients (carbohydrates and protein). Consuming carbohydrates after exercise will help replenish muscle and liver glycogen stores and stimulate muscle protein synthesis, while consuming protein immediately after exercise, rather than several hours later, results in greater muscle protein synthesis. The protein in milk, whey protein, is ideal because it contains all of the essential amino acids and is rapidly absorbed by the body.

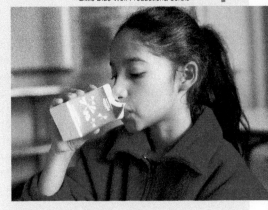
Little Blue Wolf Productions/Corbis

For hydration, electrolytes, carbohydrates, and protein, low-fat chocolate milk might be the ideal post-workout drink.

Although there are many commercial shakes and drinks available to provide the desired combination of carbohydrates and protein, low-fat chocolate milk is a cheaper alternative that will provide you with the nutrients your body needs to hydrate, repair, and recover after exercise.

Sources: Based on J. R. Karp et al., "Chocolate Milk as Post-Exercise Recovery Aid," *International Journal of Sport Nutrition and Exercise Metabolism 16*, no. 1 (2006): 78–91; T. K. Morris and E. Stevenson, "Improved Endurance Capacity Following Chocolate Milk Consumption Compared with 2 Commercially Available Sport Drinks," *Applied Physiology, Nutrition, and Metabolism 34*, no. 1 (2009): 78–82; B. D. Roy, "Milk: The New Sports Drink? A Review," *Journal of the International Society of Sports Nutrition 2*, no. 5 (2008): 15.

---

diarrhea), and a lower risk of heart disease than non-vegetarians. Preliminary evidence suggests that vegetarians may also have a reduced risk for colorectal and breast cancer. Whether these lower risks are due to the vegetarian diet per se or to a combination of lifestyle variables remains unclear.

The modern vegetarian is usually adept at combining the right types of foods to ensure proper nutrient intake. People who eat dairy products and small amounts of poultry or seafood are seldom nutrient-deficient; in fact, while vegans typically get 50 to 60 grams of protein per day, lacto-ovo-vegetarians normally consume between 70 and 90 grams per day, well beyond the DRIs. Vegan diets may be deficient in vitamins B_2 (riboflavin), B_{12}, and D. See Tables 5.2 and 5.3 for sources of these vitamins. Vegans are also at risk for calcium, iron, zinc, and other mineral deficiencies, but these nutrients can be obtained from supplements.

Strict vegans have to pay much more attention to what they eat than the average person, and by eating complementary combinations of plant products (as shown previously in Figure 5.4) they can obtain an adequate amount of essential amino acids.

EATING WELL AS A STUDENT

Post-secondary students face unique challenges when trying to maintain a healthy dietary intake. Some students live in residence and eat on their campuses where food choices might be limited. Further, most students who live in residences do not have their own—or have limited—cooking or refrigeration equipment. Others live in crowded apartments where roommates forage in the refrigerator for everyone else's food. Most students also have time constraints that make buying and preparing food a more challenging task. In addition, many lack the financial resources needed to buy the foods associated with healthier eating such as fresh vegetables and fruit, lean cuts of meat, seafood, and so on. What should a student do? We offer suggestions that may help to make healthy eating the easier and more frequent choice.

Fast Foods: Eating on the Run

Most campuses include an array of fast-food options that fit students' desires for a quick bite of food at a relatively reasonable price. Most of us know that most fast foods are high in fat and sodium—so is it possible to eat well and consume them? Yes. Not all fast foods are created equal and not all of them are "bad" for you. Keep in mind, as well, that all foods can be part of a healthy dietary intake; some simply in lesser quantities and less frequently than others. Many fast-food places offer "healthy eating" options for the discriminating consumer. The key word is *discriminating*. It is possible

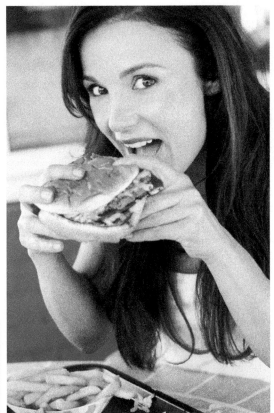

Maintaining a healthy dietary intake can be a challenge for post-secondary students, particularly with fast-food chains on most campuses.

to eat well at fast-food chains if you follow the suggestions below:

- Ask for nutritional analyses of items on the menu.
- Order it "your way"—limit mayonnaise or sauces and other add-ons. Some places have fat-free or reduced fat mayonnaise, so ask.
- Order single, small burgers. Put on your own ketchup in moderation.
- Order salads, with dressing on the side, use the dressing with moderation. Try vinegar and oil or low-fat/no-fat alternative dressings. Limit high-fat add-ons such as bacon bits, croutons, and parmesan cheese.
- Check to see what type of oil is used to cook fries if you have them. Avoid lard-based or other saturated-fat products.
- Order whole-wheat buns and bread and ask for the butter/margarine to be on the side.
- Limit fried foods in general, including hot apple pies and other crust-based fried foods.
- Choose broiled rather than fried.
- Choose low-fat or skim milk or water instead of soft drinks.

More Tips for Choosing Fast Foods Wisely

While some restaurants offer hints for health-conscious diners, you are on your own most of the time. To help you choose wisely, consider the following "best" choice options that contain fewer than 30 grams of fat. "Worst" options have up to 100 grams of fat. Keep in mind the portions often served; adjust your daily intake accordingly. The following tips can further help you to make healthier choices when eating out (American Dietetic Association, n.d.).

Fast Food

Best Grilled chicken sandwich; roast beef sandwich; single hamburger; salad with light vinaigrette

Worst Bacon burger; double cheeseburger; french fries; onion rings

Tips Order sandwiches without mayo or special sauce. Limit deep-fried items such as fish fillets, chicken nuggets, and french fries.

Italian

Best Pasta with red or white clam sauce; spaghetti with marinara or tomato-and-meat sauce

Worst Eggplant parmigiana; fettuccine alfredo; fried calamari; lasagne

Tips Stick with plain bread instead of garlic bread made with butter or oil. Ask for the server's help in avoiding cream- or egg-based sauces. Try vegetarian pizza—without extra cheese.

Mexican

Best Bean burrito (no cheese); chicken fajitas

Worst Beef chimichanga; chile relleno; quesadilla; refried beans

Tips Choose soft tortillas (not fried) with fresh salsa, not guacamole. Special-order grilled shrimp, fish, or chicken. Ask for beans made without lard or fat and for cheeses and sour cream provided on the side. Ask for low-fat or no-fat varieties.

Chinese

Best Hot-and-sour soup; stir-fried vegetables; shrimp with garlic sauce; Szechuan shrimp; wonton soup

Worst Crispy chicken; kung pao chicken; moo shu pork; sweet-and-sour pork

Tips Share a stir-fry; add steamed rice. Ask for vegetables steamed or stir-fried with less oil. Order moo shu vegetables instead of pork. Limit fried rice, breaded dishes, egg rolls, spring rolls, and items loaded with nuts. Limit high-sodium sauces.

Japanese

Best Steamed rice and vegetables; tofu as a substitute for meat; broiled or steamed chicken and fish

Worst Fried rice dishes; miso (very high in sodium); tempura

Tips Limit soy sauces. Use caution in eating sashimi and sushi (raw fish) dishes to reduce risk of bacteria or parasites.

Thai

Best Clear broth soups; stir-fried chicken and vegetables; grilled meats

Worst Coconut milk; peanut sauces; deep-fried dishes

Tips Limit coconut-based curries. Ask for steamed rice rather than fried rice.

Breakfast

Best Hot or cold cereal with 1 percent or skim milk; pancakes or French toast with syrup; scrambled eggs with whole wheat toast

Worst Belgian waffle with sausage; sausage and eggs with biscuits and gravy; ham-and-cheese omelette with hash browns and toast

Tips Ask for whole-grain cereal or shredded wheat with 1 percent or skim milk or whole wheat toast without butter or margarine. Order omelettes without cheese, and fried eggs without bacon or sausage.

Sandwiches

Best Ham and Swiss cheese; roast beef; turkey; vegetarian

Worst Tuna salad; Reuben; salami, pepperoni

Tips Ask for mustard; hold the mayo, cheese, and salt. See if turkey-ham is available, and load up on the veggies.

Seafood

Best Broiled bass, halibut, or snapper; grilled scallops; steamed crab or lobster

Worst Fried fish, fried seafood platter; blackened catfish

Tips Order fish broiled, baked, grilled, or steamed—not pan-fried, sautéed, or breaded and deep fried. Ask for fresh lemon instead of tartar sauce. Limit creamy and buttery sauces.

Understanding Nutrition and Health Claims

Understanding the terminology used by the food industry may also help you eat more healthily (Conrad, n.d.; Health Canada, n.d.b). Nutritional labelling regulations became mandatory for packaged foods distributed from larger businesses from 2005, and for smaller businesses from 2007. These regulations require pre-packaged food labels to carry a Nutrition Facts table that lists calories and 13 key nutrients in a specified amount of food (that is, a usual serving). Figure 5.5 shows an example of a Nutrition Facts label. The regulations were introduced in 2003, with many food distributors adapting their food labels to meet the regulations prior to the mandatory dates.

In addition to the labelling regulations, Health Canada updated the requirements of more than 40 nutrient content claims, resulting in the approval of only certain health claims (about the diet–health relationships) on food labels or in advertisements. It is up to the manufacturer whether to include a nutrition content or diet–health claim on the label or in the advertisement of the food. Often the claims are made—and

FIGURE 5.5

The Nutrition Facts Label

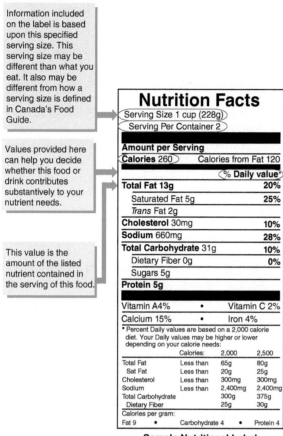

Information included on the label is based upon this specified serving size. This serving size may be different than what you eat. It also may be different from how a serving size is defined in Canada's Food Guide.

Values provided here can help you decide whether this food or drink contributes substantively to your nutrient needs.

This value is the amount of the listed nutrient contained in the serving of this food.

Sample Nutritional Label

From Office of Disease Prevention and Health Promotion, U.S. Department of Health & Human Services.

done so attractively—because they positively influence consumers' purchasing habits.

Examples of Nutrient Content Claims

Source of fibre—the food must contain at least 2 grams of dietary fibre in the amount of food specified as a serving in the Nutrition Facts table.

Low fat—the food contains no more than 3 grams of fat in the amount of food specified as a serving in the Nutrition Facts table.

Trans fat free—the food contains less than 0.2 grams of trans fat in the amount of food specified or the total amount of saturated and trans fat add up to 2 grams or less per specified serving in the Nutrition Facts table.

Cholesterol-free—the food has a negligible amount of cholesterol (less than 2 mg) in the amount of food

specified as a serving in the Nutrition Facts table. The food must also be low in saturated and trans fat.

Sodium-free—the food contains less than 5 mg of sodium in the amount of food specified as a serving in the Nutrition Facts table.

Reduced in calories—the food has at least 25 percent fewer calories than the food it is compared to.

Light—in regard to the nutritional characteristics of a product, "light" is allowed on foods reduced in fat or reduced in calories. "Light" can also be used to describe sensory characteristics associated with a particular food—so long as that characteristic is clearly identified with the claim (for example, light tasting, light coloured).

What Do the Words in Nutrient Content Claims Mean?

Free—none or hardly any

Low—a small amount

Reduced—at least 25 percent less than in a similar product

Light—allowed only on labels reduced in fat or reduced in calories. If used in reference to the characteristic of the food, the characteristic must accompany the claim.

Source—contains a useful amount

High or good source—contains a high amount

Very high or excellent source—contains a very high amount

What Are Health Claims?

Only the following diet–health claims can be made:

1. A healthy diet low in saturated and trans fats may reduce the risk of heart disease.
2. A healthy diet with adequate calcium and vitamin D, and regular physical activity helps to achieve strong bones and may reduce the risk of osteoporosis.
3. A healthy diet rich in a variety of vegetables and fruit may help reduce the risk of some types of cancer.
4. A healthy diet containing foods high in potassium and low in sodium may reduce the risk of high blood pressure, a risk factor for stroke and heart disease.

Healthy Eating on a Budget

Balancing the need for adequate nutrition with the other financial demands of college or university life can become a difficult task. However, if you take the time to plan a healthy dietary intake, you may find that you are eating better, enjoying eating more, and saving money.

You can take these steps to help ensure a quality diet:

- Do not shop when hungry; hunger influences the quantity and quality of what you buy.

- Buy vegetables and fruits in season for lower cost and higher nutrient quality. Out-of-season, flash-frozen varieties are available at a reasonable price and are a high-nutrient-quality choice, assuming you have the capacity to store frozen foods.

- Check out the flyers before shopping. Use coupons and specials for price reductions. These are only savings if they are for products you would normally buy.

- Shop whenever possible at discount warehouse food chains; capitalize on volume discounts and no-frills products.

- Plan ahead to get the most for your dollar and limit extra trips to the store. Make a menu and grocery list and then stick to it.

- Purchase meats and other products in volume, freezing portions for future needs (again, if you have the capacity to do so). Or purchase small amounts of meats and other expensive proteins and combine them with beans and plant proteins for reduced total cost, calories, and fat.

- Cook large meals and freeze smaller portions for later use, if you have the capacity to do so.

- If you find that you have no/limited money for food, check with the local food bank or social service department. Assistance may also be available on your campus as many campuses now have their own food banks.

Healthy Eating in Residence

Food services in some colleges and universities have responded positively to the new guidelines for low-fat, high-carbohydrate eating. Many offer vegetarian entrées; choices among broiled, baked, or fried foods; skim and other reduced-fat milks; nonfat yogurts; and full-service salad and pasta bars. Unfortunately, others have not changed and offer only limited choices for students, providing a limited selection of foods with primarily high- and higher-fat choices. If you find that your institution provides health-conscious food services, the guidelines and tips provided throughout this chapter should be helpful (see also Table 5.6). If not, the following are some actions you might take to help them change their food offerings and cooking practices:

- Ask if anyone has ever done a nutrient analysis of menu items at the food service or residence. If they have, find out what happened to the information obtained. If not, find out what you can do to get one done. Your student health service, health class, nutrition department, or local hospital may be a good resource.

- Once you have identified the nutrient content of these meals, take your findings to the food service provider so that changes can be made. If action does not result, contact your student newspaper and the student government to find someone willing to push for food service reform.

- If you are dissatisfied with the foods available on your campus, make your complaints known in writing to the director of student services or the food service administrator. You should also contact

TABLE 5.6

Eating Well in the Dining Hall

Choose lean meats, grilled chicken, seafood, or vegetable dishes. Limit fried chicken, fatty cuts of red meat, and dishes smothered in creamy or oily sauces.

At the salad bar, load up on leafy greens, beans, tuna, or tofu. Choose items such as avocado or nuts for a little "good" fat, and use the dressing sparingly.

Be creative in your food choices: Why not try a baked potato with salsa, or add a grilled chicken breast to your salad? Toast some bread, and top it with veggies, hummus, or grilled chicken or tuna.

When choosing foods from a made-to-order food station, ask the preparer to reduce or hold the butter, oil, mayonnaise, sour cream, or cheese or cream-based sauce. Ask for extra servings of veggies and lean meats.

Limit seconds and consuming large portions. Be careful of consuming more just because you are staying longer to be with others. Many colleges and universities limit the number of visits you make each day to the dining hall; do not view this as a reason to overeat.

If there is something you would like but it is not available in your dining hall, or if you feel your food options are limited, speak to your food services manager and provide suggestions for inclusion or greater variety.

Limit high-calorie, low-nutrient rich foods such as sugary cereals, soft-serve ice cream, waffles, and other sweet treats. Choose fruit or low-fat yogurt to satisfy your sweet tooth. Watch for added sugar in some yogurts.

the applicable student representative(s) in the Student Union. Be sure to include practical recommendations for improvements.

- Find out what is being done on other campuses in your province and throughout the country. Competition among universities and colleges often goes beyond the sports field. You might spur someone to take action.

- Use the suggestion box provided in the cafeteria. If there is not one available, try to get one set up.

- Be positive in your approach. More support is gained by providing suggestions for change than by simply criticizing current practices.

FOOD SAFETY CONCERNS

Food-Borne Illness

Most of us have experienced the characteristic symptoms of diarrhea, nausea, cramping, and vomiting that prompted us to say, "It must be something I ate." The number of cases of food poisoning in Canada has been growing, to a recent 2011 total estimated by the Government of Canada at 11 million cases per year (Canadian Food Inspection Agency, 2012). Symptoms of food-borne illness vary according to the type of organism and the amount of contaminant eaten. These symptoms can appear as early as a half hour after eating, or take several days or weeks to develop. In most people, the symptoms come on five to eight hours after eating and last only a day or two. In others, such as the very old, the very young, and those with a compromised immune system, food-borne illness can be life-threatening.

Several factors may be contributing to the increase in food-borne illnesses in Canada. One factor potentially involved is the move away from a traditional meat-and-potato dietary intake to "heart-healthy" eating with increased consumption of vegetables, fruits, and grains because it has spurred demand for fresh foods all year regardless of whether they are in season or not (American Medical Association [AMA], 2004; Centers for Disease Control and Prevention [CDC], 2002). To meet this demand, there are greater imports of fresh vegetables and fruits, increasing our risk for ingesting exotic pathogens. Although we are told when we travel to developing countries to "boil it, peel it, or don't eat it," we bring these foods into our homes and eat them, often without washing them (AMA, 2004; CDC, 2002). Food can also become contaminated by being watered with contaminated water, fertilized with "organic" fertilizers (animal manure), or not subjected to the same rigorous pesticide regulations

as Canadian-raised produce. Studies have shown that *Escherichia coli* (a lethal bacterial pathogen) can survive in cow manure for up to 70 days and multiplies in foods grown with manure unless heat or additives such as salt or preservatives are used to kill them (AMA, 2004; CDC, 2002). There are essentially no regulations that prohibit farmers from using animal manure to fertilize crops.

Other key factors associated with the increasing spread of food-borne diseases include inadvertent introduction of pathogens into new geographic regions and insufficient education about food safety (Morris, Motarjemi, & Kaferstein, 1997).

Part of the responsibility for preventing food-borne illness lies with consumers; more than 30 percent of such illnesses result from unsafe handling of food at home. The following actions may reduce your risk:

- When shopping, pick up your packaged, canned, and nonrefrigerated fresh foods first and frozen foods and perishables such as dairy products, meat, poultry, and seafood at the end.

- Check for cleanliness and food safety at the salad bar, meat, and seafood counters. Cooked shrimp, crab, or lobster lying on the same bed of ice as raw seafood can become contaminated.

- When shopping for seafood, buy from markets that get their supplies from approved sources.

- Wash your hands with soap and water before, during, and after food preparations, particularly after handling meat, seafood, or poultry. Wash your hands when returning from the grocery store or market, both before and after putting away your purchases. Wash the countertop and all utensils thoroughly with a bacteria-killing cleanser before using them for other foods.

- Most fresh meat, seafood, and poultry should be kept in the refrigerator no more than one or two days. Check the shelf life of all products before buying.

- Leftovers should be eaten within three days.

- Use a thermometer to ensure that meats are completely cooked. Beef and lamb steaks and roasts should be cooked to at least 63°C, ground meat, pork chops, ribs, and egg dishes to 71°C, chicken and other poultry breasts to 77°C, and chicken and turkey legs, thighs, and whole birds to 82°C.

- Fish is done when the thickest part becomes opaque and the fish flakes easily.

- Cooked food should never be left standing on the stove or table for more than two hours. Keep hot foods hot.

- Foods that should be refrigerated should not be left out long; if you are serving food buffet style, use dishes with ice below the serving dishes (and food contents). Keep cold foods cold.

- Do not thaw frozen foods at room temperature. Put in the refrigerator for a day to thaw, or thaw in cold water, changing the water every 30 minutes.

- When freezing raw foods, in particular meat, make sure juices cannot spill into ice cubes or other areas of the refrigerator.

- When packing lunch, ensure appropriate temperatures are maintained.

(Based on Dietitians of Canada, 2010.)

Food Additives

Additives are substances added to food to reduce the risk of food-borne illness, prevent spoilage, and enhance the look and taste. Additives can also enhance the nutrient value; for example, the fortification of milk with vitamin D and of grain products with folate add to the nutritional value of these foods. Although Health Canada regulates additives according to effectiveness, safety, and ability to detect them in foods, questions are often raised about their safety—in particular because some additives interact with medications. Generally, the fewer the chemicals, colourants, and preservatives, the better. However, it is should be noted that there is currently no hormone free meat.

Examples of common additives include

- antimicrobial agents: substances such as salt, sugar, nitrites, and others that tend to make foods less hospitable for microbes

- antioxidants: substances that preserve colour and flavour by reducing loss due to oxygen exposure. Vitamins C and E as well as the additives BHA and HHT are common antioxidants.

- artificial colours, nutrient additions, and flavour enhancers such as MSG (monosodium glutamate)

- sulfites: used to preserve vegetable colour

- dioxins: found in coffee filters, milk containers, and frozen foods

- methylene chloride: found in decaffeinated coffee

- hormones: bovine growth hormone (forbidden in Canada so far) found in animal meat and milk

In Canada, growth hormones are only approved for use in cows used for beef, not in other animals such as chickens or pigs. Hormones also occur naturally in all animals, people, and plants, so there is no hormone-free beef. The use of approved hormones and antibiotics to produce food is considered safe (Dietitians of Canada, 2016).

Food allergies Overreaction by the body to normally harmless proteins perceived as allergens. In response, the body produces antibodies, triggering allergic symptoms.

Food intolerance Adverse effects as a result of people eating particular foods that they cannot break down because they lack the needed digestive chemicals.

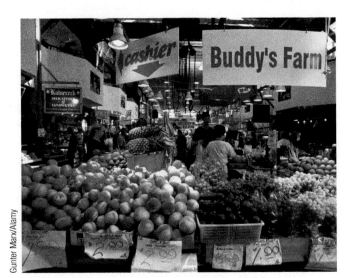

Learning to shop carefully for fresh, high-quality foods can help ensure that your food is safe and help you to attain nutritional health.

Food Allergies

Twenty to thirty percent of adults believe they are allergic to at least one food (Garzon, Kempker, & Piel, 2011). True **food allergies** occur when the body overreacts to normally harmless proteins, perceiving them as allergens. The body then produces antibodies that activate immune cells known as histamines, triggering a variety of allergic symptoms. Such allergic reactions vary tremendously and range from a case of hives or a body rash to swelling of certain body parts (especially the lips), to pain, itchiness, diarrhea, nausea, or vomiting. In more severe cases, irregularities in breathing and heartbeat are experienced, along with blood pressure fluctuations, shock, and, if untreated, death. Symptoms can occur within minutes or over a two- to three-hour period.

The most common food triggering food allergies are soybeans, legumes (including peanuts), nuts, shellfish, eggs, wheat, and milk (Garzon, Kempker, & Piel, 2011). People are often allergic to a whole family of foods; this is called "cross-reactivity." Unlike many other allergies, food allergies do not appear to be inherited. Individuals breast-fed as infants seem to have fewer food allergies (Garzon, Kempker, & Piel, 2011). If you think you have a food allergy, get tested by a trained allergist.

Some common reactions to food that may imitate allergies but do not involve the immune system are listed below (Garzon, Kempker, & Piel, 2011).

- **Food intolerance** occurs in people who lack certain digestive enzymes and suffer adverse effects when they consume substances they cannot tolerate. One of the most common examples is lactose intolerance, experienced by people without the digestive enzymes needed to digest the lactose in milk.

Another common example is gluten sensitivity or gluten intolerance, experienced by people with issues regarding the digestion of one or more of the polypeptides of wheat (Louis, 2012). Symptoms for gluten intolerance are relatively vague and cover a broad spectrum of gastrointestinal difficulties ranging from cramping and bloating to diarrhea or constipation (Louis, 2012).

- Reactions to food additives, such as sulphites and MSG.
- Reactions to substances occurring naturally in some foods, such as tyramine in cheese, phenylethylamine in chocolate, caffeine in coffee, and some compounds in alcohol.
- Unknown reactions in people who have adverse symptoms that they attribute to foods and that may actually go away when treated as allergies but for which there is no physiological basis.

Choosing Organic

Due to mounting concerns about food safety, many people refuse to buy processed foods and mass-produced agricultural products. Instead, they purchase **organically grown** foods—foods reported to be pesticide- and chemical-free. Since organic produce first came on the market, they have improved in quality, appearance, and size, although they still tend to carry a heavier price tag. A difficulty that has remained over time is in ensuring that what you buy as organic does not have "second-hand" pesticides or chemicals on it. Currently, Canadian farms can be certified as organic so long as they do not use synthetic pesticides themselves regardless of the chemicals used on neighbouring farms (Forge, 2004).

Is organic food really more nutritious? That depends on what aspect of the food is being studied and how the research is conducted. Two recent review studies, both of which examined decades of research into the nutrient quality of organic versus traditionally grown foods, reached opposite conclusions: One found organic foods more nutritious, and the other did not (Brandt et al., 2011). Moreover, little is known about the longterm benefits of consuming organic vs non-organic foods. But, we do know that pesticide residues remain on conventionally grown produce.

Locally Grown Foods

The word locavore has been coined to describe people who eat mostly food grown or produced locally, usually within close proximity to their homes. Farmers' markets or homegrown foods or those grown by independent farmers are thought to be fresher and to require far fewer resources to get them to market and keep them fresh for longer periods of time. **Locavores** believe that locally grown food is preferable to foods produced by large corporations or supermarket-based organic foods, as they make a smaller impact on the environment. The locavore movement is less concerned about foods that are grown organically as they are about buying locally grown foods. Some people argue that buying locally grown food from independent producers is more expensive then shopping at the large grocery store chains in their neighbourhood. However, if you look for in-season foods and foods available year round in your area, eating locally fits well within a restricted budget.

Eating locally has also given rise the concept of "slow foods," which is a movement reacting to the over abundance and consumption of fast foods in our modern day society. Slow foods incorporate non processed foods that are often locally grown. This concept encourages consumers to consider their overall wellness when preparing and consuming and meals. Eating a healthy diet primarily containing locally grown foods is a great option for students, the key is educating yourself about when and where to find the most affordable foods grown in your area. For students, decreasing fast food consumption and transitioning to the the slow food approach may take a little planning at first, but in the long run will simplify your life and provide many health and economic benefits.

Genetically Modified Food Crops

Genetic modification involves the insertion or deletion of genes into the DNA of an organism. In the case of **genetically modified (GM) foods**, this genetic cutting and pasting is done to enhance production; for example, by making disease- or insect-resistant plants, improving yield, or controlling weeds. In addition, GM foods are sometimes created to improve the colour and appearance of foods or to enhance specific nutrients.

The first genetically modified food crop was a tomato called the FlavrSavr, which was developed to ripen without getting soft, thereby increasing its shipping capacity and shelf life. Soybeans and cotton are the most common GM crops, followed by corn. The safety of GM foods is still a big question. In a recent report in *New Scientist,* three strains of maize (corn) showed signs of causing liver and kidney toxicity (Coghlan, 2010). These claims are refuted by producers. According to the World Health Organization, no effects on human health have been shown from consumption of GM foods in countries that have approved their use (World Health Organization, n.d.). However, the debate surrounding GM foods is not likely to end soon; see the Point of View box for more information.

Organically grown Foods grown without pesticides or chemicals.

Locavore A person who primarily eats food grown or produced locally.

Genetically modified (GM) foods Foods derived from organisms whose DNA has been altered using genetic engineering techniques.

point of view

GENETICALLY MODIFIED FOODS: Boon or Bane?

We may face food shortages if the population continues to expand and if plant diseases continue unchecked, soils are depleted, and our supply of traditional food sources is depleted by overconsumption and slow renewal. Some scientists and food producers believe that genetically modified (GM) food crops could help solve problems of matching food supply to demand, but others, including health advocates, are opposed to the further development and widespread use of genetically modified foods because of the potential for health risks and potential negative impact on the ecosystem. Below are some of the main points for and against the development of GM organisms for food.

ARGUMENTS FOR THE DEVELOPMENT OF GM FOODS

People have been manipulating food crops—primarily through selective breeding—since the beginning of agriculture. Genetic modification is fundamentally the same thing, just more precise.

Genetically modified seeds and products are tested for safety, and there has never been a substantiated claim for a human illness resulting from consumption of a GM food.

By modifying the DNA in foods that cause allergies, we may be able to prevent many food-borne allergies.

Genetically modified crops can have a positive impact on the environment. Current agricultural practices are very environmentally damaging, whereas insect- and weed-resistant GM crops will allow farmers to use far fewer chemical insecticides and herbicides.

Genetically modified crops have the potential to reduce world hunger; they can be created to grow more quickly than conventional crops, increasing productivity and allowing for faster cycling of crops, which means more food yield. Crops engineered to resist spoiling or damage allow for transportation to areas affected by drought or natural disaster.

Genetically modified crops are under development to produce and deliver vaccines. This is vitally important to protecting the health of people in developing nations and preventing epidemics.

ARGUMENTS AGAINST THE DEVELOPMENT OF GM FOODS

Genetic modification is fundamentally different from and more problematic than selective breeding because it transfers genes between species in ways that could never happen naturally.

There have not been enough independent studies of GM products to confirm that they are safe for consumption. Also, there are potential health risks if GM products approved for animal feed or other uses are mistakenly or inadvertently used in the production of food for human consumption.

The use of GM crops cannot be completely controlled, so they have the potential to damage the environment. Inadvertent cross-pollination could lead to the creation of "super weeds"; insect-resistant crops could harm insect species that are not pests; and insect- and disease-resistant crops could prompt the evolution of even more virulent species, which would then require more aggressive control measures, such as the increased use of chemical sprays.

There is the potential for genetic engineering to introduce allergens into otherwise nonallergenic foods.

Because corporations create and patent GM seeds, they will control the market, meaning that poor farmers in the developing world would become reliant on these corporations. This circumstance would be more likely to increase world hunger than to alleviate it.

Creating and patenting new life forms is unethical. The introduction of foreign genes into a plant—particularly genes taken from an animal—upsets the balance of nature.

Where Do You Stand?

○ Do you think GM foods are more helpful or harmful?

○ What are your greatest concerns over GM foods? What do you think are their greatest benefits?

○ In what ways could the creators of GM foods address the concerns of those opposed to them?

○ What sort of regulation do you think the government should have with regard to the creation, cultivation, and sale of GM foods?

○ Currently, there are no GM livestock; however, many livestock are fed GM feed or feed that includes additives and vaccines produced by GM microorganisms. Do you feel any differently about directly consuming GM crops versus eating the flesh, milk, or eggs of an animal that has been fed on GM crops?

○ If scientists were to develop GM livestock, would that alter your stance on any of these questions?

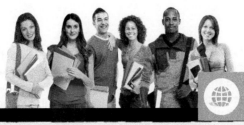
TAKING CHARGE: Managing Your Nutrition

Given the culture around food in our country, eating well and eating well consistently is not easy. It takes knowledge, careful thought and preparation, as well as the ability to put it all together to make the best decisions for your lifestyle within your budgetary limits. Still, you can improve your nutritional health if you take the time, learn more about it, and take steps to effect positive change in what, how, when, where, and why you eat. This section may help you in that regard. First, determine how much you know about eating, your 'eating quotient', then review the recommendations and put as many into action as you can immediately, saving the more challenging ones for a later date.

What Is Your EQ (Eating Quotient)?

Keeping up with the latest on what to eat—or what to eat less of—is not easy. Rate your 'eating quotient' by responding to the following questions. There is only one correct answer for each question.

1. Fresh vegetables and fruit contain more nutrients than canned or frozen varieties.

   True or False

2. While you are shopping, it makes a difference what area of the store you start in, in terms of keeping your foods safe.

   True or False

3. Fruit drinks count as a serving from the vegetable and fruit group in the Food Guide.

   True or False

4. Baked potatoes have a higher glycemic index (the ability of carbohydrates to raise blood sugar levels quickly) than sweet potatoes or apples.

   True or False

5. A late dinner is more likely to cause weight gain than eating the same meal earlier in the day.

   True or False

6. Nuts are okay to eat if you are trying to stick to a low-fat diet.

   True or False

7. Certain foods, such as grapefruit, celery, or cabbage soup, burn fat and can help you to lose weight.

   True or False

8. Which of the following has the most fibre?
   a. chuck roast
   b. dark-meat chicken with skin
   c. skinless chicken wing
   d. they are all about the same

9. Which of the following is the strongest predictor of obesity in Canada today?
   a. region of the country you live in
   b. ethnicity/culture
   c. lack of physical activity
   d. socioeconomic status

10. When you eat a meal, how long does it take for your brain to get the message that you are full?
    a. 10 minutes
    b. 20 minutes
    c. at least an hour
    d. 2 hours or more

11. Which of the following are at the top of the list in bacterial levels among domestically grown vegetables?
    a. green onions, cantaloupe, and cilantro
    b. beets, potatoes, and summer squash
    c. celery, leaf lettuce, and parsley
    d. strawberries, apples, and tomatoes

12. Which of the following foods contains the most grams of fibre per serving?
    a. 1/2 cup of strawberries
    b. 1/2 cup of kidney beans
    c. 1 cup popcorn
    d. 1 medium banana

13. Which of the following suggestions will best lead to obtaining the daily recommended level of antioxidants?
    a. Eat several dark green vegetables and orange, red, and yellow fruits and vegetables.
    b. Eat at least two servings of lean red meat per day.
    c. Eat whole-grain foods with at least 2 grams of fibre per serving.
    d. Eat several servings of tuna and salmon per week.

(continued)

14. Olive oil, one of the heart-healthy monounsaturated fats, is a great source for antioxidants. Which of the following recommendations should you follow?

    a. Buy olive oil only in amounts that you will use relatively quickly. Nutrients are lost quickly after 12 months sitting on the shelf.

    b. If you buy larger bottles of olive oil, separate it into smaller bottles and keep the lid on tightly to reduce oxidation from air contact. Refrigerate if possible. Refrigeration causes cloudiness but does not affect quality.

    c. Store olive oil in opaque airtight glass bottles or metal tins away from heat and light.

    d. All of the above.

15. Which strategy will help you identify high-fibre breads to maximize your quality carbohydrate intake?

    a. Choose whole-grain breads that list whole grains as the first ingredient.

    b. Purchase breads with 1 to 2 grams of fibre per slice.

    c. Look for bread that is dark coloured. The darker is the bread, the greater the chance that it has good-quality fibre.

    d. All of the above.

Answers

1. False: There is usually little difference between fresh, canned, and frozen vegetables and fruit in regard to nutritional value, depending on how fresh produce is handled and how quickly it reaches your super-market. Canned and frozen produce are typically picked at their peak and may contain more nutrients than fresh produce picked overripe or too early; that sat in a warehouse, spent days in transit, or sat at improper temperatures for prolonged periods. Keep in mind, however, canned or frozen vegetables and fruit may have added salt or sugar. Whenever possible, buy local produce fresh from the fields or neigh-bouring areas.

2. True: As a general rule, milk, meat, and other per-ishables that have been left at room temperature for more than two hours have an increased risk of conveying a food-borne illness. Be sure to factor in the time that you spend driving home from the store or running other errands. Start your shopping in the canned and nonrefrigerated sections of the store, leaving your meat, dairy products, and frozen foods to be picked up last. Complete your other errands before you shop for food, and if you know it will take time to get home, bring a cooler with ice to store your perishable purchases.

3. False: Even if fruit juice is an actual ingredient (often it is not, check the label), most fruit drinks consist primarily of water and high fructose corn syrup or other sweeteners, colourings, and fruit flavouring. It is always better to eat the whole fruit, because you will get added fibre, more nutrients, and other benefits. Next best are 100 percent fruit juices, preferably with added vitamin C. Lowest on the nutrient quality list are the sweetened, flavoured fruit drinks.

4. True: It is a better choice to select a sweet potato or apple instead of substituting a baked potato for fries if you are trying to keep your blood sugar levels down or manage your type 2 diabetes. For more information, check the glycemic index reference books available at most bookstores, or use the handy guide found at www.diabetesnet.com/diabetes_food_diet/glycemic_index.php.

5. False: It is not when you eat but what you eat that makes a difference in weight gain. If you ate a 500-calorie pizza at 10 p.m. in a day where your meals were light, you would not likely gain weight. However, a dietary intake that includes a big breakfast, lunch, and dinner, then a 500-calorie piece of pizza at 10 p.m. would likely provide more calories than needed and result in weight gain.

6. True: Although they are high in fat, nuts contain mostly unsaturated (good) fat and are good sources of protein, magnesium, and the antioxidants vitamin E and selenium. Moderation is the key.

7. False: No foods can burn fat or help you to lose weight. Some foods with caffeine may speed up your metabolism for a short time, but they do not cause weight loss. One of the best ways to boost your metabolism is to increase your muscle mass through resistance training and exercise—not by eating specific foods.

8. d: There is no fibre in animal foods. Fibre is found only in plants and plant-based foods such as fruits, beans, whole grains, and vegetables.

9. d: Although the other responses are all contributors to obesity, the greatest single predictor of obesity is low socioeconomic status. The poor nutritional qual-ity of foods commonly eaten when people are forced to stretch their food budget and/or have poor nutri-tional knowledge—high-fat meats, hot dogs, inex-pensive white breads and pastries, pop, chips, and other high-calorie, low-fibre foods—often increases the risk of obesity.

10. b: It takes about 20 minutes for your brain to get the message that you are full. To make sure you do not overeat, eat slowly, talk with others, put your fork down after taking a bite, take a drink of water, or do other things to delay your meal. Let your brain catch up to your fork, and slow it down!

11. a: The bad news is that in a recent government study of bacterial levels found in domestic produce, green onions, cantaloupe, and cilantro scored the highest in positive tests for two common bacteria: *Salmonella* and *Shigella*. The good news is that out of nearly 1100 samples, only 2–3 percent were contaminated. Still, washing your produce (even the bagged and prewashed variety) is a must; run a heavy stream of water over the produce while rubbing the outside under the water to remove any potential bacteria.

12. *b:* One-half cup of kidney beans provides 4.5 grams of fibre; a medium banana has 2 grams of fibre; strawberries and popcorn each have 1 gram of fibre per serving.

13. *a:* Antioxidants, particularly vitamins C and E, the mineral selenium, and plant pigments known as carotenoids (which include beta-carotene) are found in green leafy vegetables and orange, yellow, and red vegetables and fruit.

14. *d:* Olive oil loses nutrients over time, with one year being the general guesstimate of "use by" time. Keeping it in the refrigerator prolongs shelf life. If the oil smells rancid or if you note mould or other discolouration, discard the bottle.

15. *a:* A true whole-grain bread clearly says so on the label (for example, "100 percent whole wheat" or "100 percent stone-ground whole wheat"). If all the ingredients are not whole grain, then it is not a true whole-grain bread. The more fibre in each slice, the better; look for a minimum of 3 grams per slice. Colour is not a good indicator of nutrient value. Dyes and colouring can make even the whitest white bread brown.

Scoring

If you answered all of the above correctly, congratulations! You clearly have a good sense of some of the current issues and facts surrounding dietary choices. If you missed one or more questions, refer back to the corresponding section of this chapter to find out more. Recognize that nutrition information changes rapidly, and there is considerable material available.

Recommendations for Change

- *Eat lower on the food chain*. Try to substitute vegetables, fruits, nuts, or grains for animal products at least once a day.

- *Eat seasonal foods whenever possible*. By eating foods at the peak of harvest, you are most apt to avoid nutrient losses incurred by storage, freezing, canning, and so on—and are likely to obtain a lower-cost option.

- *Eat lean*. The evidence against high-fat foods mounts daily. Pay attention to labels, assess your food intake, and balance high-fat with low-fat choices. Choose leaner cuts of meat and bake, grill, boil, or broil whenever possible.

- *Eat more colour*. Generally, the more vibrant the colour in the vegetable or fruit, the more nutrients available. Eat more dark greens and oranges. Try a new vegetable or fruit each week.

- *Increase your consumption of vegetables and fruits*. Use the real thing instead of juices and get more nutrients, fibre in particular.

- *Practise responsible consumer safety*. Avoid unnecessary chemicals; buy, prepare, and store foods prudently to avoid food-borne illness.

- *Eat in moderation*. Learn to separate true hunger feelings from the food cravings that come from boredom. Recognize when your body is signalling that it is getting full, and stop eating. Moderate your caloric consumption and reduce your consumption of sugars and other dietary "extras."

- *Keep your systems functioning well*. Even the best plans are doomed to fail if life problems are dragging your systems down, particularly your digestive system.

- *Balance your dietary intake*. Consume appropriate amounts of water, proteins, carbohydrates, fats, vitamins, and minerals.

- *Pay attention to your changing nutrient needs*. Various factors in your life, such as pregnancy or illness (including stress), may require adjustments to your nutrition intake. Prepare for these changes and remain informed about reputable sources of information concerning nutrient benefits and risks.

Critical Thinking

You and your best friend chose to move into an apartment off campus this year and you have decided to make your meals together. You were raised on meals where meat was the focal point; your best friend/roommate is a lacto-ovo-vegetarian. Using the DECIDE model described in Chapter 1, decide how you two will come up with a menu that works for you both.

DISCUSSION QUESTIONS

1. What factors influence the dietary patterns, attitudes, and behaviours of the typical university or college student? Which of these factors has the greatest influence on your eating attitudes and behaviours? Why is it important that you know about your dietary influences as you think about changing your eating patterns, attitudes, and behaviours?

2. Considering your dietary intake, what improvements do you need to make to eat better? Be specific. Prioritize this list of improvements. Determine when you want to accomplish each improvement and how you can make the change(s) needed. List the actions that you can take now to enact change. List the changes that you will make in the future to enact change. What may challenge your desire to make these changes? How can you manage these challenges?

3. What are the four food groups in Eating Well with Canada's Food Guide? How many servings do you need of each? What food group(s) might you find it difficult to get enough servings from? What food group(s) do you get too many servings from? What can you do to increase or decrease your intake of selected food groups?

4. What other recommendations are made in Eating Well with Canada's Food Guide (other than servings from each food group)? Are these recommendations difficult to follow, particularly as a university or college student? Why or why not?

5. What are the major types of nutrients that you should be getting from the foods you eat? What happens if you do not get enough of one or more of these nutrients? Are vitamin and mineral supplements necessary for you individually? Why or why not?

6. Distinguish between the different types of vegetarianism. Which types are most likely to lead to nutrient deficiencies? What can be done to ensure that even the strictest vegetarian gets sufficient nutrients?

7. What are the major risks for food-borne illnesses and what can you do to protect yourself at school? At home? Why are additives added to food? What are the potential risks of these additives? How are food illnesses and food allergies different?

APPLICATION EXERCISE

Reread the "Consider This . . ." scenario at the beginning of the chapter and respond to the following:

1. Critique Ahmed's eating habits. What suggestions could you make to help him? How can you make these suggestions in a way that does not offend him?

2. Is there anything Ahmed can do to improve his eating situation? Imagine Ahmed attends your university or college; is the food available really that unhealthy or does he need more knowledge and motivation to make better choices? What specific suggestions would you make?

MASTERINGHEALTH

Go to MasteringHealth for Assignments, the eText, and the Study Area with case studies, self quizzing, and videos.

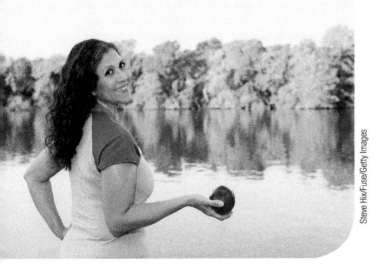

Steve Hix/Fuse/Getty Images

CHAPTER 6

MANAGING YOUR WEIGHT: FINDING A HEALTHY BALANCE

◄◉ CONSIDER THIS . . .

When Eilidh, aged 19, went home for Christmas vacation between terms at university, she weighed herself and discovered that she had gained the dreaded 'Frosh 15'. Although she knew she was not as physically active as she had been in high school and that she did not always make the healthiest choices in the Meal Hall, she did not think she had gained that much weight during her first term. She resolved then and there to not eat any sweets or junk food over the Christmas holidays and she would run every day for an hour until she lost the weight she gained. She also decided that she would not go out with her friends to the bar so that she could avoid the calories she usually consumes in the drinks and post-bar pizza stop.

Does Eilidh have the 'right' approach to managing her recent weight gain? Is her approach typical of others her age? Her sex? What might you recommend?

anadians are concerned about their body weight and shape—and should be, since more than half the population (54 percent) over the age of 18 years is classified as overweight or obese according to body mass index (BMI) calculations derived from self-reported height and weight (Statistics Canada, 2014a; 2014b). Combined, 61.8 percent of men and 46.2 percent of women are considered overweight or obese and at health risk (Statistics Canada, 2014a). Even more alarming, these population statistics regarding overweight are likely underestimated given that BMI was calculated from self-reported height and weight. When self-report is used to determine height and weight, men typically overestimate their height while women usually underestimate their weight (Statistics Canada, 2014a). Both factors of misreporting result in lower estimates for BMI and thus, potentially, an underreporting of the percentage of the population classified as overweight or obese.

The lowest rates of overweight and obesity are found in British Columbia (48 percent) while the highest rates of overweight and obesity are found in Newfoundland and Labrador. Unfortunately rates of overweight and obesity continue to rise among adults across Canada (Statistics Canada, 2014a; 2014b).

Equally alarming is the high percentage of Canadian youth considered overweight or obese. In 2014, 23.1 percent of boys and girls ages 12 to 17 years were classified as overweight or obese based upon parent-reported data (Statistics Canada, 2014b). This represented a increase from 20.4 percent in 2011. Previous research on BMI in children and youth indicated an increase in overweight and obesity as well (Tremblay & Willms, 2000), potentially indicating that the rise in the percentage of children and youth classified as obese continues unabated.

Health Risks of Overweight and Obesity

Given the attention to overweight and obesity in the media, you are likely aware of the associated health risks (see also Figure 6.1). Briefly, individuals classified as overweight or obese are at increased risk of heart

FIGURE 6.1

Potential Negative Health Effects of Obesity

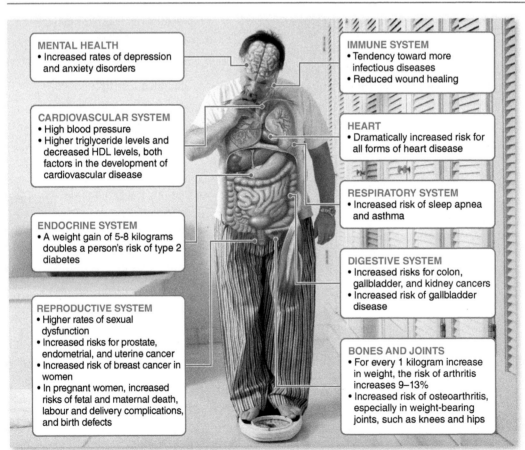

MENTAL HEALTH
• Increased rates of depression and anxiety disorders

CARDIOVASCULAR SYSTEM
• High blood pressure
• Higher triglyceride levels and decreased HDL levels, both factors in the development of cardiovascular disease

ENDOCRINE SYSTEM
• A weight gain of 5-8 kilograms doubles a person's risk of type 2 diabetes

REPRODUCTIVE SYSTEM
• Higher rates of sexual dysfunction
• Increased risks for prostate, endometrial, and uterine cancer
• Increased risk of breast cancer in women
• In pregnant women, increased risks of fetal and maternal death, labour and delivery complications, and birth defects

IMMUNE SYSTEM
• Tendency toward more infectious diseases
• Reduced wound healing

HEART
• Dramatically increased risk for all forms of heart disease

RESPIRATORY SYSTEM
• Increased risk of sleep apnea and asthma

DIGESTIVE SYSTEM
• Increased risks for colon, gallbladder, and kidney cancers
• Increased risk of gallbladder disease

BONES AND JOINTS
• For every 1 kilogram increase in weight, the risk of arthritis increases 9–13%
• Increased risk of osteoarthritis, especially in weight-bearing joints, such as knees and hips

Big Cheese Photo LLC/Alamy

disease, stroke, high blood pressure, some types of cancer, type 2 diabetes, gallbladder disease, and osteoarthritis (Katzmarzyk, 2002). Of equal concern are the emotional, spiritual, and social health risks associated with overweight and obesity partly due to the stigma surrounding them. You are also likely aware of the "simple" solution to obesity often depicted in the media: eat less, move more. However, it is not that simple—if it was, our population, and others all around the world, would not be experiencing the current levels of overweight and obesity.

This chapter describes overweight and obesity, the factors that lead to their development, and the importance of a healthy weight maintenance for overall health. It also includes practical strategies for maintaining your weight and learning to appreciate your body size and shape.

OVERWEIGHT AND OBESITY

Confusion exists in the understanding of the terms *overweight* and *obesity*. Part of the confusion relates to measurement and another part is the inconsistent and often inappropriate use of each term. **Overweight** refers to a weight greater than expected for a specific height (and is usually determined from height–weight charts or calculating BMI). **Obesity** refers to an excessive accumulation of body fat such that the individual is at increased risk for developing health problems (see Figure 6.1). Interestingly, a person can be overweight and not obese. For example, a male weightlifter or football athlete may be overweight according to a height–weight chart and BMI classification because of his high level of lean body or muscle mass even though he has a low level of body fat. Similarly, a person can be obese without being overweight. A 160-centimetre woman who weighs 54 kilograms has a BMI of 21, which is considered 'weight appropriate' (see Figure 6.2), but she can be 'soft and squishy'. Although she has a 'weight appropriate' BMI classification, she can have more than 30 percent of her weight coming from body fat if she does little physical activity, spends most of her time in sedentary activities, and, thus, has a low level of lean body or muscle mass. Weight by itself or in combination with height is not a valid indicator of obesity or fatness.

As previously mentioned, there are physical health risks associated with obesity or an excessive accumulation of body fat, include, but should not be limited to, an increased chance of developing atherosclerosis, coronary artery disease, hypertension, colon cancer, postmenopausal breast cancer, type 2 diabetes, gallbladder disease, and osteoarthritis (Katzmarzyk, 2002). Equally important are the mental health risks of excessive fatness, including poor body image and reduced self-esteem. Table 6.1 provides more specific guidelines regarding level of body percentage according to age groups for men and women from ages 20 to 80 years.

Overweight A weight greater than expected for a specific height.

Obesity An excessive accumulation of body fat associated with health risk.

TABLE 6.1

Body Fat Percentage Norms for Men and Women

Men						
Age	Very Lean	Excellent	Good	Fair	Poor	Very Poor
20–29	< 7%	7%–10%	11%–15%	16%–19%	20%–23%	>23%
30–39	<11%	11%–14%	15%–18%	19%–21%	22%–25%	>25%
40–49	<14%	14%–17%	18%–20%	21%–23%	24%–27%	>27%
50–59	<15%	15%–19%	20%–22%	23%–24%	25%–28%	>28%
60–69	<16%	16%–20%	21%–22%	23%–25%	26%–28%	>28%
70–79	<16%	16%–20%	21%–23%	24%–25%	26%–28%	>28%
Women						
Age	Very Lean	Excellent	Good	Fair	Poor	Very Poor
20–29	<14%	14%–16%	17%–19%	20%–23%	24%–27%	>27%
30–39	<15%	15%–17%	18%–21%	22%–25%	26%–29%	>29%
40–49	<17%	17%–20%	21%–24%	25%–28%	29%–32%	>32%
50–59	<18%	18%–22%	23%–27%	28%–30%	31%–34%	>34%
60–69	<18%	18%–23%	24%–28%	29%–31%	32%–35%	>35%
70–79	<18%	18%–24%	25%–29%	30%–32%	33%–36%	>36%

Source: Based on data from American College of Sports Medicine, ACSM's *Guidelines for Exercise Testing and Prescription*. 8th ed. (Baltimore, MD: Lippincott Williams & Wilkins, 2010).

FIGURE 6.2

What is your weight status? To find out, find your height (either at the top [in feet and inches] or bottom [in centimetres]) and your weight (at the right [in kilograms] or left [in pounds]) and find where these two intersect.

Legend:
- Underweight
- Weight appropriate
- Overweight
- Obese

Body Mass Index — Height (feet/inches) / Height (centimetres) — Weight (pounds) / Weight (kilograms)

Weight (lb)	5'0"	5'1"	5'2"	5'3"	5'4"	5'5"	5'6"	5'7"	5'8"	5'9"	5'10"	5'11"	6'0"	6'1"	6'2"	6'3"	6'4"	Weight (kg)
100	20	19	18	18	17	17	16	16	15	15	14	14	14	13	13	12	12	45
105	21	20	19	19	18	17	17	16	16	16	15	15	14	14	13	13	13	47
110	21	21	20	19	19	18	18	17	17	16	16	15	15	15	14	14	13	50
115	22	22	21	20	20	19	19	18	17	17	17	16	16	15	15	14	14	52
120	23	23	22	21	21	20	19	19	18	18	17	17	16	16	15	15	15	54
125	24	24	23	22	21	21	20	20	19	18	18	17	17	16	16	16	15	57
130	25	25	24	23	22	22	21	20	20	19	19	18	18	17	17	16	16	59
135	26	26	25	24	23	22	22	21	21	20	20	19	18	18	17	17	16	61
140	27	26	26	25	24	23	23	22	21	21	20	20	19	18	18	17	17	63
145	28	27	27	26	25	24	23	23	22	21	21	20	20	19	19	18	18	66
150	29	28	27	27	26	25	24	23	23	22	22	21	20	20	19	19	18	68
155	30	29	28	27	27	26	25	24	24	23	22	22	21	20	20	19	19	70
160	31	30	29	28	27	27	26	25	24	24	23	22	22	21	21	20	19	72
165	32	31	30	29	28	27	27	26	25	24	24	23	22	22	21	21	20	75
170	33	32	31	30	29	28	27	27	26	25	24	24	23	22	22	21	21	77
175	34	33	32	31	30	29	28	27	27	26	25	24	24	23	22	22	21	79
180	35	34	33	32	31	30	29	28	27	27	26	25	24	24	23	22	22	82
185	36	35	34	33	32	31	30	29	28	27	27	26	25	24	24	23	23	84
190	37	36	35	34	33	32	31	30	29	28	27	26	26	25	24	24	23	86
195	38	37	36	35	33	32	31	31	30	29	28	27	26	26	25	24	24	88
200	39	38	37	35	34	33	32	31	30	30	29	28	27	26	26	25	24	91
205	40	39	37	36	35	34	33	32	31	30	29	29	28	27	26	26	25	93
210	41	40	38	37	36	35	34	33	32	31	30	29	28	28	27	26	26	95
215	42	41	39	38	37	36	35	34	33	32	31	30	29	28	28	27	26	98
220	43	42	40	39	38	37	36	34	33	32	32	31	30	29	28	27	27	100
225	44	43	41	40	39	37	36	35	34	33	32	31	31	30	29	28	27	102
230	45	43	42	41	39	38	37	36	35	34	33	32	31	30	30	29	28	104
235	46	44	43	42	40	39	38	37	36	35	34	33	32	31	30	29	29	107
240	47	45	44	43	41	40	39	38	36	35	34	33	33	32	31	30	29	109
245	48	46	45	43	42	41	40	38	37	36	35	34	33	32	31	31	30	111
250	49	47	46	44	43	42	40	39	38	37	36	35	34	33	32	31	30	114

Height (feet/inches)	5'0"	5'1"	5'2"	5'3"	5'4"	5'5"	5'6"	5'7"	5'8"	5'9"	5'10"	5'11"	6'0"	6'1"	6'2"	6'3"	6'4"
Height (centimetres)	150.0	152.5	155.0	157.5	160.0	162.5	165.0	167.5	170.0	172.5	175.0	177.5	180.0	182.5	185.0	187.5	190.0

point of view

OBESITY: Is It a Disability?

There is no question that obesity can lead to health problems and difficulty performing activities of daily living. A person who is 50 to 100 kilograms overweight can have difficulty walking, running, getting out of a chair, and doing simple daily tasks. But does that mean that his or her level of obesity constitutes a disability? Although obesity was recently classified as a disease in the United States, it is generally not considered a disability under the federal Americans with Disabilities Act (ADA), which defines *disability* as "a physical or mental impairment that substantially limits one or more of the major life activities of [an] individual." To be covered by the ADA, a person who is obese must be at least 45 kilograms overweight or have a body mass index (BMI)

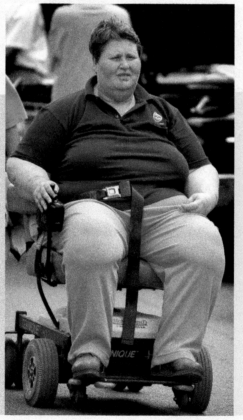

of over 40, as well as an underlying disorder that caused the obesity. These strict criteria mean that the ADA currently receives few complaints. However, some people believe obesity should be considered a disability that legally entitles individuals to health benefits and other accommodations. Other people believe that labelling obesity as a disability would add to its stigma and create more problems than it would solve.

In 2007, the Supreme Court of Canada ruled that disability is no longer predicated on no responsibility for the disability or an inability to change the circumstances of that disability. Thus under this ruling those considered to be obese (BMI of 30 or more) are considered to have a disability (Obesity Network of Canada, 2009).

ARGUMENTS FAVOURING DISABILITY STATUS FOR PEOPLE WHO ARE OBESE

○ Labelling obesity as a disability provides individuals who are obese with better medical insurance (more of an issue in the United States).

○ A disability label would protect the rights of individuals who are obese against discrimination based on their weight.

○ Obesity can involve physical disability: A person who is obese can have many related medical conditions including arthritis, elevated blood pressure, type 2 diabetes, diabetic-related vascular diseases, and a weakened cardiovascular system. All of these conditions can lead to the need for walkers, wheelchairs, and other mobility devices, as well as special health accommodations at home or in the workplace.

ARGUMENTS OPPOSING DISABILITY STATUS FOR PEOPLE WHO ARE OBESE

○ Doctors are worried that defining obesity as a disability would make them vulnerable to lawsuits from patients who are obese and do not want their weight discussed. The threat of such lawsuits would prevent doctors from discussing obesity with their patients and recommending specific actions (again, more of an issue in the United States).

○ Rather than labelling obesity as a disability and adding to its stigma, issues of unfair insurance or job practices could be handled with antidiscrimination laws.

○ Not all people who are obese are disabled by their weight, so labelling them as such would be discriminatory.

Dennis MacDonald/PhotoEdit

Where Do You Stand?

○ In your opinion, what positive results could come from classifying individuals who are obese as disabled?

○ What negative consequences do you foresee from classifying individuals who are obese as disabled?

○ How would you determine whether an individual is disabled because of his or her weight?

○ Are there legitimate situations where a person who is obese should be labelled as disabled?

○ Do you think labelling obesity as a disability would alter the way our society behaves toward and perceives individuals who are obese? If so, in what way?

Determining the Right Weight for You

The answer to whether you are at a healthy weight depends on your body structure and how your weight is distributed. Traditionally, people compared their weight to the range given on height-and-weight charts. These charts usually give the "ideal" weight for males and females of a given height and frame size. If you were above your ideal weight, you would then be classified as overweight.

More common today is to determine your weight status based on calculating your **BMI**. BMI (body mass index) is obtained by dividing your weight (in kilograms) by your height (in metres) squared. Weight should be taken without shoes or clothing, and height should be measured without shoes. Figure 6.2 can be used to determine your BMI and weight status (Health Canada, 2003). In general, a BMI below 18.5 is considered underweight. A BMI between 18.5 and 24.9 is considered weight appropriate. BMI values between 25.0 and 29.9 refer to overweight and are associated with increased health risk. Although not a measure of fatness per se, a BMI greater than 30 results in an "obese" classification because of the associated health risks found in the population at this level of BMI and greater. Further degrees of health risks are noted with BMIs above 30. Specifically, a BMI between 30.0 and 34.9 refers to Obese Class I with high health risk, a BMI between 35.0 and 39.9 refers to Obese Class II and is associated with a very high health risk, and a BMI greater than 40.0 is classified as Obese Class III with extremely high health risk.

What is the reason for the difference in acceptable fat levels between men and women (referred to in Table 6.1)? Much of it can be attributed to genetics and, more specifically, related to the natural structure of the female and male bodies and to sex hormones. Body composition is most often broken down into two main components: fat-free mass and fat mass (Malina, Bouchard, & Bar-Or, 2004). Fat-free mass is made up of all the body's components other than fat—that is, the structural and functional elements in cells, body water, muscle, bones; and other body organs such as the heart, liver, and kidneys. Compared with men, women have a lower ratio of fat-free mass to fat mass, in part due to the genetic differences in bone size and mass, muscle size, and other variables. Although there is a slight difference in body composition between boys and girls prior to the pubertal growth spurt, the differences exacerbate following it (Malina, Bourchard, & Bar-Or, 2004). Pubertal development leads to a substantive increase in fat-free mass in boys and in fat mass in girls. Women also experience greater weight and fat fluctuation due to hormonal changes, pregnancy, and menopause.

Body mass index (BMI) A relationship of weight to height.

FIGURE 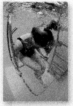 6.3

Body Fat Percentage Norms for Men and Women

Underwater (hydrostatic) weighing:
Measures the amount of water a person displaces when completely submerged. Fat tissue is less dense than muscle or bone, so body fat can be computed within a 2 to 3 percent margin of error by comparing weight underwater and out of water.

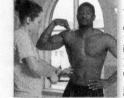

David Madison/Photographer's Choice/Getty Images

Skinfolds:
Involves "pinching" a person's fold of skin (with its underlying layer of fat) at various locations of the body. The fold is measured using a specially designed caliper. When performed by a skilled technician, it can estimate body fat with an error of 3 to 4 percent.

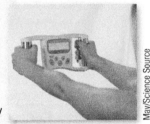

Gilles Daigle/PhotoCanada Moncton

Bioelectrical impedance analysis (BIA):
Involves sending a very low level of electrical current through a person's body. As lean body mass is made up of mostly water, the rate at which the electricity is conducted gives an indication of a person's lean body mass and body fat. Under the best circumstances, BIA can estimate body fat with an error of 3 to 4 percent.

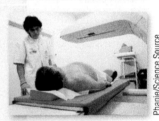

May/Science Source

Dual-energy X-ray absorptiometry (DXA):
The technology is based on using very-low-level X ray to differentiate between bone tissue, soft (or lean) tissue, and fat (or adipose) tissue. The margin of error for predicting body fat is 2 to 4 percent.

Phanie/Science Source

BOD POD:
Uses air displacement to measure body composition. This machine is a large, egg-shaped chamber made from fiberglass. The person being measured sits in the machine wearing a swimsuit. The door is closed and the machine measures how much air is displaced. That value is used to calculate body fat, with a 2 to 3 percent margin of error.

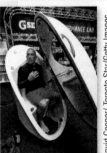

David Cooper/Toronto Star/Getty Images

Body fat is composed of two types: essential fat and storage fat. Essential fat is necessary for normal physiological functioning, such as nerve conduction. Essential fat makes up approximately 3 to 7 percent of total body weight in men and approximately 10 to 15 percent in women. Storage fat, which serves to insulate, pad, and protect the body from cold and trauma, makes up the remainder of our fat. It accounts for only a small percentage of total body weight for very lean people and between 5 and 25 percent of body weight for most healthy Canadian adults. Female body-builders, who are among the leanest of female athletes, may have a healthy body fat percentage in the range of 8 to 13 percent, nearly all of which is essential fat.

Similar to too much fat increasing your health risk, too little fat also can relate to poor health (Gronke et al., 2007). A minimal amount of fat is necessary for insulating the body, for cushioning between parts of the body and vital organs, and for maintaining several body functions. Although tremendous variation exists, it is generally suggested that in men this lower limit is approximately 3 to 4 percent and for women, 8 percent. Excessively low body fat in females may lead to amenorrhea or oligomenorrhea, a cessation or disruption of the menstrual cycle, respectively (Polotsky & Santero, 2010). The critical level of body fat necessary to maintain normal menstrual flow is believed to be between 8 and 13 percent, with exceptions to this rule given the many factors that affect the menstrual cycle. Under extreme circumstances, such as starvation diets and certain diseases, the body exhausts available fat reserves and begins breaking down muscle tissue in a last-ditch effort to obtain sufficient nourishment.

Assessing Your Body Fat Content

Since too little and too much body fat each pose a health risk, it may be important to determine an estimate of your body fat. How can it be measured? Body fat—or more correctly, body composition—can be estimated using several techniques. These techniques are far more in-depth than the simplicity of measuring height and weight as is done with height–weight charts and calculations of BMI. Cost and access are two factors to consider regarding the techniques available, particularly since some are relatively expensive and difficult to access. Another factor to consider is your reason for wanting to know your body fat content and whether or not it is essential for you to have a precise measure. At the most basic level, if your previously well-fitting jeans are now too tight, you know you have gained weight/fat and ought to take action to prevent further weight gain. Similarly, if your well-fitting jeans continue to fit well, you have maintained your weight. Or if your well-fitting jeans are a bit loose, you have lost weight and may need to take action to prevent further unneeded weight loss.

Although assessments of body composition generally quantify body weight into its basic components—that is, fat-free mass and fat mass (Malina, Bourchard, & Bar-Or, 2004)—estimates of body fat are considered most important. Further, keep in mind that with each of the techniques used to measure body composition,

there are limits to their accuracy, even when the technicians are skillful and well trained. Before agreeing to any procedure, be aware of the expense, risks, measurement error, and training/experiences of the technician. Further, consider what you will do with the value, once known, and if that value is actually needed for you to make healthier choices that influence your body composition

Dual-Energy X-Ray Absorptiometry

Dual-energy X-ray absorptiometry (DXA) measures bone mineral content and lean and fat tissue (Malina, Bourchard, & Bar-Or, 2004). This technique requires a low radiation exposure from a low-energy and high-energy photon beam. Based on appropriate computer algorithms and the amount of absorption of the photon beams by the atoms in bone mineral and soft tissues, an estimate of bone mineral, fat-free soft tissue, and fat tissue is made. A strength of the DXA method is that total body fat can be determined as well as regional body fat distribution. Given the technology and usefulness of the DXA, some consider it the most accurate or "gold standard" assessment of body composition.

Hydrostatic Weighing

Hydrostatic weighing was previously considered the gold standard for measuring body composition. This method measures the amount of water a person displaces when completely submerged. Because fat tissue has a lower density than muscle or bone tissue, body fat can be computed using a person's underwater and out-of-water weights once the density of the body is determined.

Air Displacement Plethysmography

Air displacement plethysmography (ADP) is based on the same premises as hydrostatic weighing; total body volume is measured—this time from air displacement—from which an estimate of body fat can be made. Estimates of total body volume (either in water or air) use the formula: density = mass ÷ volume (Malina, Bourchard, & Bar-Or, 2004). The major assumption and limitation of these two methods is that the density of fat and fat-free mass (fat-free mass being all components of the body except fat) is considered constant. The limitation, then, relates to bone mineral content and density, which is known to vary throughout the life cycle.

Dual-energy X-ray absorptiometry (DXA) A method of body composition assessment in which estimates are made of bone mineral content and lean and fat mass.

Hydrostatic weighing A method of determining body fat by estimating total body volume from the amount of water displaced when a person is completely submerged.

Air displacement plethysmography (ADP) A method used to determine body fat from estimates of total body volume from the amount of air displaced

Skinfold Measurements

A commonly used method to estimate body fat is **skinfold measurements**. In this procedure, a person grasps folds of skin and the underlying tissue with the thumb and index finger and then a specially calibrated instrument called a "skinfold" caliper is applied to take the measurement. The eight sites most commonly measured on the right side of the body are the triceps (back of the arm), biceps (front of the arm), subscapular (on the back), iliac crest (on the side of the body—near the "love handles"), supraspinale (along the front of the body over the hip), abdominal (next to the umbilicus—belly button), front thigh (middle of the upper leg), and medial calf (middle, inside of the lower leg). In the hands of trained technicians, this procedure can be fairly accurate. However, the fatter a person is, there is more likelihood of measurement error. Also, most skinfold calipers do not expand far enough to obtain measurements from the moderately obese (between 20 and 40 percent fat) or morbidly obese (more than 40 percent fat). Once these sites are measured, formulas are used to predict total body fat (Durnin & Womersley, 1974; Jackson & Pollock, 1978, 1980; Sloan & Weir, 1970). Caution is warranted in using these formulas as they were primarily developed on young, white, healthy males.

An alternative to predicting percentage of body fat from skinfold measurements is to simply total them. In this way a "sum of skinfolds" allows for comparison of "before" and "after" measurements. Since approximately 50 percent of body fat lies below the skin (that is, as subcutaneous fat), a loss in total sum of skinfolds indicates a loss of total body fat. Similarly, a gain in sum of skinfolds indicates a gain in total body fat.

Waist Circumference

Abdominal body fat can be estimated from **waist circumference**. A simple measuring tape is used to take the girth, or circumference, measurement at the superior border or top of the iliac crest or hip bones. Regardless of where measured (for example, at the smallest point of the torso, at the level of the umbilicus [that is, belly button], or the top of the hip bones), a larger waist circumference is associated with greater health risk (Jacobs et al., 2010). Specifically, a waist circumference greater than 102 centimetres in men and 88 centimetres in women indicates increased risk of heart disease, type 2 diabetes,

Skinfold measurements A method of assessing body fat where folds of skin and the underlying fat tissue are measured with skinfold calipers.

Waist circumference A method of assessing abdominal fat where a measuring tape assesses the girth or circumference at the top of the iliac crest.

Bioelectrical impedance analysis (BIA) A technique of body fat assessment in which the resistance to a weak electrical current is measured.

metabolic syndrome, hypertension, and hyperlipidemia (Flint et al., 2010; Reeder et al., 1997).

Bioelectrical Impedance Analysis

Another method of determining body fat percentage, **bioelectrical impedance analysis (BIA)**, involves sending a weak electric current through the body. The premise for this technique is based on the greater electrolyte and water content of fat free mass versus fat mass (Malina, Bourchard, & Bar-Or, 2004). The amount of resistance to the current, along with the person's age, sex, and other physical characteristics, are then fed into a computer that uses a special formula to determine the total amount of fat-free mass. Fat mass is deduced and a percentage of total body fat determined. In recent years, this technique has increased in use, likely because of its convenience, low cost, noninvasiveness, and quick estimate of body fat. It is important to note that for more accurate assessments when using this technique, the body should be normally hydrated because even small fluctuations in body water content alter the assessment. Even with adequate hydration and nutritional status, significant error can result in body composition estimates from BIA.

MANAGING YOUR WEIGHT

At some point in your life, you are likely to decide you need to do something about your weight. You might choose to go on a diet, with initially successful results, but not likely a long-term weight loss. The problem is that dieting, or reducing your calorie intake, is considered helpful only for the short term, not permanently. Even if combined with increased exercise or physical activity, the change is still viewed as temporary—a diet that you will go on until XX weight is lost, or you head south for a vacation. What is needed instead is a lifetime approach to eating well, being physically active, and managing your behaviours around food, physical activity, and sedentary activities. This approach is not a quick fix, nor simple to accomplish. It takes time and effort as well as careful planning and adjusting for our cultural reality.

Keeping Weight Loss in Perspective

As mentioned previously, it is often believed that losing weight is simple: you just need to expend more calories than you consume. Putting this principle into practice, however, is far from simple given our cultural attitudes and behaviours toward food, physical activity, and sedentary behaviours. More specifically, to keep your weight and potential for weight loss in perspective, you need a better understanding of how, where, why, what, and when you eat and how, where, why, what, and when you are—or are not—physically active. Other factors are involved too—factors such as stress, food availability and accessibility, depression, and sleep. To reach and maintain the weight that is right for you—the weight at which you will be most healthy—you need to develop a lifelong approach to healthy eating, physical activity, and sedentary behaviours. Your eating habits should reflect a lifetime approach to eating well, something that happens over days, weeks, and months and is not based on what you eat or do not eat one meal at a time. It is important that your approach is not to go "on" a diet, where you eat well for a short time, because then you will eventually go back "off" your diet. Similarly, your approach to being physically active must also be for your lifetime—a choice to be physically active every day, not just for a short time until your graduation or spring break vacation, but because it is something you should do on a daily basis, while recognizing that there will be days when you will be more or less physically active.

More recently, we have become aware that for overall health, we must also consider the amount of time spent in sedentary activities (DeNoon, 2010). When you are sedentary for more than six hours per day, regardless of meeting the recommended guidelines for physical activity, you are at greater health risk than if you sat for less than three hours (DeNoon, 2010). When sedentary, your metabolism slows, particularly when you watch TV. Thus, it is prudent when sedentary, such as when studying or writing papers, to make the effort to get up and move at least once each hour, even if it is just to stand up and stretch—though a five to ten minute walk break would be better. In regards to weight management, you should also manage the amount of sleep you get. Recent research indicates that people who are sleep deprived eat more than those who sleep for longer periods of times (Tremblay & Chaput, 2008). The mechanism for the greater caloric input may relate to the hormones that regulate hunger and satiety. When sleep deprived, as discussed later in this chapter, the regulation of these hormones is out of balance with a greater release of ghrelin, the hormone that stimulates appetite, and reduced release of leptin, the hormone that signals we are full or have eaten enough (Tremblay & Chaput, 2008).

What Is a Calorie?

A calorie is a unit of measurement that indicates the amount of energy obtained from a particular food. A half of a kilogram of body fat contains approximately 3500 calories (Thompson, Manore, & Sheeshka, 2007). So, each time you consume 3500 calories more than your body needs, you gain 0.5 kilogram (or, roughly, one pound). Conversely, each time your body expends 3500 calories more than it takes in, you lose 0.5 kilograms. If you add a 375 mL can of regular pop (140 calories) to your daily caloric intake and make no other changes to your dietary intake or physical activity, you would gain 0.5 kilogram in approximately 25 days (3500 calories ÷ 140 calories/day = 25 days). Conversely, if you walked for half an hour each day at a pace of 9 minutes per kilometre (172 calories is expended), you would lose 0.5 kilogram in about 20 days (3500 calories ÷ 172 calories/day = 20.3 days), again assuming you make no other changes to your dietary intake or physical activity habits.

Physical Activity

Most of your daily calorie expenditures occur as a result of your **resting metabolic rate (RMR)**. RMR is greater than BMR (or **basal metabolic rate**, which is the amount of energy your body requires at complete rest; this will be discussed at greater length later in the chapter). RMR includes BMR plus any additional energy expended through daily sedentary activities, such as food digestion, sitting, studying, or standing.

Exercise metabolic rate (EMR) and the **Thermic Effect of Food (TEF)** account for your remaining caloric needs. EMR refers to the energy expenditure as a result of physical activity and is quite variable, representing 20 to 35 percent of our caloric needs (Thompson, Manore, & Sheeshka, 2007). For most of you, this caloric expenditure comes in the form of light to moderate intensity physical activities, such as walking to class, climbing stairs, doing the dishes, running the vacuum, and doing the laundry. If you increase the level and intensity of your physical activity to moderate or vigorous, your EMR can contribute substantially more to your energy needs. The TEF refers to the energy expended eating and drinking (Thompson, Manore, & Sheeshka, 2007). The digestion, absorption, transportation, metabolization, and storage of nutrients require about 5 to 10 percent of the energy content of the food or drink consumed (Thompson, Manore, & Sheeshka, 2007).

Resting metabolic rate (RMR) The energy expenditure of the body while at rest, which includes basal metabolic rate (the metabolic rate of the body at complete rest) plus the energy required by sedentary activities, such as food digestion, sitting, studying, or standing.

Basal metabolic rate (BMR) The energy expenditure of the body under resting conditions at normal room temperature.

Exercise metabolic rate (EMR) The energy expenditure of physical activity.

Thermic Effect of Food (TEF) The energy required to digest, absorb, transport, metabolize, and store nutrients.

Increasing BMR, RMR, or EMR levels leads to a greater caloric requirement for weight maintenance. An increase in the intensity, frequency, and time or duration of your daily physical activities will have a significant impact on your total calorie expenditure and ability to manage your weight. It may even lead to weight loss, should you not alter your caloric intake. Current recommendations indicate that at least 60 minutes of moderate-intensity physical activity each day are required for weight management (Ontario Ministry of Health, n.d.). Note that this recommendation is different than the physical activity recommendations in Chapter 4, where a minimum 150 minutes of moderate or more intense physical activity are advocated per week for overall health benefits. Thus, preventing weight gain may actually require a higher level of physical activity. Similarly, to achieve weight loss, a higher level of physical activity may be needed. For weight management, emphasis should be placed on cardiorespiratory and strength-related physical activities. Cardiorespiratory activities, such as brisk walking, swimming, cycling, jogging, and so on, elevate EMR and RMR during the activity and for several hours afterwards, with a positive impact on caloric requirements. Resistance training or other activities such as yoga, tai chi, and others that involve core body training with an emphasis on building strength also have a positive impact on EMR and RMR. The impact on EMR is considerably less than cardiorespiratory training; however, the impact on RMR due to increased muscle mass is considerable.

Physical activity makes a greater contribution to EMR when larger muscle groups are used. The energy spent on physical activity includes the energy used to move the body's muscles—the muscles of the arms, back, abdomen, legs, and so on—and the extra energy required to increase heartbeat, respiration rate, blood pressure, body cooling, and so on. The number of calories expended depends on three factors:

1. the amount of muscle mass being moved
2. the amount of weight being moved
3. the amount of time the activity takes

For example, an activity involving the arms and the legs (e.g., running) burns more calories than one involving only the legs (e.g., cycling), an activity performed by a heavy person burns more calories than one performed by a lighter person, and an activity performed for 40 minutes requires twice as much energy as the same activity performed by the same person for 20 minutes.

Is Dieting Healthy?

The ultimate goal of a weight-loss program should be improved quality of life and lifetime weight maintenance (Robison et al., 1993). Weight goals should be

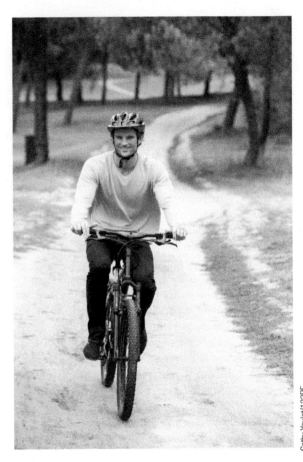

Cathy Yeulet/123RF

Engaging in regular physical activity is important for many reasons, including enhancing the 'caloric output' side of the energy balance equation.

set to reduce health risks and address medical problems and help you improve your ability to perform daily tasks without undue stress and strain—rather than to achieve an "ideal" weight or shape. In addition, weight-loss programs that promote qualitative, rather than quantitative, changes in food intake improve health and long-term weight maintenance and are more easily sustained than those that force you to severely restrict intake of calories or specific foods (Robison et al., 1993). In other words, qualitative changes such as reducing fat intake and increasing vegetable, fruit, and fibre intake, rather than simply eating less and eliminating favourite foods, is more likely to be adhered to in the short and long term. Most weight-loss programs fail to follow these basic premises. What happens when you get caught up in the false promises of "lose weight fast and furiously?" Some of the concerns are listed below:

- dieting to lose weight may be more harmful than helpful in promoting physiological and psychological health (French & Jeffery, 1994)
- because dieting only rarely results in long-term weight loss, the physiological and psychological

stress, damage to self-esteem, and other emotional disturbances are without purpose (Wilson, 1993)

- dieting causes repeated cycles of weight loss and regain, changes in metabolic rates, increased risk for cardiovascular problems, and other conditions adverse to health (Lissner et al., 1991)
- dieting contributes to the development of eating disorders such as anorexia and bulimia nervosa, and compulsive eating or binge eating disorder (Horm & Anderson, 1993)

Most health authorities recommend that, rather than going on a diet, a person should adopt a lifetime approach to healthy eating, physical activity, and sedentary activities aimed at enhancing metabolic rates and maintaining muscle mass.

Improving Your Eating Habits

Before you can change a given behaviour, you must first determine the how, what, where, when, and why of it. Your eating is influenced by a number of things including individual and environmental determinants (Raine, 2005). Individual determinants include our physiological state (that is, whether or not we are hungry), food preferences, nutritional knowledge, perceptions of healthy eating, and psychological factors. Environmental factors include the interpersonal environment created by our family and peers; the physical environment, which determines food accessibility and availability; the economic and social environment; and the cultural milieu surrounding food choices. Further, food policy has an overarching influence on the individual and environmental factors influencing our eating behaviours.

You might assess your eating behaviours using a chart that identifies where, what, when, how much, why, with whom, as well as other activities you do while eating (watching television, reading, or something else). If you keep a detailed log each day for a week, you will discover useful clues about what in your environment or in your emotional makeup relates to your eating habits. Typically, these "triggers" centre on issues related to everyday living rather than on real hunger/need to eat. As you record this information, your reasons for eating often become apparent. You might discover that you eat compulsively when reacting to stress or when there are problems in your relationships. It may also be the smell of a particular food (for example, popcorn) or a routine (for example, eating while studying) that causes you to eat, rather than hunger itself.

Once you recognize the factors related to your eating, remove the triggers or substitute other activities so that you develop healthier eating behaviours. Some

suggestions to help you manage your eating better are included below. More suggestions are included at the end of the chapter.

1. When eating, turn off all distractions, including the television, radio, and your computer. You should put your cellphone away too.
2. Include physical activity in your breaks. (Though not related to dietary intake, physical activity may take the place of "eating for something to do.")
3. Instead of gulping your food, chew slowly, putting your fork down between each bite. Speak with those around you.
4. Instead of eating by the clock, eat when you are hungry. The only meal that does not necessarily follow this rule is breakfast. It is important to break your fast each day to stimulate your metabolism or RMR.
5. Eat frequently throughout the day—three smaller meals per day plus snacks—rather than loading up at one meal and skipping others. This too boosts your RMR.
6. If you find that you generally eat all that is on a plate, use smaller plates, or serve smaller portions. Serve your plate at the counter/stove rather than having pots/bowls on the table where you are eating. You then have to consciously choose to have seconds and make more of an effort to get them.
7. If you find that you are continually seeking your favourite foods, buy them in smaller quantities, serve them in smaller portions, and store them in an inconvenient spot. It is okay to have these 'extras' provided you have them in smaller quantities and preferably not on a daily basis.
8. Eat breakfast every day.
9. Replace soft drinks and other high-fat, high calorie fluids with water.

Choosing to Eat Well

Once you learn about the factors that influence your eating, if you plan for your success and make choices accordingly, you are on your way to successful weight maintenance. Registered dietitians, holistic physicians (only holistic physicians have strong backgrounds in nutrition, which includes some MDs), health educators, exercise physiologists with nutritional backgrounds, and other health professionals can provide reliable information regarding dietary intake should you choose to seek an expert's opinion. Avoid quick weight-loss programs that promise miracle results. The majority of these programs are expensive, and most people regain their lost weight soon after completing them. Any diet that requires radical behaviour changes or cannot be followed for a lifetime is doomed to fail. Dietary plans that do not ask you to sacrifice what you enjoy and that allow you to make choices are usually the most successful. A reliable, practical, and useful tool to help you to choose to eat well is *Eating Well with Canada's Food Guide* (Health Canada, n.d.), which is described in detail in Chapter 5.

"Miracle" Diets

Fasting, starvation diets, and other forms of **very low-calorie diets (VLCDs)** are related to significant health risks (National Institutes of Health, 2008). Typically, when you deprive your body of food for prolonged periods, it makes adjustments to save you from inevitable organ shutdown. First, it depletes its energy reserves to maintain its supply of glucose. One of the first reserves the body turns to is lean body mass. When this occurs, you lose weight rapidly because significant water is lost as well. Over time, the body begins to run out of liver tissue, heart muscle, blood, and so on, as these readily available substances are used to supply energy. Only after the readily available proteins from these sources are depleted will your body begin to use fat reserves. In this process, known as **ketosis**, the body adapts to prolonged fasting or carbohydrate deprivation by converting body fat to ketones, which can be used as fuel for some brain cells. About 10 days after the typical adult begins a complete fast, the body has used most of its energy stores and death can occur (Kaye, Fudge, & Paulus, 2009).

In VLCDs, powdered formulas are usually given to patients under medical supervision (National Institutes of Health, 2008). These formulas range from 400 to 700 calories plus vitamin and mineral supplements. Although these diets may be beneficial for people who face severe threats to their health complicated by their obesity and who have failed at conventional weight-loss methods, they should never be undertaken without close medical supervision. Problems associated with fasting, VLCDs, and other forms of severe calorie deprivation include blood sugar imbalances, cold intolerance, constipation, decreased BMR, dehydration, diarrhea, emotional problems, fatigue, headaches, heart irregularity, ketosis, kidney infections and failure, loss of lean body tissue, weakness, and potential weight gain due to the yo-yo effect and other problems (Baker et al., 2012; National Institute of Health, 2008).

Very-low-calorie diets (VLCDs) Diets with caloric value of 400 to 700 calories per day.

Ketosis A condition in which the body adapts to prolonged fasting or carbohydrate deprivation by converting body fat to ketones, which can be used as fuel for some brain activity.

Low-Carbohydrate Diets

Over the years, various forms of low-carbohydrate diets have attracted millions of people with promises of quick, substantial weight loss. Bookstores struggle to keep the latest editions of low-carbohydrate diet and recipe books on their shelves. Restaurants have "low-carb" items on their menus, and there is a multimillion dollar industry of low-carb food products. In this 'low-carb' craze, you are led to believe that if you eliminate nearly all of the bread, pasta, sweets, and high-carbohydrate foods from your diet, eat red meat and other high-protein and high-fat foods until you are satisfied, you will lose weight.

Although many health professionals criticize low-carb diets as dangerous, ineffective, and unhealthy, several well-designed clinical trials indicated that low-carbohydrate diets were as good as—and, in many cases, better than—low-fat diets in leading to weight loss (Foster et al., 2003; Samaha et al., 2003). In these studies, more people complied with the low-carbohydrate than the low-fat diets, and, although they ate more fat, they did not experience the expected harmful changes in blood cholesterol (Foster et al., 2003; Samaha et al., 2003).

However, these benefits were short term, and reports of problems with low-carb diets eventually surfaced. Another study found that although low-carbohydrate diets resulted in weight loss, it was the total caloric reduction and the duration of the reduction that caused the loss, not the reduction in carbohydrate intake per se (Bravata et al., 2003). The take-home message was that any low-calorie diet that a person can stay on long enough will have similar results. Further in this study, people had difficulty complying with the rigid dietary requirements (Bravata et al., 2003). When they lost weight, they gained it back nearly as quickly as they had lost it. People with diabetes had problems because whole grains, beans, and other fibre-rich foods were not allowed. And, rather than remembering to cut back on saturated fats, people were eating bacon and eggs, huge steaks, and feeling good about the guilt-free diet.

A major problem with these low-carbohydrate diets is that they suggest that all carbohydrates are bad for you (Conner & Conner, 2004). In other words, these low-carbohydrate diets do not account for the vast difference in nutrient value among carbohydrates and their glycemic index. The glycemic index provides a ranking of foods according to how quickly their sugars are released into the bloodstream. The body converts a food's sugars into glucose, which is released slowly or rapidly into the bloodstream. Insulin is secreted to counter glucose levels and return the body to healthy levels. The amount of insulin a food triggers is referred to as *glycemic load,* which considers both a food's glycemic index and how much carbohydrate the food delivers at one time in a single serving.

Most vegetables, fruits, beans, and whole grains have low glycemic loads; their sugars enter the bloodstream gradually and trigger only a moderate rise in insulin. Sugar on its own causes insulin levels to rise more abruptly, triggering a chain of reactions that ultimately make you sluggish, bloated, and hungry, resulting in eating more and continuing the cycle. Ultimately, these high insulin levels can lead to diabetes.

To help you choose well regarding glycemic load, try following these general guidelines:

- **Choose plants.** Pick the fruit rather than its sugar-laden juice counterpart. Eating the skin of apples adds fibre and slows the entry of glucose into the bloodstream. If you eat potatoes, eat them with the skin on and cut back on other starches. Instead of potatoes and corn, try sweet potatoes and yams.

- **Forgo meat in favour of beans.** It is not necessary to cut all meat-based protein from your diet. However, when you eat meat, opt for the leaner cuts and choose poultry over pork or beef. Learn to cook and flavour beans; they are high in protein and other nutrients and have very little effect on blood sugar and insulin.

- **Go nuts several times a week.** Almonds, hazelnuts, peanuts, pecans, and others are healthy low-carbohydrate alternatives to snacking on chips and desserts made from white flour. They are not calorie free, though, so manage your intake based on your calorie needs.

- **Mix your carbs with other foods.** Eating carbohydrates with other foods such as monounsaturated oils (olive or canola) can slow the rate of carbohydrate absorption. Milk or yogurt with cereal is one example; bananas and cottage cheese in cereal is another.

- **Make whole-grain breads a staple.** Avoid white bread and look for brown breads with 100 percent whole wheat or other grains. Consider options such as brown rice and whole-wheat pizza dough and pasta. These are good choices for lowering your blood sugar.

- **Participate regularly in physical activity.** Most people would be shocked if they ate a normal meal, measured their blood sugar, then noted how dramatically their blood sugars go down after a 30-minute walk. It may seem simple, but one of the best ways to keep yourself healthy and still consume the carbs you want is through physical activity.

Trying to Gain Weight

For a variety of metabolic, hereditary, psychological, and other reasons, you may not be able to gain weight no matter how hard you try. If gaining weight is difficult for you, you must determine why you have difficulty—just like someone who has difficulty managing his or her weight. Once you have determined your how, why, where, what, and when of your dietary intake, there are several things you can do:

- Monitor your physical activity. It is important to also consider incidental movements in your monitoring (that is, active transportation, fidgeting behaviours, and so on) as these contribute to caloric needs as well. Keep a careful record of calories expended; perhaps you are not eating enough to compensate.

- Eat more. Eat more often. It is possible that you are not eating enough calories to support your body's needs. In addition to EMR, you may genetically have a higher RMR. Eat more frequently, spend more time eating, and eat high-calorie, nutrient-dense foods first if you tend to fill up fast. Take time to shop and to cook, and eat slowly. Make your sandwiches with extra-thick slices of bread and add more filling such as peanut butter, cream cheese, or cheese. Eat second helpings whenever possible and eat high-calorie, nutrient-dense snacks during the day.

- Drink more of your calories; instead of water, choose milk (chocolate and/or 2% white milk) or juice.

- Try to relax. Many people who struggle to gain weight tend to be fidgety and are continuously on the go. Slow down and try to quiet your behaviours.

RISK FACTORS FOR OBESITY

It would seem that the cause of obesity is simple: when you take in more calories than you expend, you gain weight—most often in the form of fat. If you do this frequently enough, you will become obese. If we know what the cause is, we should be able to offer a simple solution, right?

Wrong. Although the calorie balance equation (that is, if calories in equals calories out, there is no weight gain) explanation of weight management is valid, it offers only two simple reasons for a person's weight gain: we eat too much and do too little. Although ultimately that may be true, it is an oversimplification of our eating, physical activity, and sedentary behaviours. In other words, it does not include the many other sociocultural factors surrounding dietary intake and our physical activity and sedentary behaviours that contribute to excessive and less healthy food consumption, low levels of physical activity, and lengths of time being sedentary. It also fails to answer many other critical questions. If we know that eating too much will cause us to gain weight, why do we continue to eat so much? If we know we should be more physically active, why don't we simply get out there and "do it?" If we know we should sit less, why don't we get up and move? Is there a metabolic explanation for obesity? Why is there limited success for long-term weight loss from dieting?

Heredity and Genetic Factors

Are some people born to be fat? Many factors influence why one person becomes obese and another remains thin; genes seem to interact with many of these factors. More than 250 gene markers have been identified as related to obesity in more than 400 studies (Rankinen et al., 2006).

Body Type and Genes

In some animal species, the shape and size of the individual's body is largely determined by the shape and size of its parents' bodies. Heredity plays a more subtle role than most think. It is argued that obesity has a strong genetic determinant (it tends to run in families) with 40 percent of children with one obese parent and 80 percent of children with two obese parents likely to also be obese (Stunkard, 1985). However, it is difficult to distinguish between the genetic and environmental contributors to obesity in these children. Does the child become obese because his or her parents are? Or does the child become obese because he or she eats and participates in physical activity and sedentary behaviours as his or her parents do? In other words, the question remains, is obesity a result of nature or nurture?

Obesity Genes?

Although a genetic link to obesity may exist, the reality is that what has been found only accounts for 1 percent of the variance noted (Hofker & Wijmenga, 2009). Rather than inheriting a particular body type that predisposes us to become overweight or obese, it may be that our genes predispose us toward certain satiety and feeding behaviours. This "I need to eat" gene may account for up to one-third of your risk for obesity (Rankinen et al., 2006). The most promising candidate is the GAD2 gene. For some individuals, a variation in this gene increases the production of a chemical that boosts appetite and signals a person to eat (Rankinen et al., 2006). Another gene

Adaptive thermogenesis Theoretical mechanism by which the brain regulates metabolic activity according to caloric intake.

getting a lot of attention is an Ob gene (for obesity) that is believed to disrupt the body's "I've had enough to eat" signalling system and may prompt individuals to keep eating past the point of being comfortably full. Research on Pima Indians, a group with an estimated 75 percent obesity rate and 90 percent rate of overweight, points to an Ob gene that is a "thrifty gene." It is theorized that because the ancestors of the Pima Indians struggled through centuries of famine, during which the Ob gene prompted them to eat as much as possible when food was available and to conserve when not, their BMR slowed, which allowed them to store fat. Survivors may have passed their genes onto their descendants, which may explain their lower metabolic rates and tendency toward obesity today (Loos & Bouchard, 2003).

Endocrine Influences: The Hungry Hormones

Over the years, many people attributed obesity to problems with their thyroid gland and resultant hormonal imbalances. They believed that an underactive thyroid impeded their ability to burn calories. Theories abound concerning the mechanisms that regulate food intake. Some sources indicate that the hypothalamus (the part of the brain that regulates appetite) closely monitors levels of certain nutrients in the blood. When these levels begin to fall, the brain signals us to eat. In people who are obese, it is possible that the monitoring system does not work as well and that the cues to eat are more frequent and intense than in people of a healthy weight. Other sources indicate that people who are at a healthy weight may send more effective messages to the hypothalamus. This concept, known as **adaptive thermogenesis**, states that some people can consume extra calories without gaining weight because the appetite centre of their brains speeds up metabolic activity to compensate for the increased consumption. Research indicates that less than 2 percent of the population that is obese can trace their weight and/or fat problems to their thyroid or metabolic or hormonal imbalances (Mayo Clinic, 2005).

Recognizing the role of the hormones involved in energy regulation can help you to better understand your hunger, satiety, and eating behaviours. These hormones include acylated ghrelin, leptin, and insulin, among others (Hagobian & Braun, 2010). Ghrelin is believed to be involved in appetite stimulation. Leptin is believed to be involved with the satiety signal from the brain, which tells us to stop eating because we are full. Given their effect on appetite, energy intake, and energy expenditure, these hormones are classified as energy-regulating hormones and are further classified as episodic or short term and tonic or long term

(Hagobian & Braun, 2010). Ghrelin is classified as episodic given its influence on appetite, while leptin and insulin are tonic in that they regulate overall energy balance over days and weeks rather than from meal to meal (Hagobian & Braun, 2010).

Leptin and ghrelin are believed to be influenced by lack of sleep. More specifically, fewer hours of sleep in standardized experimental sleeping conditions resulted in an increase in hunger accompanied by a decrease in leptin and an increase in ghrelin (Tremblay & Chaput, 2008). In other words, your appetite is likely to be stimulated and your ability to recognize that you have had enough to eat is reduced when you do not have enough sleep.

Another hormone involved in slowing the passage of food through the intestines is called GLP-1. GLP-1 may stimulate insulin production, a key factor in preventing and controlling type 2 diabetes and obesity (Williams, Baskin, & Schwartz, 2006). It is further speculated that leptin and GLP-1 play complementary roles in weight control, where leptin regulates body weight and fat levels over the long term, calling on the fast-acting appetite suppressants GLP-1 when needed.

Hunger, Appetite, and Satiety

Scientists distinguish between **hunger**, an inborn physiological response to nutritional needs, and **appetite**, a learned response to food tied to an emotional or psychological craving for food often unrelated to nutritional need. It is possible that some people who are obese may be more likely than others at a healthy weight to satisfy their appetite and eat for reasons other than nutrition.

In some instances, the problem with overconsumption may be more related to **satiety** than to appetite or hunger. People generally feel satiated, or full, when they have satisfied their nutritional needs and their stomach signals "no more." For undetermined reasons, some people who are obese may not feel full until much later than people who are at a healthy weight.

Developmental Factors

Some people who are obese may have an excessive number of fat cells. **Hyperplasia**, which refers to an increase in the number of cells, normally occurs during specific periods of the growth process (Malina, Bouchard, & Bar-Or, 2004). Fat cells normally only increase in number during infancy and the rapid growth period of puberty. Fat cells may also increase in number when individuals are under chronic positive energy balance (that is, they continuously consume more calories than they expend) and their current fat cells are "full." Fat cells also have the ability to increase in size. This process is called **hypertrophy**, and can occur at any time

FIGURE 6.4
The figure depicts one person with various levels of fat. Note that the number of fat cells remains constant but the cells' size decreases.

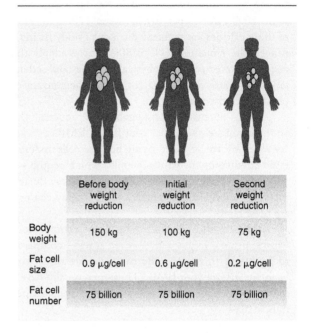

	Before body weight reduction	Initial weight reduction	Second weight reduction
Body weight	150 kg	100 kg	75 kg
Fat cell size	0.9 μg/cell	0.6 μg/cell	0.2 μg/cell
Fat cell number	75 billion	75 billion	75 billion

in childhood, adolescence, and adulthood—if calorie intake exceeds calorie output. Thus, fat gain is tied to the number of fat cells in the body (during infancy and puberty) and the capacity of the fat cells to increase in size (childhood, adolescence, and adulthood).

An adult of average weight and fat levels has approximately 30 to 50 billion fat cells (Malina, Bouchard, & Bar-Or, 2004), while an adult who is moderately obese has about 60 billion to 100 billion, and an adult who is extremely obese may have as many as 200 billion fat cells. The size of fat cells in a young adult of a healthy weight is about 80 to 100 micrometres (μm) (see Figure 6.4).

People who are obese and have a large number of fat cells may have difficulty attaining long-term fat loss because there may be a trigger released once they have substantially decreased the size of each fat cell, resulting in an increase in appetite.

Hunger An inborn physiological response to nutritional needs.

Appetite A learned response tied to an emotional or psychological craving for food often unrelated to nutritional need.

Satiety The feeling of fullness or satisfaction after eating.

Hyperplasia An increase in the number of cells.

Hypertrophy An increase in the size of cells.

Metabolic Rates and Weight

Even at rest, your body needs a certain amount of energy. As previously noted, the amount of energy your body requires at complete rest is called basal metabolic rate (BMR). In physically active individuals, about 60 to 70 percent of all the calories consumed support basal metabolism, which provides the energy (that is, calories) needed for bodily functions such as heartbeat, breathing, maintaining body temperature, and so on. So if you consume 2000 calories per day, between 1200 and 1400 of those calories are required for regular body maintenance. The remaining 600 to 800 calories supply the energy required for your physical activities and sedentary behaviours. The key factor here is the amount of physical activity you do.

BMR fluctuates considerably. In general, the younger you are, the higher your BMR. BMR is greatest when we are younger, partly because cells undergo rapid subdivision in young people, which requires a good deal of energy. Thus, BMR is highest during infancy, puberty, and pregnancy, when bodily changes are most rapid.

BMR is also influenced by body composition. Muscle tissue is highly active—even at rest—compared to fat tissue. In essence, the more muscle tissue you have, the greater your BMR. Thus, men usually have a higher BMR than women, because they have a greater muscle mass.

Age is another factor that affects BMR. After the age of 30, BMR slows down by about 1 to 2 percent per year. Therefore, people over 30 commonly find that they either have to eat less or do more physical activity to maintain their body weight. "Middle-aged spread," a reference to the tendency to gain weight or fat after the age of 30, is partly related to this change. A slower BMR, coupled with an inclination to be less physically active, puts many middle-aged people's weight over healthy limits.

In addition, your body has a number of self-protective mechanisms that signal BMR to speed up or slow down. For example, when you have a fever, the energy needs of your cells increase, and this increased activity generates heat and increases your BMR. In starvation situations, your body protects itself by slowing your BMR to conserve energy. Thus, if you choose to eat a very low-calorie diet, your body will "reset" your BMR to a lower rate. **Yo-yo dieting**, which involves repeatedly gaining and losing weight, lowers BMR in the process. When you begin to eat again after weight loss, your BMR is set lower, making it almost certain that you will regain the weight lost—especially if your previous dietary habits are resumed. After repeated cycles of such dieting/regaining, you will find it increasingly difficult to lose weight and increasingly easy to regain it, and are

Yo-yo diet Cycles in which people repeatedly gain and lose weight. This lowers their BMR, and typically leads to weight gain.

Setpoint theory A theory that suggests fat storage is determined by a thermostatic mechanism in the body that acts to maintain a specific amount of body fat.

likely to become fatter with each subsequent attempt. Besides an increase in fat, weight-cycling may also have a negative effect on your risk for heart disease and type 2 diabetes. Research indicated that middle-aged men who maintained a steady weight (even if overweight) had a lower risk of heart attack than men whose weight cycled in a yo-yo pattern (Brownell, 1993). Furthermore, it was noted that smaller, maintained weight losses were more beneficial for reducing cardiovascular risk than larger, poorly maintained weight losses (Brownell, 1993).

Related to metabolic rate is a highly controversial theory called the **setpoint theory**. It states that your body has a setpoint for weight at which it is programmed to be comfortable (Speakman et al., 2011). In other words, if your setpoint is 70 kilograms, you will gain and lose weight fairly easily within a given range (usually within 1 to 2 kg) around that setpoint. Can you change this predetermined setpoint? Proponents of this theory argue that it is possible to raise your setpoint over time by continually gaining weight and failing to engage in regular physical activity. Conversely, reducing caloric intake and being physically active over a long period of time may slowly decrease your setpoint.

Psychosocial Factors

The relationship of weight problems to deeply rooted emotional insecurities, needs, and wants remains uncertain. Food is often used inappropriately as a reward for good behaviour in childhood. As adults face various stresses in their lives, food is often also used as a comforting mechanism. Again, the research underlying this theory is controversial. What is certain is that in Canada, eating tends to be a focal point of our lives—a major part of our socialization; a social ritual associated with companionship, celebration, and enjoyment.

Eating Cues

At least one major factor in your thinking about food is the pressure placed on you by the highly sophisticated, heavily advertised "eating" campaigns launched by the food industry. Although lower-fat, lower-calorie options are available at most, if not all, fast-food restaurants, you still have the gauntlet of starchy, meaty delights and tasty high-fat fries to choose from. Food-related messages permeate the media, particularly for children and youth (Wadsworth & Berenbaum, 2001; Wadsworth & MacQuarrie, 2002). Compared to the foods recommended in *Eating Well with Canada's Food Guide,* most advertised foods are lower in nutrient density, fibre, and complex carbohydrates and higher in fat, sodium, simple carbohydrates (i.e., sugar), caffeine, and alcohol.

A large percentage of the foods Canadians eat are convenience foods or come from fast-food restaurants. We eat at fast-food restaurants for a number of reasons, including the relatively low cost and the perceived time saved. It should be kept in mind however that: (1) fast food is typically high in calories, fat, sodium, and simple carbohydrates; (2) it tends to all be eaten, even though portions are often much bigger than needed; and (3) it tends to be eaten quickly, so there is not enough time for the "I am full" signal to be acknowledged before the last bite of food is consumed (Elmer-Dewitt, 1995). This is a particular problem for post-secondary students, who encounter fast-food restaurants on campus, in addition to the all-you-can-eat buffets at food hall, combined with a perceived time shortage to focus on a sit-down, healthier, family meal.

Dietary Myth and Misperception

You have likely heard someone say, "I eat like a bird, but I can't lose weight." Should you believe the person who says this? Probably not, according to a study that analyzed the self-reported and actual caloric intakes and physical activity expenditures of a group of adults who were obese (Lichman et al., 1992). Though the individuals in this study claimed to consume fewer than 1200 calories per day, they were actually eating nearly twice as much as they indicated and engaging in only three-quarters as much physical activity as they reported. In other words, these individuals underestimated their dietary intake and overestimated their caloric output. Does this mean that obesity is simply the result of gluttony and sloth? No. In fact, many studies indicate that individuals who are obese do not eat more than their counterparts at a healthy weight. However, the majority of individuals who are obese are less physically active than people at a healthy weight. Further, if these individuals are not able to accurately assess what they eat and how much they do for physical activity, it should not be surprising that they do not know how to alter their behaviours to better manage their weight.

Lifestyle

Of all the factors affecting obesity, perhaps the most critical one relates to lifestyle. As noted in Chapter 4, 85 percent of Canadians do not meet the recommendation to obtain at least 150 minutes of moderate or more intense physical activity per week (Colley et al., 2011). One of the reasons for low levels of physical activity participation may relate to poor or inadequate experiences in physical education classes.

Currently, physical education is most often optional in high school and is seldom offered daily in elementary and junior schools. Furthermore, many children and youth are transported to and from school. This may limit the desire for active transportation later in life, as well as leading to the attitude that one must you have to be transported to your activities. Another cultural issue regarding our level of physical activity relates to how we perceive it; many believe that they have to 'exercise' and exercise is viewed as work, not as something to be enjoyed. Further, this exercise is believed to require a wellness or fitness centre to be done. See Chapter 4 for more details regarding the common barriers to physical activity.

You probably know someone who seems to be able to eat a lot and does not appear to do any more physical activity than you, yet never seems to gain weight. It is hard to understand how this person maintains his or her weight. With few exceptions, if you were to follow this person around for a typical day and monitor his or her level and intensity of physical activity, you would discover the answer to your question. Although the person's day might not include scheduled exercise, it probably includes a high level of physical activity. Walking up a flight of stairs, speeding up the pace while walking between classes, parking further away, and doing housework vigorously expend more calories than their alternatives. A major cause of low physical activity levels is the abundance of labour-saving devices in the modern household, as well as inactive modes of transportation. Using a blender instead of chopping vegetables or pushing remote-control buttons on the television as well as on garage doors results in a reduced caloric expenditure compared to previous generations. The automobile is a great convenience, but using it has significantly reduced our daily physical activity. As a result, we must choose to be physically active in a variety of ways on a daily basis.

SOCIAL BIAS AGAINST THE OVERWEIGHT

Although much has been written about the potentially devastating physical consequences of being obese, the social consequences of excessive weight and/or fat are rarely discussed. Difficulty in finding a suitable job, workplace discrimination, and problems in most every aspect of their social life have been noted by people who are obese.

Research increasingly points to a nation of weight bias. **Weight bias** refers to negative attitudes that have a detrimental effect on

Weight bias Negative attitudes that have a harmful effect on a person's interpersonal interactions and activities with people who are obese.

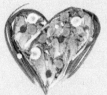

Student
Health
TODAY

Making the Link Between Your Social Networks and Your Weight

Social interactions have been shown to influence and reinforce lifestyle choices and behaviours such as smoking, alcohol use, physical activity participation, and dietary patterns. Learned behaviours acquired through social interactions with family and friends also are factors contributing to overweight and obesity. According to a 2007 study published in the *New England Journal of Medicine*, researchers found that friends can influence your body weight (Christakis & Fowler, 2007). These results were verified in a 2011 follow up study published in the *American Journal of Public Health* which reported that if you have heavier friends, family members, and colleagues, it is more likely that you will be heavier, too (Hruschka

et al., 2011). The stronger the relationship between the two people, the stronger is the link between their weights. Researchers investigated three possible pathways through which friends influence your body weight: collaboration, peer pressure, and monkey see, monkey do. The third pathway (monkey see, monkey do) was found to significantly influence behaviours linked to unhealthy weights. Although you may not necessarily share your friends' ideals for body size, your friends' body size might subconsciously shape your own ideals, which could influence or change your physical and healthy eating behaviours differently in an attempt to achieve a certain body shape or weight.

It makes sense that we are more likely to become obese if those around us are engaging in behaviours and habits that contribute to obesity, such as consuming a high-calorie diet, participating in low levels of physical activity, and spending a significant amount of time participating in sedentary activities. However, even if those around

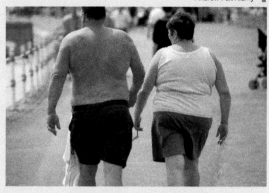

Andrew Fox/Alamy

Is your relationship affecting your weight?

you are engaging in behaviours that promote unhealthy weights, you have the power and ability to control your personal behaviours. By focusing on common goals to maintain weight, and engaging friends as potential supporters, you may be able to increase your chances of achieving a healthy weight.

Sources: Christakis, N. A., & Fowler, J. H. (2007). The Spread of Obesity in a Large Social Network over 32 Years. *New England Journal of Medicine, 357*(4), 370-379; Hruschka, D. J., Brewis, A. A., Wutich, A., & Morin, B. (2011). Shared Norms and Their Explanation for the Social Clustering of Obesity. *American Journal of Public Health, 101*(S1), S295-S300; Junge, C. (2011). How your friends make you fat --the social network of weight. Harvard Health Publications. Retrieved from www.health.harvard.edu/blog/how-your-friends-make-you-fat%E2%80%94the-social-network-of-weight-201105242666.

---

interpersonal interactions and activities with individuals who are obese. The stigma against fat people may come in several forms, including verbal types of bias (such as ridicule, teasing, insults, stereotypes, derogatory names, or pejorative language), physical stigma (such as touching, grabbing, or other aggressive behaviours), or other barriers and obstacles for people who are obese, such as the inadequate size of the seats in movie theatres, stadiums, and airplanes. In an extreme form, this stigma results in subtle and overt forms of discrimination, such as the denial of a promotion or a raise (North American Association for the Study of Obesity [NAASO], 2007).

Bias and stigmatization can lead to social isolation and a host of other problems for individuals who are obese. People who experience bias and stigma have higher rates of depression, poorer psychological adjustment, and higher rates of suicide. They may feel that they are "unlovable" and have difficulties in

relationships. They also may have higher rates of disordered eating (discussed in the next section), issues with self-esteem, more difficulties in obtaining health care, and a host of other problems (NAASO, 2007).

THINKING THIN: BODY IMAGE DISORDERS

Most think the obsession with thinness is a phenomenon of recent years. However, women have been pressured for generations to look and dress a certain way. During the Victorian era, corsets were used to achieve unrealistically tiny waists—recall Kate Winslett in the movie *Titanic*? In the 1960s, women wanted to look like Twiggy; in the 1990s, it was supermodel Kate

Moss; now we aspire to look like Joan Smalls, Karlie Kloss, or Arizona Muse, three top models according to Models.com's list of top 50 models (anonymous, n.d.). Regardless of who it is, the thin look has dominated fashion ads for years. And not only that: television, movies, the internet, and magazines constantly project images of lean, fit bodies. As a female, you are expected to believe that if you are thin, with shapely curves or well-defined muscles, you will be more desirable. Beautiful female models and underweight beauty pageant contestants typically range in size from a 0 to 2, delivering the subtle message that thin is in, desirable, and successful.

EATING DISORDERS

Obesity itself is neither a psychiatric disorder nor an **eating disorder**. Eating disorders involve severe disturbances in eating behaviours, unhealthy efforts to control body fat and weight, as well as abnormal and unrealistic attitudes about a person's body weight and shape. In general, individuals who develop eating disorders have low self-esteem and excessive concern about their body weight and shape.

Eating disorders, regardless of type, occur more frequently in females, with 95 percent of all diagnosed cases occurring in women (Raftis, 2010). Further, it tends to be younger women who are most often diagnosed—the majority of diagnoses occurring between the ages of 13 to 18 years, although diagnosis can occur in the early 20s and 30s as well (Raftis, 2010). Eating disorders are not restricted to middle-class white females with overprotective or overperfectionist parents; they span social classes and ethnic groups. They occur with similar frequencies in most industrialized countries, including Canada, the United States, Europe, Australia, Japan, New Zealand, and South Africa. Emigrants from cultures where eating disorders are rare and who come to cultures where they are more prevalent can develop eating disorders as they assimilate to the sociocultural pressures surrounding body weight and shape in their adopted culture.

Anorexia Nervosa

Anorexia nervosa is characterized by an obsession with controlling eating. Some people believe that if they can control their eating, they can control the rest of their life as well (Jones et al., 2001). This obsession usually leads them to self-starvation motivated by an intense fear of gaining weight, along with an inability to see their body the way it really is. When anorexia nervosa develops in childhood or early adolescence, one of the first signs can be the failure to gain weight associated with normal growth rather than actual weight loss. About 1 percent of females in late adolescence or early adulthood meet the diagnostic criteria of anorexia nervosa, while only about 0.3 percent of men are affected (Lydecker et al., 2012).

The following characteristics are recognized in an individual with anorexia nervosa:

- significant weight loss (approximately 15 to 25 percent of body weight)
- an inability to maintain a weight considered healthy for age and height
- an obsessive desire to be thinner
- an intense fear of becoming fat
- distorted body image (that is, the inability to see your body the way it really is; generally, the perception is that the body is fat, even though emaciated)
- weight and shape (and/or number on the bathroom scale) dictates how you feel about yourself
- strong desire to control life; believed to be done through dietary (and exercise) manipulation
- significant reduction in eating, along with repeated denials of hunger (National Eating Disorder Information Centre [NEDIC], 2008)

The medical problems associated with anorexia nervosa are many. Starvation damages the bones, the muscles, and the organs; as well as the immune, nervous, and digestive systems (Kaye, Fudge, & Paulus, 2009). People with anorexia nervosa often lose their hair or develop excessive fine facial and body hair. A woman's menstrual cycle usually stops as well (that is, amenorrhea occurs). Between 10 and 15 percent of individuals with anorexia nervosa die as a result of the disorder (Bulimia Anorexia Nervosa Association, n.d.).

Bulimia Nervosa

Bulimia nervosa involves cycles of binge eating and purging. Purging behaviours include self-induced vomiting, using laxatives, enemas, or diuretics, excessive exercising, or fasting (NEDIC, 2008). As with anorexia nervosa, the eating behaviours of individuals with bulimia nervosa are

Eating disorder A term used to describe a collection of psychiatric diseases that involve severe disturbances in eating behaviours, unhealthy efforts to control body fat and weight, and abnormal attitudes toward a person's body weight and shape.

Anorexia nervosa Eating disorder characterized by excessive preoccupation with food, self-starvation, and/or extreme exercising to achieve weight loss.

Bulimia nervosa Eating disorder characterized by cycles of binge eating and purging.

range. One frequent health issue often experienced by individuals with bulimia nervosa relates to the acid in vomit, which causes tooth enamel to dissolve. Calluses may also appear on the outer fingers/knuckles from frequent scraping along the teeth when inducing vomiting by putting one or more fingers down the throat.

Binge Eating Disorder

People with a **binge eating disorder (BED)** engage in recurrent binge eating but, unlike those with bulimia nervosa, do not purge. Binge eating occurs in about 1 to 4 percent of the population and in about 30 percent of individuals who are obese and in a weight management program (Wang et al., 2011). Most people with a BED binge because they are very hungry as a result of restrictive eating or dieting or to comfort themselves, avoid uncomfortable situations, or numb their feelings. Generally, individuals with BED do not have abnormal attitudes about dieting or body weight and shape. BED is often referred to as "compulsive overeating."

Eating Disorder Not Otherwise Specified

When individuals cannot be clearly diagnosed with one of the eating disorders previously described yet still have obvious problems with their eating and body image, they are said to have an Eating Disorder Not Otherwise Specified (ED-NOS). For example, women who meet some of the criteria for anorexia nervosa but continue to menstruate would fit in this category, as do men and women who lose a lot of weight but remain within the weight appropriate range despite their abnormal eating behaviours. Common behaviours of individuals with ED-NOS include

- purging after normal eating
- chewing food repeatedly and then spitting it out (rather than swallowing)
- binge eating and purging (but not with the regularity required for a bulimia nervosa diagnosis) (NEDIC, 2008)

Disordered Eating

Although not clinically diagnosed, disordered eating refers to a wide range of abnormal eating behaviours including various actions seen in individuals with anorexia nervosa, bulimia nervosa, and BED. These

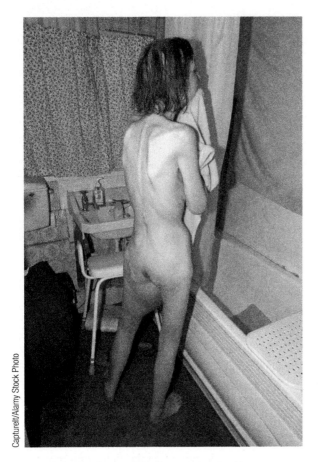

The self-starvation associated with eating disorders like anorexia nervosa can damage bones, muscles, and organs and create a host of other serious and, in some cases, life-threatening medical problems.

CaptureIt/Alamy Stock Photo

strongly influenced by a desire to be in control of their body weight and shape. The cycle begins with a binge—or the rapid ingestion of a large amount of food at one time—then continues with some sort of purging behaviour. Usually the eating feels automatic and the person feels helpless since his or her eating may initially placate feelings of anger or sadness. Due to the ingestion of a large number of calories, the binge causes considerable physical discomfort and a worry about weight gain. The cycle then continues with efforts to prevent calorie absorption with some form of purging.

Binge eating usually occurs in secrecy and is accompanied by a lack of control; it is difficult for a person to stop a binge once it has started. About 1 to 3 percent of adolescent and young adult females have bulimia nervosa; the rate among men is about 10 percent of that among females (Lydecker et al., 2012). Unlike individuals with anorexia nervosa, the body weight of individuals with bulimia nervosa is typically within the weight appropriate

Binge eating disorder (BED) Eating disorder characterized by recurrent binge eating without any purging behaviours.

168 PART 2 CHOOSING HEALTHY LIFESTYLES

behaviours include chronic restrained eating, compulsive eating, habitual dieting, and irregular chaotic eating patterns where hunger and satiety are ignored. Similar to other eating disorders, disordered eating has negative health implications for overall and emotional, spiritual, social, and physical health. Further, disordered eating is highly prevalent in our culture, with most young women exhibiting one or more of these behaviours at one or more times in their lives. For example, in a study, 27 percent of Ontario girls aged 12 to 18 reported severely problematic food and weight behaviour (Jones et al., 2001).

Anorexia Athletica

Similar to disordered eating, anorexia athletica is not a recognized psychiatric diagnosis. Many people preoccupied with food and weight exercise compulsively to control their weight in misguided attempts to gain a sense of power, control, and self-respect.

Symptoms of anorexia athletica include

- exercising beyond the requirements for good health
- being fanatical about weight and dietary intake
- stealing time from work, school, and relationships to exercise
- focusing on calorie burning and forgetting that physical activity and/or exercise can be fun
- defining self-worth in terms of performance
- rarely or never being satisfied with athletic achievements
- always pushing on to the next physical challenge
- justifying excessive behaviours by defining oneself as an athlete or insisting that current exercising behaviours are healthy (NEDIC, 2008)

Who Is at Risk?

Disordered eating patterns are the result of many factors, and there is no simple explanation for why intelligent, often highly accomplished individuals spiral downwards into the destructive behaviours that lead to eating disorders. One potential factor is the desperate need to win social approval or gain control of their lives with food.

Many persons with disordered eating patterns also suffer from other problems such as clinical depression, alcohol abuse, compulsive stealing, gambling, or other addictions (Harvard Women's Health Watch, 1996). Some studies using identical twins have shown a possible association between heredity and eating disorders, as have others that point to the proportionally large number of persons with an eating disorder who have a mother or sister similarly affected (Kaye, Fudge, & Paulus, 2009). The question of nature versus nurture can also be raised here.

Treating Eating Disorders

People can and do recover from eating disorders, though the likelihood of success is greatest when the diagnosis is early and the individual acknowledges the need for treatment. The most effective treatments combine different approaches, are individualized, and involve the patient and his or her family and friends. People with eating disorders usually come to the attention of medical personnel because someone else shows concern. Often the individual requires hospitalization, with the first goal of treatment being to restore near-normal body weight. Concurrently, individual and group psychotherapy provide an opportunity to enhance self-confidence, self-esteem, and feelings of power and control. At this time, the person learns new, more effective ways to handle stress and gain a measure of control over her or his life, so that it is no longer necessary to turn to or away from food as the solution.

Helping Someone with an Eating Disorder

As previously noted, people can, and do, recover from eating disorders, although professional help is almost always required. Recovery is more difficult the longer symptoms are denied or ignored. It is not easy to approach someone who you think has an eating disorder. What should you say? What should you do? The following are suggestions from the National Eating Disorder Information Centre (NEDIC, 2008) to direct your efforts to help someone you think may be at risk.

Be patient: When you first approach the individual, do not be surprised if your expression of concern is rejected and treated with anger and denial. Shame and pain tend to go along with an eating disorder. It is also important not to rush and to accept that it will take time for the person to recognize that he or she has an eating disorder and needs to change.

Be knowledgeable: It is important to understand that an eating disorder results from a misguided coping strategy to deal with deeper issues around control. In other words, eating disorders are about more than just not eating or being thin! Learn more about eating disorders and in particular the eating disorder you think this individual has.

Be compassionate: Eating disorders are complex problems where issues with food and body weight and shape result. It is important to understand that the person might prefer to use healthier coping mechanisms, but simply does not know how.

Be encouraging: Encourage the person to define himself or herself in ways that do not involve the eating disorder. Do this by talking about other aspects of his or her life, and of life more generally. Affirm strengths and interests unrelated to food or physical appearance.

Be nonjudgmental: It is important to express your needs in the relationship, without blaming or shaming the other person. Remember that the individual with the eating disorder will have to decide on when and how to get help, and what kind. Provide support by validating healthy changes, no matter how small they may be.

Take care of yourself: Seeing someone you care about struggling with an eating disorder might make you scared, angry, frustrated, and helpless. Still, be careful not to blame this person for his or her condition. Try to understand that eating disorders result from the behaviours used to deal with painful emotions or experiences and are a result of an attempt to gain control. The person with an eating disorder may know that his or her condition is upsetting other people, but may not be ready for or capable of change.

Do not take on the role of a therapist: Do only what you feel capable of. Get support for yourself. You need to take care of yourself while dealing with your friend or family member. Remember, you need to put on your own oxygen mask before helping others with theirs. Also remember that this person can only get better at his or her own pace. You can be supportive and gently share information. You can help this person to see and consider alternatives to his or her current behaviours. You cannot make the person get better; you cannot even force him or her to seek treatment.

Conversation Guide

Focus on feelings and relationships:

- Express concern about the person's health, yet respect his or her privacy.
- Do not comment on how the person or any others look, how fat or thin they are, how much they eat, and so on. The person is already aware of his or her body, eating habits, and likely has a distorted view of his or her body, exercise, and eating behaviours. Even if you use compliments, comments about weight or appearance reinforce the obsession with body image and weight.

- Be positive. Find neutral, comfortable places and times to talk. For example:

  Instead of saying, "You could control/stop this if you wanted to," say, "I know how hard it is for you. Let's talk about how we can find ways to make things better."

- Keep calm, focused, and respectful during difficult conversations. Set caring and reasonable limits. Be firm and consistent. For example, know how you will respond when the person wants to skip meals or eat alone, or when the person gets angry if someone eats his or her "special" food.

- Avoid power struggles about eating. Do not demand change. Do not criticize eating habits. People with eating disorders are trying to gain control because they do not feel in control of other aspects of their life. Trying to trick or force them to eat can make things worse.

- Examine your attitudes about food, weight, body image, and body size. Think about the way you personally are affected by body-image pressures, and how it is that you speak about your body, your eating, and the pressures you experience.

- Do not convey any fat prejudice, or reinforce the desire to be thin. If the person says he or she feels fat or wants to lose weight, do not say, "You are not fat." Instead, suggest that the person explore his or her reasons for dieting, and what he or she thinks weight loss can achieve. Encourage him or her to reflect on the pressure to look a certain way in society, and how this makes us feel about ourselves.

CREATING A PERSONALIZED PLAN FOR ACHIEVING YOUR HEALTHY WEIGHT

Now that you have determined that you are ready to manage your weight, the next step is an honest self-assessment of where you are. You do not need sophisticated body fat measurement techniques to know where you are. What you need is a scale and/

or a mirror. You also know if your favourite jeans are too tight! Next, you need to set a realistic goal. Ask yourself, why do I want to meet this goal? What will I do when I reach this goal? Then create a plan to reach your goal. Keep in mind what you enjoy doing. If you like taking walks, you might make walking part of your plan. If you absolutely love chocolate chip cookies, you might consider having only one or two cookies per day or every other day. Find a way to make it all fit without leading to feelings of self-deprivation or being burdened by having to be physically active. The following suggestions might help you reach your goals:

- Design your plan to meet your needs. Your plan must fit your personality, your priorities, and your study, work, and recreation schedules. It should also allow for sufficient rest and relaxation.

- Chart your progress. For many people, the daily "weigh-in" is a critical factor in maintaining their program. However, for others, the daily monitoring of weight negatively influences self-esteem. If you choose to weigh yourself daily, keep in mind that body weight normally fluctuates throughout the week and a once per week "weigh-in" is more appropriate.

- Chart your eating setbacks. Rather than thinking in terms of failure and punishment, think in terms of temporary setbacks or relapses and how to accommodate them. Review the information on Behaviour Change in Chapter 1. Carefully record your emotional states when eating, eating habits, environmental cues, and feelings regarding what and how much you eat. Better understanding your attitudes and behaviours toward food will help you to manage them effectively. Successful weight maintenance accommodates hormonal fluctuations and their potential influence on dietary habits.

- Be physically active. Different people benefit from different types of physical activities. Just because your friends are into jogging or yoga does not mean that those types of physical activities are best for you. Select physical activities that you consider fun, not a daily form of punishment for overeating. Variety may be the key here. Planning physical activities that include your friends and family may also improve your chances of success.

- Chart your physical activity or lack thereof. Similar to monitoring your setbacks in dietary intake, you should keep track of your challenges in regard to your physical activity behaviours. Once again, carefully recording how you felt prior to missing your physical activity as well as the environmental cues around you will help you to successfully overcome those sorts of challenges in the future.

- Become aware of your feelings of hunger and fullness. It may be that your eating is time-dependent or you stop eating only when the food is gone (the "clean your plate" syndrome). You need to become more aware of the eating process, by learning to recognize your hunger and the first signals that you have eaten enough.

- Accept yourself. This may be the most important aspect of successfully managing your weight. It is important to keep your weight and body shape in perspective.

- Develop stress-management skills that do not involve eating. Some people overeat in response to stress or choose less healthy foods.

- Get enough sleep—at nighttime; individuals with a "sleep debt" tend to eat more than those who are well rested.

- Try not to allow yourself to get too hungry before eating. When you are really hungry, you may overeat because you ingest large amounts of food quickly.

assess
YOURSELF

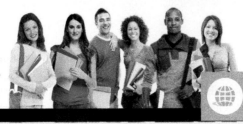

Go to MyHealthLab to complete this questionnaire with automatic scoring

TAKING CHARGE: Managing Your Weight

Managing your weight is not an easy task. For successful weight management, you need to consider it a lifelong commitment rather than a temporary diet—that is, something you intend to do for the rest of your life rather than sticking with for a few weeks and then returning to previous dietary behaviours. Complete the questionnaire below to determine if you are 'ready' to manage your weight.

Are You Ready to Manage Your Weight Effectively?

How well do your attitudes suit your ability to manage your weight? For each question, circle the answer that best describes your attitude. Be honest. As you complete Sections 2 to 5, tally your score and analyze it according to the scoring guide.

1 Diet History

A. How many times in the past year have you been on a diet?

0 times   1–3 times   4–10 times   11–20 times   More than 20

B. What is the most weight you lost on any of these diets?

0 lb   1–5 lb   6–10 lb   11–20 lb   More than 20 lb

C. How long did you stay at the new lower weight?

Less than 1 mo   2–3 mo   4–6 mo   6–12 mo   Over 1 yr

D. Put a check mark by each dieting method you have tried:

_____ Skipping breakfast	_____ Skipping lunch or dinner	_____ Taking over-the-counter appetite suppressants
_____ Counting calories	_____ Cutting out most fats	_____ Cutting out most carbohydrates
_____ Increasing regular physical activity	_____ Taking weight-loss supplements	_____ Cutting out all snacks
_____ Using meal replacements such as Slim Fast	_____ Taking prescription appetite suppressants	_____ Taking laxatives
_____ Inducing vomiting	_____ Other _____	

2 Readiness to Start a Weight-Management Program

If you are thinking about doing something different to manage your weight, answer questions A–F.

A. How motivated are you to change your eating habits?

1	2	3	4	5
Not at all motivated	Slightly motivated	Somewhat motivated	Quite motivated	Extremely motivated

B. How certain are you that you will commit to a lifetime approach to eating well?

1	2	3	4	5
Not at all certain	Slightly certain	Somewhat certain	Quite certain	Extremely certain

C. Taking into account other stresses in your life (school, work, and relationships), to what extent can you tolerate the effort required to change your eating habits?

1	2	3	4	5
Cannot tolerate	Can tolerate somewhat	Uncertain	Can tolerate well	Can tolerate easily

D. If your change in eating habits leads to a caloric deficit, you may lose weight. Are you prepared for the length of time it may take to reach a healthier weight for you?

1	2	3	4	5
Very prepared	Somewhat prepared	Moderately prepared	Somewhat prepared	Very prepared

E. If you change your eating habits, will you fantasize about eating your favourite foods?

1	2	3	4	5
Always	Frequently	Occasionally	Rarely	Never

F. If you change your eating habits, will you feel deprived, angry, or upset?

1	2	3	4	5
Always	Frequently	Occasionally	Rarely	Never

Total Your Scores from questions A–F and circle your score category.

6 to 16: This may not be a good time for you to change your eating habits. Inadequate motivation and commitment and unrealistic expectations could block your progress. Think about what contributes to your unreadiness. What are some of the factors?

Consider changing these factors before undertaking a change in how you eat.

17 to 23: You may be nearly ready to change your eating habits, and you should think about ways to boost your readiness.

24 to 30: The path is clear—you can decide how to change your eating habits in a safe, effective way.

3 Hunger, Appetite, and Eating

Think about your hunger and the cues that stimulate your appetite or eating, and then answer questions A–C.

A. When food comes up in conversation or in something you read, do you want to eat, even if you are not hungry?

1	2	3	4	5
Never	Rarely	Occasionally	Frequently	Always

B. How often do you eat for a reason other than physical hunger?

1	2	3	4	5
Never	Rarely	Occasionally	Frequently	Always

C. When your favourite foods are around the house, do you succumb to eating them between meals?

1	2	3	4	5
Never	Rarely	Occasionally	Frequently	Always

Total Your Scores from questions A–C and circle your score category.

3 to 6: You might occasionally eat more than you should, but it is due more to your own attitudes than to temptation and other environmental cues. Controlling your own attitudes toward hunger and eating may help you.

7 to 9: You may have a moderate tendency to eat just because food is available. Changing your eating habits

may be easier for you if you learn to address external cues and eat only when you are physically hungry.

10 to 15: Some or much of your eating may be in response to thinking about food or exposing yourself to temptations to eat. Think of ways to minimize your exposure to temptations so you eat only in response to physical hunger.

(continued)

4 Controlling Overeating

How good are you at controlling overeating? Answer questions A–C.

A. A friend talks you into going out to a restaurant for a midday meal instead of eating a brown-bag lunch. As a result, for the rest of the day, you:

1	2	3	4	5
Would eat much less	Would eat somewhat less	Would make no difference	Would eat somewhat more	Would eat much more

B. You "break" your healthier eating plans by overconsuming a food that is high in fat and/or sugar. As a result, for the rest of the day, you:

1	2	3	4	5
Would eat much less	Would eat somewhat less	Would make no difference	Would eat somewhat more	Would eat much more

C. You have been following your new eating plan faithfully and decide to test yourself by taking a bite of something that is high in fat and/or sugar. As a result, for the rest of the day, you:

1	2	3	4	5
Would eat much less	Would eat somewhat less	Would make no difference	Would eat somewhat more	Would eat much more

Total Your Scores from questions A–C and circle your score category.

3 to 7: You recover rapidly from mistakes. However, if you frequently alternate between out-of-control eating and very strict dieting, you may have a serious eating problem and should get professional help.

8 to 11: You do not seem to let unplanned eating disrupt your program. This is a flexible, balanced approach.

12 to 15: You may be prone to overeating after an event breaks your control or throws you off track. Your reaction to these problem-causing events could use improvement.

5 Emotional Eating

Consider the effects of your emotions on your eating behaviours, and answer questions A–C.

A. Do you eat more than you should when you have negative feelings such as anxiety, depression, anger, or loneliness?

1	2	3	4	5
Never	Rarely	Occasionally	Frequently	Always

B. Do you eat more than you should when you have positive feelings (i.e., do you celebrate feeling good by eating)?

1	2	3	4	5
Never	Rarely	Occasionally	Frequently	Always

C. When you have unpleasant interactions with others in your life or after a difficult day at work, do you eat more than you should?

1	2	3	4	5
Never	Rarely	Occasionally	Frequently	Always

Total Your Scores from questions A–C and circle your score category.

3 to 8: You do not appear to let your emotions affect your eating.

9 to 11: You sometimes eat in response to emotional highs and lows. Monitor this behaviour to learn when and why it occurs, and be prepared to find alternative activities to respond to your emotions.

12 to 15: Emotional ups and downs can stimulate your eating. Try to deal with the feelings that trigger this eating and find other ways to express them.

6 Physical Activity Patterns and Attitudes

Engaging in regular, daily physical activity is key for weight maintenance. Think about your physical activity attitudes and behaviours, and answer questions A–D.

A. How often do you engage in physical activity?

1	2	3	4	5
Never	Rarely	Occasionally	Somewhat frequently	Daily

B. How confident are you that you can be regularly physically active?

1	2	3	4	5
Not at all confident	Slightly confident	Somewhat confident	Highly confident	Completely confident

C. When you think about physical activity, do you develop a positive or negative picture in your mind?

1	2	3	4	5
Completely negative	Somewhat negative	Neutral	Somewhat positive	Completely positive

D. How certain are you that you can work regular physical activity into your daily schedule?

1	2	3	4	5
Not at all certain	Slightly certain	Somewhat certain	Quite certain	Extremely certain

Total Your Scores from questions A–D and circle your score category.

4 to 10: You're probably not as physically active as you should be. Determine whether it is your attitude about physical activity or your lifestyle that is blocking your way, then change what you must and put on those walking shoes!

11 to 16: You need to feel more positive about physical activity so you can do it more often. Think of ways to be more active that are rewarding and easily fit in your day.

17 to 20: The path is clear for you to be physically active. Now think of ways to get motivated.

Other Tips that May Help You to Manage Your Weight

In your plan, you should also consider your eating habits at home and when eating out.

When Eating at Home

- Eat only in the kitchen or dining room. Keep food out of the living room, bedroom, and study spaces.
- Spread your caloric intake throughout the day by eating smaller meals four to five times a day (this enhances RMR).
- Use smaller bowls and plates when eating.

- Choose low-calorie, nutrient-dense foods such as salad without dressing or with a small amount of dressing on the side, and pasta with a low-fat sauce more often.
- Take more time to eat; at least 20 minutes per meal is recommended. Chew your food carefully, setting your fork down between bites and enjoying the taste.
- Drink a glass of water before your meal.
- Drink a glass of water when you think you are hungry; thirst is often mistaken for hunger.
- Brush your teeth after eating to signify the end of your meal.
- Limit your purchases of high-calorie, high-fat, low-nutrient foods, even for guests or holidays.
- When having desserts, limit yourself to a small taste. Choose lower-calorie, lower-fat options for dessert, such as apple crisp or berries and yogurt more often.
- Limit the amount you eat immediately before going to bed.
- Put serving dishes on the counter or stove while you are eating. Leaving them on the table encourages second helpings even when you are no longer hungry.

When Eating Out

- Ask for it "your way." Request that the cheese be left off, the sauce cut in half, salad dressing on the side, and so on.
- Ask that entrées be broiled, steamed, baked, grilled, poached, or roasted, with only a small amount of fat used for the cooking process.

(continued)

- When ordering omelettes, ask for a one- or two-egg-yolk version containing only the whites of the other eggs. Limit meat and cheese fillings. Choose vegetable fillings whenever possible.
- Reduce portion size. Order à la carte if possible, with a salad or fresh vegetable on the side.
- Limit how frequently you eat at an all-you-can-eat restaurant.
- Drink at least one glass of water before starting your meal. Try to relax while eating and make your mealtime last. Talk more, put your fork down more frequently, chew more, and generally slow down.

- Order fresh fruits and low- or no-fat yogurts in place of heavy desserts.
- Frequent restaurants that offer low-fat, high-complex-carbohydrate meals.
- Choose water or low-fat milk as your beverage.

Source: Adapted from "Are You Ready for Weight Loss?" by K. Brownell, copyright year © 1989. Published by Tribune Media Services, Inc.

DISCUSSION QUESTIONS

1. Differentiate the terms *overweight* and *obese*.
2. How is it possible that a person can be classified as obese (BMI of 30 or greater) and not be overfat (that is, percentage of body fat within the healthy range)? Similarly, how can a person be overfat (that is, percentage of fat above the healthy range) and not be classified as obese (that is, BMI < 30)? What is a better method of determining excessive fatness?
3. List the risk factors for developing obesity. Identify the factors that seem to be most important in determining whether you will become obese. Why consider these factors and not others?
4. Discuss the pressures, if any, you feel to change your body shape. Where do these pressures come from? How has the media influenced your thoughts about your body? What can you do to combat those pressures?
5. Create a plan for weight management. In what way would you have to modify this plan for your best friend? Your sister? Your brother? Your partner?
6. Differentiate the eating disorders discussed in this chapter. Identify why women are more prone to eating disorders than men. Why university students?
7. Why are popular diets not the best method for weight management?

APPLICATION EXERCISE

Reread the "Consider This . . ." scenario at the beginning of the chapter and answer the following questions.

1. How common is Eilidh's situation? How common is her response? Do you think Eilidh will be successful over her Christmas vacation in making the changes she has proposed? Why or why not?
2. How can *Eating Well with Canada's Food Guide* and *Canada's Physical Activity Guide* help Eilidh to manage her weight? What other suggestions would you give her?
3. Why is it important to include all foods in your diet when trying to lose weight (i.e., to not eliminate certain foods)? Is it okay to consume alcohol when trying to lose weight? Why or why not?

MASTERINGHEALTH

Go to MasteringHealth for Assignments, the eText, and the Study Area with case studies, self quizzing, and videos.

focus On

Body Image

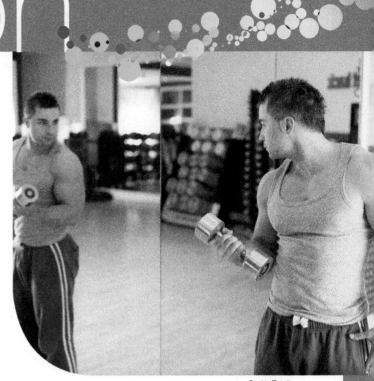

Punkie/Fotolia

As he began his arm curls, Mira checked his form in the full-length mirror on the weight-room wall. Although he realized that his biceps were bigger than when he started weight training six months ago, he still expected more. His pecs, too, still lacked definition, and he still did not have the six-pack abs he really wanted. So, after a 45-minute upper-body workout, he added 200 curl-ups. Then he left the gym to shower back at his apartment—no way was he going to risk any of the gym regulars seeing what he thought was a flabby torso unclothed. By the time Mira got home and looked in the mirror; his frustration turned to anger. He was just too fat! And when would he look physically fit? When would he have a sculpted body worth showing off? To punish himself for his slow progress, instead of taking a shower, he put on his running shoes and went for a 10-kilometre run.

When you look in the mirror, do you like what you see? Do you feel disappointed, frustrated, or even angry like Mira? Do your reactions differ when you work out regularly? Or when you are on holidays? If so, you are not alone. Most adults, children and adolescents too, are dissatisfied with their bodies. One study found that 93 percent of the women reported that they had had negative thoughts about their appearance during the past week (University of the West of England, 2011). In this study, approximately 79 percent of the women also reported that they would like to lose weight, despite the fact that the majority of the women sampled (78.4 percent) were actually within the underweight or healthy weight ranges. Although the perception of what is the 'ideal' shape may differ, most North American women, regardless of ethnic background, are dissatisfied with their body weight and shape (Webb et al., 2013). Men also experience a negative body image, with the numbers rising for recent generations (Tylka, 2013). Negative feelings about your body weight or shape can contribute to behaviours that can

threaten your health—and your life. Having a healthy body image is a key indicator of self-esteem and can contribute to reduced stress, an increased sense of personal empowerment, and more joyful living.

WHAT IS BODY IMAGE?

There are several components to your **body image**:

- How you see yourself in your mind; or the picture you have of yourself from the top of your head to the tip of your toes.

- What you believe about your own appearance (including your real perceptions about your body).

- The feelings, attitudes, and perceptions you have about your body, including your height, shape, weight, and physical appearance (Womenshealth. gov, 2009).

A *negative body image* is defined as either a distorted perception of your shape, or feelings of discomfort, shame, or anxiety about your body. You may be convinced that other people look better than you; that they are much more attractive, and your body is a sign of personal failure. Does this sound like Mira as he clearly exhibits signs of a negative body image?

Body image The picture you have of yourself in your mind, how you see yourself when you look in a mirror or and how you feel about your body.

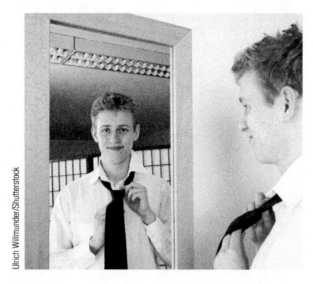

Ulrich Willmunder/Shutterstock

A healthy or positive body image allows you to look in the mirror and see how you really look as well as to appreciate who you are, what you can do, and so on, rather than how you look.

In contrast, a *positive body image* is a true perception of your appearance: You see yourself as you really are and, more importantly, you accept (or at the very least tolerate) yourself for who you are and what you look like. You understand that everyone is different—and should be different. You celebrate your uniqueness including your "flaws," which you know have nothing to do with your value as a person. Figure 1 shows a Body Image Continuum. The continuum reflects levels of positive and negative thinking regarding your body that reflect the reality of how you may think about your body.

Many Factors Influence Body Image

You are not born with a body image, but rather develop one at an early age as you compare yourself against images and others you see in the world around

FIGURE 1

This is part of a two-part continuum, the second part of which is shown in Figure 2. Individuals whose responses fall to the far left side of the continuum have a highly negative body image, whereas responses to the right indicate a positive body image.

Body hate/ dissociation	Distorted body image	Body preoccupied/ obsessed	Body acceptance	Body ownership
I often feel separated and distant from my body—as if it belongs to someone else.	I spend a significant amount of time exercising and dieting to change my body.	I spend a significant amount of time viewing my body in the mirror.	I base my body image equally on social norms and my own self-concept.	My body is beautiful to me.
I don't see anything positive or even neutral about my body shape and size.	My body shape and size keep me from dating or finding someone who will treat me the way I want to be treated.	I spend a significant amount of time comparing my body to others.	I pay attention to my body and my appearance because it is important to me, but it only occupies a small part of my day.	My feelings about my body are not influenced by society's concept of an ideal body shape.
I don't believe others when they tell me I look OK.	I have considered changing or have changed my body shape and size through surgical means so I can accept myself.	I have days when I feel fat.	I nourish my body so it has the strength and energy to achieve my physical goals.	I know that the significant others in my life will always find me attractive.
I hate the way I look in the mirror and often isolate myself from others.		I am preoccupied with my body.		
		I accept society's ideal body shape and size as the best body shape and size.		

Source: From Campus Health Service. Original continuum, C. Schislak, Preventive Medicine and Public Health. Copyright © 1997. Used with permission of Arizona Board of Regents.

you, the world in which you are immersed, and interpret the responses of family members and peers to your appearance.

The Media and Popular Culture

The images and celebrities, whether actors, singers, athletes, and so on, in the media set the standard for what our culture depicts as attractive, leading some people to engage in dangerous behaviours and practices to have the biggest biceps or fit into size 2 jeans. This obsession with appearance has long been part of our culture. As described in Chapter 6, women have been doing various things to alter their appearance over the years. Men too have been and continue to be pressured to look a particular way. All you need to do is look at the magazine rack at the checkout stand at your local grocery store to read the headlines and to see the unrealistic male and female body shapes currently promoted. Although you likely recognize that these photographs and others throughout the magazine have been 'touched up' or 'computer enhanced', you may still wish to look like them.

As mentioned in Chapter 6, more than 52 percent of Canadians are overweight or obese (Statistics Canada, 2012); thus, a significant disconnect exists between the media's idealized images and the average Canadian or North American body. At the same time, the media is a more powerful and pervasive presence than ever before, bombarding us with messages that imply that we are not good enough, and that we do not look the way we should. Not surprisingly, a significantly positive association was found between body weight ideals and body dissatisfaction in a study with more than 7400 participants from 26 countries (Swami et al., 2010).

Family, Community, and Cultural Groups

The people with whom we most often interact—our family members, friends, and others—strongly influence the way we see ourselves. Parents are especially influential in body image development. For instance, it is common and natural for adolescent girls' fathers to experience feelings of discomfort related to their daughters' changing bodies. If fathers are able to navigate these feelings successfully, and validate the acceptability of their daughters' appearance throughout puberty, it is likely that they will help their daughters maintain a positive body image. In contrast, if fathers verbalize or indicate even subtle judgments about their daughters' changing bodies, girls may begin to question how members of the opposite sex view their bodies in general. In addition, mothers who model body acceptance or body ownership may be more likely to foster a similar positive body image in their daughters, whereas mothers who are frustrated with or ashamed of their bodies may have a greater chance of fostering these attitudes in their daughters (see also Figure 1).

Interactions with your peers, teachers, co-workers, and others can also influence body image development. For instance, peer harassment (teasing and bullying) is widely acknowledged to contribute to a negative body image. Moreover, associations within your cultural group appear to influence your body image. Studies have found that females with a European ancestry experience the highest rates of body dissatisfaction, and as individuals from a minority group become more acculturated into the mainstream of Western society, the body dissatisfaction levels of women in that group increase (Swami et al., 2010; Webb et al., 2013).

Physiological and Psychological Factors

People who have been diagnosed with a body image disorder show differences in their brain's ability to regulate chemicals called *neurotransmitters,* which are linked to mood (Mayo Clinic Staff, 2010). Poor regulation of neurotransmitters is also involved in depression and anxiety disorders, including obsessive-compulsive disorder. Distortions in body image, particularly regarding the face, were linked through MRI scanning to a malfunctioning in the brain's visual processing region (Feusner et al., 2009).

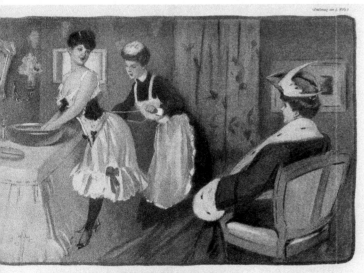

Im „Cabinet de Toilette" einer Pariserin.

Women have taken various measures to 'enhance' their body over the years.

Mary Evans Picture Library/Alamy

HOW CAN YOU DEVELOP A MORE POSITIVE BODY IMAGE?

If you want to develop a more positive body image, your first step should be to challenge the commonly held attitudes in contemporary society regarding the ideal body image for women and men and how much you may subscribe to them (University of Kansas Student Health, n.d.). Four common attitudes are noted below.

Myth 1: How you look is more important than who you are. Do you weigh yourself frequently? If so, when you do, does the value on the scale affect you and the choices you make each day? How much does it matter to you to have friends who are thin and attractive? How important do you think being thin is in trying to attract your ideal partner?

Myth 2: You can be slender and attractive if you have willpower. When you see someone who is thin, what assumptions do you make about that person? When you see someone who is overweight or obese, what assumptions do you make? Have you ever berated yourself for not having the willpower to change some aspect of your body? Have you ever berated yourself for eating or drinking something? Do you think to be thin you need to have the willpower to not eat?

Myth 3: Dieting, including various methods of fasting, are effective weight-loss strategies. Do you believe in fad diets or quick-weight-loss products? Do you think it is okay to drastically restrict calories or eliminate certain foods from your diet in the short–term to achieve weight loss? How far would you be willing to go to attain the "perfect" body?

Myth 4: Appearance is more important than health. How can you tell whether a person is healthy? Is there a certain size he or she needs to be? Is it possible for overweight people to be healthy? What motivates you to lose weight—your health or your appearance?

The National Eating Disorder Foundation recommends the following 10 steps for developing a positive body image. Keep in mind that it takes time to replace your negative thoughts with positive ones, and there is a continuum of thinking that you may have to cross.

- **Step 1.** Appreciate all that your body can do. Every day your body lets you live your dreams. Celebrate all of the amazing things your body does for you—moving, dancing, breathing, laughing, dreaming, and more.

- **Step 2.** Keep a list of things you like about yourself—things that are not related to how much you weigh or how you look. Read your list often. Add to it as you become aware of more things to like about yourself.

- **Step 3.** Remind yourself that true beauty is not simply skin deep. When you feel good about yourself and who you are, you carry yourself with a sense of confidence, self-acceptance, and openness that makes you beautiful. Beauty is a state of mind, not a state of your body.

- **Step 4.** Look at yourself as a whole person. When you see yourself in a mirror or in your mind, choose not to focus on specific body parts. See yourself as you want others to see you—as a whole person. See yourself as you see others—for the good they do or the good person they are.

- **Step 5.** Surround yourself with positive people. It is easier to feel good about yourself and your body when you are around others who are supportive and who recognize the importance of liking yourself just as you naturally are.

- **Step 6.** Shut down those voices in your head that tell you your body is not "right" or that you are a "bad" person because of how you look. You can overpower those negative thoughts with positive ones. When you think negative thoughts, stop yourself and focus on a recent success you experienced.

- **Step 7.** Wear clothes that are comfortable and that make you feel good about your body. Do not purchase the latest fashions if they do not feel comfortable or you do not feel comfortable in them. Work with your body, not against it.

- **Step 8.** Become a critical viewer of social and media messages. Pay attention to images, slogans, or attitudes that make you feel bad about yourself or your body. Protest these messages in as many ways as you can. Talk about these advertisements with others; write a letter to the advertiser or sponsoring company.

- **Step 9.** Do something nice for yourself—something that reminds you that you appreciate your body. Take a bubble bath, make time for a nap, go for a walk or run, or find a peaceful place outside to relax.

- **Step 10.** Use the time and energy that you might have spent worrying about food, calories, and your weight to do something to help others. Reaching out to other people helps you feel better about yourself and can make a positive change in our world. (Reprinted with permission from the National Eating Disorders Association, www.nationaleatingdisorders.org/nedaDir/files/documents/handouts/TenSteps.pdf.)

Some People Develop Body Image Disorders

Although most women and many men are dissatisfied with some aspect of their appearance, very few have a true body image disorder. Diagnosable body image disorders affect a small percentage of the population.

Approximately 1 percent of people in the United States suffer from **body dysmorphic disorder (BDD)** (Ahmed, Genen, & Cook, 2010). Precise rates are currently not known in Canada; however, a 2002 survey did find that approximately 1.5 percent of Canadian women between the ages of 15 and 24 did suffer from an eating disorder (Statistics Canada, 2002). People with BDD are obsessively concerned with their appearance and have a distorted view of their body shape, body size, weight, perceived lack of muscles, facial blemishes, size of body parts, and so on. Although the precise cause of the disorder is not known, an anxiety disorder such as obsessive-compulsive disorder is often present as well. Contributing factors may include genetic susceptibility, childhood teasing, physical or sexual abuse, low self-esteem, and rigid sociocultural expectations of beauty (Mayo Clinic Staff, 2010).

People with BDD may try to fix their perceived flaws through use of steroids, excessive bodybuilding, repeated cosmetic surgeries, extreme tattooing, or other appearance-altering behaviours. It is estimated that 7 to 15 percent of people seeking dermatology or cosmetic treatments have BDD (Ahmed, Genen, & Cook, 2010).

An emerging problem, seen in young men and women, is **social physique anxiety (SPA)**. SPA refers to the anxiety experienced at the real or perceived evaluation of your body by others (Fitzsimmons-Craft et al., 2012). People with high SPA may spend a disproportionate amount of time fixating on their bodies, working out, and performing tasks that are ego centred and self-directed in attempts to present their body favourably (Bratrud et al., 2010; Mülazimoglu-Balli, Koka, & Asci, 2010). SPA, like body image disturbance, relates to risk for developing an eating disorder (Fitzsimmons-Craft et al., 2012; Thompson & Chad, 2003).

WHAT IS DISORDERED EATING?

If you have a negative body image, you might fixate on a wide range of physical "flaws," ranging from thinning hair to flat feet. The "flaws" that cause the greatest distress are most often related to body weight and shape, regardless of whether you are at a healthy weight, overweight,

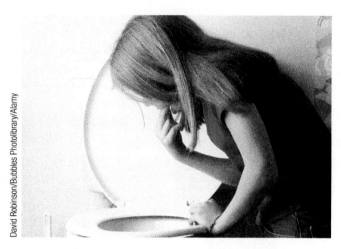

David Robinson/Bubbles Photolibrary/Alamy

People engage in various less-than-healthy behaviours to reduce their caloric intake.

or underweight. Figure 2 presents a continuum ranging from a healthy acceptance of your body to thoughts and behaviours associated with **disordered eating**. These behaviours include chronic dieting, use of diet pills and laxatives, self-induced vomiting, and others.

Some People Develop Eating Disorders

Some people who exhibit disordered eating patterns progress to a clinically diagnosable **eating disorder**. The diagnostic criteria for eating disorders are defined by the American Psychiatric Association (APA) and include *anorexia nervosa, bulimia nervosa, binge-eating disorder,* and a cluster of less distinct conditions collectively referred to as *eating disorders not otherwise specified (ED-NOS).*

Although anorexia nervosa and bulimia nervosa affect people primarily in their teens and twenties, and more frequently women, as mentioned in Chapter 6, all segments of the population have potential for developing an eating disorder. Statistics Canada, in their Mental Health Survey conducted in 2002, collected self-reported data regarding being diagnosed with an eating disorder in the past 12 months (Public Health Agency of Canada, 2011). Results indicated that 0.5 percent of Canadians over the age of 15 reported a diagnosis of an eating disorder. The rates

Body dysmorphic disorder (BDD) Psychological disorder characterized by an obsessive concern with appearance, including a distorted view of oneself.

Social physique anxiety (SPA) Refers to the nervousness or anxiety experienced at the real or perceived evaluation of your body by others.

Disordered eating A pattern of atypical and less healthy eating behaviours used to achieve or maintain a lower body weight.

Eating disorder A term used to describe a collection of psychiatric diseases that involve severe disturbances in eating behaviours, unhealthy efforts to control body fat and weight, and abnormal attitudes toward one's body weight and shape.

FIGURE 2

Eating Issues Continuum. This second part of the continuum shown in Figure 1 suggests that the progression from normal eating to eating disorders occurs on a continuum.

Eating disordered	Disruptive eating patterns	Food preoccupied/ obsessed	Concerned well	Food is not an issue
I regularly stuff myself and then exercise, vomit, or use diet pills or laxatives to get rid of the food or calories. My friends and family tell me I am too thin. I am terrified of eating fatty foods. When I let myself eat, I have a hard time controlling the amount of food I eat. I am afraid to eat in front of others.	I have tried diet pills, laxatives, vomiting, or extra time exercising in order to lose or maintain my weight. I have fasted or avoided eating for long periods of time in order to lose or maintain my weight. I feel strong when I can restrict how much I eat. Eating more than I wanted to makes me feel out of control.	I think about food a lot. I feel I don't eat well most of the time. It's hard for me to enjoy eating with others. I feel ashamed when I eat more than others or more than what I feel I should be eating. I am afraid of getting fat. I wish I could change how much I want to eat and what I am hungry for.	I pay attention to what I eat in order to maintain a healthy body. I may weigh more than I would like, but I enjoy eating and balance my pleasure with eating with my concern for a healthy body. I am moderate and flexible in goals for eating well. I try to follow the guidelines in Eating Well with Canada's Food Guide for healthy eating.	I am not concerned about what others think regarding what and how much I eat. When I am upset or depressed, I eat whatever I am hungry for without any guilt or shame. Food is an important part of my life but only occupies a small part of my time.

Source: From Campus Health Service. Original continuum, C. Schislak, Preventive Medicine and Public Health. Copyright © 1997. Used with permission of Arizona Board of Regents.

of past-year diagnoses were higher in women than men (0.8 vs. 0.2 percent) and highest in 15- to 24-year-old females (1.5 percent). Data for prior periods does not reflect that percentage of the population living with an eating disorder at any point in time.

It was further reported by the Public Health Agency of Canada (2011) that anorexia nervosa and bulimia nervosa are most predominant among adolescent girls and young women (5 to 15 percent). Binge eating disorder affects about 2 percent of the population.

Disordered eating and eating disorders are also common among athletes, affecting up to 62 percent of college and university athletes in sports such as gymnastics, wrestling, swimming, figure skating, and others with an emphasis on body weight and shape or aesthetics in performance (Beals & Hill, 2006; Ronco, 2007).

Eating disorders are on the rise among men. However, many men suffering from eating disorders fail to seek treatment, perhaps because these disorders have traditionally been thought of as a women's issue. This rise in eating disorders in men might be linked to the increased pressure for men to achieve the ideal male body incessantly promoted in the media.

What factors put individuals at risk? Eating disorders are complex and, despite scientific research to try to understand them, their biological, behavioural, and social underpinnings remain elusive. It is important to remember that eating disorders are psychological disorders. Further, you do not choose to get an eating disorder any more than you can simply eat more to recover from one. When you have an eating disorder, you often feel disempowered in other aspects of your life, and try to gain a sense of control through food—what, how much, where, with whom, and so on, you eat. When you have an eating disorder, you may also be clinically depressed, suffer from obsessive-compulsive disorder, or have other psychiatric problems. Further, you are at greater risk for an eating disorder when you have low self-esteem, negative body image, and a high tendency for perfectionism (Forsberg & Lock, 2006).

Anorexia Nervosa

Anorexia nervosa is a persistent, chronic eating disorder characterized by deliberate food restriction and severe, life-threatening weight loss. It involves self-starvation motivated by an intense fear of gaining weight along with a distorted body image. Individuals with anorexia nervosa eventually progress to restricting their intake of almost all foods. The little they do eat, they may purge through vomiting or using laxatives or they may exercise to extremes, that is, they exercise until they burn the calories consumed. Although emaciated, people with anorexia nervosa do not feel thin enough and easily identify body parts that they think are "too fat."

It is estimated that between 0.5 and 3.7 percent of females in Canada will suffer from anorexia nervosa in their lifetime (Public Health Agency of Canada, 2011). The revised APA (2010) criteria for anorexia nervosa are as follows:

- Refusal to maintain body weight at or above a minimally normal weight for age and height
- Intense fear of gaining weight or becoming fat, even though considered underweight by all medical criteria
- Disturbance in the way in which one's body weight or shape is experienced, undue influence of body weight or shape on self-evaluation, or denial of the seriousness of the current low body weight

Figure 3 illustrates the physical and mental consequences of anorexia nervosa. In essence, individuals with anorexia nervosa are starving themselves to death. The causes of anorexia nervosa are complex and variable. Many people with anorexia nervosa have other coexisting psychiatric problems, including low self-esteem, depression, an anxiety disorder, and substance

> **Anorexia nervosa** Eating disorder characterized by excessive preoccupation with food, self-starvation, or extreme exercising to achieve weight loss.

FIGURE 3

What Anorexia Nervosa Can Do to Your Body

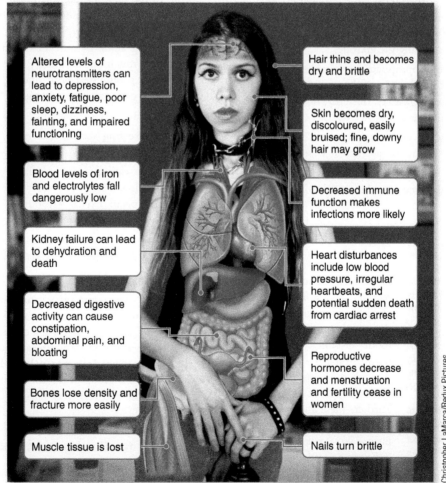

- Altered levels of neurotransmitters can lead to depression, anxiety, fatigue, poor sleep, dizziness, fainting, and impaired functioning
- Blood levels of iron and electrolytes fall dangerously low
- Kidney failure can lead to dehydration and death
- Decreased digestive activity can cause constipation, abdominal pain, and bloating
- Bones lose density and fracture more easily
- Muscle tissue is lost
- Hair thins and becomes dry and brittle
- Skin becomes dry, discoloured, easily bruised; fine, downy hair may grow
- Decreased immune function makes infections more likely
- Heart disturbances include low blood pressure, irregular heartbeats, and potential sudden death from cardiac arrest
- Reproductive hormones decrease and menstruation and fertility cease in women
- Nails turn brittle

Christopher LaMarca/Redux Pictures

abuse. Potential physical factors include an imbalance of neurotransmitters and genetic susceptibility (Eating Disorder Institute, 2009; National Association of Anorexia Nervosa and Associated Disorders, n.d.).

Bulimia Nervosa

Individuals with **bulimia nervosa** binge on huge amounts of food and then engage in some kind of purging, or compensatory behaviour, such as vomiting, taking laxatives, or exercising excessively to lose the calories they consumed. People with bulimia nervosa are obsessed with their bodies, weight gain, and appearance, but unlike those with anorexia nervosa, their problem is often hidden from the public eye because their weight is usually in the healthy range or they may be slightly overweight.

Between 1.1 and 4.2 percent of women will experience bulimia nervosa in their lifetime (Public Health Agency of Canada, 2011). The revised APA (2010) diagnostic criteria for bulimia nervosa are as follows:

- Recurrent episodes of binge eating (defined as eating, in a discrete period of time, an amount of food that is larger than most people would eat during a similar period of time and under similar circumstances, and experiencing a sense of lack of control over eating during the episode)

- Recurrent inappropriate compensatory behaviour to prevent weight gain, such as self-induced vomiting; misuse of laxatives, diuretics, or other medications; fasting; or excessive exercise

- Binge eating and inappropriate compensatory behaviour occurs on average at least once a week for three months

- Body shape and weight unduly influence self-evaluation

- The disturbance does not occur exclusively during episodes of anorexia nervosa

Figure 4 illustrates the physical and mental consequences of bulimia nervosa. For those who choose to purge using vomiting, the most common symptom is tooth erosion, which results from stomach acids passing through the mouth along with the contents of the stomach. Further, these individuals who vomit as their method of purging are also at risk for electrolyte imbalances and dehydration, both of which can contribute to a heart attack and sudden death.

Bulimia nervosa Eating disorder characterized by binge eating followed by inappropriate measures, such as vomiting, laxative use, or excessive exercise to prevent calorie absorption.

Binge-eating disorder A type of eating disorder characterized by binge eating once a week or more, but not typically followed by a purge.

Eating disorders not otherwise specified (ED-NOS) Eating disorders that are a psychiatric illness but do not fit the diagnostic criteria for anorexia nervosa, bulimia nervosa, or binge-eating disorder.

A combination of genetic and environmental factors is thought to relate to bulimia nervosa (National Alliance on Mental Illness, 2010). A family history of obesity, an underlying anxiety disorder, and an imbalance in neurotransmitters are all possible contributing factors.

Binge-Eating Disorder

Individuals with **binge-eating disorder** gorge in a way similar to those who have bulimia nervosa, but do not purge. Thus, these individuals are often clinically obese. As in bulimia nervosa, binge-eating episodes are characterized by eating large amounts of food rapidly, even when not feeling hungry, and feeling guilty or depressed afterwards (National Association of Anorexia Nervosa and Associated Disorders, 2011).

The Public Health Agency of Canada (2011) reported that 2 percent of the population is affected by binge eating disorders. The revised APA (2010) criteria for binge-eating disorder are as follows:

- Recurrent episodes of binge eating

- The binge-eating episodes are associated with three (or more) of the following:
  1. eating much more rapidly than normal;
  2. eating until feeling uncomfortably full;
  3. eating large amounts of food when not feeling physically hungry;
  4. eating alone because of embarrassment over how much one is eating;
  5. feeling disgusted with oneself, depressed, or very guilty after overeating

- Marked distress regarding binge eating is present

- The binge eating occurs, on average, at least once a week for three months

- The binge eating is not associated with inappropriate compensatory behaviours (e.g., purging) and does not occur exclusively during the course of bulimia nervosa or anorexia nervosa

Some Eating Disorders Are Not Easily Classified

The APA (2010) recognizes that some patterns of disordered eating qualify as a legitimate psychiatric illness but do not fit into the strict diagnostic criteria for anorexia nervosa, bulimia nervosa, or binge-eating disorder. These are the **eating disorders not otherwise specified (ED-NOS)**. This group of disorders can include night eating syndrome and recurrent purging in the absence of binge eating.

Treatment for Eating Disorders

Because eating disorders are caused by a combination of many factors, there are no quick or simple solutions.

FIGURE 4

What Bulimia Nervosa Can Do to Your Body

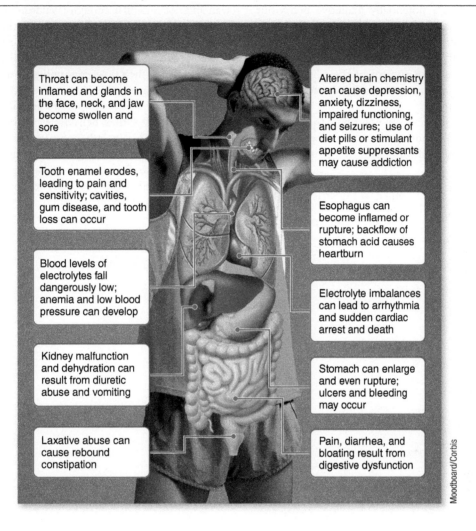

Throat can become inflamed and glands in the face, neck, and jaw become swollen and sore

Tooth enamel erodes, leading to pain and sensitivity; cavities, gum disease, and tooth loss can occur

Blood levels of electrolytes fall dangerously low; anemia and low blood pressure can develop

Kidney malfunction and dehydration can result from diuretic abuse and vomiting

Laxative abuse can cause rebound constipation

Altered brain chemistry can cause depression, anxiety, dizziness, impaired functioning, and seizures; use of diet pills or stimulant appetite suppressants may cause addiction

Esophagus can become inflamed or rupture; backflow of stomach acid causes heartburn

Electrolyte imbalances can lead to arrhythmia and sudden cardiac arrest and death

Stomach can enlarge and even rupture; ulcers and bleeding may occur

Pain, diarrhea, and bloating result from digestive dysfunction

Moodboard/Corbis

Without treatment, approximately 20 percent of people with an eating disorder will die from it; with treatment, long-term full recovery rates range from 44 to 76 percent for anorexia nervosa and from 50 to 70 percent for bulimia nervosa (Franco, 2011; Mirasol Eating Disorder Recovery Centers, 2010).

When a person with an eating disorder seeks treatment—or is forcibly placed in treatment—the first focus is on reducing threat to life. This involves various efforts aimed at calorie intake, including intravenous or feeding tubes when necessary. If the patient is stabilized, long-term therapy is then employed, which focuses on the psychological, social, environmental, and physiological factors involved. Therapy allows the patient to work on adopting new eating attitudes and behaviours, building self-confidence, and finding other ways to deal with life's problems. Support groups can help the family and the individual learn to foster positive actions

and interactions. Treatment of an underlying anxiety disorder or depression may also be a focus.

SOME PEOPLE DEVELOP EXERCISE DISORDERS

Although exercise is generally beneficial to health, in excess it can cause problems. A recent study of almost 600 college students revealed that 18 percent met the criteria for **compulsive exercise** (Guidi et al., 2009). Also called *anorexia athletica,* compulsive exercise is characterized by a *compulsion* to

Compulsive exercise Disorder characterized by a compulsion to engage in excessive exercise, and feelings of guilt and anxiety if the level of exercise is perceived as inadequate.

exercise rather than a *desire* to do so. That is, the person struggles with guilt and anxiety if he or she does not work out. Compulsive exercise is also discussed in Chapter 9 as a potentially addictive behaviour. People who exercise with compulsion, similar to people with eating disorders, often define their self-worth externally. These individuals over-exercise in order to feel more in control of their lives. Disordered eating or a diagnosable eating disorder is often part of the picture.

Compulsive exercise can contribute to a variety of injuries. It can also put significant stress on the heart, especially if combined with disordered eating.

Muscle dysmorphia Body image disorder in which men believe that their body is not lean or muscular enough.

Muscle Dysmorphia

Muscle dysmorphia, sometimes referred to as "reverse anorexia," appears to be a relatively new form of body image disturbance and exercise disorder among men in which a man believes that his body is insufficiently lean and not muscular enough (Waldron, 2011). Men with muscle dysmorphia believe that they look "puny," when in reality they look normal or may even be considerably muscular. As a result of their adherence to a meticulous diet, their time-consuming workout schedule, and their shame over their perceived appearance flaws, they may neglect important social or occupational activities. Other behaviours characteristic of muscle dysmorphia include comparing oneself unfavourably to others, checking one's appearance in the mirror, and camouflaging one's appearance. Men with muscle dysmorphia also are likely to abuse anabolic steroids and dietary supplements (Silverman, n.d.).

assess YOURSELF

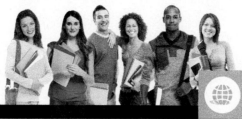

Go to MasteringHealth to complete this questionnaire with automatic scoring

TAKING CHARGE: Managing Your Body Image

Determining whether or not your eating and exercising behaviours are putting you at risk of an eating disorder is not black and white. Weighing yourself, counting calories, or working out every day does not mean you have health problems. Still, some of the efforts you might make to lose a few pounds could spiral out of control. It has been said that every eating disorder began with a diet, but that every diet does not lead to an eating disorder. To find out whether your efforts to be thin are harmful to you, take the following quiz from the National Eating Disorders Association (NEDA).

Are Your Efforts to Be Thin Spinning Out of Control?

1. I constantly calculate numbers of fat grams and calories.

   T   F

2. I weigh myself often and find myself obsessed with the number on the scale.

   T   F

3. I exercise to burn calories and not for health or enjoyment.

   T   F

4. I sometimes feel out of control while eating.

   T   F

5. I often go on extreme diets.

   T   F

6. I engage in rituals to get me through meal-times and/or secretively binge.

   T   F

7. Weight loss, dieting, and controlling my food intake have become my major concerns.

   T   F

8. I feel ashamed, disgusted, or guilty after eating.

   T   F

9. I constantly worry about the weight, shape, and/or size of my body.

   T   F

10. I feel my identity and value are based on how I look or how much I weigh.

    T   F

If any of these statements is true or partly true for you, you could be dealing with disordered eating. If so, talk about it! Tell a friend, parent, teacher, coach, youth group leader, doctor, counsellor, or nutritionist what you are going through.

Source: National Eating Disorders Association.

The above Assess Yourself activity gave you the chance to evaluate your feelings about your body and to determine whether or not you might be engaging in eating or exercise behaviours that may have a negative impact on your overall health. Below are suggestions to consider to improve your body image:

- Talk back to the media. Write letters to advertisers and magazines that depict unhealthy and unrealistic body types. Boycott their products or start a blog commenting on harmful body image messages in the media.
- Rather than count calories, eat the minimal number of servings from each food group. Aim for variety from each food group. Enjoy what you eat, how it tastes and how it feels, rather than thinking about how many calories you consumed.
- Find a photograph of a person you admire not for his or her appearance, but for his or her contribution to humanity. Paste it up next to your mirror to remind yourself that true beauty comes from within and benefits others.
- Start a diary. Each day, record one thing you are grateful for that has nothing to do with your appearance. At the end of each day, record one small thing you did to make someone's world a little brighter.
- Establish a group of friends who support you for who you are, not what you look like, and who get the same support from you. Form a group on a favourite social-networking site, and keep in touch, especially when you start to feel troubled by self-defeating thoughts or have the urge to engage in unhealthy eating or exercise behaviours.
- Borrow from the library or purchase one of the many books on body image now available, and read it!

CHAPTER 7
COMMITTING TO RELATIONSHIPS AND SEXUAL HEALTH

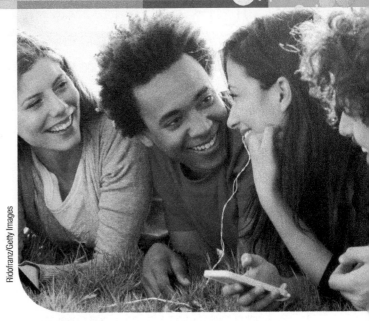

Ridofranz/Getty Images

LEARNING OUTCOMES

- Describe effective communication and the role it plays in intimate and nonintimate relationships.

- Clarify the characteristics of intimate relationships, the potential barriers to healthy relationships, and the factors important in maintaining intimate relationships.

- Describe the warning signs of a failing relationship, where you can get help, and factors that ultimately lead to the relationship failing.

- Differentiate sexual and gender identity. How are they developed? How does society help and/or hinder their development?

- Identify the various sexual dysfunctions as well as the treatment of each.

◄●● CONSIDER THIS . . .

Jorge and Yasmin have been dating exclusively for more than two years and have talked about moving in together. Over time, Yasmin has noticed that Jorge has become possessive of her and jealous of time she spends with others—regardless of whether they are male or female. As a result, they fight regularly about who she does things with, potential threats to their relationship, and so on. Recently, Jorge took a weekend to go hunting with the guys while Yasmin stayed home to get caught up on her work. When Yasmin's friends called her to ask her to go to a party, she decided to go. When Jorge called her on her cellphone later and asked her how her night was going, she lied and said it was quiet and that she was getting lots of work done. Jorge, hearing the noise in the background, called her a liar and asked where she really was.

What should Yasmin say? What should she do? Why do you think she lied? Is dishonesty in a relationship justified? Why or why not? Is Jorge's jealousy a healthy, normal part of their relationship? Is Yasmin's response to it normal? Can a relationship based on mistrust, half-truths, and possessiveness survive? Why or why not?

As a human, you are a social being—you have a basic need to belong and feel loved, appreciated, and wanted. You cannot live without relating to others in some way. In fact, research indicates that the ability to relate well with people, as well as give and receive love and support throughout your life, can have almost as much impact on your health as regular physical activity and consuming a diet that follows Eating Well with Canada's Food Guide (MayoClinic.com, 2003; Uberg et al., 2005). All relationships involve a degree of risk, and by taking these risks we grow and truly experience all that life has to offer. By looking at your intimate and nonintimate relationships, components of sexual identity, gender roles, and sexual orientation, you will come to better understand who you are and increase your capacity to relate effectively with others and build better, stronger relationships.

COMMUNICATING: A KEY TO ESTABLISHING RELATIONSHIPS

From the moment of birth, we struggle to be understood. We flail our arms, cry, scream, smile, frown, and make sounds and gestures to attract attention, get a reaction from someone, or have someone understand what we want or need from them. By the time you enter adulthood, you have developed a unique way of communicating using gestures, words, expressions, and body positions. No two of you communicate in the exact same way or have the same need to connect with others. Some of you are outgoing and quick to express emotions and thoughts. Others are quiet, reluctant to talk about feelings, and prefer to spend time alone.

Different cultures have not only distinct languages and dialects but also unique ways of expressing themselves and using body language to communicate (Snapp & Leary, 2001). Some cultures gesture wildly; others maintain a closed and rigid means of speaking. Some cultures are offended by apparent "fixed and dilated" staring, while others welcome a steady look in the eyes. Although people differ in the way they communicate, this does not mean that one sex, culture, or group is better or should be a model for the others regarding their approach to communication. You have to be willing to accept differences and work to keep communication lines open and fluid. Appearing interested, actively engaged in the interaction, and open and willing to exchange ideas and thoughts is something that you typically learn with practice and hard work.

Self-disclosure Sharing personal information with others.

Communicating How You Feel

Do you find it easy to express how much you care about friends and family members with hugs, kisses, and verbal expressions? If you are comfortable telling them you love them and that they mean a lot to you, chances are that you also will be able to tell them when you are feeling sad, disappointed, angry, or frustrated. However, it is important to realize that some people were not raised in affectionate families or a culture supportive of open expressions, do not readily discuss feelings or emotions, and sometimes struggle to find the right words for expressing what they feel.

When two people begin a relationship, they bring their communication styles with them (Manusov & Harvey, 2001). How often have you heard someone say, "We just cannot communicate," or "You are sending mixed messages?" These exchanges occur regularly as people start relationships or work through communication problems in an existing relationship. Because communication is a process, every action, word, facial expression, gesture, or body posture becomes part of your shared history and part of the evolving impression you make on others and others make on you. If you are angry in your responses, others will be reluctant to interact with you. Similarly, when others are angry or abrupt in their responses to you, you are not likely to want to continue to interact with them. If you bring "baggage" from past negative interactions to new relationships, you may be cynical, distrustful, and guarded in your exchanges with others. If you are positive, happy, and share openly with others, they will be more likely to communicate openly with you. This ability to communicate assertively is an important skill in relationships (see the suggestions that follow). When you are an assertive communicator, you are in touch with your feelings and values and able to directly and honestly communicate your needs or defend your decisions in a positive manner.

Improving Communication Skills

Because people have such different ways of communicating, there is no recipe for how to communicate effectively in a given situation. At times, silence might be the best approach. However, there are things that you can do to become better communicators and to encourage and assist others in their attempts to interact with you.

Learning Appropriate Self-Disclosure

Sharing personal information with others is called **self-disclosure**. If you are willing to share personal information with others, they will likely share personal information with you. In other words, if you want to learn more about someone, you have to be willing to share parts of yourself with that person. Self-disclosure is not storytelling or sharing secrets; rather, it is revealing how you are reacting to the present situation and giving information about the past relevant to the other person's understanding of your current reactions (Caputo, Hazel, & McMahon, 1994).

Self-disclosure can be a double-edged sword, as there is risk in divulging personal insights and feelings. If you sense that sharing feelings and personal thoughts will result in a closer relationship, you will likely take the risk. But if you believe that self-disclosure will result in rejection or alienation, you are not so likely to take that risk. If the confidentiality of previously shared information has been violated, you are likely to hesitate to disclose yourself in the future.

Becoming a Better Listener

You can likely quite easily think of someone who "never listens" and monopolizes the entire conversation. Although it is easy to recognize poor listening skills in others, it is much more difficult to acknowledge our own deficiencies. Listening is a vital part of interpersonal communication; it allows you to share feelings, express concerns, communicate wants and needs, and let your thoughts and opinions be known. If you want to communicate effectively, you must work at improving your speaking and listening skills. Improving these skills will enhance your relationships, improve your understanding of what you want to say, and allow you to interpret more effectively what others say. You listen best when (1) you believe that the message is important and relevant to you; (2) the speaker holds your attention through humour, dramatic effect, use of media, or other techniques; and (3) you are in the mood to listen (free of distractions and worries). When you listen effectively, you try to understand what people are thinking and feeling from their perspective. You not only hear the words, but you also try to understand what is really being said.

On a daily basis, you likely have times when you simply "tune out." When a professor drones on about a subject you do not relate to or are not very interested in, you may begin doodling and/or daydreaming. You may even pull out your cellphone and start texting! When a friend or colleague tells the same story again and again, you might say "uh-huh"—and worry that you will be caught and asked a question about it. You might grimace or smile when you see a particular person approach you depending upon how eager you are to talk to him or her. What is the difference? Why do you tune out when some people speak and tune in for others? You likely gravitate toward those who seem to understand and agree with you and with whom you have fun and interesting interactions. Sometimes, this

tuned-out behaviour is a result of lack of sleep, stress, preoccupation, drunkenness, or being under the influence of drugs. Other times, it is because the speaker is a person who talks for the sake of talking or you find the speaker and/or what he or she is talking about boring. Still, many of the most common listening difficulties are things that you can work to improve.

What does it take to be a very good or excellent listener? Practise the following skills and consciously use them on a daily basis to improve your communication skills.

- Be present in the moment. Contrary to popular thought, good listeners do not just sit back with their mouths shut. They participate and acknowledge what the speaker is saying. (Nodding, smiling, saying "yes" or "uh-huh," and asking reflective questions at appropriate times are part of this. Take care, however, not to say "uh-huh" too frequently since it can be distracting and convey insincerity.)

- Nonverbal communication is key when listening to others. Use positive body language and voice tone. Show that you are "with" the speaker by turning toward him or her and staying focused (wandering eyes are a sure sign that your mind is elsewhere). Avoid barrier gestures such as shaking your head "no," negative faces, or folding your arms; smile at appropriate times and maintain eye contact without staring. Your tone of voice, posture, and attitude should convey interest.

- Express empathy, not necessarily sympathy. Watch for verbal and nonverbal clues to the other person's feelings and try to relate to them. For example, saying, "That must have been really hard for you" can encourage the speaker to talk and feel more comfortable with you as an understanding and caring listener.

- Ask for clarification. If you are not sure what the speaker means, ask for clarification or paraphrase what you think you heard. This kind of feedback is invaluable in avoiding misinterpretation and lapses in overall communication. As a speaker, you might ask, "What did you think I was just saying?" so long as it is said in a nonthreatening manner.

- Control the desire to interrupt. Some people start nodding and gesturing before you even get a word out. If you are like that, squelch it, even if you have to put an inconspicuous—or conspicuous—hand over your mouth. Try taking a deep breath for two seconds, then hold your breath for another second and really listen to what is being said as you slowly exhale. Try not to be so enthusiastically empathetic that you finish speakers' sentences or put words in people's mouths.

- Avoid snap judgments based on what people look like or what they say. If you notice some strange mannerism, try to focus on what is being said, not on how it is being said. Avoid stereotyping or labelling, particularly with people who have a background different from yours.

- Resist the temptation to "set the other person straight." Control your urge to correct errors, be right, or react defensively. Listen without reacting or trying to rationalize what the speaker is trying to say.

- Try to focus on the speaker. Sometimes it is tough to listen to someone who is talking about a painful situation, especially if we are experiencing or have recently experienced something similar. Hold back the temptation to "tell all" about your own negative experience. Each person reacts to his or her situations in his or her own way. Give the speaker the moment and later, after he or she has finished talking, you can talk about your own experience as a way of validating the feelings expressed. Do not tell someone how to feel or react to a particular situation. Also refrain from telling this person that you know exactly how he or she feels.

- Be tenacious. Stick with the speaker and try to stay on the topic. If he or she wanders, gently nudge him or her back by saying, "You were just saying. . . ." Offer your thoughts and suggestions, and remember to advise only up to a certain point. Clarify with "this is my opinion" as a reminder that you are offering your thoughts, rather than a fact.

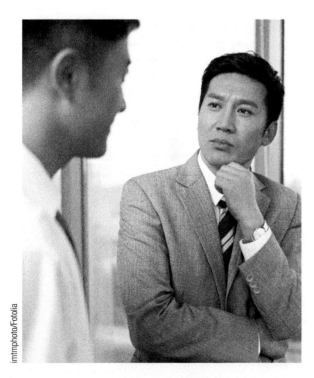

imtmphoto/Fotolia

Listening is a key component of communication.

CHARACTERISTICS OF INTIMATE RELATIONSHIPS

There are many definitions of **intimate relationships**. One definition is that "intimacy involves feelings of emotional closeness and connectedness with another person and the desire to share each other's innermost thoughts and feelings. Intimate relationships are characterized by attitudes of mutual trust, caring, and acceptance" (Options for Sexual Health, 2012, n.p.). In this context, friends, family, lovers, partners, and even people you work with or interact with at the grocery store may be included in the sphere of intimate interactions. For the purposes of this chapter, we define intimate relationships in terms of three characteristics: behavioural interdependence, need fulfillment, and emotional attachment. Each of these characteristics can be related to interactions with family, close friends, and romantic relationships (Brehm, 1992).

Behavioural interdependence refers to the mutual impact that people have on each other as their lives and daily activities become intertwined. What one person does might influence what the other person might want and can do. Such interdependence can become stronger over time to the point that each person would find a void in his or her life if the other person left.

Another characteristic of intimate relationships is that they fulfill psychological needs and, as such, are a means of need fulfillment. These needs, which can often be met only through relationships with others, are as follows:

- The need for approval and for a sense of purpose in life—requiring the sense that what you say and do matters.

- The need for intimacy—requiring someone with whom you can share your feelings freely.

- The need for social integration—requiring someone with whom you can share your worries and concerns.

- The need for nurturing—requiring someone whom you can take care of.

- The need for being nurtured—requiring someone who can take care of you.

- The need for reassurance or affirmation of your worth—requiring someone to tell you that you matter.

In other words, rewarding, intimate relationships, partners, or friends meet each other's needs. They disclose feelings, share confidences, and discuss

Intimate relationships Close relationships with other people in which you offer, and are offered, validation, understanding, and a sense of being valued intellectually, emotionally, and physically.

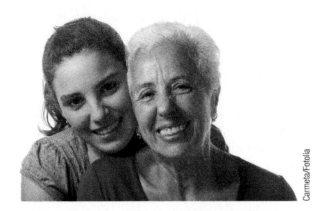
Carmeta/Fotolia

Emotional bonding and other elements of intimate relationships are rooted in a caring, supportive family environment.

practical concerns; they help each other and provide reassurance. They serve as major sources of social support and reinforce your feelings that you are important and serve a purpose in life.

In addition to behavioural interdependence and need fulfillment, intimate relationships involve strong bonds of emotional attachment, or feelings of love and attachment. The intimacy level experienced by any two people cannot easily be judged by those outside the relationship. Although sex can often be an important part of an intimate relationship, a relationship can also be very intimate without it. In fact, many satisfying and lasting intimate relationships go well beyond the need for sexual contact.

Emotional availability, the ability to give to and receive from others emotionally without fear of being hurt or rejected, is another characteristic of intimate relationships. At times, you may need to protect yourself psychologically by making yourself unavailable emotionally. For example, if a relationship ends, you might close down emotionally and carefully avoid letting yourself feel too much. This gives you the time to regroup and heal before reaching out to people again. It also reduces the risk of a rebound romance that is often doomed to failure as a result of unresolved personal hurts and issues.

FORMING INTIMATE RELATIONSHIPS

Throughout your life, you go through predictable patterns of relationships. In your early years, your most significant relationships are most often with your family. Gradually, your relationships widen to include friends, co-workers/classmates, and acquaintances.

Emotional availability The ability to give to and receive from other people emotionally without being inhibited by fears of being hurt.

You are also likely to develop one or more romantic or sexual relationships with another person over your lifetime. Each of these relationships plays a significant role in your emotional, social, spiritual, and physical health.

Families: The Ties That Bind

Although many people consider the family the foundation of Canadian society and talk about a return to "family values" as a desirable objective, it is clear that the modern Canadian family looks quite different from families of previous generations. The *Leave It to Beaver* family model that was held up during the 1950s—Mom with her apron, staying at home, content in her role as mother and spouse; Dad with his briefcase, trying to move up the corporate ladder; and two or three happy, well-adjusted children—is no longer the norm. In Canada today, it is quite common for both parents to work outside of the home and children can be raised not only by a Mom and Dad but also by single parents, same-sex parents, grandparents, relatives, stepparents, nannies, day-care centre workers, and other "parents."

Regardless of the form or structure of each family, all families should care for, protect, love, and socialize with one another. Whether the family is related by birth or simply connected by a high level of love and regard, their living arrangement, or some other factor, the family network often provides the sense of security needed to develop into healthy adults. The definition of family changes dramatically from culture to culture and from place to place over time.

The Vanier Institute of the Family (n.d.) defines family as "any combination of two or more persons bound together over time by ties of mutual consent, birth or adoption/placement and who, together, assume responsibilities for variant combinations of the following: physical maintenance and care of group members; addition of new members through procreation or adoption; socialization of children; social control of members; production, consumption and distribution of goods and services; affective nurturance – love."

Today's Family Unit

The United Nations defines eight basic types of families:

- nuclear families
- single-parent families
- cross-generational families
- adopted/foster families
- never-married families

- blended families

- grandparents as parents

- same-sex parent families (American Academy of Pediatrics, 2013)

You might think of family in terms of the "family of origin." Your family of origin includes the people present in the household during a child's first years of life—usually parents and siblings. However, as noted, given the various families identified above, the family of origin might also include a stepparent, parents' lovers, or significant others such as grandparents, aunts, or uncles. The family of origin has a tremendous impact on the child's emotional, social, and spiritual development. The nuclear family accounts for about half of all families with children under the age of 18 years and consists of two biological parents (usually, but not necessarily, married) and their children (American Academy of Pediatrics, 2013).

If parents are comfortable in sharing feelings, affection, and love with each other and their offspring, their children are likely to become emotionally connected adults. If the home environment provides stability and seems a safe place to be, it is likely that the children will learn to express feelings and develop intimacy skills. Given the amount of time typically spent together, sibling interactions have an important role in children's social-cognitive development (Whiteman, Becerra Bernard, & Jensen, 2010). In particular, unique opportunities for social and emotional development arise from various conflict situations as siblings are sensitive to one another's reactions, behaviours, and emotions. The family of origin has the potential to encourage significant positive interactions and growth. People can learn and practise positive behaviours as well as the

rights and wrongs of negative behaviours in a safe and nonjudgmental environment when the family itself is healthy. However, if the family is mentally or physically unhealthy, regardless of type, it can pose significant barriers to later relationships.

Establishing Friendships

> A friend is one who knows you as you are
> understands where you've been
> accepts who you've become,
> and still gently invites you to grow.
>
> —*Author Unknown*

Although you likely have a clear idea of the distinction between a friend and a lover, this difference is not always easy to verbalize. You might think the major difference is that there is no intimate physical involvement between friends. You may see the difference in terms of level of intimacy as, often, intimacy levels are much lower between friends than between lovers. But, as stated previously, people can be intimate with each other without being sexually involved. Confused? You are probably not alone. Surprisingly, there has not been much research to clarify these terms. Beyond the fact that two people participate in a relationship as equals, friendships include the following (see also Figure 7.1):

- Enjoyment. Friends enjoy each other's company, although there may be temporary states of anger, disappointment, or mutual annoyance.

- Acceptance. Friends accept each other as they are, without trying to change one another.

FIGURE 7.1

Common Bonds of Friends and Lovers

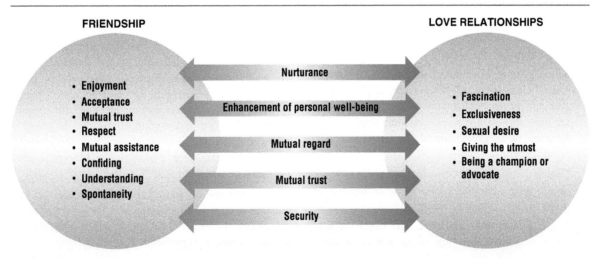

- Trust. Friends have mutual trust; each assumes that the other will act in his or her friend's best interests.

- Respect. Friends respect each other; each assumes that the other uses good judgment in making life choices.

- Mutual assistance. Friends are inclined to help and support one another. They can count on each other in times of need or duress as well as in positive times, worthy of celebration.

- Confiding. Friends share experiences and feelings with each other that they do not share with other people.

- Understanding. Friends know what is important to each other and usually understand each other's behaviour.

- Spontaneity. Friends feel free to be themselves in the relationship rather than play a role, wear a mask, or refrain from revealing their true self (Turner & Rubinson, 1993).

Significant Others, Partners, Couples

Although family and friends provide necessary intimate relationships, you are likely to choose at some point whether or not to enter into an intimate sexual relationship with another person. Most couples fit into one of four categories of significant relationships: married heterosexual couples, cohabiting heterosexual couples, married lesbian or gay couples, and cohabiting lesbian or gay couples. Love relationships in each of these four groups typically include the characteristics of friendship as well as the following related to passion and caring:

- Fascination. Lovers tend to pay attention to the other person even when they should be involved in other activities. They think often of the other person and want to think about, look at, talk to, touch, or merely be with him or her.

- Exclusiveness. Lovers have a special relationship that usually precludes having the same relationship with a third party.

- Sexual desire. Lovers want physical intimacy with their partner and desire to touch, hold, kiss, and engage in sexual activities. However, lovers may choose not to act on their sexual desire because of religious, moral, or other practical considerations.

- Giving the utmost. Lovers care enough to give the utmost when the other is in need, sometimes to the point of extreme self-sacrifice.

- Being a champion/advocate. The depth of lovers' caring may show up as an active, unselfish championing of each other's interests and a positive attempt to ensure that the other succeeds (Turner & Rubinson, 1993).

For obvious reasons, the best love relationships share friendships, and the best friendships include several love components. Both types of relationships share common bonds of nurturance; enhancement of personal well-being; and a genuine sense of mutual regard, trust, and security.

This Thing Called Love

Love is a gift, not an obligation.

—*Author Unknown*

What is love? Defining love is more difficult than simply listing characteristics of a loving relationship. Love has been written about and engraved on walls; it has been the theme of countless novels, poems, movies, songs, and plays. There is no one definition of love, and the word means different things depending on cultural values, age, sex, education, experiences, and situation.

Love most often exists as one of two kinds: companionate and passionate. Companionate love is a secure, trusting attachment, similar to what you often feel for family members or close friends (Hatfield, 1988). In companionate love, two people are attracted, have much in common, care about each other's well-being, and express reciprocal liking and respect. Passionate love involves a state of high arousal filled with the ecstasy of being loved or the agony of being rejected (Hatfield, 1988). The person experiencing passionate love tends to be preoccupied with his or her partner and to perceive the loved person as perfect (Baron & Byrne, 1994). Passionate love will not occur unless the following three conditions are met:

- The person must live in a culture in which the concept of "falling in love" is idealized.

- A "suitable" person to love must be present. If the culture a person is immersed in—including influence from parents, movies, books, songs, peers, and the like—projects the need to seek a particular partner with a certain level of attractiveness or belonging to a certain ethnic or age group or with a certain socioeconomic status, and none is available, the "seeker" may find it difficult to allow him- or herself to find "love."

- There must be some type of physiologic arousal that occurs when a person is in the presence of the object of desire. Sexual excitement is often the way this arousal is expressed.

In the "triangular theory of love," love is clarified by isolating three key ingredients:

- Intimacy. The emotional component, which involves feelings of closeness

- Passion. The motivational component, which reflects romantic, sexual attraction

- Decision/commitment. The cognitive component, which includes the decisions you make about being in love and the degree of commitment to your partner (Acevedo & Aron, 2009)

According to this model, the greater the intimacy, passion, and commitment, the more likely a person is to be involved in a healthy, positive loving relationship. It is also noted in this theory that different types of love exist when not all three components are combined (Acevedo & Aron, 2009). For example, passionate love results from the combination of intimacy and passion without commitment; passion without commitment or intimacy is defined as infatuated love; and fatuous love results from passion and commitment without intimacy. Further, it is argued that over time in successful relationships, passion decreases, intimacy increases, and commitment level becomes stable.

A second theory of love and attraction based on brain circuitry and chemistry is quite different from the triangular theory just discussed. In this theory, in regard to attraction and the process of falling in love, a fairly predictable pattern is followed based on:

- Imprinting, in which our evolutionary patterns, genetic predispositions, and past experiences trigger romantic reaction

- Attraction, in which neurochemicals produce feelings of euphoria and elation

- Attachment, in which endorphins—natural opiates—cause lovers to feel peaceful, secure, and calm

- Production of a "cuddle chemical"—the brain secretes the chemical oxytocin, thereby stimulating sensations during lovemaking and eliciting feelings of satisfaction and attachment (Fisher, 1993).

Lovers who claim to be swept away by passion may not, therefore, be far from the truth (Toufexis & Gray, 1993).

A meeting of the eyes, a touch of the hands, or a whiff of scent may set off a flood that starts in the brain and races along the nerves and through the blood. The familiar results—flushed skin, sweaty palms, heavy breathing—are identical to those experienced when under stress. Why? Because the love-smitten person is secreting chemical substances such as dopamine, norepinephrine, and phenylethylamine (PEA) that are chemical cousins of amphetamines.

Although attraction may in fact be a "natural high," with PEA levels soaring, this hit of passion loses effectiveness over time as the body builds tolerance to it, as it does to any other drug. Needing a continual fix, some people may become attraction junkies, seeking the intoxication of love in a way similar to a drug user who seeks a chemical high (Toufexis & Gray, 1993). It has been speculated that PEA levels drop significantly over a three- to four-year period, thus eliciting the "four-year itch" that shows up in the peaking fourth-year divorce rates present in more than 60 cultures. Those romances that last beyond the four-year decline of PEA are influenced by another set of chemicals known as endorphins, soothing substances that give lovers a sense of security, peace, and calm (Fisher, 1993).

In another theory, researchers describe the first stage as the lust phase, in which our biological and genetic histories converge to pique our interest and intensity of response. In the lust phase, if someone comes into our range of awareness, a chemical surge triggers our enthusiastic response. Known as pheromones and said to be as unique as our fingerprints, these triggers are scent-infused chemicals found in perspiration under the arm (McLoughlin, 2003). These pheromones trigger a unique sensory reaction in the nose and result in attraction if the producer is a match for you (McLoughlin, 2003). It is believed that following these pheromone triggers comes the attraction phase, often labelled the "falling in love" phase, and then the attachment phase. Keep in mind that we do not all react to pheromones in the same way and ought to be careful about presuming we do; our reactions are individual and complex even though they may follow a similar pattern (Kippenberger et al., 2012). The two hormones most important in the attachment phase are oxytocin and vasopressin (Baskerville & Douglas, 2010; Kagerbauer et al., 2013). Oxytocin increases the bond between lovers, is released by both sexes during orgasm, and is one of the chemicals responsible for contractions during childbirth and milk expression when breastfeeding. Scientists suspect that vasopressin is the chemical responsible for creating the desire to be monogamous with another person. One theory suggests that the more sex a couple has, the greater the bond between them.

In addition to the possible chemical influences, your past experiences may significantly affect your attraction to others. Your parents' modelling of traits you believe to be desirable or undesirable may play a role in drawing us to people with similar traits. Many researchers investigated the possible link between heterosexual males seeking partners similar to their mothers and heterosexual females seeking partners similar to their fathers. For heterosexual males and females, it may be that you are attracted to what you are familiar with.

GENDER ISSUES

In any relationship, understanding and communication are important ingredients for success. Sometimes it may seem that the relating styles of men and women are so different that obtaining true understanding and open communication may be next to impossible. Men's and women's social conditioning are so different that it is almost as if they are raised in two different cultures (Tannen, 1990). Women are brought up to feel comfortable and share freely in their intimate relationships. As a result, they tend to be more nurturing and less afraid to share their fears, anxieties, and emotions. It is okay if they cry, scream, or express wide emotional swings. Men are not supposed to cry—at least according to popular belief in Western culture. Unlike their female counterparts, they should not show emotions and are brought up believing that being strong and independent is more important than close friendships. As a result, there are differences in the way men and women communicate and interact (Figure 7.2).

FIGURE 7.2

He Says/She Says

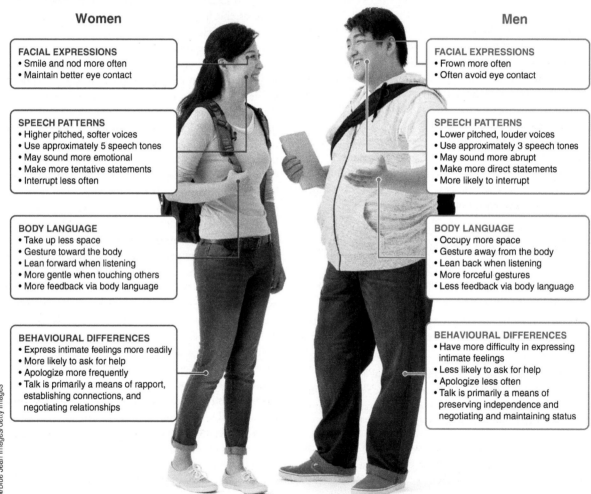

Women

FACIAL EXPRESSIONS
• Smile and nod more often
• Maintain better eye contact

SPEECH PATTERNS
• Higher pitched, softer voices
• Use approximately 5 speech tones
• May sound more emotional
• Make more tentative statements
• Interrupt less often

BODY LANGUAGE
• Take up less space
• Gesture toward the body
• Lean forward when listening
• More gentle when touching others
• More feedback via body language

BEHAVIOURAL DIFFERENCES
• Express intimate feelings more readily
• More likely to ask for help
• Apologize more frequently
• Talk is primarily a means of rapport, establishing connections, and negotiating relationships

Men

FACIAL EXPRESSIONS
• Frown more often
• Often avoid eye contact

SPEECH PATTERNS
• Lower pitched, louder voices
• Use approximately 3 speech tones
• May sound more abrupt
• Make more direct statements
• More likely to interrupt

BODY LANGUAGE
• Occupy more space
• Gesture away from the body
• Lean back when listening
• More forceful gestures
• Less feedback via body language

BEHAVIOURAL DIFFERENCES
• Have more difficulty in expressing intimate feelings
• Less likely to ask for help
• Apologize less often
• Talk is primarily a means of preserving independence and negotiating and maintaining status

BJI/Blue Jean Images/Getty Images

There are some gender-specific communication patterns and behaviours that are obvious to the casual observer (see graphic). However, according to Dr. Cynthia Burggraf Torppa at Ohio State University, the bigger difference is the way in which men and women interpret or process the same message. She indicates that women are more sensitive to interpersonal meanings "between the lines," and men are more sensitive to subtle messages about status or social hierarchy. Recognizing these differences and how they make us unique is a good first step in avoiding unnecessary frustrations and miscommunications.

Sources: C. Burggraf Torppa, Family and Consumer Sciences, Ohio State University Extension, "Gender Issues: Communication Differences in Interpersonal Relationships," 2010, http://ohioline.osu.edu/flm02/pdf/fs04.pdf; J. Wood, *Gendered Lives: Communication, Gender, and Culture*, 10th ed. (Belmont, CA: Cengage, 2013).

Why the Differences?

Although there are various theories about why males and females relate the way they do, the basic difference likely lies in the development patterns of men and women (Martin & Ruble, 2010). Men may be less able to express emotions and achieve intimacy owing to the process of identity development in infancy, which is often more difficult for males than females. Boys initially achieve intimacy with a female caregiver, usually a mother, at a preverbal stage. By the time they develop verbal skills, boys have physically separated from their caregiver. Thus, for men, intimacy may consist of physical proximity rather than verbal sharing. Because girls do not need to separate themselves from a female caregiver, they do not separate their feelings of intimacy from their verbal constructs. As a result, women are often able to express intimacy verbally, whereas men often are not. This male/female disparity in the ability to express emotions is the single greatest difference between the sexes and the greatest threat to intimacy in many relationships. This theory has received widespread acceptance among sociologists and psychologists. The disparity in the ability to express emotions may account for common female complaints about male attitudes toward sex; generally, emotion generates sexual feelings in women, whereas sexual feelings generate emotion in men. Sex, it seems, is one area in which men are allowed to contact deeper emotional states that may be hard for them to access in other circumstances. In fact, sexual activity carries the major burden of emotional expression for many males and may explain the urgency with which some men approach sex.

Picking Partners: Similarities and Differences between Genders

Just as males and females may find different ways to express themselves, the process of partner selection is also distinct. In males and females, more than chemical and psychological processes influence the choice of partners (Hendricks & Hendricks, 1992). One factor is proximity, or being in the same place at the same time. The more you see a person in your hometown, at social gatherings, or at work, the more likely an interaction will occur. Thus, if you live in Winnipeg, you will probably choose another Winnipegger. If you live on Prince Edward Island, you will probably choose another Islander.

You also pick a partner on the basis of similarities (attitudes, values, intellect, experiences, interests); the adage that "opposites attract" usually is not true. Even though you may initially be attracted to someone extremely different from you, time tends to reveal that your lack of commonalities is too big a barrier to overcome. If your potential partner expresses interest or liking, you may react with mutual regard, known as reciprocity. The more you express interest, the safer it is for someone else to return the regard, and the cycle spirals onward.

Another factor that apparently plays a significant role in selecting a partner is physical attraction. Whether such attraction is caused by a chemical reaction or a socially learned behaviour, males and females appear to have different attraction criteria. Men tend to select their mates primarily on the basis of youth and physical attractiveness. Although physical attractiveness is an important criterion for women in mate selection, they tend to place greater emphasis on partners who are somewhat older, have good financial prospects, and are dependable and industrious. Good grooming is an almost universally desirable trait for all. If you smell or appear less than squeaky clean, you may have problems in the partner arena regardless of your sex or sexual orientation.

BARRIERS TO INTIMACY

Obstacles to intimacy include lack of personal identity, emotional immaturity, and a poorly developed sense of responsibility. The fear of being hurt, low self-esteem, mishandled hostility, chronic "busyness" (and its attendant lack of emotional presence), a tendency to "parentify" loved ones, and a conflict of role expectations can be equally detrimental. In addition, individual insecurities and difficulties in recognizing and expressing emotional needs can lead to an intimacy barrier. These barriers to intimacy have many causes, including the different emotional development of men and women and/or an upbringing in a dysfunctional family.

Dysfunctional Families

As noted earlier, the ability to sustain genuine intimacy is largely developed in the family of origin. Unfortunately, sharing, trust, and openness do not always occur in the family. In fact, the assumption that such intimacy exists in the family of origin might actually be unrealistic. As adults, we may discover that although we thought our family encouraged emotional intimacy, it was actually judgmental, full of expectations, controlling, and, in many ways, dysfunctional. A **dysfunctional family** is one in which the interaction between family members inhibits psychological growth rather than encouraging self-love, emotional expression, and individual growth. If you were to examine even the most pristine family under a microscope,

Dysfunctional family A family in which the interaction between family members inhibits rather than enhances psychological growth.

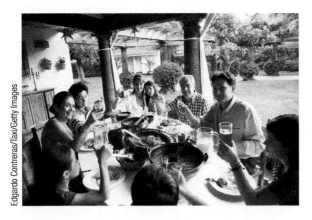

Healthy families that encourage emotional intimacy are generally able to avoid the damage to self-esteem and limited psychosocial growth that often happens in dysfunctional families.

abuse varies from spanking to violent beatings. Sexual abuse refers to any suggestive conversations, inappropriate kissing, touching, petting, oral, anal, or vaginal sex, or any other kinds of sexual interaction between a child and an older child, adolescent, or adult. Emotional abuse includes name-calling, teasing, and other tactics that damage a child's self-esteem.

Jealousy in Relationships

Jealousy is an aversive reaction evoked by a real or imagined relationship involving your partner and another person. Jealously can be experienced in response to the real or perceived loss of a meaningful and sexual relationship with your partner because of another person (Dijkstra, Barelds, & Groothof, 2010). Contrary to what many believe, jealousy is not a sign of intense devotion or of passionate love. Instead, jealousy is a sign of underlying problems that are a significant barrier to a healthy, intimate relationship. The roots of jealous feelings and behaviours may run deep and typically include:

- Overdependence on the relationship. People who have few social ties and rely exclusively on their significant others tend to be excessively fearful of losing them.

- High value on sexual exclusivity. People who believe that sexual exclusiveness is a crucial indicator of a love relationship are more likely to become jealous.

- Severity of the threat. People may feel uneasy if a person with a fantastic body, stunning good looks, and a great personality appears interested in their partner.

- Low self-esteem. The underlying question that torments people with low self-esteem is, "Why would anyone want me?" People who feel good about themselves are less likely to feel unworthy and to fear that someone else is going to snatch their partner.

- Fear of losing control. Some people need to feel in control of the situation. Feeling that they may be losing the attachment of or control over a partner can cause jealousy.

you would likely find some type of dysfunction. No group of people who live together day in and day out can interact perfectly all the time. However, many people have begun to overuse the term *dysfunctional* to refer to even the smallest problems in the family unit. True dysfunctionality refers to settings where negative interactions are the norm rather than the exception. Children raised in these settings face tremendous obstacles to growing up to be healthy. Coming to terms with past hurts can take years. However, with careful planning and introspection, support from loved ones, and counselling when needed, children from even the worst homes have proved to be remarkably resilient. Many are able to leave the past and focus on the future, developing into healthy, well-adjusted adults. It is important to note that dysfunctional families are found in every social, ethnic, religious, and economic group.

For more than a decade, social scientists studied the impact of the alcoholic home environment on the sexual and intimate behaviours of adult children of alcoholics (ACOAs). A number of intimacy problems were identified as typical of ACOAs. Many ACOAs claim that they become involved in unhealthy relationships and have difficulty trusting others, problems in communicating with partners, and difficulty defining a healthy relationship (Klausner & Hasselbring, 1990).

Another large group of people struggling with intimacy problems originating in the family of origin are survivors of childhood emotional, physical, or sexual abuse. Experiencing or witnessing physical, sexual, or emotional abuse as a child can have an impact on a person's intimate relationships as an adult (Lassri & Shahar, 2012). Domestic violence, whether directed at a child or another family member, can affect a child's ability to trust others and to maintain an intimate relationship later in life (Moylan et al., 2010). Physical

For men and women, jealousy is related to the expectation that it would be difficult to find another relationship if the current one ends. For men, jealousy is related to self-evaluative dependence—that is, the degree to which the man's self-esteem is affected by his partner's judgments. A certain amount of jealousy is expected in any relationship. Communicating effectively about it will prevent the jealousy from causing any lasting damage.

Jealousy An aversive reaction evoked by a real or imagined relationship involving a person's partner and another person.

COMMITTED RELATIONSHIPS

Feelings of love or sexual attraction do not always equal commitment in a relationship. There can be love—with or without sex—without commitment. Commitment in a relationship refers to an intent to act over time in a way that perpetuates the well-being of the other person, you, and the relationship. A committed relationship involves tremendous diligence on the part of both partners. Over the years, partners learn about one another and adjust their relationship accordingly. What separates committed from uncommitted relationships is the willingness of the partners to dedicate themselves to acquiring and using the skills that will ensure a lasting relationship.

Marriage

Marriage is the traditional committed relationship in many societies around the world. For many people, marriage is the ultimate expression of an intimate relationship. When two people marry in Canada, they enter into a legal agreement that includes shared financial plans, property, and responsibility in raising children (should children become part of the relationship). For religious people, marriage is also a sacrament of spirituality, rights, and obligations of each person.

In 2012, of the total population in Canada 39.7 percent were legally married, 8.6 percent were living common law, 2.2 percent were legally separated, 39.5 percent were single, 4.8 percent were divorced, and 5.2 percent were widowed (Statistics Canada, 2012).

Most people believe that marriage involves **monogamy**, or exclusive sexual involvement with one partner. The lifetime pattern for many Canadians appears to be **serial monogamy**, which means that a person has a monogamous sexual relationship with one partner for the duration of a relationship before moving on to another monogamous relationship. Some people prefer to have an **open relationship**, or open marriage, in which the partners agree that each person may be sexually involved outside their relationship.

Humans are not naturally monogamous; that is, most of us are capable of being sexually or emotionally involved with more than one person at a time. Yet Canadian society frowns on involvement with another person when in a committed relationship. Many people find themselves attracted to others while in a relationship and consciously try to stop subsequent interactions. Others find themselves involved unintentionally. Still others actively seek out extra-relationship affairs. Whether by choice or chance, sexual infidelity is a common factor in many divorces and break-ups. It seems that only people with exceptionally strong self-images and a dedication to the principles of open relationships are able to maintain non-monogamy over a period of time.

As with all relationships, there are marriages that work well and bring satisfaction to the partners, and there are marriages that are unhealthy for the people involved. A good marriage can yield support and stability, not only for the couple but also for those involved in the couple's life. Considerable research also indicates that married people live longer, are happier, remain mentally alert longer, and suffer fewer bouts of physical and mental ailments (McIntyre, 2013). However, traditional marriage does not work for everyone and is not the only path to a happy and successful committed relationship.

Cohabitation

Cohabitation or common-law is defined as two unmarried people with an intimate connection who live together in the same household. The relationship can be stable, with a high level of commitment between the partners. In the latest Canadian census data available (2012), common-law couples comprised 17.1 percent of all legally married couples, including same-sex couples (Statistics Canada, 2012). The length of time living in a married-like condition required to be defined as 'common-law' varies according to province, the type of law, and whether or not there are children (Common Law Relationships, n.d.). In general, at least six months is required. The number of couples living common-law has risen steadily over the past 50 or 60 years such that there are now approximately three million couples.

The increase in living common-law may be partly attributed to questioning of traditional values and the recognition that marriage may not be the only legitimate basis for sexual relations. The availability of cheaper, more effective birth control has probably been another factor, as has the notion that marriage is no longer a prerequisite for childbearing (Clark & Crompton, n.d.). Many couples also believe that living together simply because they choose to may be more important than being bound by a legal document.

Although living common-law is a viable alternative for some, many cohabitors eventually marry because of pressures from parents and friends, difficulties in obtaining insurance and tax benefits, legal issues over property, and a host of other reasons. The disadvantage of living common-law lies in the lack of societal validation for the relationship and, in some cases, in the societal disapproval of living together without being married. Cohabiting partners do not usually experience the

Monogamy Exclusive sexual involvement with one partner.

Serial monogamy Monogamous sexual relationship with one partner before moving on to another.

Open relationship A relationship in which partners agree that there can be sexual involvement outside the relationship.

Cohabitation Living together without being married.

social incentives to stay together that they would if they were married. This type of living arrangement is common among many religious communities and various ethnic groups. If they decide to separate, however, they do not experience the legal and financial problems involved in obtaining a divorce. In most provinces, cohabitation that lasts more than six months is viewed as a **common-law marriage** in the eyes of the court on issues of child care and spousal support. It is not the same, however, as becoming legally married. Some laws treat common-law spouses the same as married spouses. For example, parents' responsibilities to their children are the same whether the parents are married to each other or not. On the other hand, some laws apply to married people and not to common-law couples, such as the one that divides matrimonial property. In addition, employee benefits often cover common-law spouses. In still other situations, how the law treats a common-law couple depends on how long they have lived together. For example, Service Canada considers moving to be with a spouse a valid reason to quit a job, and, for this purpose, considers a couple who have been living together for at least one year to be spouses (Statistics Canada, 2002).

Gay and Lesbian Partnerships

People seek intimate, committed relationships during their adult years whether they are heterosexual or homosexual. Lesbians and gay men are socialized like others in our culture and place a high value on relationships. They seek the same things in their primary relationships as heterosexual partners: friendship, communication, validation, companionship, and a sense of stability. Studies of lesbian couples indicate high levels of attachment and satisfaction and a tendency toward monogamous, long-term relationships. Gay men, too, tend to form committed, long-term relationships, especially as they age (Freidman & Downey, 1994).

Challenges to successful homosexual relationships often stem from the discrimination they face and from difficulties dealing with social, legal, and religious doctrines. On July 19, 2005, Canada redefined the legal and social boundaries of marriage to include same-sex couples.

SUCCESS IN COMMITTED RELATIONSHIPS

Because the traditional marriage ceremony includes the vow "till death do us part," the definition of success in a relationship tends to be based on whether a couple stays together over the years.

Common-law marriage Cohabitation lasting at least six months.

Marriage has become the model to which relationships must conform to be considered stable or healthy. One reason for the increase in cohabitation or living common-law and other alternative relationships is the need for new forms in which people can express their love and commitment to one another and still have individual needs met adequately. Success in relating to another human being may have more to do with the quality of the interaction between two people than with the number of years they live together. Many social scientists agree that the ideal in relating to another person is to develop a committed bond, the boundaries and form of which can—and should—change to allow the maximum degree of growth over time.

Partnering Scripts

Most parents love their children and want them to be happy. They often believe that their children will achieve happiness by living in a way similar to how they have.

Accordingly, children are raised with a very strong script for what is expected of them as adults. Each group in society has its own partnering script that prescribes standards regarding sex, age, social class, ethnicity, religion, physical attributes, and personality types. By adolescence, boys and girls generally know exactly what type of person they are expected to befriend or to date.

Society provides constant reinforcement for traditional couples. People who choose an "appropriate" partner usually have plenty of validation for the relationship. The love and support they feel from friends and family is genuine. It also comes with expectations of what will occur within the relationship. Decisions that the couple feels should be exclusively theirs may provoke unsolicited advice from friends and family.

As Canadian society becomes increasingly multicultural, there is more frequent mixing of cultures, backgrounds, and ethnicities. A relationship between people of different cultural and ethnic backgrounds often brings increased tension partly because of the lack of societal reinforcement. In addition to a lack of recognition given to nontraditional couples, friends and family often blame the nontraditional nature of the pairing if the relationship does not survive.

The Importance of Self-Nurturance

It is often stated that you must love yourself before you can love someone else. What does this mean? Learning how you function emotionally and how to nurture yourself through all life's situations is a lifelong task. There seems to be a certain level of individual maturity that needs to be reached before a successful intimate relationship becomes possible. You can look to age of marriage and divorce rates for support. Someone marrying in his or her teens faces a risk of marital breakdown twice as high as someone who marries between the ages of 25 and 29 years (Canadian Encyclopedia, 2012). People who wait until their mid-30s to marry have a considerably reduced risk of marital break-up.

Two concepts especially important to knowing yourself and maintaining a good relationship are accountability and self-nurturance. **Accountability** means that both partners see themselves as responsible for their decisions and actions. In other words, your partner is not held responsible for the positive or negative experiences in life. Each and every choice is your own responsibility. When two people are accountable for their own emotional states, partners can be angry, sad, or frustrated without their partner taking it personally. When you are accountable, you might say something like, "This has nothing to do with you; I just happen to be angry right now."

Self-nurturance goes hand-in-hand with accountability. In order to make good choices in life, you need to maintain a balance of sleeping, healthy eating, being physically active, working, relaxing, and socializing. When the balance is disrupted, as it will inevitably be, when you are self-nurturing you will be patient with yourself and sort these things out to get back on track. When you make poor choices, as all people do, you learn from the experience when you are self-nurturing. Learning to live in a balanced and healthy way is a lifelong process. Two people on a path of accountability and self-nurturance together have a much better chance of maintaining a satisfying relationship.

Elements of Good Relationships

Satisfying and stable relationships share certain elements. Some of these are achieved through conscious efforts and communication; others evolve over time. People in healthy, committed relationships trust one another. Without trust, intimacy will not develop and your relationship will experience trouble and possible failure. **Trust** can be defined as the degree of confidence felt in a relationship. Trust includes three fundamental elements: predictability, dependability, and faith.

- Predictability means that you and your partner can predict one another's behaviours. This sense of predictability is based on the knowledge that you and your partner act in consistently positive ways.

- Dependability means that you and your partner can rely on one another to give support in all situations, particularly in those in which either of you feel threatened with hurt or rejection.

- Faith means that you and your partner feel absolutely certain about one another's intentions and behaviours.

Trust and intimacy are the foundation of healthy, committed relationships. Spouses who like and enjoy one another as people and find each other interesting frequently are happier than those who do not. Many spouses describe their partners as their best friends. Although most marriages have their share of ups and downs, successful couples are able to communicate and touch one another in an atmosphere of caring. They value a good sense of humour and exhibit communication, cooperation, and the ability to resolve conflicts constructively.

Sexual intimacy is also a major part of healthy relationships, but sex is not the major reason the relationship exists. Some couples admit to sexual dissatisfaction but feel their relationship is more important. Rather than seek an outlet in an extramarital affair, those who are dissatisfied with their sex lives adjust and spend little energy worrying about it because the relationship is satisfying in other, important ways. Many couples report that as communication and trust increase in a long-term, committed relationship, their sexual relationship also improves.

STAYING SINGLE

While many people choose to marry and have children, increasing numbers of young and older adults remain single. As previously noted, 39.5 percent of the population is single; 53.6 percent of which is male (Statistics Canada, 2012). While many of these people seek or have sought committed relationships, they find being single preferable. Singles clubs, social outings arranged by communities and churches, extended-family environments, and a large number of social services support the single lifestyle. Although some research indicates that single people live shorter lives, are less happy, are more likely to be financially distressed, and are more prone to illnesses than their married counterparts, other studies contradict these findings. It should be noted that it may be social isolation (as measured by the social network index), not marital status, that has an impact on self-reported health (White et al., 2009).

Accountability Accepting responsibility for personal decisions, choices, and actions.

Self-nurturance Taking care of yourself as needed.

Trust The degree of confidence felt in a relationship.

HAVING CHILDREN

When a couple decides to have children, their relationship changes. Resources of time, energy, and money are split many ways, and the partners no longer have each other's undivided attention. Babies and young children do not time their requests for food, sleep, and care to the convenience of adults. Therefore, individuals or couples whose basic needs for security, love, and purpose are met make better parents. Any stresses that already exist in a relationship are further accentuated when parenting is added to the list of responsibilities. Having a child does not "fix" a bad relationship and, in fact, can compound problems that already exist. A child cannot and should not be expected to provide the parents with self-esteem and security.

Changing patterns in family life affect the way children are raised. In modern society, it is not always clear which partner will adjust his or her work schedule to provide the primary care. Remarriage creates a new family of stepparents and stepsiblings. An increasing number of individuals are choosing to have children in a family structure other than a male/female couple. Single women or lesbian couples can choose adoption or alternative (formerly "artificial") insemination as a way to create a family. Single men or gay couples can choose to adopt or obtain the services of a surrogate mother. Regardless of the structure of the family, certain factors remain important to the well-being of the unit: consistency, communication, affection, and mutual respect.

Some people become parents without a lot of forethought and some children are born into a relationship that does not last. This does not mean it is too late to do a good job of parenting. Attention, consistency, and caring can be provided by other adults if a parent cannot be physically or emotionally present for a period of time. Children are resilient and forgiving if parents show respect to them and communicate about household activities that affect their lives. Even children who grow up in a household of conflict can feel loved and respected if the parents treat them fairly. This means that parents take responsibility for any of their own conflicts and make it clear to the children that they are not the reason for the conflict. Further, these parents do not bring their children into the conflict, nor do they use them as pawns against one another.

Changes in the traditional family structure have forced society to examine alternative means of raising children. Day-care centres, extended families, and live-in babysitters or nannies are becoming important alternatives to the traditional "nuclear family" unit.

ENDING A RELATIONSHIP

The Warning Signs

The symptoms of a troubled relationship are relatively easy to recognize. However, many couples choose to ignore them until the situation erupts into some type of emotional confrontation. By then, the relationship may be beyond salvaging. Breakdowns in relationships usually begin with a change in communication, however subtle. It is difficult to precisely describe what can and what does go wrong in a relationship although it is apparent that unresolved conflicts increase, often resulting in unresolved anger. This conflict and anger might result in problems in sexual relations that add to the conflict and anger.

When a couple who previously enjoyed spending time alone together find themselves continually in the company of others, spending time apart, or preferring to stay home alone, it may be a sign that the relationship is in trouble. Of course, the need for individual privacy is not a cause for worry—it is essential to health. If, however, a partner decides to make a change in the amount and quality of time spent together without the input or understanding of the other, it may be a sign of hidden problems.

Post-secondary students, particularly those who are socially isolated because they are far from family and hometown friends, can be particularly vulnerable to remaining in unhealthy relationships. They may become emotionally dependent on a partner for everything from eating meals to recreational and study time: mutual obligations such as shared rental arrangements, transportation, and child care can make it difficult to leave. It is also easy to mistake unwanted sexual advances for physical attraction or love. Without a network of friends and supporters with whom a student can talk, obtain validation for feelings, or share concerns, he or she may feel that the relationship is all he or she has.

Honesty and verbal affection are usually positive aspects of a relationship. In a troubled relationship, however, they can be used to cover up irresponsible or hurtful behaviours. "At least I was honest" is not an acceptable substitute for acting in a trustworthy way. The words "But I really do love you" should not be used as a licence to be inconsiderate, rude, or hurtful to a partner.

Seeking Help: Where to Look

The first place some people look for help when there are problems in a relationship is a trusted friend. Although friends can offer needed support during these difficult times, few have the training and detachment necessary to help you resolve your

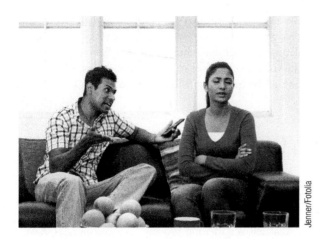

Unresolved conflicts and frequent emotional confrontations are signs of a troubled relationship. If each partner is committed to staying together, counselling might bring about positive change.

problems. Others find that they do not have the type of friendships that lend themselves to divulging these kinds of problems.

Most communities have private practitioners trained to counsel married or committed couples. Community mental health centres usually have trained counsellors as well. These practitioners may be psychiatrists, licensed psychologists, social workers, or counsellors with advanced degrees. These counsellors are often specially equipped to deal with the unique needs of young adults with relationship, sexual, emotional, financial, or other concerns. Most student health centres or counselling centres on campus have reduced student fees or no fees for students who need help. Additionally, many employers have access to Employee Assistance Program (EAP) and these benefits typically extend to students attending post-secondary studies. If you are unaware of such services, talk with your instructor and ask for his or her advice about where someone with your type of problem may get help.

Trial Separations

Sometimes a relationship becomes so dysfunctional that even counselling cannot bring about significant change. Moving apart for a period of time may allow some preliminary healing and give both parties an opportunity to reassess themselves and their commitment to the relationship. Trial separations do not guarantee that the situation will improve, nor do they mean the relationship is ending. If the couple is involved in counselling or has other support systems and mutually agree on the need for a trial separation, it may be a way to regroup and save a failing relationship.

Why Relationships End

The reasons for divorce and relationship breakdown are numerous. A unified law for divorce for Canadians was established in 1968 with divorce rates increasing ever since (Canadian Encyclopedia, 2012). Divorce rates are lowest in the first year of marriage and peak in the fourth year (Canadian Encyclopedia, 2012). The risk for divorce decreases after that, with most divorces occurring before 15 years of marriage. One contributing factor may be the lack of communication and cooperation between partners under the additional stress of tragedies such as the death of a child, serious illness of one partner, severe financial difficulties, and career failures. What about separation and divorce between people who have not experienced these tragedies? Poor communication and a lack of cooperation between partners along with unmet expectations regarding marriage or relationships in general or personal roles within the relationship are likely contributing factors. Some enter marriage with unrealistic expectations about what marriage will be like and how they and their partner will behave. Some enter relationships looking for someone to fill an empty spot in their lives. Failure to communicate such expectations to your partner can lead to resentment and disappointment. Because many premarital expectations may be unreasonable, early exploration of these expectations is important. This exploration may take place together or within a support program.

Differences in sexual needs may also contribute to the demise of a relationship. Many partners find that their spouses desire sex at different times or in different styles and frequencies than they do. Again, poor communication is at the root of these differences. Couples need to talk about their sexual differences to ensure that they both enjoy and consent to their sexual activity.

The bottom line is that if couples do not grow together, they often grow apart. Reality dictates a need to change or adapt to life's experiences as you grow older, your careers change, you develop new friendships, or your family life changes, first with the addition of children and then later when they move away from home. Without a commitment to working on your differences and continuing to build a life together, many people choose to move on, and this decision—as difficult as it is —could be the best for all concerned.

Deciding to End Your Relationship

At some point, troubled couples may feel that their relationship cannot be fixed. The decision to end their relationship is usually difficult, even for couples whose relationship was over long before the decision was made. Choosing to leave is not an easy decision, nor is formally separating and/or divorcing.

For married couples, wading through divorce or dissolution proceedings may be painful as they decide child-custody issues, alimony questions, and division of property. Finding legal assistance can be difficult, because painful emotions usually affect judgment. Couples living common-law also experience difficulty in separating. Legal problems involving property, children, and alimony are often more ambiguous for these couples than in a marriage. Some couples expend a lot of time, money, and energy working out settlements with lawyers who specialize in resolving the issues related to the end of a common-law relationship.

Aside from legal worries, many newly separated or divorced people experience emotions of anger, guilt, rejection, and unworthiness. No matter how miserable the relationship, feelings of failure are not uncommon or abnormal following a divorce or separation, and the emotional wounds take varying amounts of time to heal. Counsellors familiar with loss and grieving estimate that it takes at least a year and often longer to recover from the loss of a major relationship, whether by death or separation. With time, support from others, and community or professional help, most people do recover and establish new relationships.

Coping with Loneliness

Some people find establishing and maintaining relationships difficult. Others find that through death, illness, or distance, their relationships disappear or grow dim with time. Loneliness, or the unfulfilled desire to engage in a close personal relationship, is a difficult emotion to experience, even for the most determined person.

The loss of a committed relationship is usually too painful for a person to want to repeat. Reflecting on the beginning, the middle, and the ending of the relationship and identifying where there were problems can help you avoid similar mistakes in the future. Concentrating on the negative aspects of past behaviours of an ex-partner is a natural tendency, and may be helpful in getting in touch with your emotions or in learning from the situation. It is equally important to spend time remembering what was loved in the other person and what is lovable about yourself. Intimacy, love, and commitment between people change

Sexual identity Our recognition of ourselves as sexual beings; a composite of sex, gender, gender roles, sexual preference, body image, and sexual scripts.

Gonads The reproductive organs in a male (testes) and female (ovaries).

Puberty The period of sexual maturation.

Pituitary gland The endocrine gland controlling the release of hormones from the gonads (ovaries and testes).

Secondary sex characteristics Characteristics associated with sex developed during puberty such as vocal pitch, pubic and underarm hair, and genital development.

the lives of those involved. It is through relationships that we give and receive our greatest support and validation as worthwhile human beings. When you accept the risk and challenge of close relationships, you accept one of the greatest gifts life has to offer.

YOUR SEXUAL IDENTITY

Although you are a sexual being from birth, you are not born with complete knowledge about your sexuality. Learning about and becoming comfortable with your sexual self is a lifelong process. Taboos, morales, laws, and sexual myths abound and often hinder the process of learning about your sexuality. Family, friends, and the media—including print and electronic forms—music, religion, and educational institutions, provide you with information about your sexuality and how you should or should not express it.

In the end, it is up to you to blend all of this information with your personal experience and values to create your own sexual identity. A complex interaction of genetic, physiological, and environmental factors determines your **sexual identity**. The beginning of your sexual identity occurs at conception, with the combining of chromosomes that determine your sex. It is your biological father who determines whether you will be a boy or a girl. All eggs (ova) carry an X sex chromosome; sperm carry either an X or a Y chromosome. If a sperm carrying an X chromosome fertilizes an egg, the resulting combination of sex chromosomes (XX) creates the blueprint to produce a female. If a sperm carrying a Y chromosome fertilizes an egg, the XY combination produces a male. The genetic instructions included in the sex chromosomes lead to the differential development of male and female **gonads** at about the eighth day in utero. Once the male gonads (testes) and the female gonads (ovaries) are developed, they play a key role in all future sexual development because they are responsible for the production of sex hormones. The primary sex hormones produced by females are estrogen and progesterone. In males, the hormone of primary importance is testosterone. The release of testosterone in a maturing fetus signals the development of a penis and other male genitals. If no testosterone is produced, female genitals form.

During **puberty**, sex hormones play major roles in further development. Hormones released by the **pituitary gland**, called gonadotropins, stimulate the testes and ovaries to make appropriate sex hormones. The increased production of estrogen in females and testosterone in males leads to the development of **secondary sex characteristics**. Secondary sex characteristics in males include deepening of the voice; development of facial, pubic, and underarm hair; and genital (penis and testes) development. In females, secondary sex characteristics include growth of the breasts, menarche, widening of the hips, and the development of pubic and underarm hair.

Gender Identity and Roles

Thus far, we have described sexual identity only in terms of your sex. Sex simply refers to the biological condition of being male or female based on physiological and hormonal differences. **Gender**, on the other hand, refers to your sense of masculinity or femininity as defined by the society in which you live. Each of you expresses your maleness or femaleness to others on a daily basis through the **gender roles** you play. **Gender identity** refers to your personal sense or awareness of being masculine or feminine, a male or a female. A person's gender identity does not always match his or her biological sex; this is called being **transgendered**. There is a broad spectrum of expression among transgendered persons that reflects the degree of dissatisfaction they have with their sexual anatomy. Some transgendered persons are very comfortable with their bodies and are content simply to dress and live as the other gender. It might also be difficult for you to express your true sexual identity because you feel bound by existing gender-role stereotypes. An individual might be born one sex but their gender identity does not match their biological condition and thus they may transition to the other gender. Some individuals are comfortable simply making a change in their gender. However, others choose to undergo surgical procedures to change physical aspects of their body, allowing them to further express their sexual identity. **Gender-role stereotypes** refer to generalizations about how males and females should express themselves and the characteristics each possesses. Traditional sex roles are examples of gender-role stereotyping. Men are thought to be independent, aggressive, better in math and science, logical, and in control of their emotions. Women, on the other hand, are expected to be passive, nurturing, intuitive, sensitive, and emotional. **Androgyny** is the combination of traditional masculine and feminine traits in a single person. Androgynous people do not always follow traditional sex roles but, rather, act according to the given situation. The process by which a society transmits behavioural expectations to its individual members is called **socialization**. Gender roles are shaped or socialized by our parents, peers, education, and many forms of media including television, advertisements, the internet, music, video games, and movies. Think about the current television shows or movies you watch. In what ways do the characters in these shows or movies stereotype gender roles?

REPRODUCTIVE ANATOMY AND PHYSIOLOGY

An understanding of the functions of the male and female reproductive systems will help you derive pleasure and satisfaction from your sexual relationships, be sensitive to your partner's wants and needs, and be more responsible in your choices regarding your sexual health.

Female Reproductive Anatomy and Physiology

The female reproductive system includes two major groups of structures: the external and internal genitals (see Figures 7.3 and 7.4). The **external female genitals** include the outwardly visible structures often referred to as the vulva. The **vulva** includes the mons pubis, the labia minora and majora, the clitoris, the urethral and vaginal openings, and the vestibule of the vagina. The **mons pubis** is a pad of fatty tissue covering the pubic bone. The mons protects the pubic bone, and during puberty becomes covered with coarse hair. The **labia minora** are folds of mucous membrane and the **labia majora** are folds of skin and erectile tissue that enclose the urethral and vaginal openings. The labia minora are found just inside the labia majora.

The **clitoris** is the female sexual organ whose only known function is sexual pleasure. It is located at the upper end of the labia minora and beneath the mons pubis. Directly below the clitoris is the **urethral opening** through which urine leaves the body. Below the urethral opening is the opening of the **vagina**. In some women, the vaginal opening is covered

Gender Your sense of masculinity or femininity as defined by the society in which you live.

Gender roles Expression of maleness or femaleness.

Gender identity Your personal sense or awareness of being masculine or feminine, male or a female.

Transgendered When a person's gender identity does not match the person's biological sex.

Gender-role stereotypes Socialized generalizations concerning how males and females should be and how they express themselves.

Androgyny Combination of traditional masculine and feminine traits in a single person.

Socialization Process by which a society identifies attitudinal and behavioural expectations to its individual members.

External female genitals The outwardly visible structure or vulva.

Vulva Includes the mons pubis, labia majora and minora, clitoris, urethral and vaginal openings, and vestibule of the vagina and its glands.

Mons pubis Fatty tissue covering the pubic bone in females; in physically mature women, the mons is covered with coarse hair.

Labia minora "Inner lips" or folds of tissue just inside the labia majora.

Labia majora "Outer lips" or folds of tissue covering the female sexual organs.

Clitoris A pea-sized nodule of tissue located at the top of the labia minora.

Urethral opening The opening through which urine is released.

Vagina The passage leading from the vulva to the uterus.

FIGURE 7.3

External Female Genital Structures

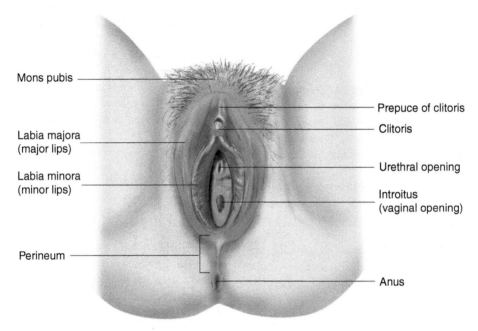

- Mons pubis
- Prepuce of clitoris
- Clitoris
- Labia majora (major lips)
- Labia minora (minor lips)
- Urethral opening
- Introitus (vaginal opening)
- Perineum
- Anus

Source: Figure from *Exploring Human Sexuality: Making Healthy Decisions* by Richard D. McAnulty, copyright © 1997. Used by permission of Richard D. McAnulty.

FIGURE 7.4

Side View of the Female Reproductive Organs

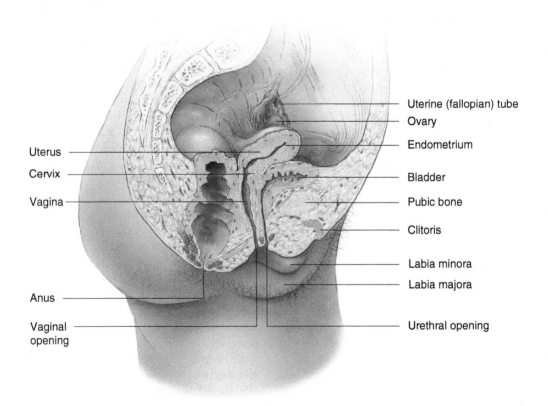

- Uterus
- Cervix
- Vagina
- Anus
- Vaginal opening
- Uterine (fallopian) tube
- Ovary
- Endometrium
- Bladder
- Pubic bone
- Clitoris
- Labia minora
- Labia majora
- Urethral opening

by a thin membrane called the **hymen**. It is a myth that an intact hymen is proof of virginity. The **perineum** is the area between the vulva and the anus. Although not technically part of the external genitalia, the tissue in this area has many nerve endings and is sensitive to touch; it can play a part in sexual excitement.

The **internal female genitals** of the reproductive system include the vagina, uterus, fallopian tubes, and ovaries. The vagina is a tubular passageway from the uterus to the outside of a female's body. This passageway allows menstrual flow to exit from the uterus during a woman's monthly cycle and serves as the birth canal. The vagina also receives the penis during intercourse. The **uterus**, also known as the womb, is a hollow, muscular, pear-shaped organ. Hormones acting on the inner lining of the uterus, called the **endometrium**, either prepare the uterus for implantation and development of a fertilized egg or signal that no fertilization has taken place, in which case the endometrium deteriorates and becomes menstrual flow.

The lower end of the uterus is called the **cervix** and extends down into the vagina. The **ovaries** are almond-sized structures suspended on either side of the uterus. The ovaries produce the hormones estrogen and progesterone and are the reservoir for immature eggs. All the eggs a female will ever have are present in her ovaries at birth. Eggs mature and are released from the ovaries in response to hormones. Extending from the upper end of the uterus are two thin, flexible tubes called the **fallopian tubes**. The fallopian tubes are where the sperm and egg meet and fertilization takes place. Following fertilization, the fallopian tubes serve as the passageway to the uterus, where the fertilized egg implants and development continues.

The Onset of Puberty and the Menstrual Cycle

During puberty, the female reproductive system matures and secondary sex characteristics transform girls into women. Under the direction of the endocrine system, the pituitary gland, the hypothalamus, and the ovaries secrete hormones that act as the chemical messengers among them. Working in a feedback system, hormonal levels in the bloodstream act as the trigger mechanism for release of more or different hormones.

At the beginning of puberty in females, the **hypothalamus** receives the message to begin secreting **gonadotropin-releasing hormone (GnRH)**. The release of GnRH in turn signals the **pituitary gland** to release hormones called gonadotropins. **Follicle-stimulating hormone (FSH)** and **luteinizing hormone (LH)** are two gonadotropins, and their role is to signal the gonads, in this case the ovaries, to start producing **estrogen** and **progesterone**.

Increased estrogen directs the development of female secondary sex characteristics. In addition, estrogen is responsible for regulating the reproductive cycle (see Figure 7.5). The usual age range for the onset of the first menstrual period, termed **menarche**, is 10 to 16 years, with the average age in Canada around 12 or 13 years (Malina, Bouchard, & Bar-Or, 2004).

The average menstrual cycle is 28 days and is divided into three phases: the proliferatory phase, the secretory phase, and the menstrual phase. During the proliferatory phase, the pituitary gland releases FSH and LH. The FSH acts on the ovaries to stimulate the maturation process of several **ovarian follicles (egg sacs)**. These follicles secrete estrogen and, in response, the lining of the uterus, the endometrium, begins to grow and develop. The inner walls of the uterus become coated with a thick, spongy lining composed of blood and mucus. In the event of fertilization, the endometrial tissue will become a nesting place for the developing embryo. The increased estrogen level also signals the pituitary to slow down FSH production and to increase LH secretion. Of the several follicles developing in the ovaries, only one each month normally reaches complete maturity. Under the influence of LH, this one ovarian follicle rapidly matures, and, on or about the fourteenth day of the proliferatory phase, it releases an ovum into the fallopian tube—a process referred to as **ovulation**. Just prior to ovulation, the mature egg's follicle begins to increase secretion of progesterone, the first function of which is to spur the addition of further nutrients to the developing endometrium.

After ovulation, the ovarian follicle is converted into the corpus luteum, or yellow body,

Hymen Thin tissue covering the vaginal opening.

Perineum Tissue extending from the vulva to the anus.

Internal female genitals The vagina, uterus, fallopian tubes, and ovaries.

Uterus (womb) Hollow, pear-shaped muscular organ whose function is to house the developing fetus.

Endometrium Soft, spongy matter that makes up the uterine lining.

Cervix Lower end of the uterus that opens into the vagina.

Ovaries Almond-sized organs that house developing eggs and produce hormones.

Fallopian tubes Tubes that extend from the ovaries to the uterus.

Hypothalamus An area of the brain located near the pituitary gland. The hypothalamus works with the pituitary gland to control reproductive functions.

Gonadotropin-releasing hormone (GnRH) Hormone that signals the pituitary gland to release gonadotropins.

Pituitary gland A gland located deep within the brain; controls reproductive functions.

Follicle-stimulating hormone (FSH) Hormone that signals the ovaries to prepare to release an egg and to begin producing estrogen.

Luteinizing hormone (LH) Hormone that signals the ovaries to release an egg and to begin producing progesterone.

Estrogen Hormones that control the menstrual cycle.

Progesterone Hormone secreted by the ovaries; helps keep the endometrium developing in order to nourish a fertilized egg; also helps maintain pregnancy.

Menarche The first menstrual period.

Ovarian follicles (egg sacs) Areas within the ovary in which individual eggs develop.

Ovulation The point of the menstrual cycle at which a mature egg ruptures through the ovarian wall.

FIGURE 7.5

Hormonal Control and Phases of the Menstrual Cycle

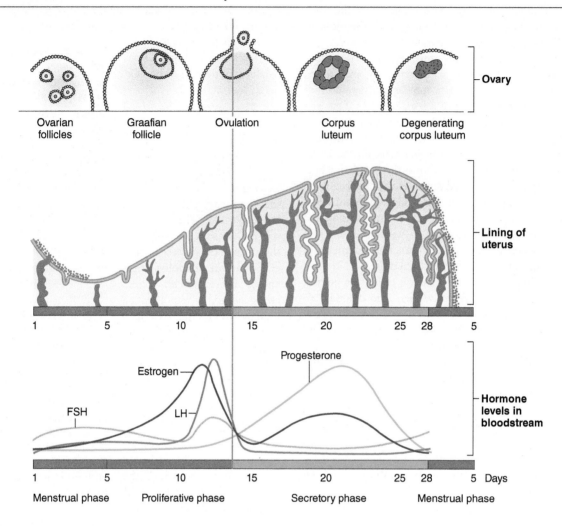

which continues to secrete estrogen and progesterone but in decreasing amounts. In addition, FSH falls back to its preproliferatory levels. Essentially, the woman's body is "waiting" to see whether fertilization occurs. During the time after ovulation, LH declines, and progesterone levels begin to rise, causing additional tissue growth in the endometrium. This phase of the cycle is called the secretory phase.

If fertilization takes place, cells surrounding the developing embryo release a hormone called **human chorionic gonadotropin (HCG)**. This hormone leads to increased levels of estrogen and progesterone secretion, which maintains the endometrium while signalling the pituitary gland not to start a new menstrual cycle. If fertilization does not occur, the egg gradually disintegrates in about

72 hours. The corpus luteum gradually becomes non-functional, causing levels of progesterone and estrogen to decline. As hormonal levels decline, the endometrial lining of the uterus loses its nourishment, dies, and is sloughed off as menstrual flow. Menstruation is the third phase of the menstrual cycle.

Menopause

Just as menarche signals the beginning of a woman's potential reproductive years, **menopause**—the permanent cessation of menstruation—signals the end. Generally, menopause occurs between the ages of 40 and 60 years and results in decreased estrogen levels. Reduced estrogen typically results in a decrease in vaginal lubrication, hot flashes, headaches, dizziness, and joint pain. Further, women may experience disrupted sleep as well as problems with their vagina and bladder such as more vaginal and urinary infections,

Human chorionic gonadotropin (HCG) Hormone that calls for increased levels of estrogen and progesterone secretion if fertilization has taken place.

Menopause The permanent cessation of menstruation.

difficulty holding urine long enough to get to the bathroom, and issues with dryness that may make vaginal intercourse uncomfortable (National Institute of Aging, 2008). As a woman's body adjusts to the decreased level of estrogen, these symptoms abate.

Hormones such as estrogen and progesterone have been prescribed as menopausal hormonal therapy (MHT) or to relieve menopausal symptoms and reduce the risk of biological changes including bone loss (National Cancer Institute, n.d.). The National Cancer Institute (n.d.) lists the following risks associated with MHT:

- urinary incontinence
- dementia
- stroke, blood clots, and heart attack
- breast cancer
- endometrial cancer
- lung cancer
- colorectal cancer

As such, a woman needs to discuss the risks and benefits of MHT with her health-care provider and come to an informed decision. Certainly lifestyle changes such as regular physical activity and a dietary intake low in fat and adequate in calcium can also help protect postmenopausal women from cancer, heart disease, and osteoporosis. Engaging in regular physical activity may also alleviate the symptoms experienced from reduced estrogen.

Male Reproductive Anatomy and Physiology

The structures of the male reproductive system can be divided into external and internal genitals (see Figure 7.6). The penis and the scrotum make up the **external male genitals**. The **internal male genitals** include the testes, epididymides, vasa deferentia, urethra, and three other structures—the seminal vesicles, the prostate gland, and the Cowper's glands—that secrete components that, with sperm, make up semen. These three structures are sometimes referred to as the **accessory glands**.

External male genitals The penis and scrotum.

Internal male genitals The testes, epididymides, vasa deferentia, ejaculatory ducts, urethra, and accessory glands.

Accessory glands The seminal vesicles, prostate gland, and Cowper's glands.

FIGURE 7.6
Side View of the Male Reproductive Organs

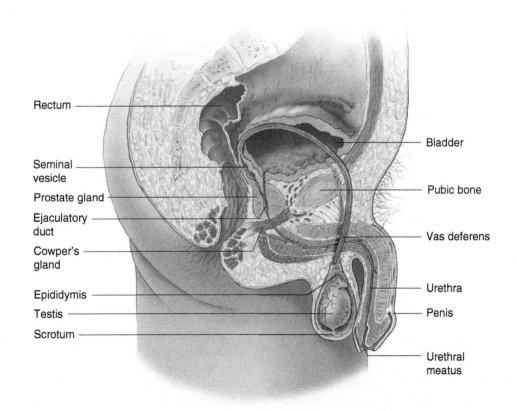

Rectum
Seminal vesicle
Prostate gland
Ejaculatory duct
Cowper's gland
Epididymis
Testis
Scrotum

Bladder
Pubic bone
Vas deferens
Urethra
Penis
Urethral meatus

The **penis** is the organ that releases sperm during ejaculation. The urethra, which passes through the centre of the penis, acts as the passageway for semen and urine to exit the body. During sexual arousal, the spongy tissue in the penis becomes filled with blood, making it erect. Further sexual excitement leads to **ejaculation**, a series of rapid spasmodic contractions that propel semen out of the penis.

Situated behind the penis outside the body is a sac called the **scrotum**. The scrotum protects the testes and helps control the temperature within the testes, which is vital to sperm production. The **testes** (singular: testis) are egg-shaped structures in which sperm are manufactured. The testes also contain cells that manufacture **testosterone**, the hormone responsible for male secondary sex characteristic development.

Spermatogenesis describes the development of sperm. Like the maturation of eggs in the female, this process is governed by the pituitary gland. Follicle-stimulating hormone (FSH) is secreted into the bloodstream to stimulate the testes to manufacture sperm. Immature sperm are released into a comma-shaped structure on the back of each testis called the **epididymis** (plural: epididymides), where they reach full maturity.

The epididymis contains coiled tubules that gradually "unwind" and straighten to become the **vas deferens**. The two vasa deferentia, as they are called in the plural, make up the tubular transportation system with the sole function of storing and moving sperm. Along the way, the **seminal vesicles** provide sperm with nutrients and other fluids that compose **semen**.

The vasa deferentia eventually connect each epididymis to the ejaculatory ducts, which pass through the **prostate gland** and empty into the urethra. The prostate gland contributes more fluids to the semen, including chemicals to aid the sperm in fertilization of an ovum, and, more importantly, a chemical that neutralizes the acid in the vagina to make its environment more conducive to sperm motility (ability to move) and potency (potential for fertilizing an ovum).

Just below the prostate gland are two pea-shaped nodules called the Cowper's glands. Their primary function is to secrete a fluid that lubricates the urethra and neutralizes any acid that may remain in the urethra after urination. Urine and semen do not come into contact with each other. During ejaculation of semen, the tube to the urinary bladder is closed off by a small valve.

Circumcision: Risk versus Benefit

Parents decide whether their male infant will be circumcised. Circumcision involves the surgical removal of the **foreskin**, a flap of skin covering the tip of the penis. Most circumcisions are performed for religious or cultural reasons or because of concerns about hygiene. In the uncircumcised male, oily secretions and sloughed-off dead cells (smegma) can collect under the foreskin and create an irritation or a breeding ground for infection. Removing the foreskin makes cleansing the penis easier. Today, infants can be given a local anesthetic, and circumcisions can be performed with little or no pain. This does not mean, however, that the procedure itself is without risk. All surgery involves some risk. If circumcision is performed later in life under a general anesthetic, the risk of complications is greater. Like all other elective surgical procedures, careful consideration of the risks and benefits of circumcision should be made prior to making a decision.

EXPRESSING YOUR SEXUALITY

Finding healthy ways to express your sexuality is an important part of developing your sexual self. Many avenues of sexual expression are available.

Human Sexual Response

Sexual response is a physiological process that involves different stages. The biological goal of the response process is the reproduction of the species. Human psychological traits greatly influence sexual desire and response. Thus, we may find relationships with one partner vastly different from those we experience with another partner.

Sexual response generally follows a pattern, though individual differences are common. Men and women each exhibit four common stages: excitement/arousal, plateau, orgasm, and resolution. In addition, some men may experience a fifth stage, the refractory period. Regardless of the type of sexual activity (stimulation by a partner or self), the response stages are the same.

Penis Male sexual organ.

Ejaculation The propulsion of semen from the penis.

Scrotum Sac of tissue that encloses the testes.

Testes Two organs, located in the scrotum, that manufacture sperm and produce testosterone.

Testosterone The male sex hormone manufactured in the testes.

Spermatogenesis The development of sperm.

Epididymis A comma-shaped structure atop the testis where sperm mature.

Vas deferens A tube that transports sperm toward the penis.

Seminal vesicles Storage areas for sperm where nutrient fluids are added.

Semen Fluid containing sperm and nutrients that increase sperm viability and neutralize vaginal acid.

Prostate gland Gland that secretes nutrients and neutralizing fluids in the semen.

Foreskin Flap of skin covering the end of the penis.

During the first stage, excitement/arousal, genital responses are caused by **vasocongestion**, or increased blood flow in the genital region. Increased blood flow to these organs causes them to swell. The vagina begins to lubricate in preparation for penile penetration and the penis becomes partially erect. Both sexes may exhibit a "sex flush," or light blush all over their bodies. Excitement/arousal can be generated by touching, kissing, talking, through fantasy, viewing films or videos, or reading erotic literature.

The plateau phase is characterized by an intensification of the initial responses. Voluntary and involuntary muscle tensions increase. The woman's nipples and the man's penis become erect. A few drops of semen, which may contain sperm, are secreted from the penis at this time. The woman's genitalia also become "wet" at this point as her vagina continues to lubricate.

During the orgasmic phase, vasocongestion and muscle tensions reach their peak, and rhythmic contractions occur through the genital regions. In women, these contractions are centred in the uterus, the outer vagina, and the anal sphincter. In men, the contractions occur in two stages. First, contractions within the prostate gland begin propelling semen through the urethra. In the second stage, the muscles of the pelvic floor, the urethra, and the anal sphincter contract. Usually, but not always, semen is ejaculated from the penis. In both sexes, spasms in other major muscle groups also occur, particularly in the buttocks and abdomen. Feet and hands may also contract, and facial features often contort.

Muscle tension and congested blood subside in the resolution phase, as the genital organs return to their pre-arousal states. Both sexes usually experience deep feelings of well-being, satisfaction, and profound relaxation.

As previously noted, some men experience a fifth phase—the refractory phase. In this phase, men experience a period of time in which their systems are incapable of subsequent arousal. This refractory period may last from a few minutes to several hours. The length of the refractory period increases with age. Following orgasm and resolution, many women are capable of being aroused and brought to orgasm again, though subsequent orgasms are typically less intense. Men and women experience the same stages in the sexual response cycle; however, the length of time spent in any one stage is variable. Thus, one partner may be in the plateau phase while the other is in the excitement or orgasmic phase. Such variations in response rates are entirely normal. Some couples believe that simultaneous orgasm is desirable for sexual satisfaction. Although simultaneous orgasm is pleasant, so are orgasms achieved at different times.

Sexual pleasure and satisfaction are also possible without orgasm or intercourse. Achieving sexual maturity includes learning that sex is not a contest with a real or imaginary opponent. The sexually mature person

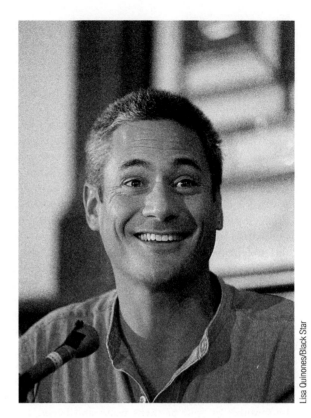

In a society where anti-homosexual attitudes prevail, a gay person's decision to make his or her sexual preference known to the public, as Olympic diver Greg Louganis did, involves courage and a strong belief in oneself.

Lisa Quinones/Black Star

enjoys sexual activity whether or not orgasm occurs. Expressing love and sexual feelings for another person involves many pleasurable activities, of which intercourse and orgasm may be only a part.

Sexual Orientation

Sexual orientation refers to a person's enduring emotional, romantic, or sexual attraction to others. You may be primarily attracted to members of the opposite sex (**heterosexual**), the same sex (**homosexual**), or both sexes (**bisexual**). Or you could be **pansexual** or **asexual**. Many homosexuals prefer the terms **gay**, queer, or **lesbian** to describe their sexual orientation. Gay and queer can apply to both men and women, but lesbian refers specifically to women.

Vasocongestion The engorgement of the genital organs with blood.

Sexual orientation A person's enduring emotional, romantic, sexual, or affectionate attraction to other persons.

Heterosexual Experiencing primary attraction to and preference for sexual activity with people of the other sex.

Homosexual Experiencing primary attraction to and preference for sexual activity with people of the same sex.

Bisexual Refers to attraction to and preference for sexual activity with people of both sexes.

Pansexual Sexual orientation involving attraction to all genders.

Asexual An individual with no sexual orientation, feelings, or desires.

Gay Sexual orientation involving primary attraction to people of the same sex; usually but not always applies to men attracted to men.

Lesbian Sexual orientation involving attraction of women to other women.

Gay and bisexual people are often targets of **sexual prejudice**—negative attitudes and hostile actions directed at members of a particular social group. Hate crimes, discrimination, and hostility toward sexual minorities are evidence of ongoing sexual prejudice (Herek & McLemore, 2013).

Most researchers today agree that sexual orientation is best understood using a model that incorporates biological, psychological, and socio-environmental factors. Biological explanations focus on research into genetics, hormones, and differences in brain anatomy. Psychological and socio-environmental explanations examine parent-child interactions, sex roles, and early sexual and interpersonal interactions. Collectively, this growing body of research suggests that the origins of homosexuality, like heterosexuality, are complex (Rosario & Schrimshaw, 2014). To diminish the complexity of sexual orientation to "a choice" is a clear misrepresentation of current research. Homosexuals do not "choose" their sexual orientation any more than heterosexuals do.

Understanding the functions of the female and male reproductive systems will help you derive pleasure and satisfaction from your sexual relationships, be sensitive to your partner's wants and needs, and make responsible choices regarding your own sexual health.

Developing Sexual Relationships

Perhaps the most important part of developing mature sexuality is learning to develop rewarding sexual relationships. Like all skills, developing relationships takes time, patience, and practice. Your sexual education begins with yourself, your family, and your close friends. You watch the significant adults in your life and pattern your attitudes and behaviours after theirs. At puberty, when extra-familial elements, such as peers and the media, become more important, you adapt some of their standards to your behaviours. Your shyness, aggressiveness or assertiveness, passiveness, and levels of comfort with your sexuality come from your personality and from what you have learned from others.

You bring not only your history to your sexual relationships, but also your peculiar chemistry. The human potential for passionate sexual love has been defined as **limerence**. Hatfield, Bensman, and Rapson (2011) provide details regarding the potential measurement of romantic and passionate love. The word *limerence* is derived from the

Sexual prejudice Negative attitudes and hostile actions directed at those with a different sexual orientation.

Limerence The quality of sexual attraction based on chemistry and gratification of sexual desire.

Celibacy Not engaging in sexual activity.

name of the portion of the brain that controls sexual response, the limbic cortex. Limerence is what makes us feel sexually "turned on" by another person. This powerful feeling can overshadow common sense. Sexual relationships based on limerence may or may not develop into long-lasting or committed relationships. Limerence is thought to last two years at most. Relationships based upon a love that has taken time to mature are much more likely to last. The following are some "symptoms" of limerence:

- Intrusive thoughts about the object of desire.
- Dependence of mood on love object's actions.
- Fear of rejection, along with an almost incapacitating shyness.
- Sharp sensitivity to interpret the desired person's actions favourably and ability to interpret any signs from the other as hidden passion.
- Buoyant, walking-on-air feeling when reciprocation is evident.
- Intensity of feelings that leaves other concerns in the background.
- Ability to emphasize what is admirable in the love object and to avoid dwelling on the negative—or even the ability to reconceptualize the negative into a positive attribute (Tennov, 1989).

Sexual Expression: What Are Your Options?

The range of human sexual expression is virtually infinite. What you find personally satisfying and enjoyable may not work for another person. Further, the ways you choose to meet your sexual needs today may be very different two weeks, two years, or twenty years from now. Knowing and accepting yourself as a sexual person with individual desires and preferences is the first step in achieving sexual satisfaction. Understanding that learning about your sexuality, including your sexual expression, is a lifelong process is another step in achieving short- and long-term sexual satisfaction.

Celibacy

Celibacy is avoidance of or abstention from sexual activities with others. A completely celibate person also does not engage in masturbation (self-stimulation), whereas a partially celibate person avoids sexual activities with others but engages in autoerotic behaviours such as masturbation. Some individuals choose to be celibate for religious or moral reasons. Others may be celibate for a period of time due to illness, the end of a long-term relationship, or lack of an acceptable partner. For some, celibacy is a lonely, agonizing state, but others find that it is a good time for introspection, value assessment, and personal growth.

Autoerotic Behaviours

The goal of **autoerotic behaviours** is sexual self-stimulation. Sexual fantasy and masturbation are the most common autoerotic behaviours. **Sexual fantasies** are sexually arousing thoughts and dreams. Fantasies may reflect real-life experiences or forbidden desires or may provide the opportunity to practice new or anticipated sexual experiences. The fact that you may fantasize about a particular sexual experience does not mean that you want to, or have to, act out that experience. Sexual fantasies are just that—fantasy. **Masturbation** is self-stimulation of the genitals. Although many people feel uncomfortable discussing masturbation, it is a common sexual practice across the life span. Masturbation is a natural, pleasure-seeking behaviour in infants and children. It is a valuable and important means for adolescent males and females, as well as adults, to explore their sexual feelings and responsiveness. In addition, masturbation is an important means of sexual expression for individuals without a partner or for individuals with a partner who is not capable of or interested in sexual activity.

Kissing and Erotic Touching

Kissing and erotic touching are two very common forms of nonverbal sexual communication or expression. Men and women have **erogenous zones**, or areas of the body that when touched lead to sexual arousal. Erogenous zones include genital as well as nongenital areas, such as the earlobes, mouth, breasts, and inner thighs. Almost any area of the body can be conditioned to respond erotically to touch. Spending time with your partner exploring and learning about his or her erogenous areas is another pleasurable, safe, and satisfying means of sexual expression.

Oral–Genital Stimulation

Cunnilingus is the term used for oral stimulation of a woman's genitals, and **fellatio** refers to oral stimulation of a man's genitals. Many partners find oral–genital stimulation an intensely pleasurable means of sexual expression. For others, oral sex is not an option because of moral or religious beliefs. It is important to remember that HIV and other sexually transmitted infections (STIs) can be transmitted via unprotected oral–genital sex. Use of an appropriate barrier device is strongly recommended if either partner's disease status is in question or unknown or if either partner is not monogamous. (See Chapter 8 for more details.)

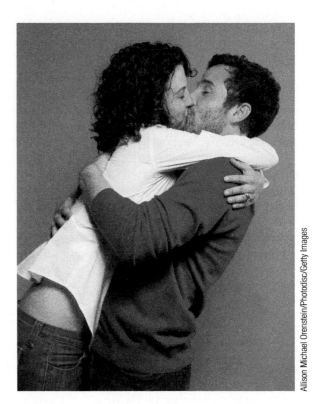

Kissing can be a nonverbal form of sexual communication.

Allison Michael Orenstein/Photodisc/Getty Images

Anal Intercourse

The anal area is highly sensitive to touch, and some find pleasure in its stimulation. **Anal intercourse** refers to the insertion of the penis or objects into the anus. Some also practise stimulation of the anus by mouth or with the fingers. If you engage in this form of sexual expression, remember to use condoms to prevent STIs. (See Chapter 8 for more details.) Also, when anal intercourse is practised heterosexually, it should be kept in mind that anything inserted into the anus should not be directly inserted into the vagina, given the potential for bacterial transmission.

Vaginal Intercourse

The term *intercourse* generally refers to **vaginal intercourse**, or insertion of the penis into the vagina. *Coitus* is another term for vaginal intercourse, the most often practised form of sexual expression between a man and a woman. A great

Autoerotic behaviours Sexual self-stimulation.

Sexual fantasies Sexually arousing thoughts and dreams.

Masturbation Self-stimulation of genitals.

Erogenous zones Areas in the body that, when touched, lead to sexual arousal.

Cunnilingus Oral stimulation of a woman's genitals.

Fellatio Oral stimulation of a man's genitals.

Anal intercourse The insertion of the penis into the anus.

Vaginal intercourse The insertion of the penis into the vagina.

variety of positions can be used during coitus. Examples include the "missionary position" (man on top facing the woman), woman on top, side by side, or man behind (rear entry). Many partners enjoy changing and experimenting with different positions. Sexual intercourse can take on different meanings under different circumstances. It can be a hurried, unplanned event involving little communication in the back seat of a car or an erotic, sensual experience including the exchange of love and mutual emotions in a private setting. Knowledge of yourself and your body, along with your ability to communicate effectively with your partner, will play a large part in determining the enjoyment or meaning of intercourse for you and your partner. Whatever your circumstance, you should practise safe sex to avoid STIs or unwanted pregnancy. (See Chapter 8 for more details.)

What Is Right for Me?

Invariably, whenever people talk about the spectrum of sexual behaviours, someone in the group will bring up the issue of normality. In *The Joy of Sex*, Comfort (1972) summarizes "normality" succinctly:

> Accordingly, if you must talk about "normality," any sex behaviour is normal which (1) you both enjoy, (2) hurts nobody, (3) is not associated with anxiety, (4) does not cut down your scope. . . . "Normal" implies there is something which sex ought to be. That is, it ought to be a wholly satisfying link between two affectionate people, from which both emerge unanxious, rewarded, and ready for more.

Many couples worry that they do not have sex often enough. Popular magazines frequently give the "average" number of times couples engage in sex every week. Such numbers are meaningless. Rather than compare yourself to these statistics, you would be wise simply to follow your own feelings. The bottom line is that you and your partner must decide what is best for the two of you.

Variant Sexual Behaviour

Variant sexual behaviour is the term used to describe sexual behaviours not engaged in by most people. Some variant sexual behaviours can be harmful to the individual, to others, or to both. Some of the following activities are illegal in Canada. For example:

Variant sexual behaviour A sexual behaviour not engaged in by most people.

Sexual dysfunction Problems associated with achieving sexual satisfaction.

- Group sex. Sexual activity involving more than two people. Participants in group sex run a higher risk of STIs, including HIV.

- Transvestitism. The wearing of clothing of the opposite sex. Most transvestites are men, heterosexual, and married.

- Fetishism. Sexual arousal achieved by looking at or touching inanimate objects, such as underclothing or shoes.

- Exhibitionism. The exposure of one's genitals to strangers in public places. Most exhibitionists seek shock or fear from their victims. Exhibitionism is illegal.

- Voyeurism. Observing other people for sexual gratification. Most voyeurs are men who attempt to watch women undressing or bathing. Voyeurism is illegal and an invasion of privacy.

- Sadomasochism. Sexual activities in which gratification is received by inflicting pain (verbal or physical abuse) on a partner or by being the object of such infliction. A sadist is a person who receives gratification from inflicting pain, and a masochist is a person who receives gratification from experiencing pain.

- Pedophilia. Sexual activity or attraction between an adult and a child. Any sexual activity involving a minor, including creating, possessing, or selling child pornography, is illegal in Canada.

- Autoerotic asphyxiation. The practice of reducing or eliminating oxygen to the brain, usually by tying a cord around one's neck, while masturbating. Tragically, some individuals accidentally hang themselves in the process.

- Sexting and internet luring. Sexting refers to creating and sharing sexual images or messages through the use of digital media such as cell phones, email, instant messaging, or social networking sites. Internet luring is when an adult communicates with a child under the age of 16 for sexual purposes.

DIFFICULTIES THAT CAN HINDER SEXUAL FUNCTIONING

There are various problems that hinder sexual functioning—these are quite common with as many as 76 percent of women and 35 percent of men experiencing some sort of dysfunction (Allahdadi, Tostes, & Webb, 2009). The label given to the various problems that interfere with sexual pleasure is **sexual dysfunction**. You should not be embarrassed if you experience a sexual dysfunction at some point in your life. Your sexuality does not come with a lifetime warranty. You can have breakdowns involving your sexual function similar to breakdowns in any of your other body systems. Sexual dysfunctions can be divided into four major classes:

College and university students often think everyone is having more sex than they are and with numerous partners. These perceptions may result in them feeling self-conscious about their own lack of sexual activity or encourage increased promiscuity in order to "measure up." In reality, most post-secondary school students' opinions about sex, relationships, and contraception/STI protection and their attitudes toward sexual activity vary greatly. Results from a recent survey answered by college and university students might help you sort through some of these misperceptions:

- Approximately 72 percent of the 1500 college students surveyed had engaged in intercourse during the past year, just 51 percent said they used a condom.

- Thirty eight percent of students cited birth control pills as their preferred contraception. This is disconcerting because birth control does not protect against contracting STIs.

- Although many students rate their sexual health knowledge as very good or excellent, nearly 75 percent scored 5 out of 10 or worse on a related quiz.

- While, 34 percent of students described their most recent sexual encounter as being casual (i.e., a "hook-up," "booty call," or "friends with benefits"), 67 percent of males and 80 percent of college females were happy or very happy with their sexual lives.

Sources: Data from American College Health Association, *American College Health Association—National College Health Assessment: Reference Group Data Report Fall 2010* (Baltimore: American College Health Association, 2011); and American College Health Association, *American College Health Association—National College Health Assessment: Reference Group Data Report Spring 2008* (Baltimore: American College Health Association, 2009). Both available at www.acha-ncha.org. http://news.nationalpost.com/health/sex-survey-reveals-nearly-a-quarter-of-canadian-university-students-abstain-but-many-others-avoid-condom-use.

---

sexual desire disorders, sexual arousal disorders, orgasm disorders, and sexual pain disorders. In most cases, sexual dysfunctions can be treated successfully if both partners are willing to work together to solve the problem.

Sexual Desire Disorders

The most frequent reason people seek a sex therapist is **inhibited sexual desire (ISD)**. ISD is the lack of a sexual appetite or simply a lack of interest and pleasure in sexual activity (Medicine Plus, 2010). In some instances, it can result from stress or boredom with sex. **Sexual aversion disorder** is another type of desire dysfunction, characterized by sexual phobias (unreasonable fears) and anxiety about sexual contact. The psychological stress of a punitive upbringing, rigid religious background, or a history of physical or sexual abuse might be a source of these desire disorders.

Sexual Arousal Disorders

The most common disorder in this category is **erectile dysfunction**. Erectile dysfunction, or impotence, refers to difficulty in achieving or maintaining a penile erection sufficient for intercourse. At some time in his life, every man experiences impotence. Causes are varied and include underlying diseases, such as diabetes or prostate problems, reactions to some medications (for example, medication for high blood pressure), depression, fatigue, stress, alcohol, performance anxiety, and guilt over real or imaginary problems (such as when a man compares himself to his partner's past lovers). Impotence generally becomes more of a problem as men age, affecting one in four men over the age of 65 (National Kidney and Urological Diseases Information Clearinghouse, n.d.).

Chronic impotence (impotence lasting more than three months) should be treated by a physician. A complete medical examination and history are necessary to rule out physical causes. Viagra (sildenafil citrate), Levitra, and Cialis are used as treatments for erectile dysfunction. Taken orally one hour before sexual activity, Viagra is reported to manage erectile dysfunction successfully in 70 to 80 percent of cases (Pfizer Labs, 2010). The most commonly reported side effects of Viagra include headache, flushing, stomach ache, urinary tract infection, diarrhea, dizziness, rash, and mild and temporary visual changes (Sairam et al., 2002). There also have been several deaths among Viagra users, prompting more caution in prescribing it to patients with known cardiovascular disease and those taking commonly prescribed short- and

Inhibited sexual desire (ISD) Lack of sexual appetite or simply a lack of interest and pleasure in sexual activity.

Sexual aversion disorder Type of desire dysfunction characterized by sexual phobias and anxiety about sexual contact.

Erectile dysfunction Also called impotence; difficulty in achieving or maintaining a penile erection sufficient for intercourse.

long-acting nitrates, such as nitroglycerin. Impotence due to psychological factors can be treated with psychotherapy. Such treatment is effective in 90 percent of cases.

Orgasm Disorders

Between 20 and 30 percent of the male population is affected by premature ejaculation at some time in their lives (Rowland et al., 2010). **Premature ejaculation** is ejaculation that occurs prior to or very soon after the insertion of the penis into the vagina. Another orgasm disorder in males is **retarded ejaculation**, or the inability to ejaculate once the penis is erect. Treatment for premature ejaculation involves a physical examination to rule out organic causes. If the cause of the problem is not physiologic, therapy is available to help a man learn how to control the timing of his ejaculation. Fatigue, stress, performance pressure, and alcohol can be contributing factors to these orgasmic disorders in men.

When a woman is unable to achieve orgasm with her partner, she often blames herself and fakes orgasm to preserve her partner's ego. Researchers reported that up to 66 percent of women have faked an orgasm at one time or another (Darling & Davidson, 1986). Until recently, societal norms were that women were not supposed to enjoy sex but rather "do it" to fulfill their "marital duty." The Kinsey reports in the 1950s and Masters and Johnson's findings in the 1960s and 1970s raised questions about these sexual myths. We recognize today that women enjoy sexual activity as much as men. In the past, women who did not experience orgasm were called "frigid." This term is no longer used because it implies that a woman is at fault. Instead, the term **preorgasmic** is used, since many women can learn to become orgasmic.

For women whose sexual pleasure is hampered, therapy is available. A physical examination to rule out organic causes is generally the first step. Masturbation is usually a primary focus in helping a woman to become orgasmic. Through masturbation, a woman can learn how her body responds sexually to various types of touch. Once a woman has become orgasmic through masturbation, she must learn to communicate her needs to her partner. The investment of time and caring by both partners is usually worth the effort as 70 percent of preorgasmic women can be helped.

Premature ejaculation Ejaculation that occurs prior to or almost immediately following penile penetration.

Retarded ejaculation The inability to ejaculate once the penis is erect.

Preorgasmic In women, the state of never having experienced an orgasm.

Dyspareunia Pain experienced by women during intercourse.

Vaginismus A state in which the vaginal muscles contract so forcefully that penetration cannot be accomplished.

Sexual Pain Disorders

Two common disorders in the category of sexual pain disorders are dyspareunia and vaginismus. **Dyspareunia** is pain experienced by a female during vaginal entry, including penile–vaginal intercourse (Furukawa et al., 2012). This pain can be caused by endometriosis, uterine tumours, chlamydia, gonorrhea, or urinary tract infections. Further, emotional, relational, and behavioural factors may contribute to this disorder (Furukawa et al., 2012). Damage to tissues during childbirth and insufficient lubrication during intercourse may also cause pain or discomfort. Dyspareunia can also be psychological in origin. As with other problems, dyspareunia can be treated with good results. The first step in treatment is a thorough pelvic examination to rule out physical disease. Diseases or disorders can usually be cured with medication or surgery. Vaginal lubricants can be purchased to help with inadequate lubrication. Psychologically caused dyspareunia is much more difficult to treat.

Vaginismus is the involuntary contraction of vaginal muscles, making penile insertion painful or impossible. Most cases of vaginismus are related to fear of intercourse or to unresolved sexual conflicts. Treatment of vaginismus involves teaching a woman to achieve orgasm through nonvaginal stimulation. Becoming orgasmic is important because research has indicated that treatment for vaginismus is more successful in orgasmic women. The woman and her partner are then taught methods for dilating the vagina, either with fingers or a vibrator. As dilation is achieved, the woman is taught to relax in order to allow penetration. Cure rates are close to 100 percent.

Drugs and Sex

Because psychoactive drugs affect our entire physiology, they affect our sexual behaviours. Promises of increased pleasure make drugs very tempting to those seeking greater sexual satisfaction. Too often, however, drugs become central to sexual activities and damage the relationship. Alcohol is notorious for reducing inhibitions and giving increased feelings of well-being and desirability (see also Chapter 10). At the same time, alcohol inhibits sexual response; thus, the mind may be willing, but not the body. Perhaps the greatest danger associated with use of drugs during sex is the tendency to blame the drug for negative or irresponsible behaviours: "I can't help what I did last night because I was drunk" is a response that demonstrates sexual immaturity. A sexually mature person carefully examines risks and benefits and makes decisions accordingly. If drugs are necessary to increase erotic feelings, it is likely that the partners are being dishonest about their feelings for each other. Good sex is not dependent on chemical substances.

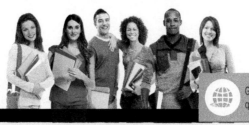

assess YOURSELF

TAKING CHARGE: Creating Better Relationships

After reading this chapter, it should be apparent that relationships involve complex interactions between individuals. To create strong and effective relationships, you must carefully assess the values you put on friendships, significant others, and other forms of interpersonal interactions. Healthy relationships involve developing intimacy in several dimensions. It may be helpful for you to take a personal inventory of your relationships. To determine how healthy they are, consider the questions below:

- What relationships are most important to you right now?
- How have these relationships affected your relationships with others? Are you giving enough time to your other relationships?
- Have you thought about how good your relationships are from an emotional perspective? A psychological perspective? A physical perspective? A spiritual perspective? Which of these factors is the most important to you? Why?
- What would an ideal set of relationships look like for you? How many close interactions would you want to make time for? What would be the nature and extent of these relationships?
- Are you comfortable with yourself sexually? Are you satisfied with your current choice(s) of sexual expression?
- What do you expect in a committed relationship? What would you be willing to accept in terms of attitudes and/ or behaviours from your committed partner? What do you expect of yourself?
- What do you think are the three most important attributes of a friend? Do you display these attributes with your friends?
- How are you limited or bound by gender-role stereotypes?
- Have you considered your values or beliefs about what is most important to you in a prospective lifelong partner? Are you asking for the same attributes that you would be able to give to a partner?
- Do you make a habit of putting yourself in the other person's shoes when discussing how your actions may have made that person feel or how that person may be feeling in general?
- Do you take time to listen to your friends? Your parents? Your acquaintances? Your professors? Do you find yourself thinking about your own problems, thoughts, or issues when someone is trying to tell you about his or her problems?
- Do you reach out to friends who are having problems in their relationships?
- Are you supportive of couples having problems in their relationship without being judgmental or taking sides?
- Do you try to work through your problems with others, or do you run from, avoid, or get angry rather than try to talk through your difficulties?
- Are you supportive of counselling services and other campus and community services that offer help for people who have troubled relationships?
- Do you listen carefully to what your legislators propose in the way of family and individual policies and programs that may unfairly harm others?

Is It Love or Infatuation?

In the early stages, love and infatuation can be very similar. They both produce a characteristic rush of excitement as well as a strong desire to have more of the loved one's time, energy, and physical contact. The primary difference is that, with love, the feelings grow deeper as you get to know the person better and come to appreciate him or her more. With infatuation or a crush, you realize that Ms. or Mr. Right was not all you had thought. Taking the following test may help you determine whether it is the real thing or an infatuation. Respond honestly YES or NO to the following statements.

(continued)

1. I knew I was in love with this person almost immediately.
2. Even though I have known this person for a while, I still really love his/her personality.
3. I wonder sometimes if the person has changed a lot since I have known him/her because he/she acts differently around me now.
4. The more I am with this person, the more I want to be around him/her.
5. I am less interested in the person sexually than I was in the beginning.
6. The more I know about this person, the more I want to know.
7. The more I know about this person, the less interested I am in him/her.
8. I feel really good associating with this person and being regarded as a couple.
9. I have begun to notice more things "wrong" with this person and spend a lot of time trying to get him/her to change.
10. Even though I have been with this person for a while, I am still as sexually interested as I was in the beginning.
11. I would just as soon do things with other people as with this person because I would probably have more fun.
12. I am able to share my feelings with this person and trust him/her completely.
13. I really love this person but do not feel good about sharing intimate feelings with him/her yet.
14. This person brings out the best in me and genuinely seems to care about me.
15. I love this person, but I do not respect him/her the way I respect others.

Interpretation

There are no right or wrong responses to these statements. Answering YES to the even-numbered statements may indicate that your feelings are more likely to be love-directed. Answering YES to the odd-numbered statements may indicate a tendency toward infatuation. Count the number of YES responses to the even-numbered statements and the number of YES responses to the odd-numbered statements. Look carefully at each statement. Are these things that you feel are important enough to work on? Or are your responses telling you that another person may be a better choice?

Building Healthy Relationships

Understanding your relationships and clarifying love or infatuation are both steps toward understanding yourself and your relationships. When you are in a short- or long-term relationship, you can also benefit from understanding what to do if your relationship is in trouble. The following set of frequently asked questions can help you in that regard.

What can I do if my relationship is in trouble?

Do not put it off—get professional help now. Often couples are afraid to admit that there is a problem and wait too long. The distancing increases and things are said and done that are hard to take back. The right time to start improving the relationship is now, not later.

What kind of help is available?

Many professionals with specialized training in couple and family therapy can help: clergy, medical doctors, psychologists, psychiatrists, and social workers. Most communities have a Community Information Service that lists social service agencies and therapists whose specialty is couple and family therapy. Marriage and family therapists are also listed online.

What do couple and family therapists do?

Talking about your situation with a therapist can help you to gain a new perspective on the issues you are dealing with. You can also improve your level of communication so that the thoughts and feelings that have previously been unspoken are brought out into the open. The tension level is lowered so that old issues can be resolved.

How do I choose a couple and family therapist?

Since you will be sharing intimate details of your relationship with your therapist, you want to make sure that there is a good match, and that you feel safe. Feel free to call several offices and get a feel for the therapist. Most therapists should be willing to have a five-minute discussion on the phone with you while you are searching for the right match.

What kind of questions should I ask?

You are looking for two things: professional competence and personal style. For competence issues you will want to know what professional training therapists have, what professional associations they belong to, and if they are registered in their profession. Couple and family therapists must have at least a master's degree in relationship counselling and have been supervised for a minimum of 1000 client hours before they can be registered. All provinces have an Association of Marriage and Family Therapists and an Association of Social Workers. They can provide you with a list of therapists in your area. You can also contact the Canadian Guidance Counsellors Association.

How long does therapy take?

Each situation is unique. Usually the therapist will set one appointment each week for the first few weeks. Each session is generally about an hour, with an average of 8 to 10 sessions. Often by that time significant changes have been made in the relationship and you are ready to make a go of it on your own.

How much does therapy cost?

Costs can vary from $50 to $125 per session. Registered psychologists usually charge more than $100 per session. Public health insurance does not cover the cost of therapy unless the therapy is provided by a psychiatrist. Many employee benefit plans will cover all or portions of the cost of couple and family therapy. Check with your service provider to see what assistance you can receive.

How long do I have to wait to get an appointment?

Usually you will be seen within a week or two. It depends, however, on how flexible you can be. Most therapists will have some evening hours, but these usually fill up quickly. If you require an evening appointment, you might have to wait a little longer.

Who should come to the appointment?

Whoever is involved! If it is a marital or couple issue, it is best if both partners attend. If it is a family issue, the therapist may ask the whole family to attend. This helps the therapist to see the situation in its full context and for each person involved to present how he or she experiences the issue.

What if my partner won't come?

The therapist may suggest some helpful strategies to lower your partner's anxiety and make it easier for him or her to attend. If, however, your partner chooses not to participate, it is still possible to continue with therapy on your own.

DISCUSSION QUESTIONS

1. What is the role of communication in nonintimate and intimate relationships? How can you become a better listener? Speaker?

2. What are behavioural interdependence, need fulfillment, and emotional attachment, and why is each of these important in subsequent relationship development?

3. What are the common types of intimate relationships? Which of these do you think is most important to you right now? Why?

4. Why are your relationships with your family important? Explain how your family unit is similar to or different from the family unit of the early 1960s. Who makes up your family of origin? Your nuclear family?

5. How can you tell the difference between a love relationship and one that is based primarily on attraction? What common characteristics do love relationships share?

6. What prevents intimacy? What can you do to reduce or remove these barriers?

7. What are the common elements of good relationships?

8. What actions can you take to improve your interpersonal relationships?

9. What are the functions of the various hormones during puberty? What physical changes are brought about by menopause?

10. What are "normal" sexual behaviours? Do men and women differ in sexual response? In their preference for sexual behaviours?

11. Do drugs and alcohol enhance sexual performance? What risks are involved in such experimentation?

APPLICATION EXERCISE

Reread the "Consider This . . . " scenario at the beginning of the chapter and answer the following questions.

1. From what you have read in this chapter, what problems do Jorge and Yasmin have in their relationship?

2. Why do you think people feel forced to tell lies or half-truths in their relationships with others?

3. Are there times with your partner when it is okay to be dishonest or to not tell the truth, or should you always be totally honest and truthful about your actions?

4. Do you believe that you should tell your partner about all of your previous sexual experiences? Why or why not?

MASTERINGHEALTH

Go to MasteringHealth for Assignments, the eText, and the Study Area with case studies, self quizzing, and videos.

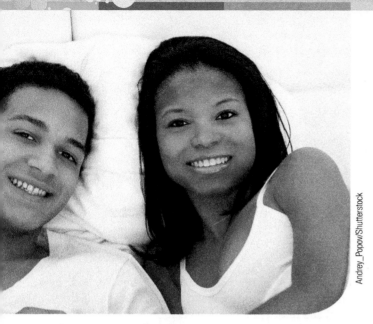

Andrey_Popow/Shutterstock

CHAPTER 8

CONSIDERING YOUR REPRODUCTIVE CHOICES

◂◉ CONSIDER THIS . . .

Jamila and Karim have been dating for several months. After a wonderful evening together, they go back to Karim's place with the intention of having sex. When they arrive at Karim's, they discover that neither of them has a condom. Karim thought that Jamila was taking the birth control pill. Jamila thought Karim would have condoms. Rather than spoil the evening, Jamila and Karim have unprotected sex. The next day, they argue over who is responsible for the birth control.

What mistakes were made in this situation? In Jamila and Karim's relationship? When should a couple talk about birth control, including whose responsibility it is? What about the issue of preventing sexually transmitted infections? Who is responsible for providing birth control? Who is responsible for protection from sexually transmitted infections? What are the risks of engaging in unprotected sex? What were the alternatives?

LEARNING OUTCOMES

- Describe the various contraceptive methods available, including their accessibility, availability, and effectiveness in preventing pregnancy and sexually transmitted infections.

- Identify the emotional health, maternal health, financial evaluation/planning, and contingency planning to be considered when planning to become a parent.

- Explain the importance of prenatal care in the process of pregnancy.

- Summarize the basic stages of childbirth as well as complications that can arise during labour and delivery.

- Review the primary causes of and possible solutions to infertility.

Fertility is a mixed blessing for women. The ability to participate in the miracle of birth is an incredible experience for many. Yet the responsibility for controlling your fertility can also be overwhelming. Through research and technology, we now have a better understanding of the intimate details of reproduction as well as the processes designed to control or enhance our fertility. Along with information and technological advance comes choice and responsibility to make the right choice for you. Choosing if and when to have children is one of the most important decisions you will make. A woman and her partner have much to consider before planning or risking a pregnancy. Children, whether planned or unplanned, change your life. Children require a lifelong personal commitment of love and nurturing.

Before you plan or risk a pregnancy, you have a responsibility to make sure you are physically, emotionally, and financially prepared to care for another human being. One measure of maturity is the ability to discuss reproduction, birth control, and sexually transmitted infection (STI) protection with your sexual partner before succumbing to sexual urges. If you cannot discuss birth control or STI protection with your partner, then you are not mature enough to engage in sex. Men often assume that their partner is taking care of birth control. Women often feel that if they bring up the subject, it implies that they are "easy" or "loose." You will find embarrassment-free discussion a lot easier when you understand human reproduction, contraception, STI protection, and thoroughly consider your attitudes toward these matters before you get into compromising situations.

MANAGING YOUR FERTILITY

Conception refers to the fertilization of an ovum by a sperm. The sperm enters the ovum. Its tail breaks off, and a protective chemical barrier secreted by the ovum surrounds the sperm and prevents other sperm from entering. A viable egg, a viable sperm, and possible access to the egg by the sperm are necessary conditions for conception.

Contraception refers to methods of preventing conception. Society has and continues to search for a simple, infallible, and risk-free method of preventing pregnancy. The present methods of contraception fall into two categories: reversible

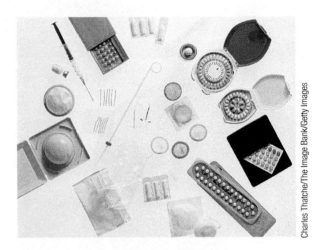

For couples who want to avoid pregnancy, a wide variety of contraceptives are available, including IUDs, cervical caps, diaphragms, different types of pills, and male and female condoms.

Charles Thatche/The Image Bank/Getty Images

methods, such as the pill, condoms, abstinence, and others; and permanent methods, such as vasectomy (for men) and tubal ligation (for women).

Reversible Contraception

Abstinence and "Outercourse"

Strictly defined, abstinence means not engaging in intercourse. Traditionally, individuals could still engage in such forms of sexual intimacy as massage, kissing, and solitary masturbation and consider themselves abstainers. However, many people today have broadened the definition of abstinence to include all forms of sexual contact, even those that do not culminate in sexual intercourse.

Couples who go a step farther than massage and kissing and engage in such activities as oral–genital sex and mutual masturbation are sometimes said to be engaging in "outercourse." Like abstinence, outercourse can be 100-percent effective for birth control as long as the male does not ejaculate near the vaginal opening. Unlike abstinence, however, there is still a risk of STIs. Oral–genital contact can result in transmission of an STI, although the risk can be reduced by using a condom on the penis or a dental dam on the vaginal opening.

Condoms

The **condom** is a strong sheath of latex rubber or other material designed to fit over an erect penis (Figure 8.1). The condom catches the ejaculate, thereby preventing sperm migration toward the egg. The condom is the only temporary means of birth control available for men and the only barrier that effectively

---

Fertility The ability to reproduce.

Conception The fertilization of an ovum by a sperm.

Contraception Methods of preventing conception.

Condom A sheath of thin latex or other material designed to fit over an erect penis to collect semen upon ejaculation.

FIGURE 8.1
How to Use a Condom

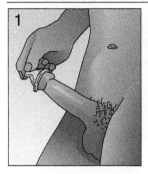
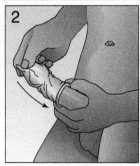
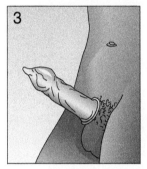
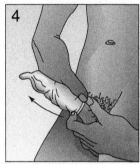

The condom should be rolled over the erect penis as soon as it is erect (even during outercourse). A small space (about 1 cm) should be left at the end of the condom to collect the semen after ejaculation. Hold the tip of the condom, and unroll it all the way to the base of the penis. Hold the base of the condom before withdrawal to avoid spilling any semen.

prevents the spread of STIs, including HIV. Regardless of your preferred method of birth control, you should always use a condom. Condoms come in a wide variety of styles: coloured, ribbed for "extra sensation," lubricated, nonlubricated, and with or without reservoirs at the tip. They also can be purchased with or without spermicide in pharmacies, in some schools, and in some public washrooms. Some health clinics, including those on many college and university campuses, provide condoms free of charge. A new condom must be used for each act of intercourse or oral sex.

Condoms help prevent the spread of some STIs, including genital herpes and HIV. They may also slow or reduce the development of cervical abnormalities in women that can lead to cancer. The theoretical **perfect-use effectiveness rate** for condoms is 98 percent, meaning that when they are used correctly and consistently, 2 out of 100 women who use them will become pregnant in one year (Hatcher et al., 2007). In reality, however, their effectiveness, or **typical-use rate**, is only 85 percent (15 out of every 100 women who use condoms will become pregnant in one year) because they are so often used incorrectly

or inconsistently (Hatcher et al., 2007). The unintended pregnancies or failure rates of contraceptives according to typical and perfect-use rates are shown in Table 8.1. Condoms should always be used for vaginal, anal, and oral sex. They must be rolled on the erect penis before the penis touches the vagina, leaving about a 1-centimetre space at the tip to collect ejaculated semen (see Figure 8.1). After ejaculation, the condom should be held at the base of the penis before withdrawal, to avoid spillage. For greatest efficacy, condoms should be used with a spermicide containing nonoxynol-9.

Another reason why condoms are not as effective in real life as they are in theory is that they can break during intercourse, especially if they are old or poorly stored. They must be stored in a cool place (not in a wallet, hip pocket, or in the glove compartment of your car!) and should be inspected before use for small tears.

Some people claim that a condom ruins the spontaneity of sex; stopping to put it on breaks the mood for them. Others report that the condom decreases sensation. These perceived inconveniences contribute to improper use. As mentioned, the condom should be put on the penis as soon as it is erect, so that should not interrupt the mood. Couples can also put the condom on together as part of foreplay, thus enhancing the mood and generally leading to more successful birth control and STI protection.

Oral Contraceptives

Oral contraceptive pills were first marketed in Canada in 1961 and quickly became the most widely used reversible method of fertility control. Most oral contraceptives work through the combined effects of synthetic estrogen and progesterone. Because the levels of estrogen in the pill are higher than those produced by the body, the pituitary gland is not signalled to produce follicle-stimulating hormone (FSH); without FSH, ova will not develop in the ovaries. Further, progesterone in the pill prevents growth of the uterine lining and thickens the cervical mucus, forming a barrier against sperm.

Pills are meant to be taken in a cycle. At the end of each three-week cycle, the user discontinues the drug or takes a placebo pill for one week. The resultant drop in hormones causes the uterine lining to disintegrate, and the user will have menstrual flow, usually within one to three days. The same cycle is repeated every 28 days. Menstrual flow is generally lighter than in a non-pill user because the hormones in the pill prevent thick endometrial build-up.

Perfect-use effectiveness rate The percentage rate of women who will become pregnant in one year when a contraceptive method is used correctly and consistently.

Typical-use effectiveness rate The percentage of women who will become pregnant in one year considered that a contraceptive method is often used incorrectly or inconsistently.

Oral contraceptive pills Pills that prevent ovulation by regulating hormones taken daily for three weeks of the menstrual cycle.

TABLE 8.1

Contraceptive Effectiveness

	Number of Unintended Pregnancies per 100 Women during the First Year of Use	
	Typical Use	Perfect Use
Continuous abstinence[*]	0	0
Female sterilization	0.5	0.5
Male sterilization	0.15	0.1
Implanon	0.05	0.05
IUD (intrauterine device)		
ParaGard (copper T)	0.8	0.6
Mirena (LNG-IUS)	0.2	0.2
Depo-Provera	3	0.3
Oral contraceptives (combined pill and progestin-only pill)	8	0.3
Ortho Evra patch	8	0.3
NuvaRing	8	0.3
Male condom[†] **(without spermicides)**	15	2
Diaphragm[†] **(with spermicidal cream or jelly)**	16	6
Sponge		
Women who have never given birth	16	9
Women who have given birth	32	20
Female condom[†] **(without spermicides)**	21	5
Fertility awareness methods	25	12
Withdrawal	27	4
Spermicides[†] **(foams, creams, gels, vaginal suppositories, and vaginal film)**	29	18
No method	85	85
Emergency contraceptive pill	Treatment initiated within 72 hours after unprotected intercourse reduces the risk of pregnancy by 75–89 percent (with no protection against STIs).	

[*]Indicates complete protection from STIs.

[†]Indicates limited protection from STIs.

Note: "Typical Use" refers to failure rates for men and women whose use is not consistent or always correct. "Perfect Use" refers to failure rates for those whose use is consistent and always correct.

Source: From *Contraceptive Technology*, 19th rev. ed. Copyright © 2007 Contraceptive Technology Communications, Inc. Used with permission of the Ardent Media, Inc.

Today's pill is different from the one introduced more than five decades ago. The original pill contained large amounts of estrogen and progestin, which increased health risk, in particular for deep vein thrombosis (Liao & Dollin, 2012). Today's versions of the pill contain considerably less estrogen and progestin with more pharmacologically specific progestins which are more focused in their drug effect in preventing pregnancy (Liao & Dollin, 2012). Some pills are progestin only (Chadwick et al., 2011). As a result of more than 50 years of research and pharmacological manipulation, today's birth control pill has less health risk than in the past. Still, there is risk for stroke due to increased chance of blood clots and with increasing age and longer term oral contraceptive use, risk of heart attack increases (Chadwick et al., 2011). Thus, women (and their partners) should consider their individual risk prior to choosing the pill as their contraceptive.

Because the chemicals in oral contraceptives change the way the body metabolizes certain nutrients, all women using the pill should check with their prescribing practitioners regarding dietary supplements. The nutrients of concern include vitamin C and the B-complex vitamins—B_2, B_6, and B_{12}, as

point of view

CONDOMS: His or Hers?

If you are part of a sexually active heterosexual couple, or even 'hooking up' regularly, preventing pregnancy may be one of your top priorities, particularly when you are in the midst of your post-secondary education and may not be prepared for the responsibilities a child brings. Condoms (as previously mentioned) can be used as a form of birth control and for STI protection too—though the women's condom is not as effective. So which one is better to use? That depends upon you and your partner. Do not both use one; the friction between the two condoms can cause one or both to break.

Read on—perhaps together—and decide which option works best for you, for now.

HERS

The female condom is a lubricated plastic tube with flexible rings at either end. One end of the tube is sealed. To use this condom, you insert it into your vagina in such a way that the sealed end of the tube covers your cervix and the open end slightly covers your labia (the outer lips of your vagina; see Figure 8.2). In this way, the condom blocks sperm from entering your womb. The female condom is about 75 percent effective at preventing pregnancy.

The female condom should be put in place prior to any genital-to-genital contact.

Female condoms, similar to male condoms, cannot be reused and should be discarded after use (whether or not he ejaculates in you).

Female condoms, again similar to male condoms, are available without a prescription at your local pharmacy.

Female condoms provide some protection against STIs, but are not as effective as male condoms.

HIS

The male condom is made of latex, plastic, or an animal membrane such as lambskin. Latex condoms are the most effective at preventing the spread of STIs. Remove it from the package and roll it on an erect penis, leaving a little room at the top for ejaculate. In this way, sperm is prevented from entering the woman's womb. Condoms on their own are about 85 percent effective in preventing pregnancy. When a spermicide is also used, their efficacy rises to about 97 percent.

The condom should be placed on the penis as soon as it is erect and prior to any oral-to-genital or genital-to-genital contact.

A new condom is needed for each ejaculation; condoms cannot be reused.

Condoms can be purchased without a prescription from your local pharmacy. They come in all shapes, sizes, colours, and materials. The standard size will fit most men; though extra-large are available as well as 'snug' sizes that fit a bit tighter. Some condoms have a predesigned nipple at the end to trap the ejaculate. Extra strength condoms are available for those who have trouble with condom breakage. Lubricated condoms can be purchased; often the lubricant contains spermicide, which may provide some protection from pregnancy should the condom break. Flavoured condoms are available and are designed primarily for oral sex.

Source: Based on Sexual Health, Birth Control, and Condoms, Birth Control Health Centre, published by WebMD, LLC.

well as folic acid—so, if you are on the pill, you have another reason to choose a nutritious diet that includes whole grains, plenty of fresh vegetables and fruit, lean meats, fish and poultry, and nonfat dairy products (see also Chapter 5). Oral contraceptives can interact negatively with other drugs (Planned Parenthood, 2013a). Some antibiotics diminish the pill's effectiveness, as can a flu virus that results in vomiting or diarrhea (Planned Parenthood, 2013a). A backup contraceptive should be used for the rest of the pill pack if these circumstances occur. Women in doubt should check with their prescribing practitioners, their pharmacists, or other knowledgeable health professionals.

Although return of fertility may be delayed after discontinuing the pill, it is not known to cause infertility. Women who had irregular menstrual cycles before going on the pill are more likely to have problems conceiving, regardless of pill use.

The perfect-use effectiveness rate of oral contraceptives is 99.7 percent, making them one of the most effective reversible methods of fertility control (Hatcher et al., 2007). Using the pill is convenient and does not interfere with sexual activity. It can lessen menstrual difficulties, such as cramps, premenstrual syndrome (PMS), dysmenorrhea, and might also clear up acne (Maguire & Westhoff, 2011). Women using oral contraceptives have lower risks for developing endometrial and ovarian cancers and, to a lesser extent, colon cancer (Maguire & Westhoff, 2011). They are also less likely than nonusers to develop fibrocystic breast disease. In addition, pill users have lower incidences of ectopic pregnancies, ovarian cysts, pelvic inflammatory disease, and iron deficiency anemia. As previously mentioned, possible serious health problems associated with the pill include the tendency for pill users' blood to form clots and an increased risk for high blood pressure in a few women. Clotting can lead to strokes or heart attacks (Chadwick et al., 2011). The risk is low for most healthy, non-smoking women under 35; it increases with age and, especially, with cigarette smoking. Although the perfect-use rate of oral contraceptives is 99.7 percent, the typical-use effectiveness is only 92 percent (Hatcher et al., 2007). The typical-use rate may relate to the fact that the pill must be taken every day. If a woman misses taking one pill, she is advised to use an alternative form of contraception for the remainder of that cycle. The cost of the pill can be a problem for some women. Finally, some younger teenagers report that the requirement to have a complete gynecological examination in order to get a prescription for the pill is an obstacle. In fact, 69 percent of female teenagers think that this requirement frightens their peers away from use of the pill (Greydanus & Shearin, 1990). Educating young women about what goes on in a gynecological exam and highlighting the importance of such exams may ease their anxiety, along with confirmation that their examination and prescription remains confidential.

Progestin-Only Pills

Progestin-only pills (or minipills) contain small doses of progesterone. Women who feel uncertain about using estrogen pills, who smoke, who suffer from side effects related to estrogen, or who are nursing may want to take these pills rather than combination pills. There is still some question about the specific ways progestin-only pills work.

Depo-Provera An injectable method of birth control that lasts for three months.

Current thought is that they change the composition of the cervical mucus, thus impeding sperm travel. They may also inhibit ovulation in some women. The perfect use effectiveness rate of progestin-only pills is 96 percent, which is lower than that of estrogen-containing pills (Hatcher et al., 2007). Also, their use usually leads to irregular menstrual bleeding.

Birth Control Patch (Ortho-Evra)

In Canada, since January 2003, women have been able to obtain a dermal patch that may be applied to the skin by prescription and use it in place of birth control pills or injections. The patch contains the hormones progestin and estrogen, two ingredients also found in birth control pills. It works like a smoking cessation patch, releasing medication through the skin into the bloodstream. The patch can be worn on the buttocks, upper outer arm, abdomen, back, or stomach. A new patch is applied every week for three weeks each month. During the fourth week, no patch is worn to allow for menstruation. If a patch falls off at any time you must replace it within a 24-hour period to maintain your normal birth control cycle.

While the patch will not protect you from STIs, it may be an alternative worth considering for those who frequently forget to take birth control pills and who do not like injections. The patch has similar effectiveness rates as the pill: perfect use is 99.7 percent effective and typical use is 92 percent (Hatcher et al., 2007). A small percentage of women may find that they are not able to use the patch because it irritates the skin.

Depo-Provera

Depo-Provera is a long-acting synthetic drug injected intramuscularly every three months. Although used in other countries for years, the Health Protection Branch did not approve it for use in Canada until 1997.

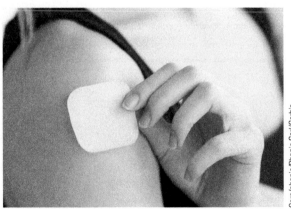

Ortho Evra, the contraceptive patch.

Garo/phanie/Phanie Sarl/Corbis

Researchers believe that the drug prevents ovulation. Its perfect use effectiveness in preventing pregnancy is greater than 99 percent, while its typical use is 97 percent (Hatcher et al., 2007). Its use may prevent menstrual blood loss, iron deficiency anemia, premenstrual tension, and endometriosis. The main disadvantage is irregular bleeding, which can be troublesome at first, but within a year most women are amenorrheic (have no menstrual cycles). Weight gain (an average of 2.5 kg in the first year) is also common and may be of concern for women who already have issues with weight maintenance. Other potential disadvantages include fatigue, mood disturbances, loss of libido, and increased risk of osteoporosis and diabetes. Dizziness, nervousness, and headache are other possible side effects. Unlike other methods of contraception, this method cannot be stopped immediately if problems arise. In addition, fertility may not return immediately after Depo-Provera use is discontinued.

NuvaRing

Introduced in 2002, this effective contraceptive offers protection for four weeks at a time when used as prescribed. Perfect use results in a 99.7 percent effectiveness rate (Hatcher et al., 2007). Typical use results in 92 percent effectiveness at preventing pregnancy (Hatcher et al., 2007). **NuvaRing** is a soft flexible ring about 5 centimetres in diameter that the user inserts into the vagina and leaves in place for three weeks. The user removes it for one week during her menstrual cycle. Once the ring is inserted, it continuously releases estrogen and progestin.

Advantages to NuvaRing include protection against pregnancy for one month, no pill to take daily, no requirement to be fitted by a clinician, no requirement to use spermicide, and the quick return of the

ability to become pregnant when no longer in use. Possible side effects include increased vaginal discharge and vaginal irritation or infection. Oil-based vaginal medicine to treat yeast infections cannot be used when the ring is in place, and a diaphragm or cervical cap cannot be used as a backup method.

Emergency Contraceptive Pills

Emergency contraceptive pills can be used when a condom breaks, after a sexual assault, or any time unprotected sexual intercourse occurs. Although often referred to as "the morning-after pill," they can be taken up to five days after unprotected intercourse to reduce the risk of pregnancy by 85 percent (Planned Parenthood, 2013b). Since pregnancy does not always immediately happen during sexual intercourse, emergency contraceptive pills can be used to prevent pregnancy, by delaying the release of an egg during ovulation. There are currently two common emergency contraceptive pills available. Plan B One Step was made accessible over the counter by the Federal Government as of June 10, 2013 (Planned Parenthood, 2013b). Preven was approved by Health Canada in November 1999. It contains two hormones that stop or delay ovulation and may prevent a fertilized egg from implanting in the uterus. Two pills are to be taken within 24 hours of intercourse and another two 12 or more hours after that. This prescription drug is intended for a woman who uses a method that fails or a woman who has experienced non-consensual sex. It is not "the abortion pill." Nor should it be considered a preferred method of contraception over the long term; it is meant to be used only in cases of emergency. Moreover, it does not protect against contracting an STI. Nausea, vomiting, menstrual irregularities, breast tenderness, headaches, abdominal pain and cramps, and dizziness are the most likely side effects for both these types of pills.

Foams, Suppositories, Jellies, and Creams

Like condoms, these contraceptive preparations are available without a prescription. Chemically, they are referred to as **spermicides**—substances designed to kill sperm.

Jellies and creams are packaged in tubes, and foams are available in aerosol cans. They must be inserted far enough into the vagina to cover the cervix, providing both a chemical barrier that kills sperm and a physical barrier that stops sperm from continuing toward an egg (Figure 8.2).

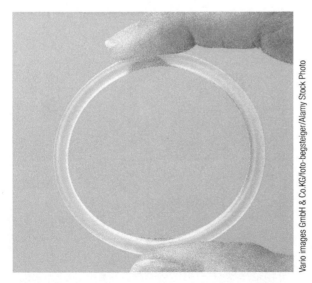

NuvaRing (actual size).

Vario images GmbH & Co.KG/foto-begsteiger/Alamy Stock Photo

NuvaRing A soft, flexible ring inserted into the vagina for three weeks at a time; prevents pregnancy in the same way that the pill does.

Emergency contraceptive pills Drugs taken up to three days after intercourse to reduce the risk of pregnancy.

Spermicides Substances designed to kill sperm.

Suppositories are waxy capsules placed deep in the vagina that melt once they are inside. They must be inserted 10 to 20 minutes before intercourse to have time to melt, but no longer than one hour prior to intercourse or they lose their effectiveness. Similar to condoms, additional contraceptive chemicals must be applied for each subsequent act of intercourse. Suppositories help prevent the spread of some sexually transmitted infections. Jellies and creams are designed to be used with a diaphragm or condom. When used with another method of contraception, their effectiveness improves. Used alone, the perfect-use effectiveness of foams, creams, gels, vaginal suppositories, and vaginal film is 82 percent (Hatcher et al., 2007). Typical use effectiveness is only 71 percent (Hatcher et al., 2007).

Female Condoms

The **female condom** is a single-use, soft, loose-fitting polyurethane sheath. It is designed as one unit, with two diaphragm-like rings. One ring, which lies inside the sheath, serves as an insertion mechanism and

Female condom A single-use polyurethane sheath for internal use by women.

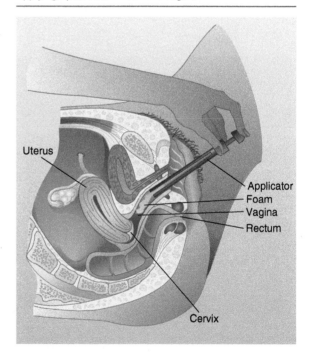

FIGURE 8.2

Applying Spermicide within the Vagina

Uterus

Applicator
Foam
Vagina
Rectum

Cervix

internal anchor. The other ring, which remains outside the vagina once the device is inserted, protects the labia and the base of the penis from infection. Perfect use effectiveness of the female condom is less than for the male condom at 95 percent (Hatcher et al., 2007). Typical use is also lower at 79 percent (Hatcher et al., 2007). Still, many women like the female condom, similar to the birth control pill, because it gives them more control over their reproduction.

Diaphragm with Spermicidal Jelly or Cream

Invented in the mid-nineteenth century, the **diaphragm** was the first widely used birth control method for women. Before that, most women relied on their partner to use a condom or to withdraw before ejaculation. The diaphragm is a soft, shallow cup made of thin latex rubber. Its flexible, rubber-coated ring is designed to fit snugly behind the pubic bone in front of the cervix and over the back of the cervix on the other side. Diaphragms are manufactured in different sizes and must be fitted to the woman by a trained practitioner. The practitioner should also be certain that the user knows how to insert her diaphragm correctly before she leaves his or her office.

Diaphragms must be used with spermicidal cream or jelly. The spermicide is applied to the inside of the diaphragm before insertion. The jelly or cream is held in place by the diaphragm, creating a physical and chemical barrier against sperm. Additional

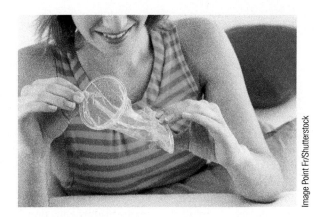

The female condom.

spermicide must be applied before each subsequent act of intercourse, and the diaphragm must be left in place for six to eight hours after intercourse to allow the chemical to kill any sperm remaining in the vagina (see Figure 8.3).

The typical-use effectiveness rate of the diaphragm with spermicidal cream or jelly is 84 percent; perfect-use effectiveness is 94 percent (Hatcher et al., 2007). Risk for **toxic shock syndrome (TSS)** increases when a diaphragm is used during menstruation or remains in place beyond the recommended time. TSS results from the multiplication of certain types of

Diaphragm A latex, saucer-shaped device designed to cover the cervix and block access to the uterus; should be used with spermicide.

Toxic shock syndrome (TSS) A potentially life-threatening disease that occurs when specific bacterial toxins multiply unchecked in wounds or through improper use of tampons or diaphragms.

FIGURE 8.3
Use and Placement of a Diaphragm

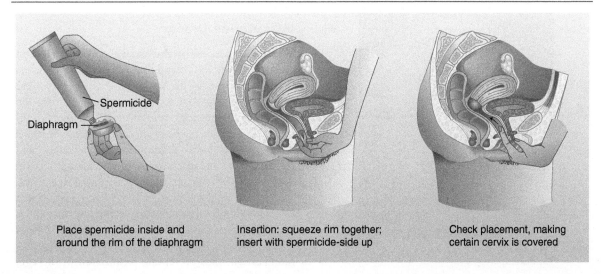

Place spermicide inside and around the rim of the diaphragm

Insertion: squeeze rim together; insert with spermicide-side up

Check placement, making certain cervix is covered

Staphylococcus bacteria that spread to the bloodstream and cause sudden high fever, rash, nausea, vomiting, diarrhea, confusion, headaches, muscle aches, and a sudden drop in blood pressure (MedlinePlus, 2013a). If not treated, TSS can be fatal. The diaphragm (as well as tampons left in place too long) creates conditions conducive to the growth of these bacteria. To reduce their risk of TSS, women should wash their hands carefully with soap and water before inserting or removing their diaphragm and tampons.

Another problem with the diaphragm is that it can put undue pressure on the urethra, blocking urinary flow and predisposing the user to bladder infections. A further disadvantage is that inserting the device can be awkward, especially if the woman is rushed. When inserted incorrectly, the effectiveness rate of the diaphragm decreases.

Contraceptive Sponge

First manufactured in 1983, the contraceptive sponge increased in popularity among young women during the 1980s and early 1990s. Plagued by reliability issues, allergic reactions, and other serious concerns, the original sponge was discontinued. In Canada, a new sponge is available called Protectaid. The sponge—as depicted in the photograph shown below—is made of a polyurethane foam and contains nonoxynol 9. It fits over the cervix and provides a physical barrier against sperm. A main advantage is convenience, as the sponge does not have to be fitted by a medical practitioner and can be purchased without a prescription.

Cervical cap A small cup made of latex designed to fit snugly over the entire cervix.

Intrauterine device (IUD) A T-shaped device implanted in the uterus to prevent pregnancy.

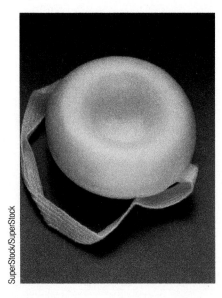

SuperStock/SuperStock

The contraceptive sponge.

Protection begins upon insertion and lasts for up to 24 hours. Unlike other methods, there is no need to reapply spermicide or insert a new sponge for subsequent acts of intercourse within the same 24-hour time frame; it must be left in place for at least six hours after the last intercourse. Disadvantages include the limited protection from STIs and limited typical-use effectiveness of 84 percent for women who have never had a child and only 68 percent for women who have given birth; perfect-use effectiveness is 91 percent for women who have not given birth and 80 percent for women who have (Hatcher et al., 2007). Allergic reactions and vaginal irritations are common side effects with the sponge. Further, when the vaginal lining becomes irritated, the risk of yeast infections and STIs increases as well. There is also an increased risk of TSS.

Cervical Cap

Cervical caps are one of the oldest methods used to prevent pregnancy. Early caps were made from beeswax, silver, or copper. The modern cervical cap was approved for use in Canada by the Health Protection Branch in 1982. The cervical cap is a small cup made of latex designed to fit snugly over the entire cervix. It must be fitted by a practitioner and is designed for use with contraceptive jelly or cream. It is somewhat more difficult to insert than a diaphragm because of its smaller size.

The cap keeps sperm out of the uterus. It is held in place by suction created during application. Insertion may take place any time up to two days prior to intercourse, and the device must be left in place for six to eight hours after intercourse. The maximum length of time the cap can be left on the cervix is 48 hours. If removed and cleaned, it can be reinserted immediately. Some women report unpleasant vaginal odours after use. Because the device can become dislodged during intercourse, placement must be checked frequently. It cannot be used during the menstrual period and there is increased risk of TSS.

Intrauterine Device

Widespread use of **intrauterine devices (IUDs)** or IUCDs, where C stand for contraceptive, for contraception began in the mid-1960s, when they were advertised as less risky and more convenient than the pill. These devices fell out of favour in the mid-1970s, following negative publicity about the Dalkon Shield, a device associated with pelvic inflammatory disease and sterility. The manufacturer stopped making Dalkon Shields in 1975. We are not certain how IUDs work, despite the fact that women have been using them since 1909. Although it was once thought that IUDs act by preventing implantation of a fertilized egg, most experts now believe that they interfere with the sperm's mobilization, thus preventing fertilization of the egg, or that they prevent the release of the egg from the ovary (Planned Parenthood, 2013c).

A physician must fit and insert the IUD (Planned Parenthood, 2013c). For insertion, the device is folded and placed into a long, thin plastic applicator. The practitioner measures the depth of the uterus with a special instrument and then uses these measurements to place the IUD accurately. When in place, the arms of the T open out across the top of the uterus. One or two strings extend from the IUD into the vagina so the user can check to make sure that her IUD is in place. The device should be replaced every five years and is removed by a practitioner.

Although IUDs have a perfect- and typical-use rate greater than 99 percent, the discomfort and cost of insertion may be a disadvantage (Hatcher et al., 2007). When in place, the device can cause heavy menstrual flow and severe cramps. There is also risk of uterine perforation. Women using IUDs have a higher risk of ectopic pregnancy, pelvic inflammatory disease, infertility, and tubal infections (Planned Parenthood, 2013c). If a pregnancy occurs while the IUD is in place, most research suggests a 50 percent miscarriage rate, though IUD manufacturers suggest 25 percent (Moschos & Twickler, 2011). Removal of the device as soon as the pregnancy is known is advised. Doctors often offer therapeutic abortion to women who become pregnant while using an IUD because of the serious risks (including premature delivery, infection, and congenital abnormalities) associated with continuing the pregnancy.

Withdrawal

The **withdrawal** method is not a very effective method of birth control that involves withdrawing the penis from the vagina just prior to ejaculation. Because there can be up to half a million sperm in the drop of fluid at the tip of the penis before ejaculation, this method is unreliable and ineffective at preventing pregnancy and the spread of STIs. Timing withdrawal is also difficult; males concentrating on accurate timing may not be able to relax and enjoy intercourse. The typical-use effectiveness rate for the withdrawal method is 73 percent; perfect-use effectiveness is 96 percent (Hatcher et al., 2007).

Oral Contraceptives for Men?

The development of an oral contraceptive for men has been slow. Evidently, the mechanisms involved in the manufacture and release of sperm are not as easy to manipulate as the female ovulatory and uterine cycles. Some oral contraceptives for men have been tested, but they produced unpleasant side effects such as diminished sex drive and impotence. At the present time, research into the development of new male contraceptives is being carried on in various countries. One compound undergoing research is gossypol, a substance derived from the cotton plant. Chinese and Canadian researchers have found that gossypol inhibits sperm production, causing infertility. Difficulties in reversing the effects of the drug are presenting problems, as are concerns over long-term health consequences and possible genetic effects.

Other researchers are investigating the possibility of using ultrasound as a male contraceptive. In this method, a high-frequency sound machine is placed in contact with the scrotum. The device emits sound waves that slow sperm production, thereby lowering sperm counts. In some cases, sperm counts have remained lowered for up to two years after the procedure. Reduced sperm count, as opposed to total destruction of sperm, may suffice as a contraceptive measure because a minimum number of sperm are needed for fertilization. Before this method can be made available, the risks for testicular cancer and genetic damage must be thoroughly explored.

Fertility Awareness Methods (FAM)

Methods of fertility control that rely upon the alteration of sexual behaviours are called **fertility awareness methods (FAM)**. These methods include observing female "fertile periods" by examining cervical mucus or keeping track of internal temperature and then abstaining from vaginal intercourse during these fertile times.

Although the "rhythm method" is often the object of ridicule because of its low effectiveness rates, it can be the only acceptable method of birth control available to women of certain religions. Current reproductive knowledge enables women and their partners to use natural methods of birth control better with fewer risks of pregnancy, although these methods still remain less effective than others previously discussed.

Fertility awareness methods of birth control rely upon basic physiology. A released ovum can survive for up to 24 hours after ovulation (Ovascience, 2013). Sperm can live for three to five days in the vagina (Harms, 2012). Natural methods of birth control help women to learn more about their bodies in addition to learning how to recognize their fertile times. Changes in cervical mucus prior to and during ovulation and a rise in basal body temperature are two indicators frequently used in natural contraceptive techniques. Another method involves charting a woman's menstrual cycle and ovulation times on a calendar. Any combination of these methods may be used to determine fertile times more accurately. The effectiveness of any of the

Withdrawal A method of contraception that involves withdrawing the penis from the vagina before ejaculation.

Fertility awareness methods (FAM) Several types of birth control that require alteration and/or abstinence of sexual behaviours based upon awareness of a woman's fertile time.

methods listed below is highly dependent upon the woman's knowledge and understanding of her body as well as diligence in following the recommended guidelines. There are numerous agencies, including churches—of which you do not necessarily need to be a member—willing to assist women in learning about these methods of fertility control.

Cervical Mucus Method

The **cervical mucus method** requires women to examine the consistency and colour of their normal vaginal secretions (Planned Parenthood, 2013d). During your period, menstrual flow covers any signs of mucus. Following your period, there are usually a few days without mucus which are classified as 'safe' days. When your egg starts to ripen, more mucus is produced—this mucus is generally yellow or white, cloudy, and sticky or tacky. Generally, there is the most mucus before ovulation and it feels slippery like raw egg white and can be stretched between your fingers. This is called the 'slippery days' and represents the peak of your fertility; any sexual activity involving penis–vagina contact must be avoided at this time and for several days after. After the slippery days will be days with less mucus that is once again cloudy and tacky. Then, there are a few more dry days before your period starts.

Body Temperature Method

The **body temperature method** relies on the fact that the female's basal body temperature rises between 0.4 and 0.8 degrees after ovulation (Planned Parenthood, 2013d). For this method to be effective, the woman must chart her temperature for several months to recognize her body's temperature fluctuations. It is recommended that women take their basal body temperature every morning before getting out of bed. This can be done using an oral thermometer or one specifically designed to measure basal body temperature. In order to ensure accuracy, women should have at least three hours of uninterrupted sleep each night. Abstinence from intercourse and any other penis–vagina contact must be observed preceding the temperature rise and until several days after the temperature rise was first noted.

Cervical mucus method A FAM that relies upon changes in cervical mucus to determine when the woman is fertile so the couple can abstain from intercourse during those times.

Body temperature method A FAM that requires a woman to monitor her body temperature for the rise that signals ovulation and to abstain from intercourse around this time.

Calendar method A FAM that requires mapping the woman's menstrual cycle on a calendar to determine presumed fertile times and abstaining from intercourse and any other penis–vagina contact during those times.

Sterilization Permanent fertility control achieved through surgical procedures.

Tubal ligation Sterilization of the female that involves cutting and tying off of the fallopian tubes.

Calendar Method

The **calendar method** requires women to record the exact number of days in their menstrual cycle. Since few women menstruate with complete regularity, a record of the menstrual cycle must be kept for 12 months, during which some other method of birth control must be used. The first day of a woman's period is counted as day one. To determine the first fertile unsafe day of the cycle, she subtracts 18 from the number of days in the shortest cycle. To determine the last unsafe day of the cycle, she subtracts 11 from the number of days in the longest cycle. This method assumes that ovulation occurs during the midpoint of the cycle (see Figure 8.4). The couple must abstain from penis–vagina contact during the fertile time. Given the assumptions of the calendar method (that is, that ovulation always occurs at midpoint of the cycle, the cycle is regular and predictable, and so on), the calendar method is the least effective of the FAM methods.

Women interested in FAM of birth control are advised to take supervised classes. The risks of an unwanted pregnancy are great for the untrained woman. Reading a book or watching a film on the subject or talking to the proprietor of the local health food store will not likely provide the necessary training to ensure maximum effectiveness. Incidentally, information on these methods can also be helpful to couples who are trying to conceive.

Permanent Contraception

Sterilization, permanent fertility control achieved through surgical procedures, has become a popular method of contraception for women and men. Although some of the newer surgical techniques make reversal of sterilization theoretically possible, anyone considering sterilization should assume that the operation is not reversible. Before becoming sterilized, people should think through such possibilities as divorce and remarriage or a future improvement in their financial status that may make them want a larger family.

Female Sterilization

One method of sterilization in females is called **tubal ligation**. It is achieved through a surgical procedure that involves tying the fallopian tubes closed or cutting them and cauterizing (burning) the edges to seal the tubes so that an egg can no longer be fertilized. The operation is usually done in a hospital on an outpatient basis. First, the abdomen is inflated with carbon dioxide gas through a small incision in the navel. The surgeon then inserts a laparoscope into another incision just above the pubic bone. This specially designed

FIGURE 8.4

The Fertility Cycle

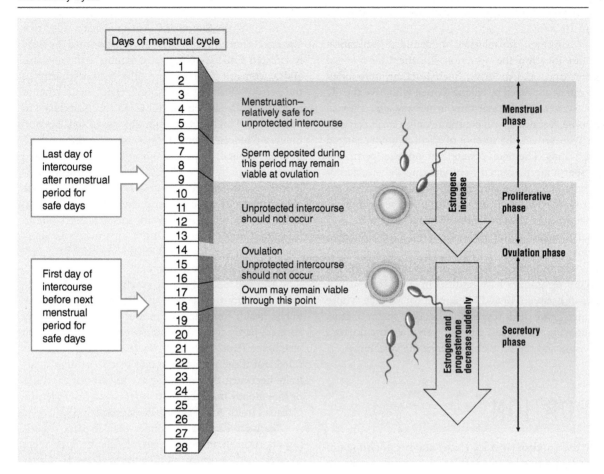

instrument has a fibre-optic light source that enables the physician to see the fallopian tubes clearly. Once located, the tubes are cut and tied or cauterized.

Ovarian and uterine functions are not affected by a tubal ligation. The woman's menstrual cycle continues, and released eggs simply disintegrate and are absorbed by the lymphatic system. As soon as her incision is healed, the woman may resume sexual intercourse with no fear of pregnancy.

As with any kind of surgery, there are risks. Some patients are given general anesthesia, which presents a small risk; others receive local anesthesia. The procedure itself usually takes less than an hour, and the patient is generally allowed to return home within a short time after waking up. Women considering a tubal ligation should thoroughly discuss all the risks with their physician before the operation.

A **hysterectomy**, or removal of the uterus, is a method of sterilization requiring major surgery. It is usually done only when the woman's uterus is diseased or damaged.

Male Sterilization

Sterilization in men is less complicated than in women. The procedure, called a **vasectomy**, is usually done on an outpatient basis using a local anesthetic. The surgeon makes an incision on each side of the scrotum. The vas deferens on each side is then located, and a piece is removed from each. The ends are often cauterized and tied or sewn shut.

After a vasectomy, there is usually some discomfort, local pain, swelling, and discolouration for about a week. In a small percentage of cases, more serious complications occur: formation of a blood clot in the scrotum (which usually disappears without medical treatment), infection, and inflammatory reactions. Because sperm are stored in other areas of the reproductive system besides the vas deferens, couples must use alternative methods of birth control for at least one month after

Hysterectomy The removal of the uterus.

Vasectomy Sterilization of the male that involves the cutting, cauterizing, and tying off of the vasa deferentia.

the vasectomy. The man must check with his physician (who will do a semen analysis) to determine when unprotected intercourse can take place. The pregnancy rate in women whose partners had vasectomies is about 15 in 10 000.

Many men are reluctant to consider sterilization because they fear the operation will affect their sexual performance and/or drive. Such fears are unfounded and can be alleviated by talking to men who have already had a vasectomy. A vasectomy in no way affects sexual response. Because sperm constitute only a small percentage of the semen, the amount of ejaculate is not changed significantly. The testes continue to produce sperm, but the sperm are prevented from entering the ejaculatory duct because of the surgery. After a time, sperm production may diminish. Any sperm manufactured disintegrate and are absorbed into the lymphatic system.

Although a vasectomy should be considered a permanent procedure, surgical reversal is sometimes successful in restoring fertility. Improvements in microsurgery techniques have resulted in annual pregnancy rates of between 40 and 60 percent for women whose partners have had reversals. The two major factors influencing the success rate of reversal are the doctor's expertise and the time elapsed since the vasectomy.

ABORTION

The law on **abortion** has seen a number of changes in Canada and much activity federally and provincially. In 1869, two years after Confederation, a law was enacted that prohibited abortion with a penalty of life imprisonment. Those who oppose abortion believe that the embryo or fetus is a human being with rights that must be protected. Others have worked to get easier access to abortion for women. In 1967, the Federal Standing Committee on Health and Welfare began considering amendments to the Criminal Code relating to abortion. Dr. Henry Morgentaler, an abortion activist and physician, appeared "on behalf of the Humanist Fellowship of Montreal, urging the repeal of the abortion law and freedom of choice on abortion" (Planned Parenthood, n.d.). In 1969, Dr. Morgentaler closed his general practice and opened a clinic in Montreal to specialize in abortion, using the vacuum aspiration method. In 1970, 1971, and 1973, 13 charges of illegal abortion were brought against Dr. Morgentaler. On November 13, 1973, a jury acquitted him. The next year, however, he was convicted by the Quebec Court of Appeal. Dr. Morgentaler appealed to the Supreme Court of Canada, but, in 1975, the appeal was dismissed and he served 10 months in jail. In 1983, Dr. Morgentaler

Abortion The medical means of terminating a pregnancy.

Vacuum aspiration The use of gentle suction to remove fetal tissue from the uterus.

opened clinics in Toronto and Winnipeg and was again charged, along with other clinic doctors and the head nurse. Appeal procedures and renewed charges continued through 1986.

In 1988, the Supreme Court of Canada ruled that Canada's abortion law was unconstitutional because it violated Canada's Charter of Rights and Freedoms and a woman's right to "life, liberty and security of the person" (Planned Parenthood, n.d.). In an attempt to recriminalize abortion, Bill C-43 was introduced in Parliament. This bill, which sought to prohibit abortion unless a physician deemed it necessary for the mother's physical, mental, or psychological health, was defeated by the Senate in 1991. Harassment and threats of violence by anti-abortion protesters have caused some physicians to stop performing abortions. On May 8, 1992, a firebomb destroyed the Morgentaler clinic in Toronto. On November 8, 1992, in Vancouver, abortion provider Dr. Garson Romalis was shot and seriously wounded while at home.

Another focus of debate is who will pay for abortions. Abortions conducted in hospitals are covered by public health insurance. Clinics, though, may be fully covered, partly covered, or not covered at all (Childbirth by Choice Trust, 1995). In 1995, the federal government ruled that if the provinces accept that abortion is medically necessary, they must pay the full cost of abortions or lose money from federal transfer payments under the Canada Health Act (Planned Parenthood, n.d.).

Statistics Canada no longer collects data regarding abortion (Statistics Canada, 2013). In 2010 there were 64 641 abortions performed in Canada (Canadian Institute for Health Information, 2010). The highest number of performed abortions were reported in Ontario (28 765); in contrast Northwest Territories only report 40 abortions and PEI had no reported abortions for 2010.

Methods of Abortion

The type of abortion procedure used is determined by how many weeks pregnant the woman is. Pregnancy length is calculated from the first day of a woman's last menstrual period. If performed during the first trimester of pregnancy, abortion presents a relatively low risk to the mother. The most commonly used method of first-trimester (weeks 1 to 12) abortion is **vacuum aspiration**. The procedure is usually performed with a local anesthetic. The cervix is dilated with instruments or by placing laminaria, a sterile seaweed product, in the cervical canal. The laminaria is left in place for a few hours or overnight and slowly dilates the cervix. After it is removed, a long tube is inserted into the uterus through the cervix. Gentle suction is then used to remove the fetal tissue from the uterine walls.

FIGURE 8.5

Vacuum Aspiration Abortion

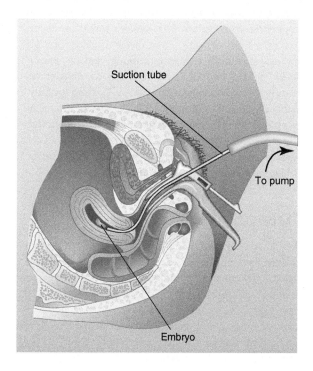

Pregnancies that progress into the second trimester can be terminated through **dilation and evacuation (D&E)**, a procedure that combines vacuum aspiration with a technique called **dilation and curettage (D&C)**. For this procedure, the cervix is dilated with laminaria for one to two days and a combination of instruments and vacuum aspiration is used to empty the uterus (see Figure 8.5). Second-trimester abortions are frequently done under general anesthetic. Both procedures can be performed on an outpatient basis (usually in the physician's office) with or without pain medication. Generally, the woman is given a mild tranquillizer to help her relax. Both procedures can cause moderate to severe uterine cramping and blood loss.

The **hysterotomy**, or surgical removal of the fetus from the uterus, may be used during emergencies or when the mother's life may be in danger and when other types of abortions are deemed too dangerous.

The risks associated with abortions include infection, incomplete abortion (when parts of the placenta remain in the uterus), missed abortion (when the fetus is not actually removed), excessive bleeding, and cervical and uterine trauma. Follow-up and attention to dangerous signs decrease the chances of any long-term problems. The mortality rate for first-trimester abortions is 0.8 per 100 000 women. The rate for second-trimester abortions is higher, at 4.3 per 100 000 women. This higher rate is due to the increased risk of uterine

perforation, bleeding, infection, and incomplete abortion due to the fact that the uterine wall becomes thinner as the pregnancy progresses.

Two other methods used in second-trimester abortions, though less commonly than the D&E method, are prostaglandin or saline **induction abortions**. In these methods, prostaglandin hormones or a saline solution is injected into the uterus. The injected solution kills the fetus and causes labour contractions to begin. After 24 to 48 hours the fetus and placenta are expelled from the uterus.

PLANNING A PREGNANCY

The technological ability to control your fertility gives you choices not available when your parents were born. The loosening of social restrictions in the areas of marriage and parenting also affords single men and women, and gay and lesbian couples, the opportunity to become parents. Regardless of your marital status, the preparation to become a parent involves similar considerations and decisions. If you are in the process of deciding whether to have children, you should take the time to evaluate your emotions, finances, and health.

Emotional Health

First consider why you want to have a child: To fulfill an inner need to carry on the family? Out of loneliness? Any other reasons? Can you care for a child in a loving and nurturing manner? Are you ready to adjust your life and give the time necessary to bear and raise a child? You can prepare yourself for this change in your life in several ways. Reading about pregnancy and parenthood, taking classes, talking to parents of children of all ages, and joining a support group are helpful forms of preparation. If you choose to adopt, you will find many support groups available to you as well.

Maternal Health

Before becoming pregnant, a woman should have a thorough medical examination. **Preconception care** should include assessment of possible

Dilation and evacuation (D&E) An abortion technique that combines vacuum aspiration with dilation and curettage; fetal tissue is sucked and scraped out of the uterus.

Dilation and curettage (D&C) An abortion technique in which the cervix is dilated with laminaria for one to two days and the uterine walls are scraped clean.

Hysterotomy The surgical removal of the fetus from the uterus.

Induction abortion A type of abortion in which chemicals are injected into the uterus through the uterine wall; labour begins and the woman delivers a dead fetus.

Preconception care Medical care received prior to becoming pregnant that helps a woman assess and address potential maternal health.

pregnancy complications. Medical problems such as gestational diabetes and high blood pressure should be discussed, as should any genetic disorders that run in either family. Additional suggestions for a healthy pregnancy include:

- Engage in regular physical activity (see also Chapter 4)
- Eat according to Eating Well with Canada's Food Guide (see also Chapter 5)
- Maintain a normal weight (see also Chapter 6)
- Do not smoke, drink alcohol, or use illicit drugs
- Reduce or eliminate caffeine intake
- Avoid exposure to X-rays and environmental chemicals such as lawn and garden chemicals
- Prior to becoming pregnant, have your annual dental X-rays and your regular checkup

Paternal Health

It is common wisdom that mothers-to-be should steer clear of toxic chemicals that can cause birth defects. Even women trying to conceive are cautioned to avoid toxic environments and to eat a nourishing diet, to stop smoking and drinking alcohol, and to avoid most medications. Similar precautions are also recommended for fathers-to-be, at least while engaged in the baby-making process. It is believed that a man's exposure to chemicals influences not only his ability to father a child but also the future health of his child.

Fathers-to-be have been overlooked in the past for several reasons. It was assumed that the genetic damage leading to birth defects and other health problems occurred while a child was in the mother's womb or was caused by random errors of nature. Scientists have recently discovered that how sperm look has little to do with how they act. Misshapen sperm can penetrate an egg, and they do not necessarily carry defective genetic goods. Moreover, sperm that look healthy and swim well can be the true genetic culprits. DNA fluorescent markers have identified normal-looking yet genetically flawed sperm that carry too many or too few chromosomes. Fathers contribute the extra chromosome 21 in about 6 percent of children with Down syndrome, which causes learning disabilities; the extra X chromosome in 50 percent of boys with Klinefelter's syndrome, which causes abnormal sexual development; and the shortened chromosome 15 in about 85 percent of children with Prader-Willi syndrome, a disorder characterized by physical and learning disabilities and obesity.

Although some birth defects are caused by the random errors of nature, some disorders can be traced to sperm damaged by chemicals. Sperm are naturally vulnerable to toxic assault and genetic damage. Many drugs and ingested chemicals can readily invade the testes from the bloodstream; others ambush sperm after they leave the testes and pass through the epididymides, where they mature and are stored. By one route or another, half of 100 chemicals studied so far (including by-products of cigarette smoke) apparently harm sperm. Some researchers believe that vitamin C is nature's way of protecting sex cells from damage. Poor dietary intake, exposure to toxic chemicals, cigarette smoking, and not enough foods rich in vitamin C are probably the biggest culprits in sperm damage (Schmidt, 1992). More recently a father's age has also been identified as a factor contributing to damaged sperm. As paternal age increases, so may the risk that fathers pass on damaged sperm that lead to gene mutations associated with the onset of autism and schizophrenia among children (Kong et al., 2012).

Financial Evaluation

You also need to evaluate your finances. Both partners should find out about their employers' policies concerning parental leave, including length of leave available and conditions for returning to work. Canadian law allows one or the other parent—natural, adoptive, or combination—to have 37 weeks of parental leave some time during the 52-week period from the day the child is born or becomes part of your care (Human Resources and Skills Development Canada, 2012).

Raising a child exacts a tremendous strain on most families' finances; expenses during the first year of life average at least $10 000. The expense of raising a child from birth to 18 years of age (in 2011 dollars) in a typical two-child family was estimated to be $243 600—not including the cost of post-secondary education (Cornell, 2011)! This comes to $1070 per month. The cost varies according to the number of children in the home; raising a lone child is more expensive for a total of $304 600, while if there are three or more children, families typically spend 22 percent less per child ($190 050) (Cornell, 2011).

Parents should decide if either of them is willing to put their career on hold and spend the formative years raising their child(ren). The financial implications of this decision should be considered as well. Alternatively, the cost and availability of quality child care should be considered. Prospective parents should realistically assess how much family assistance they can expect with a new baby, as well as the availability and cost of non-family child care should staying at home to raise their child(ren) not be considered a viable option.

Contingency Planning

A final consideration is how to provide financially and practically for your child should something happen to you and/or your partner. If both of you were to die while the child is young, do you have relatives or close friends who would raise the child?

If you have more than one child, would they have to be split up or could they be kept together? What sort of financial situation would your child(ren) be in? Unpleasant though it may be to think about, this sort of contingency planning is extremely important.

Decision Making about Unplanned Pregnancy

Even the best birth control methods can fail. Pregnancies do occur despite due diligence. Women are raped. When an unwanted pregnancy occurs, the decision whether to terminate, to carry to term and keep the baby, or to carry to term and give the baby up for adoption must be made. This is a personal decision each woman must make according to her personal beliefs, values, and resources after carefully considering the alternatives. There are resources available to help women with this decision.

Making decisions about an unplanned pregnancy is difficult (Sunnybrook and Women's Health Sciences Centre, n.d.). For many women (and men), an unplanned pregnancy can be one of the first times that they have to deal with a decision about their health and the course of their life.

If you experience an unplanned pregnancy you have three options:

* continue the pregnancy and raise the child
* continue the pregnancy and place the child for adoption
* end the pregnancy with an abortion

Consider the various aspects of your life when considering these options (Sunnybrook and Women's Health Sciences Centre, n.d.). Unplanned pregnancy can happen at different stages of a woman's life. Often the decision is about what is best at this time; at another point in your life the decision might be different.

You might:

* think about your personal beliefs—including spiritual and cultural beliefs, values, and practices, and those of others in your life
* assess your existing relationships (partner, family, friends) and the support that these relationships need and can provide
* evaluate financial and social realities
* consider your living conditions and life circumstances
* examine your feelings about becoming a parent, and parenting

As with any decision, you need to come to grips with making a decision, enacting that decision, and then accepting that decision, once made. It is very common for women—and their partners—to have a variety of emotional reactions to an unplanned pregnancy. Dealing with your feelings is an important part of making a decision you can live with. Each couple is unique and the time and effort needed to make a decision will be different for everybody. Weighing the pros and cons of such a personal decision can be stressful and challenging (Sunnybrook and Women's Health Sciences Centre, n.d.). You may wish to seek advice before making this decision. Whom you choose to talk to varies; each of you has individual needs for privacy and for emotional, physical, economic, and spiritual support. You should look for people to help you in the decision-making process who are:

* knowledgeable (able to provide information or referrals)
* nonjudgmental
* able to provide support whatever your decision, regardless of what it is
* people you feel comfortable talking to

You may only want to talk to health-care providers or you may prefer talking to your partner or family member, a friend, or a member of the clergy. Whomever you talk to, you should never feel coerced or forced to make a decision that is not your own.

PREGNANCY

Prenatal Care

A successful pregnancy requires the mother's ability to take care of herself and her unborn child. It is essential to have regular checkups with a doctor or midwife, beginning as soon as possible (certainly within the first three months). Early detection of fetal abnormalities and identification of high-risk mothers and infants are the major purposes of prenatal care. On the first visit, the practitioner should obtain a complete medical history of the mother and her family and note any hereditary conditions that could put a woman or her fetus at risk.

Regular appointments to measure weight gain and blood pressure and monitor the size and position of the fetus should continue throughout the pregnancy. This early care reduces infant mortality and low birthweight. Experts recommend obstetrical visits once a month to 28 weeks, biweekly to 36 weeks, and weekly to 40 weeks.

Additional concerns include the mother's physical condition, her level of nutrition, her confidence in her ability to give birth, her use of drugs and medications, and the availability of a skilled practitioner (midwife or doctor) who can oversee the pregnancy and delivery. A woman planning a pregnancy also needs a support system (spouse or partner, family, friends, community groups) willing to give her and her child the love and emotional support needed during and after her pregnancy. In most areas, prenatal classes are available, including some for pregnant teens.

Choosing a Practitioner

A woman should carefully choose a practitioner who will attend her pregnancy and delivery, although in some localities physicians, midwives, and specialists may be in short supply. If possible, this choice should be made before you become pregnant. Your family physician may also be able to recommend a midwife or specialist. The pregnant woman needs to find a practitioner she can trust with her own life and that of the baby and with whom she can communicate freely.

When choosing a practitioner, parents should ask a number of questions concerning credentials and professional qualifications. Besides this information, a pregnant woman must ask questions specific to her condition. Prospective parents should also inquire about the practitioner's experience in handling various complications, commitment to being at the mother's side during delivery, and beliefs and practices concerning the use of anesthesia, fetal monitoring, induced labour, and forceps delivery. What are the practitioner's attitudes toward circumcision and alternative birthing procedures? Finally, the parents should learn under what circumstances the practitioner would perform a Caesarean section.

Two types of physicians can attend pregnancies and deliveries. The obstetrician-gynecologist (ob-gyn) is an MD who specializes in obstetrics (pregnancy and birth) and gynecology (care of women's reproductive organs). These practitioners are trained to handle all types of pregnancy- and delivery-related emergencies. A family

Teratogenic Causing birth defects; may refer to drugs, environmental chemicals, X-rays, or diseases.

practitioner is a licensed MD who provides comprehensive care for people of all ages. Most family practitioners have obstetrical experience and will refer a patient to a specialist if/when necessary. Unlike the ob-gyn, the family practitioner can serve as the baby's physician after attending the birth.

A third option many women are choosing is to have their prenatal, delivery, and postnatal care given by a midwife, who is also an experienced practitioner trained to attend pregnancies and deliveries. Some of the reasons for choosing midwifery care are

- knowing that the person who has cared for you throughout your pregnancy will be with you during the labour and delivery (if you go into labour when your family practitioner is not on call, you are likely to have a different physician deliver your baby)

- having more time to ask questions and express your concerns during appointments (midwives typically schedule a longer time for appointments and are willing to discuss any concerns, personal or medical, that arise during pregnancy)

- the ability to reach your midwife with questions or problems between visits

- a postpartum home visit and other home visits if necessary

- breastfeeding support

Midwives are trained to recognize situations that call for the opinion—or the intervention—of a physician and will refer their clients to specialists or even ask a physician to take over care (for instance, if an emergency C-section is required) when necessary. So a woman may go for one or more consultations with a doctor (about her blood sugar, her weight, or age-related concerns, for instance) while still having the care of a midwife throughout her pregnancy. Further, many midwives have "admitting privileges" at a hospital, which means they can supervise hospital births as well as home births.

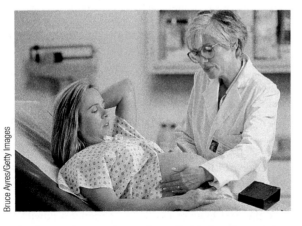

Good prenatal care involves regular medical checkups by a practitioner with whom the mother feels she can communicate freely.

Alcohol and Drugs

A woman should avoid all drugs as much as possible during pregnancy unless prescribed or advised by a doctor—and then she should ask whether the medication is really necessary and whether there is a safer alternative. Always tell a physician, dentist, or other practitioner if you are pregnant or think you might be pregnant. Even common over-the-counter medications such as Aspirin and beverages such as coffee and tea can damage a developing fetus. The fetus is particularly susceptible to the **teratogenic** (birth-defect-causing) effects of some chemical substances during the first three months of pregnancy. The fetus can also develop an addiction to or tolerance for drugs that the mother is using.

Of particular concern to medical professionals is the use of tobacco and alcohol during pregnancy. Women who drink heavily may have normal first babies and then subsequently deliver children with a fetal alcohol spectrum disorder (May & Gossage, n.d.). **Fetal alcohol spectrum disorder (FASD)** describes a number of disorders related to alcohol consumption during pregnancy, including fetal alcohol syndrome, fetal alcohol effects, partial fetal alcohol effects, alcohol-related neurodevelopmental disorders, and neurobehavioural disorder–alcohol exposed. FASD manifests in lifelong developmental and cognitive disabilities in children. The exact amount of alcohol necessary to cause FASD is not known and thus, a safe recommendation is to refrain from all alcohol consumption when trying to get pregnant. Table 8.2 provides a list of teratogenic effects of alcohol and other drugs ingested by the mother.

Cigarette smoking during pregnancy has more predictable effects than alcohol. Studies indicate a 25 to 50 percent higher rate of fetal and infant deaths among women who smoke during pregnancy than among those who do not (U.S. Department of Health and Human Services, 1990). Women who smoke more than

Fetal alcohol spectrum disorders (FASD) A number of disorders related to alcohol consumption during pregnancy—including fetal alcohol syndrome, fetal alcohol effects, partial fetal alcohol effects, alcohol-related neurodevelopmental disorders, and neurobehavioural disorder–alcohol exposed—that result in lifelong developmental and cognitive disabilities in children.

TABLE 8.2
Teratogenic Effects of Drugs

Drug	Effects
Isotretinoin (Acutane)	• Ear abnormalities, including small or absent ears • Facial abnormalities, including small jaw; sharply sloping, narrow forehead; wide spaced eyes; small chin; and flat, depressed nasal bridge • Heart defects
Alcohol	• Cognitive disabilities • Physical delays in growth • Increased risk of spontaneous abortion (i.e., miscarriage) • Fetal alcohol syndrome
Amphetamines	• Damage to nervous system
Acetylsalicylic acid	• Fetal cardiovascular system damage, specifically closure of the ductus arteriosus • Alterations in fetal hemostasis • Fetal intrauterine growth retardation
Barbiturates	• Congenital malformation such as cleft lip, hypertelorism (very widely spaced eyes) • Cardiac abnormalities • Neural tube defects
SSRIs	• Congenital malformations to the respiratory, motor, and central nervous systems • Gastrointestinal symptoms
Corticosteroids	• Cleft lip • Low birth weight • Intrauterine growth retardation • Small risk of stillbirth
Cocaine hydrochloride	• Uncontrolled jerking motions after birth • Infant paralysis • Depressed interactive behaviours
Opioids	• Immediate withdrawal in newborns • Permanent learning disabilities
Streptomycin sulfate	• Cranial nerve damage • Deafness
Vaccines	• Live virus could infect the placenta and developing fetus

Sources: Gunatilake, R., & Avinash, P. (2016). Drugs in pregnancy. *MSD Manual*. Retrieved from www.msdmanuals.com/professional/gynecology-and-obstetrics/drugs-in-pregnancy/drugs-in-pregnancy; Bánhidy F., Lowry R. B., & Czeizel A. E. (2005). Risk and benefit of drug use during pregnancy. *Int J Med Sci*, 2(3), 100–106; Adam M. P., Polifka J. E., & Friedman J. M. (2011). Evolving knowledge of the teratogenicity of medications in human pregnancy. *Am J Med Genet Part C*,157, 175–182; https://www.drugs.com/pregnancy/isotretinoin.html.

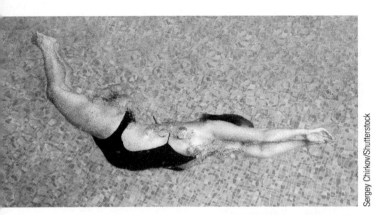

Physical activity during pregnancy helps the mother control her weight and contributes to easier deliveries and healthier babies.

Sergey Chirkov/Shutterstock

TABLE 8.3
Nutrient Deficiency Effects

Nutrient	Deficiency Effect in Infants
Vitamin A	Premature birth, intrauterine growth retardation, low birth weight
Vitamin B12	Miscarriage and possibly to adverse infant neurobehavioural development
Vitamin D	Fetal rickets and abnormal teeth development
Folic Acid	Miscarriage and neural tube defects
Iodine	Miscarriage, stillbirths, and mental retardation of the newborn infant
Iron	Low infant birth weight, premature death
Zinc	Congenital abnormalities, miscarriage, intrauterine growth retardation, premature birth

Source: Ladipo, O. (2000). Nutrition in pregnancy: mineral and vitamin supplements. *American Journal of Clinical Nutrition, 72*(1), 280s–290s.

10 to 15 cigarettes a day during pregnancy have higher rates of miscarriage, stillbirth, premature births, and low-birthweight babies than nonsmokers. Fetal research on the effects of "secondhand" or sidestream smoke (inhaling smoke produced by others) is inconclusive, but babies whose parents smoke can be twice as susceptible to pneumonia, bronchitis, and related illnesses as other babies.

X-Rays

X-rays present a clear danger to the fetus. Although most diagnostic X-rays produce minimal amounts of radiation, even low levels of radiation may cause birth defects or other problems, particularly if several low-dose X-rays occur over a short time period. Thus, women who are pregnant are advised to avoid X-rays unless absolutely necessary.

Nutrition and Physical Activity

Women who are pregnant have additional needs for water, protein, calories, and certain vitamins and minerals, so their dietary intake should be carefully monitored by a qualified practitioner. Special attention should be paid to obtaining sufficient folic acid (found in dark leafy greens and fortified grains), iron (dried fruits, meats, legumes, liver, egg yolks), calcium (nonfat or low-fat dairy products, some canned fish), and fluids. Vitamin supplements can alleviate some deficiencies, but there is no substitute for a well-balanced dietary intake. Babies born to mothers whose nutrition has been poor run high risks of substandard mental and physical development (see Table 8.3).

Weight gain during pregnancy helps nourish a growing baby. For a woman of normal weight before pregnancy, the recommended weight gain during pregnancy ranges from 11 to 16 kilograms (25 to 35 pounds); a woman carrying twins should gain about 16 to 20 kilograms (35 to 45 pounds). Usually, the mother can expect to gain about five kilograms (~12 pounds) during the first 20 weeks and about 0.5 kilograms (approximately 1 pound) per week during the rest of the pregnancy.

Of the total number of kilograms gained during pregnancy, about three to four are the baby's weight. The baby's birthweight is important, since a low weight can lead to health problems during labour and the baby's first few months. Eating well and gaining enough weight help reduce the chances of having a low-birthweight baby. If a woman gains an appropriate amount of weight while pregnant, chances are that her baby will gain weight properly, too.

As in all other stages of life, physical activity is an important factor in overall maternal health, as well as in attaining an appropriate weight gain during pregnancy. Guidelines for women who are pregnant were developed by the Society of Obstetricians and Gynaecologists of Canada and the Canadian Society for Exercise Physiology (Davies et al., 2003). The recommendations are as follows:

1. *All women without contraindications should be encouraged to participate in aerobic and strength-conditioning exercises as part of a healthy lifestyle during their pregnancy.*

2. *Reasonable goals of aerobic conditioning in pregnancy should be to maintain a good fitness level throughout pregnancy without trying to reach peak fitness or train for an athletic competition.*

3. *Women should choose activities that will minimize the risk of loss of balance and fetal trauma.*

4. *Women should be advised that adverse pregnancy or neonatal outcomes are not increased for exercising women.*

5. *Initiation of pelvic floor exercises in the immediate postpartum period may reduce the risk of future urinary incontinence.*

6. *Women should be advised that moderate exercise during lactation does not affect the quantity or composition of breast milk or impact infant growth* (Davies et al., 2003, p. 331).

More general safety considerations for physically active pregnant women include:

- Avoid prolonged or strenuous exertion during the first trimester.
- Avoid isometric exercise or straining while holding your breath.
- Maintain adequate nutrition and hydration—drink liquids before, during, and after exercise.
- Limit exercise in warm or humid environments.
- Avoid exercise while lying on your back past the fourth month of pregnancy.
- Avoid exercises that involve physical contact or danger of falling.
- Periodic rest periods may help to minimize possible low oxygen or temperature stress to the fetus.
- Know the reasons to stop exercise and consult a qualified physician immediately if they occur (Davies et al., 2003).

Other Factors

A pregnant woman should avoid exposure to toxic chemicals, heavy metals, pesticides, gases, and other hazardous compounds. She should not clean cat-litter boxes because cat feces can contain organisms that cause a disease called toxoplasmosis. If a pregnant woman contracts this disease, her baby might be stillborn or have cognitive disabilities or other birth defects.

Before becoming pregnant, a woman should be tested to determine if she has had rubella (German measles). If she has not had it, she should be immunized for it and wait the recommended length of time before becoming pregnant. A rubella infection can kill the fetus or cause blindness or hearing disorders in the infant. If a woman has ever had genital herpes, she should inform her midwife or physician. Contact with an active herpes infection during birth can be fatal to the infant. If a pregnant woman knows she has herpes, she may be prescribed anti-virals before delivery to reduce the likelihood of her having an outbreak; if she has active lesions at the time of delivery, the practitioner will recommend delivering the baby by Caesarian section.

A Woman's Reproductive Years

More than half of the average Canadian woman's expected life span is spent between menarche (first menses) and menopause (last menses), a period of approximately 40 years. During this 40-year period, she must make many decisions about her reproductive health.

Today, a pregnant woman over 35 has plenty of company. While births to women in their 20s are declining, the rate of first births to women between the ages of 30 and 39 has doubled in the past decade, and births to women over 39 have increased by more than 50 percent. Many women who wait until their 30s to consider having a child find themselves wondering, "Am I too old to have a baby?" Researchers believe that there is a decline in the quality and viability of eggs produced after age 35, which has resulted in an increase in the number of women struggling with fertility issues and a concomitant increase in the use of fertility clinics. Statistically, the chances of having a miscarriage or a baby with birth defects do rise after the age of 35. **Down syndrome**, a genetic anomaly where a baby is born with an extra chromosome, characterized by mild to severe cognitive disabilities and a variety of physical abnormalities, is the most common birth defect found in babies born to older mothers (Centers for Disease Control and Prevention, 2011a). The incidence of Down syndrome in babies born to mothers aged 20 is 1 in 10 000 births; it rises to 1 in 365 births when the mother is 35, to 1 in 109 when she is 40, and to 1 in 32 when she is 45. Women who choose to delay motherhood until their late 30s also worry about their physical ability to carry and deliver their babies. For these women, regular moderate-intensity physical activity will help to maintain good posture and promote a successful delivery.

Pregnancy Testing

A woman might suspect she is pregnant before she has a pregnancy test. A typical sign is a missed menstrual period, though this is not always an accurate indicator. A woman can miss her period for a variety of reasons: stress, excessive physical activity without an adequate dietary intake, or emotional upset. Another common sign of pregnancy is sore breasts. This too, can be caused by other health issues. Confirmation of a pregnancy should be obtained from a pregnancy test scheduled in a medical office or birth control clinic.

Women who wish to know immediately whether or not they are pregnant can purchase home pregnancy test kits. These kits, sold over the counter in drugstores, are about 85 to 95 percent reliable. A positive test is based on the secretion of **human chorionic gonadotropin (HCG)** found in the woman's urine. Home test kits come equipped with a small sample of red blood cells coated with HCG antibodies, to which the user adds a small amount of urine. If the concentration of HCG is great enough, it will clump together with the HCG antibodies, indicating that the user is pregnant.

Down syndrome A genetic anomaly characterized by cognitive disabilities and a variety of physical abnormalities.

Human chorionic gonadotropin (HCG) Hormone detectable in blood or urine samples within the first few weeks of pregnancy.

If taken too early in the pregnancy, the test may show a false negative. Other causes of false negatives are unclean test tubes, ingestion of certain drugs, and vaginal or urinary infections. Accuracy also depends on the quality of the test itself and the user's ability to perform it and interpret the results. Blood tests administered and analyzed by a medical laboratory give more accurate results.

The Process of Pregnancy

Pregnancy begins the moment a sperm fertilizes an ovum in the fallopian tubes (see Figure 8.6). From there, the single cell multiplies, becoming a sphere-shaped cluster of cells as it travels toward the uterus, a journey that can last three to four days. Upon arrival, the embryo burrows into the thick, spongy endometrium and is nourished from this carefully prepared lining.

Early Signs of Pregnancy

The first sign of pregnancy is usually a missed menstrual period (although some women "spot" in early pregnancy, and such spotting may be mistaken for a period). Other signs of pregnancy include

Trimester A three- month segment of pregnancy, useful in describing different developmental stages.

Embryo The fertilized egg from conception until the end of two months' development.

Fetus The name given the developing baby from the third month of pregnancy until birth.

- breast tenderness
- extreme fatigue
- sleeplessness
- emotional upset
- nausea
- vomiting (especially in the morning)

A pregnancy typically lasts 40 weeks. The due date is calculated from the expectant mother's last menstrual period. Pregnancy is typically divided into three phases, or **trimesters**, of approximately three months each.

The First Trimester

During the first trimester, there are few noticeable changes in the maternal body. The expectant mother may urinate more frequently and experience morning sickness, swollen breasts, and fatigue. These symptoms may not be frequent or severe, so she may not realize she is pregnant at this time unless she has a pregnancy test.

During the first two months after conception, the **embryo** differentiates and develops its various organ systems, beginning with the nervous and circulatory systems. At the start of the third month, the embryo is called a **fetus**, indicating that all organ systems are in place. For the rest of the pregnancy, growth and refinement occur in each major body system so that they can function independently, yet in coordination, at birth.

The Second Trimester

At the beginning of the second trimester, physical changes in the mother become more visible. Her breasts swell and her waistline thickens. During this time, the

FIGURE 8.6

Fertilization

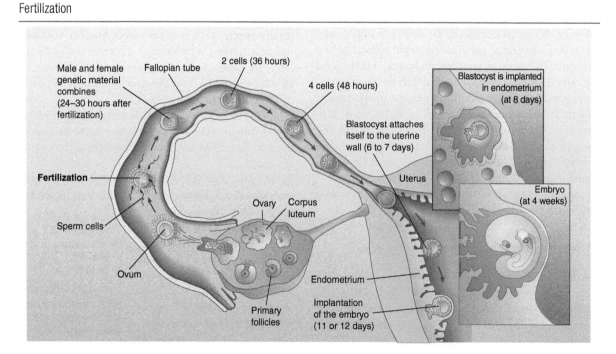

fetus makes greater demands upon the mother's body. In particular, the **placenta**, the network of blood vessels that carry nutrients and oxygen to the fetus and fetal waste products to the mother, becomes well established.

The Third Trimester

This is the period of greatest fetal growth. The fetus gains most of its weight during these last three months. During the third trimester, the fetus needs large amounts of calcium, iron, and nitrogen and obtains these from the food the mother eats. Approximately 85 percent of the calcium and iron the mother digests goes into the fetal bloodstream. Although the fetus may live if it is born during the seventh month, it needs the layer of fat usually acquired during the eighth month and time for the organs (especially the respiratory and digestive organs) to develop to their full potential. Babies born prematurely—depending upon the level of prematurity—usually require intensive medical care.

Prenatal Testing and Screening

Modern technology enables medical practitioners to detect health defects in a fetus as early as the 14th to 18th weeks of pregnancy. One common testing procedure, **amniocentesis**, which is strongly recommended for women over the age of 35, involves inserting a long needle through the mother's abdominal and uterine walls into the **amniotic sac**, the protective pouch surrounding the baby (see Figure 8.7). The needle draws out 15 to 20 mL of fluid, which is analyzed for genetic information about the baby (Mount Sinai Hospital, n.d.). This test can reveal the presence of 40 genetic abnormalities, including Down syndrome, Tay-Sachs disease (a fatal disorder of the nervous system common among Jewish people of Eastern European descent), and sickle-cell anemia (a debilitating blood disorder found primarily

FIGURE 8.7
Amniocentesis

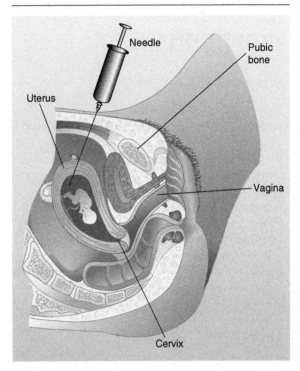

The process of amniocentesis can detect certain congenital problems as well as the sex of the fetus.

among individuals of African descent). Amniocentesis can also reveal the sex of the child. Although widely used, amniocentesis is not without risk. Chances of fetal damage and miscarriage as a result of testing are 1 in 200 (Mount Sinai Hospital, n.d.).

Another procedure, ultrasound (or sonography), uses high-frequency sound waves to determine the size and position of the fetus. Ultrasound can also detect defects in the central nervous system and digestive system of the fetus. Knowing the position of the fetus assists practitioners in performing amniocentesis and in delivering the child.

A third procedure, chorionic villus sampling (CVS), involves snipping tissue from the developing fetal sac. CVS can be used at 10 to 12 weeks of pregnancy with the results available in 12 to 48 hours. This test is an attractive option for couples at high risk for having a baby with Down syndrome or a debilitating hereditary disease.

Parents are usually referred for genetic counselling before such tests, so they will understand the test and the potential significance of the results beforehand and have a chance

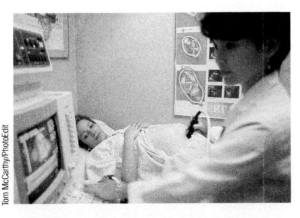

Ultrasound testing can reveal defects in the developing fetus, and, as the time of delivery nears, it can provide useful information about the size and position of the unborn child.

Placenta The network of blood vessels that carries nutrients to the developing infant and carries wastes away; it connects to the umbilical cord.

Amniocentesis A medical test in which a small amount of fluid is drawn from the amniotic sac; usually used to detect genetic diseases.

Amniotic sac The protective pouch surrounding the baby.

to ask questions and understand their options, particularly should the test reveal a serious birth defect.

CHILDBIRTH

Where to Have Your Baby

Today's prospective mothers have many delivery options. These range from hospital birth supervised by a physician to home birth with a midwife, with a number of options in between. When considering birthing alternatives, parental values are important. Many couples, for instance, feel that the modern medical establishment has dehumanized the birth process; thus, they choose to deliver at home or at a birthing centre, a homelike setting outside a hospital where women can give birth and receive postdelivery care from a team of professional practitioners, including midwives or physicians and registered nurses.

Labour and Delivery

The birth process has three stages. The exact mechanisms that signal the mother's body that the baby is ready to be born are unknown. During the few weeks preceding delivery, the baby normally shifts and turns to a head-down position, and the cervix begins to dilate (open up). The junction of the pubic bones also loosens to permit expansion of the pelvic girdle during birth (see Figure 8.8).

In the first stage of labour, the amniotic sac breaks, causing a rush of fluid from the vagina (commonly referred to as "breaking of the waters"). Contractions (initially similar to what cramps feel like when a woman has her menstrual cycle) in the abdomen and lower back also signal the beginning of labour. Early contractions push the baby downward, putting pressure on the cervix and thereby causing it to dilate further. The first stage of labour may last from a couple of hours to more than a day for a first birth, and is usually shorter during subsequent births.

The end of the first stage of labour, called **transition**, is the part of the process when the cervix becomes fully dilated and the baby's head begins to move into the vagina, or the birth canal. Contractions, these ones much stronger, more intense, and forceful, usually come quickly during transition. Transition usually lasts 30 minutes or less.

The second stage of labour follows transition when the cervix has become fully dilated. Contractions become rhythmic, stronger, and more painful

Transition The process during which the cervix becomes nearly fully dilated and the head of the fetus moves into the birth canal.

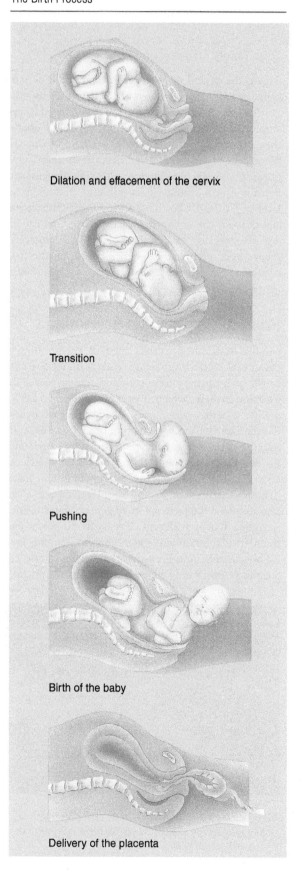

FIGURE 8.8
The Birth Process

Dilation and effacement of the cervix

Transition

Pushing

Birth of the baby

Delivery of the placenta

as the uterus works to push the baby through the birth canal. The second stage of labour (called the expulsion stage) may last between one and four hours (though it is shorter for some women) and concludes when the infant is finally pushed out of the mother's body.

After delivery, the attending practitioner cleans the baby's mucus-filled breathing passages, and the baby takes its first breath, generally accompanied by a loud wail. (The traditional "slap" on the baby's buttocks, often romanticized in movies, is no longer a common practice.) In the meantime, the mother continues into the third stage of labour, during which the placenta, or afterbirth, is expelled from the womb. This stage is usually completed within 30 minutes of delivery. The umbilical cord is then tied and severed. The stump of cord attached to the baby's navel dries up and drops off within a few days.

Prenatal Education

In terms of facilities and professionals, expectant parents in Canada can receive a variety of services for prenatal education in the community where they live. Most prenatal programs inform parents of what to expect during labour and delivery, encourage them to participate in the planning and decision-making around labour and delivery (where to have the birth, who will be at the birth, choice of pain control methods, and so on), and include instruction in a range of comfort measures including breathing techniques.

Drugs in the Delivery Room

Choosing whether or not to use painkilling drugs during the birthing process is another decision to consider prior to labour and delivery—though your decision may be altered given the reality of the pain experienced. Drug-free labour involves the use of physical activity, massage, and controlled rhythmic breathing to control pain. Many women who choose "natural" childbirth mistakenly believe that the activities taught in their classes will make their labour and delivery painless. When it comes time to give birth, they may feel inadequate because they experience the normal pain associated with childbirth. Pain is to be expected, and, if it becomes too intense, you have the option of receiving medication to provide some relief.

This is an issue that the mother should discuss with her practitioner before the birth of her baby. It is important to know your practitioner's position on the use of painkilling drugs during delivery and to understand if it is in keeping with your own. A woman's partner should know her wishes beforehand so that he or she can advocate for her during the labour. Women should also understand that they may change their mind about pain management during labour and that this is okay.

Breastfeeding and the Postpartum Period

Although the new mother's milk will not begin to flow for two or more days following delivery, her breasts secrete a yellowish substance called colostrum. Because this fluid contains vital antibodies to help fight infection, it is beneficial for the newborn to suckle. Given the overwhelmingly supportive research for breastfeeding from a variety of perspectives, it is strongly recommended that full-term newborns be breastfed (Public Health Agency of Canada, 2009). This recommendation does not mean that breast milk is the only adequate method of nourishing a baby. Prepared formulas also provide nourishment that allows a baby to grow and thrive.

In addition to being perfectly suited to a baby's nutritional needs, there are other advantages to breastfeeding (Public Health Agency of Canada, 2009). Babies who are breastfed have fewer illnesses and a much lower hospitalization rate because breast milk contains maternal antibodies and immunological cells that stimulate the infant's immune system. When breastfed babies do get sick, they recover more quickly. They are also less likely to become obese than babies fed formulas, and they have fewer allergies.

For some mothers and babies, breastfeeding is established easily, but for others it is difficult and may require support from a lactation consultant or breastfeeding clinic.

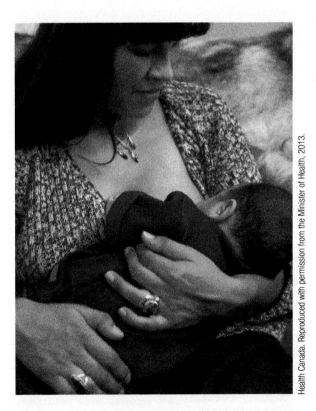

In addition to being perfectly suited to the infant's needs, breastfeeding enhances the closeness between mother and child.

Health Canada. Reproduced with permission from the Minister of Health, 2013.

This is normal and mothers who want to breastfeed and are having problems should not hesitate to ask for help. The Public Health Agency of Canada (2009) provides "10 valuable tips for breastfeeding" on its website.

When deciding whether to breast- or bottle-feed, mothers should consider their own desires and preferences. Both feeding methods can supply the physical and emotional closeness essential to the parent–child relationship.

The postpartum period typically lasts four to six weeks after delivery. During this time, the mother's reproductive organs revert to a nonpregnant state. Many women experience energy depletion, anxiety, mood swings, and depression during this period. This experience, known as **postpartum depression**, appears to be a normal end-product of the birth process. For most women, the symptoms gradually disappear as their bodies return to normal. For others, the symptoms, coupled with the stresses of managing a new family, can lead to more severe depression that lasts for several months. Either way, this needs to be assessed by a health-care practitioner immediately.

Complications

Various complications can occur during labour and delivery, even following a relatively easy and uneventful pregnancy. Such possibilities should be discussed with the practitioner prior to labour so the mother and her partner understand what medical procedures may be necessary for the mother's safety and for that of her child.

Caesarean Section (C-Section)

If labour lasts too long, if a baby is presenting incorrectly (about to exit the uterus in any way other than head first), or if the baby is in distress, a **Caesarean section (C-section)** may be necessary. This surgical procedure involves making an incision across the mother's abdomen and through the uterus to remove the baby. This operation is also performed in cases in which labour is extremely difficult, maternal blood pressure falls rapidly, the placenta separates from the uterus too soon, the mother has diabetes, or other problems occur.

A Caesarean section can be traumatic for the mother if she is not prepared. Risks to the mother are the same as for any major abdominal surgery, and recovery from birth takes considerably longer. Although a C-section may be necessary

Postpartum depression The experience of energy depletion, anxiety, mood swings, and depression that women may feel in the first four to six weeks after delivery.

Caesarean section (C-section) A surgical procedure in which a baby is removed through an incision made in the mother's abdominal and uterine walls.

Miscarriage Loss of the fetus before it is viable; also called spontaneous abortion.

Ectopic pregnancy Implantation of a fertilized egg outside the uterus, usually in a fallopian tube.

in certain cases, some physicians and critics feel that the option has been used too frequently in Canada. The World Health Organization (cited by Chaillet et al., 2007) recommends that the Caesarean section rate should not be higher than 10 to 15 percent, but the Caesarean delivery rate in Canada increased steadily from 17.5 to 23.7 percent of deliveries between 1994–1995 and 2002–2003. The guidelines dealt with three scenarios: breech presentation, prolonged labour, and previous Caesarean section. The adage was formerly "Once a Caesarean, always a Caesarean." Now, however, surgical techniques allow many women who had a C-section to deliver subsequent children vaginally.

Miscarriage

One in ten pregnancies does not end in delivery. The spontaneous loss of the fetus before it is viable, before the 20th week of pregnancy, is called a **miscarriage** (also referred to as spontaneous abortion) (MedlinePlus, 2013b). About half of all fertilized eggs are aborted spontaneously within the first seven weeks, usually before a woman knows she is pregnant; about 15 to 20 percent of women are aware of their miscarriage (MedlinePlus, 2013b). An estimated 70 to 90 percent of women who miscarry eventually become pregnant again. Reasons for miscarriage vary. In some cases, the fertilized egg fails to divide correctly. In others, genetic abnormalities, maternal illness, or infections are responsible. Maternal hormonal imbalance, a weak cervix, or toxic chemicals in the environment can also cause a miscarriage. In most cases, the cause is not known. However, risk is greater after women turn 30 and where there have been previous miscarriages (MedlinePlus, 2013b).

Another cause of miscarriage is **ectopic pregnancy**, or implantation of a fertilized egg outside the uterus. A fertilized egg can implant itself in the fallopian tube or, occasionally, in the pelvic cavity. Because these structures are not capable of expanding and nourishing a developing fetus, the pregnancy cannot continue. Such pregnancies are surgically terminated. Most often, the affected fallopian tube is also removed.

Ectopic pregnancy is generally accompanied by pain in the lower abdomen or an aching feeling in the shoulders as the blood flows toward the diaphragm. If bleeding is significant, blood pressure drops and the woman can go into shock. If an ectopic pregnancy goes undiagnosed and untreated, the fallopian tube ruptures, and the woman is then at significant risk of hemorrhage, peritonitis (infection in the abdomen), and death.

The incidence rate of ectopic pregnancy has escalated in Canada in recent years—estimated to occur in 1 of 40 to 1 of 100 pregnancies—and no one really understands why (MedlinePlus, 2013b). We do know that ectopic pregnancy is a potential side effect of pelvic inflammatory disease (PID), which has become increasingly common in recent years, because the scarring or blockage of the fallopian tubes characteristic of this disease prevents the fertilized egg from passing to the uterus. Though they are at a higher risk of another ectopic pregnancy, about 50 percent of women who have had an ectopic pregnancy conceive again.

A blood incompatibility between mother and father can cause **Rh factor** problems, and sometimes miscarriage. Rh is a blood protein. Rh problems occur when the mother is Rh-negative and the fetus is Rh-positive. During a first birth, some of the baby's blood passes into the mother's bloodstream. An Rh-negative mother may manufacture antibodies to destroy the Rh-positive blood introduced into her bloodstream at the time of birth. Her first baby will be unaffected, but subsequent babies with positive Rh factor will be at risk for a severe anemia called hemolytic disease because the mother's Rh antibodies will attack the fetus's red blood cells.

Medical advances now offer prevention and treatment; the mother and fetus can be tested and, if Rh incompatibility is found, intrauterine transfusions can be given or an early delivery by C-section can be performed, depending upon the individual case. Prevention of the problem is preferable to treatment. All women with Rh-negative blood should be injected with a medication called RhoGAM within 72 hours of any birth, miscarriage, or abortion. This injection will prevent them from developing the Rh antibodies.

No matter what the cause of a miscarriage (even if the pregnancy was unwanted), it can be an emotional experience, and the woman may need support for some time afterwards.

Stillbirth

Stillbirth is one of the most traumatic events a couple can face. A stillborn baby is one that is born dead, often for no apparent reason. The grief experienced following a stillbirth is usually devastating and can last for years. In many cases, no amount of reassurance from the attending physician, relatives, or friends can assuage the grief or guilt. In Canada, there were 2734 stillbirths reported during 2009 (Statistics Canada, 2009). The highest rates of stillbirth occur in women ages 25 to 29 (2.0) and 30 to 34 (2.0).

Sudden Infant Death Syndrome

The sudden death of an infant under one year of age for no apparent reason is called sudden infant death syndrome (SIDS). SIDS is the leading cause of death for Canadian infants between 28 days and one year of age, with 17.2 percent of deaths attributed to it (Public Health Agency of Canada, 2012). Although the number of deaths attributed to SIDS has decreased over the years, it remains a public health concern with the risk higher in males, infants who are born premature or are of low birthweight, infants who are socioeconomically disadvantages, as well as in Aboriginal infants (Public Health Agency of Canada, 2012). SIDS, also referred to as "crib death," is not a disease itself but rather is designated the cause of death after all other possibilities are ruled out. A SIDS death is sudden and silent; the death occurs quickly, often associated with sleep and with no signs of suffering.

Because SIDS is a diagnosis of exclusion, we do not know what causes it. However, several risk factors have been identified:

- Risk is greater in males.
- Risk is greater in infants two to four months.
- Risk is greater in infants from families of lower socioeconomic status.
- Risk is greater when infants sleep on their front rather than their back or in a prone position.
- Risk is greater with maternal smoking during pregnancy.
- Risk is greater when the infant is exposed to secondhand smoke in the home.
- Risk is greater if the infant's head is covered during sleep.
- Risk is greater with overheating.
- Risk may be greater when the infant shares a bed with his or her parents.
- Risk appears to be reduced through breastfeeding (Public Health Agency of Canada, 2012).

Given these risk factors, the Public Health Agency of Canada makes the following recommendations:

1. For *every* sleep, infants should be placed on their backs.
2. To reduce risk for SIDS, prevent exposure to tobacco smoke before and after birth.
3. Infants are safest and at lowest risk for SIDS when placed to sleep in a crib, cradle, or bassinet that meets Canadian regulations.
4. Room sharing is advocated because the risk for SIDS is lower when infants share a room with their caregiver. Room sharing refers to the infant's cradle, crib, or bassinet being placed in the caregiver's room and close to the caregiver's bed.
5. All mothers should be encouraged and helped to breastfeed their babies (Public Health Agency of Canada, 2012).

The death of an infant—whether a result of a known cause or not—is traumatic for parents, siblings, family, and

Rh factor A blood protein related to the production of antibodies. If an Rh-negative mother is pregnant with an Rh-positive fetus, the mother will manufacture antibodies that can kill the fetus.

Stillbirth The birth of a dead baby.

friends. The lack of a discernible cause, the suddenness of the tragedy, and the involvement of the legal system make a SIDS death especially difficult, leaving a great sense of loss and a need for understanding. Some communities have support groups to help parents and other family members through this grieving process. On a more positive note, infant mortality rates in Canada have been declining with current rates (2009—the last year with data reported) at 4.9 per 1000 (Statistics Canada, 2012). The highest rates of infant mortality are in the Northwest Territories (15.5) and the Nunavut (14.8), while the lowest rates are in Prince Edward Island (3.4) and Nova Scotia (3.4) (Statistics Canada, 2012).

INFERTILITY

An estimated one in six Canadian couples experiences **infertility**, or difficulties in conceiving a number that has doubled since the 1980s (Government of Canada, 2013). The reasons for this phenomenon include the trend toward delaying childbirth (as a woman gets older, she is less likely to conceive), the use of IUDs, and the rise in the incidence of pelvic inflammatory disease.

Causes in Women

As noted, one cause of infertility in women is **pelvic inflammatory disease (PID)**, a serious infection that scars the fallopian tubes and blocks sperm migration. Women often develop PID as a result of a gonorrhea or chlamydia infection that progresses to the fallopian tubes and the ovaries. The risk of infertility after one bout of PID is 12 percent. After two bouts, it doubles to nearly 25 percent, and following three bouts, it increases to higher than 50 percent (Centers for Disease Control and Prevention, 2011b).

Endometriosis is a major cause of infertility. In this disorder, parts of the endometrial lining of the uterus implant themselves outside the uterus—in the fallopian tubes, lungs, intestines, outer uterine walls, ovarian walls, or on the ligaments that support the uterus. The disorder can be treated surgically or with hormonal preparations. Success rates vary. Between 30 and 50 percent of women diagnosed with endometriosis are infertile (Bulletti et al., 2010).

Polycystic ovary syndrome, an endocrine disorder that affects between 6 and 10 percent of women, regardless of ethnicity, is a leading cause of infertility (Canadian Women's Health Network, 2013). It is a hormonal disorder that causes the ovaries to produce excessive amounts of the androgens (male hormones), which then interfere with egg production (Canadian Women's Health Network, 2013). One study found that a 12-week exercise intervention, combined with nutritional counselling, was effective in improving hormonal profile in the women who participated (Bruner, Chad, & Chizen, 2006). Further research is needed to confirm this exploratory research.

Causes in Men

Among men, the single largest fertility problem is low sperm count (Sharpe, 2012). Compounding low sperm count is sperm quality—that is, sperm that cannot move quickly enough and die before they reach the egg (Sharpe, 2012). Although only one viable sperm is needed for fertilization, research indicates that the other sperm in the ejaculate aid in the fertilization process. There are normally 60 to 80 million sperm per millilitre of semen. When the count drops below 20 million, fertility declines. Low sperm count can be attributable to environmental factors, such as exposure of the scrotum to intense heat or cold, radiation, or altitude, or even to wearing excessively tight underwear or outerwear. The mumps virus damages the cells that make sperm. Varicose veins above one or both testicles can also render men infertile. Male infertility problems account for approximately 30 percent of infertility cases (Government of Canada, 2013).

Treatment

The road to parenthood may be long and frustrating for the couple wishing to conceive. Fortunately, medical treatment can identify the cause of infertility in about 90 percent of affected couples. The chances of becoming pregnant range from 30 to 70 percent, depending on the specific cause of the infertility. The countless tests and the invasion of privacy that characterize some couples' efforts to conceive can put stress on an otherwise strong, healthy relationship. Before starting fertility tests, it is recommended that the couple reassess their priorities. Some will choose to undergo counselling to clarify their feelings about the fertility process. A good physician or fertility team will take the time to ascertain the couple's level of motivation.

Fertility tests for men include a sperm count, sperm motility, and analysis of any disease processes present. Women are thoroughly examined by an obstetrician/gynecologist for the composition of cervical mucus, the presence and extent of tubal scarring, and evidence of endometriosis. Complete fertility

---

Infertility Difficulties in conceiving.

Pelvic inflammatory disease (PID) An infection that scars the fallopian tubes and consequently blocks sperm migration, leading to infertility.

Endometriosis A disorder in which uterine lining tissue establishes itself outside the uterus.

---

testing may take four to five months and can be emotionally stressful. In some cases, surgery can correct structural problems such as tubal scarring. In others, administering hormones can improve the health and number of ova and sperm. Sometimes pregnancy can be achieved by collecting the male's sperm from several ejaculations and inseminating the female at a later time. Many couples also seek "alternative" methods of improving fertility, such as acupuncture, naturopathy, and "fertility yoga."

When all surgical and hormonal attempts to restore a couple's natural fertility fail, there are still some techniques available that may allow them to have a child. **Fertility drugs** can be used to stimulate ovulation in women. Ninety percent of women who use these drugs will begin to ovulate, and half will conceive. Fertility drugs are associated with a number of side effects, including headaches, irritability, restlessness, depression, fatigue, edema (fluid retention), abnormal uterine bleeding, breast tenderness, vasomotor flushes (hot flashes), and visual difficulties. Women using fertility drugs are also at increased risk of multiple ovarian cysts (fluid-filled growths) and liver damage. The drugs sometimes trigger the release of more than one egg. Thus, a woman treated with one of these drugs has a 1 in 10 chance of having multiple births. Most multiple births are twins, but triplets and even quadruplets are not uncommon.

Alternative insemination of a woman with her partner's sperm (as mentioned above) is another treatment option. If this procedure fails, the couple may choose insemination by an anonymous donor from a "sperm bank." Many men donate their sperm to such banks. The sperm are classified according to the physical characteristics of the donor (for example, blond hair, blue eyes), and then frozen for future use. Sperm can survive in this frozen state for up to five years. The woman being inseminated usually chooses sperm from a man whose physical characteristics resemble those of her partner or match her own personal preferences. Given the concern about the possibility of transmitting the AIDS virus and other diseases through alternative insemination, all donors are routinely screened for diseases before they donate.

In vitro fertilization, often referred to as "test tube" fertilization, involves collecting a viable ovum from the prospective mother and transferring it to a nutrient medium in a laboratory, where it is fertilized with sperm from the woman's partner or a donor. After a few days, the embryo is transplanted into the mother's uterus, where, it is hoped, it will develop normally.

In **gamete intrafallopian transfer (GIFT)**, the egg is "harvested" from the woman's ovary and placed in the fallopian tube with her partner's or a donor's sperm. Less expensive and time-consuming than in vitro fertilization, GIFT mimics nature by allowing the egg to be fertilized in the fallopian tube and to migrate to the uterus according to the normal timetable. The success rate for this procedure is approximately 20 percent.

In **nonsurgical embryo transfer**, a donor's egg is fertilized by the man's sperm and then implanted in the woman's uterus. This procedure may also be used in cases involving the transfer of an already-fertilized ovum into the uterus of another woman.

Embryo transfer is another treatment for infertility. In this procedure, an ovum from a donor's body is artificially inseminated by the man's sperm, allowed to stay in the donor's body for a time, and then transplanted into the prospective mother's body. Some laboratories are experimenting with **embryo freezing**, in which a fertilized embryo is suspended in a solution of liquid nitrogen. When desired, it is gradually thawed and implanted into the prospective mother. The first birth of a frozen embryo in the United States was reported in June 1986. In the future, this technique may make it possible for young couples to produce an embryo and save it for later implantation when they are ready to have a child, thus reducing the risks of fertilization of older eggs.

Surrogate Motherhood

Between 60 and 70 percent of infertile couples are able to conceive after treatment. The rest decide to live without children, adopt, or attempt surrogate motherhood. Surrogate motherhood is also a consideration for male homosexual couples. In this option, the couple arranges for a woman to be alternatively inseminated by one of the partners' sperm. The surrogate then carries the baby to term and surrenders it at birth to the couple. Although it is illegal in Canada to pay a surrogate mother for having a child, she can be compensated for the expenses involved. It has been estimated that legal and medical expenses can run as high as $30 000. Couples considering surrogate motherhood are advised to consult a lawyer regarding contracts among the involved parties.

Fertility drugs Hormones that stimulate ovulation in women not ovulating.

Alternative insemination Fertilization accomplished by depositing a partner's or a donor's semen into a woman's vagina.

In vitro fertilization Fertilization of an egg in a nutrient medium and subsequent transfer back to the mother's body.

Gamete intrafallopian transfer (GIFT) The harvesting of an egg from the female partner's ovary, which is then placed with the male partner's sperm in her fallopian tube, where it is fertilized and then migrates to the uterus for implantation.

Nonsurgical embryo transfer In vitro fertilization of a donor egg by the male partner's (or a donor's) sperm and subsequent transfer to the female partner's or another woman's uterus.

Embryo transfer Alternative insemination of a donor with the male partner's sperm; after a time, the embryo is transferred from the donor to the female partner's body.

Embryo freezing The freezing of an embryo for later implantation.

TAKING CHARGE: Ensuring Your Sexual Health

This chapter describes your reproductive and sexual health. As a sexually healthy adult, you have many decisions to make. Careful reflection and consideration of your personal values will help you to decide first if you are ready to engage in sex. Before you actually engage in sex, you must consider your contraceptive options as well as how you will protect yourself from STIs. This chapter concludes with the opportunity to consider your values and practices regarding contraceptive use in the 'Assess Yourself' below. Be honest as you respond to each of the questionnaires and reflect upon the suggestions made. This section is followed by some suggestions regarding choosing a contraceptive and another section about talking to your partner regarding condom use. As you will note, communication is key in taking the steps to protect yourself from unplanned pregnancy and STIs.

Contraceptive Comfort and Confidence Scale

These questions will help you assess whether the method of contraception you are using now or may consider using in the future will be effective for you. Answering yes to any of these questions predicts potential problems. If you have more than a few yes responses, you should talk to a health-care provider, counsellor, partner, or friend to decide whether to use this method or how to use it so that it will be effective. In general, the more yes answers you have, the less likely you are to use this method consistently and correctly with every act of intercourse and therefore be at risk of pregnancy.

Method of contraception you use now or are considering: _____

Length of time you have used this method: _____

Answer Yes or No to the Following Questions	Yes	No
1. Have you ever had problems using this method?	☐	☐
2. Have you ever become pregnant while using this method?	☐	☐
3. Are you afraid of using this method?	☐	☐
4. Would you really rather not use this method?	☐	☐
5. Will you have trouble remembering to use this method?	☐	☐
6. Will you have trouble using this method correctly and consistently?	☐	☐
7. Do you still have unanswered questions about this method?	☐	☐
8. Does this method make menstrual cycles longer, heavier, or more painful?	☐	☐
9. Does this method cost more than you can afford?	☐	☐
10. Could this method cause serious complications?	☐	☐
11. Are you opposed to this method because of any religious or moral beliefs?	☐	☐
12. Is your partner opposed to this method?	☐	☐
13. Are you using this method without your partner's knowledge?	☐	☐
14. Will using this method embarrass your partner?	☐	☐
15. Will using this method embarrass you?	☐	☐
16. Will you enjoy intercourse less because of this method?	☐	☐
17. If this method interrupts lovemaking, will you or your partner avoid using it?	☐	☐
18. Has a nurse or doctor ever told you not to use this method?	☐	☐

19. Is there anything about your personality that could lead you to use this method incorrectly? ☐ ☐

20. Are you at risk of being exposed to HIV (the human immunodeficiency virus) or other sexually transmitted infections (STIs) if you use this method? ☐ ☐
Total number of yes answers: _____

Make It Happen

The following example shows you how the previous questionnaire can be used effectively.

Micha had been using a diaphragm as her form of birth control. When she completed the self-assessment, she discovered that there were several aspects of it that made her uncomfortable. The questions to which she answered "yes" showed that she sometimes forgot to bring her diaphragm when she planned to see her boyfriend, Luke, and she disliked using it because it interrupted her sexual activity. She also was embarrassed to use it because she did not like inserting it in front of Luke. Micha decided she should investigate other birth control options and discuss them with Luke. Her first step was to visit her student health centre and, based on her likes and dislikes, to choose one or two alternatives. Among the options suggested to Micha were the contraceptive patch (Ortho Evra) and the vaginal ring (NuvaRing), both of which she would not have to remember to use and would not interrupt sexual activity. Micha's next step was to talk to Luke about his likes and dislikes and then to make a final decision based on her confidence in the method, its convenience, and its cost.

Consider your responses again. What will you do differently? What will you do the same?

Source: From *Contraceptive Technology*, 17th ed. Copyright © 1998 Contraceptive Technology Communications, Inc. Used with permission of the Ardent Media, Inc.

Choosing a Contraceptive

Part of sexual maturity is taking responsibility for your personal health regarding contraceptives and STI protection. Aside from simply worrying about contraceptive effectiveness and convenience, you need to consider the effects that your birth control method may have on your health now and in the future. Here are some things to keep in mind when you decide on your contraceptive method:

1. Talk to your medical professional about your and your family's medical history. Is there anything that would encourage the use of one method over another? Some contraceptive methods may have serious side effects according to your medical history (for example, if there is a history of high blood pressure in your family, you may choose not to use oral contraceptives).

2. Learn about the potential side effects. If you experience the side effects of a contraceptive, you should talk to your doctor immediately. Your doctor may suggest switching to a different contraceptive or may simply assure you that the "side effects" do not appear related to contraceptive use.

3. Devise a method to ensure that you cannot miss using it. If you take the pill, take it at the same time every day. Associating it with a certain time or event (for instance, taking a morning shower) will reinforce your memory. If you use condoms, you might keep some in your coat pocket so they will be there when you need them. Or you might keep your diaphragm packed in your overnight bag.

4. Learn how to talk to your partner about your choice of contraception and STI protection. Decisions about contraceptives should be made as a couple, taking each person's health and desires into account.

5. Learn about drug interactions with your birth control method. While we will discuss this in more detail in Chapter 9, it is important to know what medications might interact with your method of birth control. For example, interactions can occur between alcohol and contraceptive pills or between antibiotics and contraceptive pills. Specifically, alcohol and antibiotics may diminish the effectiveness of birth control pills in some women. Ask your doctor or pharmacist about drug interactions if you receive a prescription drug. If there is a potential for diminished effectiveness of your contraceptive, ask when you can resume normal sexual relations without taking added precautions.

Talking with Your Partner about Using Condoms

Knowing what is best for your health and doing something about it can be two different things—particularly when it relates to your sexuality and sexual behaviours. Talking with your partner about

(continued)

condoms can be hard—especially the first time. It is a sign of maturity and readiness for sexual activity if the two of you can bring the subject up and talk effectively about it. Here are some suggestions:

1. Think about what you want to say ahead of time. Sort out your feelings about using condoms before you talk with your partner.
2. Choose a time to talk before your first intimate moment. Getting things straight before you engage in sexual activity means you will both be prepared and relaxed.
3. Decide how you want to start the conversation. You might say, "I need to talk with you about something that is important to both of us," or,

"I have been hearing a lot lately about safer sex. Have you ever used condoms?" or, "I feel kind of embarrassed, but I care too much about you and myself not to talk about this."
4. Remember, starting to talk is the hardest part. Do not be surprised if your partner responds with, "I am glad you brought it up. I was worried too," or, "I like sharing the responsibility of sex. I appreciate a woman who is willing to let me."
5. Once you have agreed to use condoms, do something positive and fun. Go to the store together. Buy lots of different brands and colours. Plan a special day when you can experiment. Just talking about how you will use all those condoms can be a turn-on.

DISCUSSION QUESTIONS

1. Create a list of the five most effective contraceptive methods. What are the pros and cons for their use? Which would you choose and why?
2. When considering having a child, what sort of planning should take place? What aspects of maternal and paternal health should be considered?
3. What are some of the most important decisions that your parents made about raising you? How would you raise your child differently? The same?
4. Describe the growth of the fetus through the three trimesters. How does the mother keep herself and her baby healthy? What medical checkups or tests should be done during each trimester?
5. Identify the decisions parents face when thinking about childbirth, including where and how to have the child. How does the first-time parent decide what to do?
6. If you and your partner were having difficulty getting pregnant, what would your options be? If you were infertile, what would your options be then?

APPLICATION EXERCISE

Reread the "Consider This . . ." scenario at the beginning of the chapter and answer the following questions:

1. What concerns you most about Jamila and Karim's relationship? Why? Is it realistic that two people can date for several months and never discuss sex? What would you have done differently from Jamila and Karim? Why?
2. If you could tell incoming first-year students three suggestions about using birth control and protection from sexually transmitted infections, what would they be? Why these suggestions? What would you say about your campus culture around sex?

MASTERINGHEALTH

Go to MasteringHealth for assignments, the eText, and the study Area with case studies, self-quizzing, and videos.

focus On

Sexually Transmitted Infections (STIs)

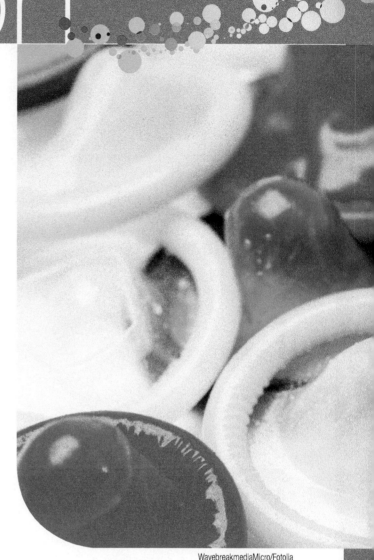

WavebreakmediaMicro/Fotolia

Kareem and about 100 other students are on a celebratory trip at an all-inclusive resort in the Caribbean. He (and the others) are enjoying the 'all-inclusive' nature of this trip, including the food, alcohol, and various other amenities. After spending hours in the sun and enjoying several local cocktails, he finds himself considerably aroused. He has been conversing and flirting with one of the bartenders who also seems to have an interest in Kareem. When this bartender is off work, he suggests that Kareem meet him for a drink and perhaps an adventure around the island. Kareem, eager to see where this situation goes, happily accepts. Once off the resort, the bartender suggests to Kareem that they go to his place. Kareem agrees and the two engage in unprotected sex. In addition to the risk of STIs, what other risks might Kareem face? How likely is it for students to engage in unprotected sex when on an all-inclusive vacation like this?

Sexually transmitted infections (STIs), previously called sexually transmitted diseases or STDs, have been around since human's earliest recorded times. Despite what we know about STIs and how to prevent them, infection rates are currently on the rise, especially in university- and college-aged students. (See Tables 1 and 2 for the most recent data regarding rates of 'reported' STIs.) As such, many students are leaving their post-secondary institution with more than just a diploma or degree (The Canadian Press, 2011).

It is possible that the increase in STI rates is partly due to improved and more effective STI testing and reporting (Public Health Agency of Canada, 2012). However, it is naïve to think that that is the real culprit accounting for the rise in STIs noted in young people today. The attitude and 'culture' regarding sex are strong contributing factors. For example, the perception that 'hooking up' is prevalent and expected on campus, as well as a more casual attitude some college and university students have toward sex, is likely contributing to the rise noted in STIs today. Although 'hooking up' is a relatively ambiguous term ranging from kissing to vaginal, oral, or anal sex, the commonality is that it refers to a casual encounter between two people (Kinstler, 2012). Further, hooks ups only have as little or as much meaning as individuals put into them—with this meaning seldom discussed prior to, during, or following the encounter. This casual attitude, whether real or not, has resulted in some students feeling pressured to have sex, often times unprotected sex with the potential for increasing the spread of STIs. Stories of casual sex among students are plentiful, particularly around celebratory events, including graduation trips where hooking up also seems to be the norm, not the exception, particularly given the amount of alcohol typically consumed at the all-inclusive resorts.

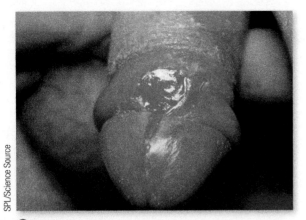

SPL/Science Source

ⓐ Primary syphilis

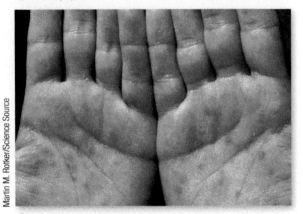

Martin M. Rotker/Science Source

ⓑ Secondary syphilis

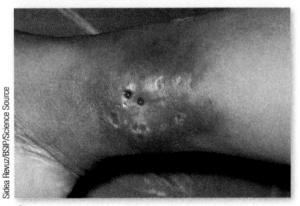

Sidea Revuz/BSIP/Science Source

ⓒ Latent syphilis

Syphilis

(a) A chancre on the site of the initial infection is a symptom of primarily syphilis

(b) A rash is characteristic of secondary syphilis

(c) Lesions called 'gummas' are often present in latent syphilis

TABLE 1

Reported Rates[1] of Chlamydia, Gonorrhea, and Syphilis
By Province/Territory for 2009.[2]

		Males	Females
Chlamydia	15–19 yrs	394.4	1720.3
	20–24 yrs	900.7	1871.4
Gonorrhea	15–19 yrs	61.1	145.6
	20–24 yrs	141.2	149.0
Syphilis	15–19 yrs	3.4	1.2
	20–24 yrs	13.0	3.4

Source: Data from Public Health Agency of Canada, copyright year
2012. Published by Public Health Agency of Canada.

[1]Rate per 100 000 population. Population estimates provided by
Statistics Canada. (Source: Statistics Canada, Demography Division, Demographic Estimates Section, July Population Estimates,
1997–2005 final intercensal estimates, 2006 final postcensal estimates, 2007-2008 updated postcensal estimates, 2009 preliminary
postcensal estimates.)

[2]2009 data are preliminary and changes are anticipated. Data were
verified with provinces and territories as of November, 2010.

TABLE 2

Reported Rates of Chlamydia, Gonorrhea, and Syphilis, by
Province and Territory, 2010

	Chlamydia	Gonorrhea	Syphilis
BC	261.9	30.1	3.4
AB	352.9	31.9	4.5
SK	484.0	72.6	3.4
MB	516.0	79.5	1.4
ON	253.4	30.0	5.9
QC	219.1	26.1	6.8
NB	242.8	8.1	4.5
NS	237.3	9.2	1.9
PE	149.7	9.2	1.9
NL	126.3	2.4	0.8
YT	666.2	89.8	2.9
NT	2086.4	502.8	18.3
NU	4193.3	1950.6	0.0

Source: (2012). Report on Sexually Transmitted Infections, Retrieved
from http://publications.gc.ca/collections/collection_2013/aspc-phac/
HP37-10-2010-eng.pdf.

Alcohol may be another contributing factor to the current rise in STIs. As will be noted in Chapter 10, alcohol reduces inhibitions; thus, individuals are likely to say and do things when under its influence that they might not if they were sober. In other words, students may be more likely to have casual sex, even unprotected sex, when their inhibitions are reduced because of their alcohol consumption. Support for this notion comes from surveys with Bowdoin students who self-reported having sex when they were drunk (67 percent) (Kinstler, 2012). Further, these students said they were more likely to flirt (34 percent) when they had been drinking.

It is important to keep the culture of your campus community in mind given its potential to influence your decisions regarding your choice to have sex or to not have sex. Further, you should recognize which attitudes and behaviours put you at a greater or lesser risk of contracting STIs (see also Figure 1). The obvious most protective behaviour is to not have sex with another person—the only way STIs can be transmitted is through fluid contact. So, if you do not engage in partner sex, then you cannot contract, nor spread, an STI. You can be abstinent, masturbate, or engage in phone sex or other forms of 'dirty' talk without risk of contracting an STI. The riskiest behaviour is to engage in unprotected anal, vaginal, or oral sex with another person who has had previous sexual experiences. Suggestions for safer sex practices are given in the next section.

PRACTISING SAFE (SAFER) SEX

Along with Health Canada, the American College of Obstetricians and Gynecologists (ACOG, 2008) and the American Social Health Association (2011) suggest that practising the following behaviours will help you to reduce your risk of contracting a sexually transmitted infection (STI):

- Avoid casual sexual partners. All sexually active adults who are not in a lifelong monogamous relationship should practise safer sex. The only guarantee that your potential sexual partner is 'clean' is if he or she has not had any sexual relations in the past—none at all.

- Always use a latex condom or a dental dam (a sensitive latex sheet, about the size of a tissue, that can be placed over the female genitals to form a protective layer) correctly and consistently during vaginal, oral, or anal sex. A new condom should be used after each ejaculate (see also Chapters 8 and 12).

- Postpone sexual involvement until you are assured that you and your partner are not infected; discuss past sexual history and, if necessary, get tested for any potential STIs.

- Avoid injury to body tissue during sexual activity. Some pathogens can enter the bloodstream through microscopic tears in anal or vaginal tissues.

- Avoid sexual activity in which semen, blood, or vaginal secretions could penetrate mucous membranes or enter through breaks in the skin.

- Avoid using drugs and alcohol, which can dull your senses and affect your ability to take responsible precautions with potential sex partners.

- Wash your hands before and after sexual encounters. Urinate after all sexual activity and, if possible, wash your genitals.

- Total abstinence is the only absolute way to prevent the transmission of STIs. Abstinence can be a difficult choice to make. If you have any doubt about the potential risks of having sex, consider other means of intimacy—massage, dry kissing, hugging, holding and touching, and masturbation (alone or with a partner).

FIGURE 1

High-risk behaviours	Moderate-risk behaviours	Low-risk behaviours	No-risk behaviours
Unprotected vaginal, anal, and oral sex—any activity that involves direct contact with bodily fluids, such as ejaculate, vaginal secretions, or blood—are high-risk behaviours.	Vaginal, anal, or oral sex with a latex or polyurethane condom and a water-based lubricant used properly and consistently can greatly reduce the risk of STI transmission. Dental dams used during oral sex can also greatly reduce the risk of STI transmission.	Mutual masturbation, if there are no cuts on the hand, penis, or vagina, is very low risk. Rubbing, kissing, and massaging carry low risk, but herpes can be spread by skin-to-skin contact from an infected partner.	Abstinence, phone sex, talking, and fantasy are all no-risk behaviours.

There are different levels of risk for various behaviours and various sexually transmitted infections (STIs); however, no matter what, any sexual activity involving direct contact with blood, semen, or vaginal secretions is high risk.

- Think about and plan for situations ahead of time to avoid risky behaviours, including settings with alcohol and drug use.
- If you are worried about your own HIV or STI status, have yourself tested. Do not risk infecting others.

COMMUNICATING WITH YOUR PARTNER ABOUT STIs

The more you know about STIs and the more you internalize personal susceptibility, the greater the chance that you will adopt safer behaviours. Yet, despite large-scale public awareness and education programs, infection continues to rise. In addition to the previously discussed casual attitudes and behaviours towards sexual activity, many medical, education, and youth officials feel that the major obstacle to preventing STIs among young people is the discomfort most have about discussing personal needs and feelings regarding these infections and practising safer sex behaviours. For many young people, discussing STI status and safer sex practices, such as condom use, can be uncomfortable. Some fear that raising the issue suggests lack of trust in the partner, others worry that safer behaviours will hinder their sexual enjoyment, and still others fail to recognize their personal vulnerability for contracting an STI. As a result, many people put themselves at risk for infection rather than hurt the other person's feelings. Therefore, a major goal in the fight against STIs is to improve one-on-one communication between young people. Perhaps it is useful to keep in mind that if you are mature enough to be engaging in sex, you should also be mature enough to discuss that sex before it happens. This conversation should include your interests and limits as well as a discussion regarding pregnancy prevention (assuming heterosexual sexual activity) as well as STI protection. The following tips can help open the lines of communication.

- Remember that you have a responsibility to your partner to disclose your STI status. Your partner also has a responsibility to disclose his or her STI status to you too. You also have a responsibility to yourself to do what needs to be done to stay healthy and infection free. Do not be afraid to ask about your partner's or potential partner's STI status. If either person's status is unknown, suggest going through the testing together—before engaging in any sexual activity—as a means of sharing something important with each other.
- Be direct, honest, and determined in talking about sex before you become involved. Do not be silly or evasive. Get to the point, ask clear questions, and do not be put off receiving a satisfactory response. Remember, a person who does not care enough to talk about sex or seems embarrassed to be talking about sex probably is not mature enough or does not care enough to take responsibility for his or her actions.
- Discuss your potential sexual activity, pregnancy, and STI prevention without sounding defensive or accusatory. Develop a personal comfort level with each of these topics prior to raising the issues with your partner. Be prepared with complete information and articulate your feelings clearly. Reassure your partner that your reasons for desiring abstinence or safer sex arise from respect rather than distrust. Sharing feelings is easier in a calm, suspicion-free environment in which both people feel comfortable, so be sure to create a calm environment free of interruptions to have this conversation.
- Encourage your partner to be honest and to share feelings. This will not happen overnight. If you have never had a serious conversation with this person before you get into an intimate situation, you cannot expect honesty and openness when the lights go out.

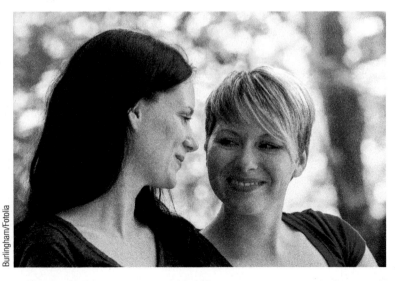

Burlingham/Fotolia

Talking to your partner about sex and STI protection is the mature thing to do.

- Analyze your beliefs and values ahead of time. It is not wise to get yourself into an awkward situation before you have had time to think about what is important to you, what you believe in, and what is right for you. Know where you will draw the line, and be very clear with your partner about what you expect. If you believe that using a condom is necessary, make sure you communicate this to your partner. Further, you should ensure you have condoms available for when the time is right to have sex.

- Decide what you will do if your partner does not agree with you. Anticipate your partner's potential objections or excuses and prepare your responses accordingly. Regardless of your partner's objections, do not engage in unprotected sex unless you both have been tested and both remain monogamous (and do not inject illegal drugs).

- Ask questions about past history. Although it may seem as though you are prying into another person's business, your current and future health depends upon knowing basic information about your partner's past. An idea of your partner's past sexual practices and use of injected drugs is valuable. Again, it is important to let your partner know why you are concerned and that you are not inquiring due to jealousy or other ulterior motives.

- Discuss the significance of monogamy for you and your partner in your relationship. A basic question to ask before becoming involved in a sexual relationship is: "How important is a committed relationship to you?" You may even need to discuss what a committed relationship means to you. You will need to decide early how important this relationship is to you and how much you are willing to work to arrive at an acceptable compromise on lifestyle.

COMPLICATIONS OF STIs: PID IN WOMEN, EPIDIDYMITIS IN MEN

If left untreated, many STIs can lead to serious complications for men and women. Without diagnosis and medical treatment, up to 40 percent of women who are infected with *Neisseria gonorrhoeae* or *Chlamydia trachomatis* may develop pelvic inflammatory disease (PID) (Centers for Disease Control and Prevention, 2010). Pelvic inflammatory disease is "an infection of the female upper genital tract involving any combination of the endometrium, fallopian tubes, pelvic peritoneum and contiguous structures" that can result from complications resulting from an untreated STI (Public Health Agency of Canada, 2013a).

Symptoms of PID vary but generally include lower abdominal pain, fever, unusual vaginal discharge, painful intercourse, painful urination, and irregular menstrual bleeding. The vague symptoms associated with chlamydial and gonococcal PID cause 85 percent of women to delay seeking medical care, thereby increasing the risk of permanent damage and scarring that can lead to infertility and ectopic pregnancy (MedlinePlus, 2011). It is estimated that there are 100 000 new cases of PID each year in Canada, though the exact numbers are not known because PID is not reported nationally (Public Health Agency of Canada, 2013a). It is further estimated that 10 to 15 percent of women of reproductive age have had at least one episode of PID (Public Health Agency of Canada, 2013a). Among women with PID, ectopic pregnancy (in which an embryo begins to develop outside of the uterus, usually in a fallopian tube) occurs in 9 percent, and chronic pelvic pain in 18 percent (MedlinePlus, 2011). Chances of ectopic pregnancy, pelvic pain, and tubal factor infertility increase proportionally with number of PIDs (Public Health Agency of Canada, 2013a).

Epididymitis is swelling (inflammation) of the epididymis, and is most common among young men ages 19 to 35 (U. S. National Library of Medicine, 2010). More specifically, epididymitis is defined as "inflammation of the epididymis manifested by a relatively acute onset of unilateral testicular pain and swelling often with tenderness of the epididymis and vas deferens and occasionally with erythema and edema of the overlying skin" (Public Health Agency of Canada, 2013b). Epididymitis is most commonly caused by the spread of *Neisseria gonorrhoeae* or *Chlamydia trachomatis* from the urethra or the bladder. Symptoms can include blood in the semen, swollen groin area, discharge from the urethra, discomfort in the lower abdomen or pelvis, and pain during ejaculation or during urination. A physical examination along with other medical tests, including a testicular scan and tests for chlamydia and gonorrhea, can diagnose the condition. Treatment usually involves pain medications and anti-inflammatory medications (Centers for Disease Control and Prevention, 2011). During the seven-day drug treatment, the patient and his sexual partners should refrain from any sexual activity (Public Health Agency of Canada, 2013b).

The serious complications that can result from untreated STIs further illustrate the need for early diagnosis and treatment. Regular screening and testing is particularly important, because many STIs are often asymptomatic, increasing the risk of complications such as PID and epididymitis.

assess YOURSELF

Go to MasteringHealth to complete this questionnaire with automatic scoring

TAKE CHARGE: Managing Your Sexual Self

To reduce your risk of STIs, you need to understand your sexual self—including your knowledge of, attitudes toward, and behaviours around the risks of contracting STIs, as well as to the prevention of STIs. Once you better understand your sexual self, you also need to take actions so that you are prepared physically, mentally, and emotionally for the sexual activity you will or will not engage in. The following quiz will help you evaluate whether your beliefs and attitudes about sexually transmitted infections (STIs) lead you to behaviours that increase your risk of infection.

STIs: Do You Really Know What You Think You Know?

Indicate whether you believe the following items are true or false, then consult the answer key that follows.

	True	False
1. You can always tell when you have an STI because the symptoms are so obvious.	☐	☐
2. Some STIs can be passed on by skin-to-skin contact in the genital area.	☐	☐
3. Herpes can be transmitted only when a person has visible sores on his or her genitals.	☐	☐
4. Oral sex is safe sex.	☐	☐
5. Condoms reduce your risk of both pregnancy and STIs.	☐	☐
6. As long as you do not have anal intercourse, you cannot get HIV.	☐	☐
7. All sexually active females should have a regular Pap smear.	☐	☐
8. Once genital warts have been removed, there is no risk of passing on the virus.	☐	☐
9. You can get several STIs at one time.	☐	☐
10. If the signs of an STI go away, you are cured.	☐	☐
11. People who get an STI have a lot of sex partners.	☐	☐
12. All STIs can be cured.	☐	☐
13. You can get an STI more than once.	☐	☐

Answer Key

1. **False.** The unfortunate fact is that many STIs show no symptoms. This has serious implications: (a) you can be passing on the infection without knowing it, and (b) the pathogen may be damaging your reproductive organs without you knowing it.

2. **True.** Some viruses are present on the skin around the genital area. Herpes and genital warts are the main culprits.

3. **False.** Herpes is most easily passed on when the sores and blisters are present, because the fluid in the lesions carries the virus. But the virus is also found on the skin around the genital area. Most people contract herpes this way, unaware that the virus is present.

4. **False.** Oral sex is not safe sex. Herpes, genital warts, and chlamydia can all be passed on through oral sex. Condoms should be used on the penis. Dental dams should be placed over the female genitals during oral sex.

5. **True.** Condoms significantly reduce the risk of pregnancy when used correctly. They also reduce the risk of STIs. It is important to point out that abstinence is the only behaviour that provides complete protection against pregnancy and STIs.

6. **False.** HIV is present in blood, semen, and vaginal fluid. Any activity that allows for the transfer of these fluids is risky. Anal intercourse is a high-risk activity, especially for the receptive (passive) partner, but other sexual activity is also a risk. When you do not know your partner's sexual history and you are not in a long-term monogamous relationship, condoms are a must.

7. **True.** A Pap smear is a simple procedure involving the scraping of a small amount of tissue from the surface of the cervix (at the upper end of the vagina). The sample is tested for abnormal cells that may indicate cancer. All sexually active women should have regular Pap smears.

8. **False.** Genital warts, which may be present on the penis, the anus, and inside and outside the vagina, can be removed. However, the virus that caused the warts will always be present in the body and can be passed on to a sexual partner.

9. **True.** It is possible to have many STIs at one time. In fact, having one STI may make it more likely that a person will acquire more STIs. For example, the open sore from herpes creates a place for HIV to be transmitted.

10. **False.** The symptoms may go away, but your body is still infected. For example, syphilis is characterized by various stages. In the first stage, a painless sore called a *chancre* appears for about a week and then goes away.

11. **False.** If you have sex once with an infected partner, you are at risk for an STI.

12. **False.** Some STIs are viruses and therefore cannot be cured. There is no cure at present for herpes, HIV/AIDS, or genital warts. These STIs are treatable (to lessen the pain and irritation of symptoms), but not curable.

13. **True.** Experiencing one infection with an STI does not mean that you can never be infected again. A person can be reinfected many times with the same STI. This is especially true if a person does not get treated for the STI and thus keeps reinfecting his or her partner with the same STI.

Source: Based on "STD Quiz." Published by Jefferson County, 2009.

CHAPTER 9
RECOGNIZING USE, MISUSE, ABUSE, AND ADDICTION TO DRUGS AND BEHAVIOURS

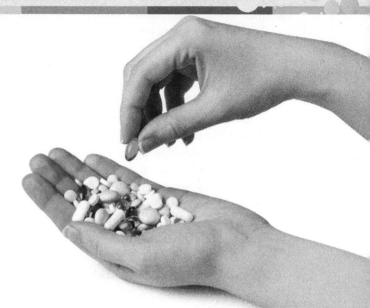

Graphia76/Getty Images

LEARNING OUTCOMES

- Define drug use, misuse, abuse, and addiction.

- Describe the influence of set and setting on response to drugs and potentially addictive behaviours.

- Clarify the physiology and psychology of addiction.

- Identify drug interactions.

- Describe the various methods of administering or taking drugs.

◄◉ CONSIDER THIS ...

A bacterial flu is going around your campus; part of the treatment is an antibiotic prescription. All of Tracey's roommates have had the flu already. When Tracey finally succumbs to this flu, rather than waste her time and effort going to the doctor for her own prescription, she starts taking the leftover prescription her roommate Laken did not finish.

▌ dentify the misuse of drugs in this scenario for Tracey and Laken. What should be done differently for and by both young women?

Substance and behavioural dependency challenges the health of many Canadians. The effect of these dependencies goes beyond the individual users/participants and extends to their families, friends, and communities. In recent years, it has also become increasingly clear that chemical or drug dependency, such as on nicotine, alcohol, and other drugs, represents only one part of Canada's health issues with addiction. Indeed, many Canadians struggle with compulsive and harmful behaviours that are not only conventional, but enhance the lives of people who can engage in them moderately. For example, some people become addicted to gambling, shopping, or exercising, while others engage in these behaviours without personal, social, or financial harm.

DRUG USE, MISUSE, AND ABUSE

Although drug abuse is usually defined in connection with illicit (i.e., illegal) and psychoactive drugs, many people abuse and misuse prescription and over-the-counter drugs as well as legal substances such as coffee, tobacco, alcohol, and herbal preparations. While **drug use** is considered taking a drug for the reason it was intended, **drug misuse** is considered the use of a drug for a purpose for which it was not intended (U.S. Food and Drug Administration, 2013). For example, taking an over-the-counter pain reliever when you have a headache is an example of drug use, while taking a friend's prescription painkiller for your headache is misuse (because it was not prescribed for you and you are therefore taking it in a way for which it was not intended). Drug misuse also includes, among other things, not taking prescription or over-the-counter drugs according to the directions and not completing the full dose of a prescription (U.S. Food and Drug Administration, 2013). **Drug abuse** is defined as the excessive use of a drug. Excessive use, however, is difficult to quantify, partly because what is excessive for one person may not be for another, given the various factors involved including body size, sex, previous use, and so on. Drug abuse is also defined according to your motivations for taking the drug, for example, if you are taking a higher than prescribed dose of a prescribed medication for the euphoric effect (Barrett, Meisner, & Stewart, 2008; U.S. Food and Drug Administration, 2013).

There are risks and benefits to the use of any chemical substance. Intelligent and conscious decision making requires a clear-headed evaluation of these risks and benefits and the realization that unforeseeable reactions or problems can arise. Your decision to use or not use a particular drug should be made to best suit your needs for those particular circumstances. In order to compare risks to benefits, you might want to create a profile for each drug you use or are considering using. A drug profile identifies the active ingredients in the drug, receptor sites that will be affected, main effects, side effects, potential interactions with other drugs you use, and any potential adverse reactions. You could then consider your rationale for using the drug and make your decision accordingly, keeping in mind the potential personal, social, and, perhaps, legal consequences of your choice.

Individual Response: Set and Setting

Individuals differ in how they respond to drugs and behaviours that are potentially addictive. Furthermore, responses to drugs and behaviours can be different within an individual as well depending upon a number of things, including mental and physical health. More than the drug or behaviour is involved in your mental and physical responses to them. Your responses also involve more than the amount of drug or behaviour involved. Set and setting are two factors that can influence the main and side effects of drugs. The **main effect** of a drug refers to the general purpose of the drug, while the **side effect** refers to other effects, often not desired, from the drug or behaviour (Hanson, Ventruelli, & Fleckenstein, 2012). For example, the main effect of an analgesic such as Advil or Aspirin is to relieve pain, while a side effect may be stomach discomfort. Tylenol is usually prescribed for people with gastrointestinal issues because it does not cause stomach discomfort. **Set** refers to the total internal environment, or mindset, of a person at the time a drug is taken or behaviour is engaged in. Various physical, emotional, and social factors interact to influence the effect of a drug or behaviour on you. Your expectations of what the drug will or will not do are also part of the set. For example, if you read about the potential side effects for a particular drug, you may experience more side effects when taking that drug than someone who chose not to read this information or who glanced over it quickly. Another example is that if you are told and believe a particular drug should solve your health issue, you are more likely to experience that effect, including relief of your various symptoms. This can happen even when you take a

Drug use Taking a drug in the way it was intended.

Drug misuse Using a drug in a way it was not intended. For example, using someone else's prescription, whether for the same malady or for the effect of the drug.

Drug abuse The excessive use of a drug, where excessive use is individually determined.

Main effect The intended reaction(s) to a drug; the reason for which the drug was taken.

Side effect Unintended reaction(s) to a drug.

Set Your total internal environment, or mindset, at the time you take a drug or engage in a behaviour.

sugar pill. The ability to get better without an actual drug because you believe you are taking something to help you recover is called the placebo effect (Placebo Effect, 2012). In other cases, set may be related to your mood. If you are "pumped" for a party and plan to get drunk, it is likely that you will feel the effects of alcohol faster than when you are not in as much of a mood to party. Although all individuals respond to their 'set', the elderly are particularly susceptible. In fact, the elderly often experience more placebo and side effects with their prescription and over-the-counter drug use than other populations (Fabian, 2013).

Whereas *set* refers to the drug user's internal environment, **setting** refers to the drug user's total external environment. It encompasses the physical and social aspects of your environment at the time you take the drug or engage in the particular behaviour. If you are surrounded by a group of friends, loud rap music, and a noisy crowd, the drug will generally produce a greater effect than when you take it in a quiet place with soft music, comfortable furniture, low lights, and relaxed company.

DEFINING ADDICTION

Addiction is defined as "a persistent, compulsive dependence on a behaviour or substance" (The Free Dictionary, n.d.). In the past, addiction was used only to describe dependence on a drug or substance. The definition has now been extended to include mood-altering behaviours or activities. Generally, if you are addicted to a substance or behaviour, your academic performance or work suffers; relationships deteriorate; economic hardships develop; and there are negative effects on your physical, emotional, and social health. If you are addicted to a drug or behaviour, you likely exhibit at least three of the following:

- excessively uses a substance or engages in a behaviour—that is, you use a greater quantity of a drug or persist with a behaviour over a longer period of time than intended

- expresses a persistent desire, or makes unsuccessful efforts to cut down or control use of the substance or engagement in the activity

- spends a great deal of time getting or using the substance or engaging in the behaviour or recovering from its effects and after-effects

- is frequently too intoxicated or incapacitated by the after-effects of the drug or behaviour to fulfill major obligations

- gives up regular activities to use the substance or engage in the behaviour

- continues to use the substance or participate in the activity despite having problems with it

- develops a physical tolerance to the substance (therefore needs more to get the same effect) or behaviour (therefore needs to engage in more of the activity) to get the same effect

- exhibits withdrawal when not using the substance or engaging in the behaviour

- uses the substance or engages in the behaviour to relieve or avoid withdrawal symptoms

Physiologic dependence is only one indicator of addiction. Psychological dynamics play an important role, which explains why behaviours not related to the use of chemicals—gambling, for example—can also be addictive. In fact, psychological and physiological dependence are so intertwined that it is not possible to separate the two. For every psychological state, there is a corresponding physiological state. In other words, everything you feel is tied to a chemical process or reaction occurring in your body (Doweiko, 1993), even when there is no drug ingested, as when, for example, engaging in a potentially addictive behaviour.

Chemicals or drugs are responsible for the most profound addictions, not only because they produce

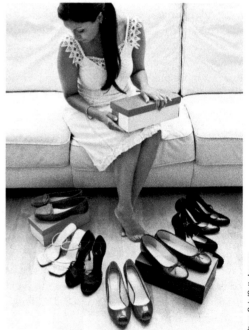

Steve Cole/Getty Images

What makes an addiction different from a habit? Once a person recognizes a habit and decides to change it, the habit can usually be broken; with an addiction, there is such a strong sense of compulsion to engage in the behaviour that the person cannot control his or her choice of whether or not to engage in it.

Setting Your total external environment, or mindset, at the time you take a drug or engage in a behaviour.

Addiction A persistent, compulsive dependence on a behaviour or substance.

dramatic mood changes, but also because they cause cellular changes to which the body adapts so well that it eventually requires the chemical in order to function normally (National Institute of Drug Abuse, 2010). Thus, for a particular behaviour to be addictive, it must have the potential to produce a positive mood, which results in a chemical change in the body such that engaging in the behaviour is needed to simply feel normal.

Since behaviours such as gambling, spending/shopping, working, exercise, sex, and internet or other technology use also create changes at the cellular level along with positive mood changes, a person can become addicted to them. Although the mechanism is not well understood, all forms of addiction likely reflect a dysfunction of certain biochemical systems in the brain (Nakken, 1988).

The Physiology of Addiction

Virtually all mental, emotional, and behavioural functions occur as a result of biochemical interactions between nerve cells in the body. Biochemical messengers, called neurotransmitters, exert their influence at specific receptor sites on nerve cells. Drug use and chronic stress (see also Chapter 3) can alter these receptor sites and cause the production and breakdown of neurotransmitters.

Mood-altering chemicals, for example, fill up the receptor sites for the body's natural "feel-good" neurotransmitters (endorphins) so that nerve cells are fooled into believing they have enough neurotransmitters and therefore shut down production of these substances temporarily. When the drug use is stopped, those receptor sites become emptied, resulting in uncomfortable feelings that remain until the body resumes neurotransmitter production or more of the drug is consumed. Some people's bodies always produce insufficient quantities of these neurotransmitters, so they naturally seek chemicals like alcohol as substitutes, or they pursue behaviours like vigorous physical activities/exercise or thrill-seeking activities such as sky diving or riding a rollercoaster that increase natural production. Thus, we may be "wired" to seek substances or experiences that increase pleasure or reduce discomfort.

Generally, when a drug is consumed regularly or a behaviour is engaged in consistently, tolerance develops. **Tolerance** is a phenomenon in which progressively larger doses of a drug or more intense involvement in an experience is needed to obtain the desired effects (Sussman & Sussman, 2011). All of us develop some degree of tolerance to drugs and mood-altering behaviours. The difference between those who do and do not become addicted may relate to the quantity and frequency of their use or engagement, as well as the negative effects as a result of their use. However, it should be pointed out that some drugs have a particularly profound effect and tolerance develops even when only small quantities are consumed.

Withdrawal is another phenomenon associated with drugs and mood-altering experiences. The drug or activity replaces or causes an effect that the body normally creates on its own. If the experience is repeated often enough or the substance ingested frequently enough, the body makes an adjustment and, as a result, requires the drug or experience to obtain the effect it previously produced itself. In other words, the drug or behaviour is required to simply feel normal. Stopping the behaviour or no longer ingesting the drug will therefore result in physiological and psychological symptoms of withdrawal (Sussman & Sussman, 2011). Withdrawal symptoms of chemical dependencies are generally the opposite of the effects of the drug taken and may require medical support. For example, withdrawal from cocaine includes a characteristic "crash" (depression and lethargy), while withdrawal from barbiturates involves trembling, irritability, and convulsions. Withdrawal symptoms for addictive behaviours, although usually less dramatic, are still a profound experience. Common withdrawal symptoms for discontinued addictive behaviours include discomforts such as anxiety, depression, irritability, guilt, anger, and frustration, along with an underlying preoccupation with or craving for another experience (Hanson, Venturelli, & Fleckenstein, 2012). Withdrawal symptoms from drugs or behaviours range from mild to severe. The severest form of withdrawal is delirium tremens (DTs), which occurs in approximately 5 percent of individuals withdrawing from alcohol, and involves hallucinations, disorientation, tachycardia, hypertension, fever, agitation, and diaphoresis (Hoffman & Weinhouse, 2013). DTs commonly affect people addicted to alcohol for 10 or more years, as well as individuals when they stop after a period of several months of heavy drinking (MedlinePlus, 2013).

The Addictive Process

Addiction is a process that evolves over time. It begins when a person repeatedly seeks relief from unpleasant feelings or situations. This pattern is known as **nurturing through avoidance** and is a maladaptive way of taking care of emotional needs (Johnson, 1986). As a person becomes increasingly dependent on the

---

Tolerance Phenomenon in which a progressively larger dose of a drug or more intense involvement in a particular behaviour is needed to produce the desired euphoric effects.

Withdrawal Experienced by individuals addicted to a drug or behaviour when the drug is not consumed or behaviour not engaged in. Generally, the withdrawal symptom experiences are directly opposite to the effects experienced when engaging in the substance or behaviour.

Nurturing through avoidance Repeatedly seeking the illusion of relief from the drug or behaviour to avoid unpleasant feelings or situations until it becomes an addiction.

addictive behaviours or drug, there is a corresponding deterioration in relationships with family, friends, and co-workers, in performance at work or school, and in personal life. Eventually, these individuals do not find the addictive behaviours or drug pleasurable but still consider it preferable to the unhappy realities they seek to escape, as well as the withdrawal symptoms they experience when they do not take the drug or engage in the behaviour.

Signs of Addiction

Although different opinions exist as to the cause, most experts agree that there are universal signs of addiction. Addictions are characterized by four commonalities (Sussman & Sussman, 2011): (1) **compulsion**, which is described by obsession, or excessive preoccupation, with the behaviour or drug and an overwhelming need for it; (2) **loss of control** or the inability to predict reliably whether any isolated occurrence of the behaviour or use of a drug will be healthy or damaging; (3) **negative consequences**, such as physical damage, legal trouble, financial problems, academic failure, relationship difficulties, and family dissolution; and (4) **denial**, or the inability to perceive that the behaviour or drug use are self-destructive. These four components are present in all addictions, whether chemical or behavioural.

Traditionally, diagnosis of an addiction was limited to drug addiction and based on three criteria:

- the presence of an abstinence syndrome or withdrawal;
- an associated pattern of pathologic behaviours (deterioration in work or academic performance, relationships and social interaction, and other personal circumstances); and
- **relapse**, the tendency to return to the addictive behaviour or drug after a period of abstinence.

Furthermore, until recently, health professionals were unwilling to diagnose an addiction until medical symptoms appeared in the patient. We now know that although withdrawal, pathological behaviours, relapse, and medical symptoms are valid indicators of addiction, they do not characterize all addictive behaviours.

Compulsion Obsessive preoccupation with a behaviour or substance and an overwhelming need for it.

Loss of control Inability to predict reliably whether any isolated involvement with the addictive substance or behaviour will be healthy or damaging.

Negative consequences Difficulties such as physical damage, legal trouble, financial ruin, academic failure, relationship difficulties, family dissolution, and others as a result of continued engagement with a substance or behaviour.

Denial Inability to recognize that there is a problem resulting from current use of a drug or engagement in a particular behaviour.

Relapse The tendency to use or re-engage in the addictive behaviour or drug after a period of abstinence.

ADDICTIVE BEHAVIOURS

You likely have little difficulty understanding addiction to drugs because a chemical is ingested, but you may find addiction to a behaviour more difficult to understand, particularly when the behaviour is essential to healthy living (e.g., exercise or eating) or a normal part of life (e.g., sex or shopping). Although there are a number of behaviours that we can become addicted to, only four common addictive behaviours are profiled here: compulsive gambling, shopping, exercise, and use of technology.

Gambling

Gambling is a form of recreation and entertainment for many Canadians—67 percent of households report at least one gambling incident in the past year (Marshall, 2011). The most common gambling activities are ticket lotteries, charities, and Scratch/Instant Win (Responsible Gambling Council, Canadian Partnership for Responsible Gambling, 2012). Most people who gamble do so casually and moderately. In Canada the average amount of money spent on gambling per person 18 years and over in 2013–2014 was $536. Among the provinces the amount ranged from a low of $350 in Nova Scotia to a high of $799 in Saskatchewan (Canadian Partnership for Responsible Gambling, 2014). For some, however, it is not just a fun and exciting recreational activity, but rather a compulsive or pathological behaviour. Pathological or compulsive gambling continues to be considered a mental disorder by the American Psychiatric Association in the revised *Diagnostic and Statistical Manual of Mental Disorders*, 5th Edition published in May, 2013. An individual who exhibits at least 4 of the following 9 behaviours over a 12-month period is considered to have a gambling addiction:

1. Needs to gamble with increasing amounts of money in order to achieve the desired excitement.

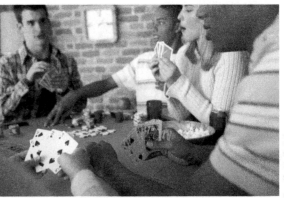

One form of behavioural addiction is gambling.

2. Is restless or irritable when attempting to cut down or stop gambling.

3. Has made repeated unsuccessful efforts to control, cut back, or stop gambling.

4. Is often preoccupied with gambling (e.g., having persistent thoughts of reliving past gambling experiences, handicapping or planning the next venture, thinking of ways to get money with which to gamble).

5. Often gambles when feeling distressed (e.g., helpless, guilty, anxious, depressed).

6. After losing money gambling, often returns another day to get even ("chasing" one's losses).

7. Lies to conceal the extent of involvement with gambling.

8. Has jeopardized or lost a significant relationship, job, or educational or career opportunity because of gambling.

9. Relies on others to provide money to relieve desperate financial situations caused by gambling.

People addicted to gambling or drugs describe similar cravings and highs. Research shows that individuals addicted to gambling have decreased blood flow to a key section of the brain's reward system as well as lower levels of serotonin and dopamine (Gambling as Addiction, 2005). As with people addicted to drugs, it is thought that individuals addicted to gambling compensate for this deficiency by overdoing it and then getting hooked. Most individuals addicted to gambling gamble for the excitement, not the money-making possibility, placing increasingly larger bets to achieve the desired level of excitement or euphoric feeling—similar to what a person who uses drugs seeks.

Men are more likely to gamble than women, as are individuals who are divorced, of lower income, of African-Canadian heritage, older, and living within 100 kilometres of a casino (Welte et al., 2004). Unsurprising given increased access to online gambling venues and use of technology by college or university students, gambling is increasing in prevalence, particularly gambling online. Further, students have easier access to gambling opportunities given the growing number of casinos, scratch tickets, lotteries, and sports betting networks. Poker playing, in particular, has increased in popularity among students. Access to poker on the internet and televised poker tournaments are likely factors in the large number of young people who now spend an increased, and potentially unhealthy, amount of time and money playing poker.

Combined data from provincial and national surveys, both of which used the Canadian Problem Gaming Index, indicates that 2.5 to 3.8 percent of the Canadian adult population (ages 15+ years) are at moderate risk or are problem gamblers (Responsible Gambling Council, Canadian Partnership for Responsible Gambling, 2012). Young people are two to three times more likely than adults to develop gambling problems (Turner, MacDonald, & Somerset, 2007). Similar to their older male counterparts, male students are more likely to gamble than female students. Other common characteristics include spending more time watching TV, using computers for non-academic purposes, spending less time studying, earning lower grades, participating in intercollegiate athletics, and engaging in frequent binge drinking and using illicit drugs in the past year (The Annenburg Public Policy Center, 2005).

Most people who gamble do so casually—that is, for entertainment—and can stop any time they want to and are able to see the importance of being able to stop of their own volition. However, individuals addicted to gambling are not able to control their urge to gamble even when faced with devastating consequences such as high debt, legal problems, and the loss of most meaningful things, including homes, families, jobs, health, and even their lives. Negative effects of gambling on health include a greater risk of cardiovascular problems as well as an increased rate of suicide.

Shopping and Borrowing

Although compulsive spending has been a pervasive problem for some time in Canada, a more insidious form of addiction lurks in the new "plastic generation." Credit card companies entice people, even students, to have it all right now—whether or not you can afford it. As a result, we have become a 'buy now, pay for it later' society.

Credit card companies are succeeding, with millions of MasterCards, VISAs, and other forms of credit in existence. Further, many students have relatively easy access to lines of credit. Opportunities to overspend are expanded by the increased acceptance and availability of online shopping. The resulting debt is phenomenal with the potential for lasting effects. Although most people manage their debt with careful planning, others do not. Some individuals spend money to meet emotional needs not fulfilled elsewhere, while anxiety, self-doubt, and anger can lead to spending as a way of coping with daily stressors. Addiction has taken over a person's shopping behaviours when his or her needs are only met by shopping and spending and the person only feels normal when engaging in these behaviours. College and university students may be particularly vulnerable to overspending and meeting their emotional needs through shopping because advertisers and credit card companies target them heavily.

Compulsive gambling and shopping frequently lead to compulsive borrowing to support the addiction.

Irresponsible investments and purchases lead to debts that the individual who is addicted tries to repay by borrowing more. Compulsive debtors borrow money repeatedly from family, friends, or institutions despite the problems this causes. Whereas most people incur overwhelming debt through a combination of hardship and lack of understanding regarding financial management, compulsive debtors incur debt primarily to support their habits of compulsive and excessive buying or gambling behaviours, which they engage in for the pleasurable feelings that result and/or to relieve painful feelings of withdrawal.

Exercise Addiction

It may seem odd that a behaviour that we need to engage in on a daily basis (see Chapter 4) also has the potential for addiction. Yet, exercise is a powerful mood enhancer that can be addictive. Firm statistics on the incidence of exercise addiction are not available, but one indication of its prevalence is that a large portion of individuals with the eating disorders anorexia nervosa and bulimia nervosa use exercise to purge instead of, or in addition to, self-induced vomiting (Cook & Hausenblas, 2008). Individuals addicted to exercise do so compulsively to try to meet their needs—for nurturance, intimacy, self-esteem, and self-competency—that an object or activity cannot truly meet. Some warning signs of exercise addiction include always or usually working out alone; following the same rigid exercise pattern; exercising for more than two hours daily, repeatedly; fixation on weight loss or calories burned; exercising when sick or injured; exercising to the point of pain and beyond; and skipping work, class, or social plans for workouts. Addictive exercise results in negative consequences similar to those found in other addictions: alienation of family and friends, injuries from overdoing it, and a craving for more.

Technology Addictions

As technology becomes integrated more and more into your daily life, your risk of overexposure grows as it does for people of all ages. Some people, in fact, become addicted to new technologies, such as smart phones, video games, networking sites, and the online world in general. Have you ever opened your web browser to quickly check something, and an hour later found yourself still blogging or checking your Facebook page? Do you have friends who seem more concerned with texting or surfing than with eating, going out, studying, or having a face-to-face conversation? These attitudes and behaviours are not unusual; many experts suggest that technology addiction is real and can present serious problems for those addicted. An estimated one in eight internet users will likely experience internet addiction (The Center for Internet Addiction, 2010). Younger people are also more likely to be addicted to the Internet than middle-aged users (Morrison & Gore, 2010).

What is normal internet use? Some college students average eight hours or so per week, while other web surfers average 20 hours online without having major problems. What you do online may be as important as how long you spend there. Some online activities, such as gaming and cybersex, seem to be more compelling and potentially addictive than others.

Individuals addicted to the internet, similar to individuals addicted to a drug or other behaviour, typically exhibit symptoms such as general disregard for their health, sleep deprivation, neglecting family and friends, lack of physical activity, euphoria when online, lower grades in school, and poor job performance. Individuals addicted to the internet may feel moody or uncomfortable when they are not online. These individuals may be using their behaviour to compensate for feelings of loneliness, marital or work problems, a poor social life, or financial problems.

MANAGING AN ADDICTION

Due to individual denial, recognizing that a problem exists is one of the most difficult steps in the process of managing and treating an addiction. An **intervention** is a planned process of confrontation by significant others to break down denial compassionately so that an individual can see the destructive nature of his or her addiction. The individual must learn that his or her addiction is destructive and requires treatment. Once this has been accomplished, treatment and recovery can begin. If this step does not occur, treatment and recovery are not possible.

Treatment and recovery for any addiction begins with abstinence—refraining from the addictive behaviours or substance. Abstinence, however, does little to change the personality and psychological dynamics or the biological and environmental influences behind the addictive behaviours. Recovery also involves learning new ways of looking at oneself, others, and the world. It may involve replacing addictive habits and behaviours with less harmful or addictive ones. It may require exploration of a traumatic past so that psychological wounds can heal. It requires new

Intervention A planned process of confrontation by significant others to break down denial compassionately so that an individual can see the destructive nature of his or her addiction.

ways of taking care of oneself, physically and emotionally, and involves developing communication skills and new ways of having fun. Recovery programs are the fuel that gives individuals who are addicted to a substance or behaviour the energy to resist relapsing. For a large number of individuals who have an addiction, recovery begins with a period of formal treatment. An effective program has the following characteristics:

- Professional staff familiar with the specific addictions for which help is being sought
- A flexible schedule of inpatient and outpatient services
- Access to medical personnel who can assess the medical status of an individual with an addiction and provide treatment for all medical concerns as needed
- Medical supervision of individuals with an addiction at high risk for a complicated detoxification process, such as that found with withdrawal from alcohol
- A team approach to treatment of the addictive disorders (for example, medical personnel, counsellors, psychotherapists, social workers, clergy, educators, dieticians, physical activity promoters, and family members)
- Group and individual therapy options
- Integration of peer-led support groups and encouragement to continue involvement with support groups even after treatment ends
- Structured after-care and relapse-prevention programs
- A clean and attractive environment
- A cordial and helpful staff

Highly structured treatment programs help their clients get started on a lifetime program of personal recovery. They include wellness programs to teach critical self-care skills, educational programs to formulate a deep understanding of the addiction, self-help groups to provide a foundation of support after treatment, and several forms of therapy, including these:

- **Individual therapy.** Individuals with an addiction can identify and experience feelings they have been chronically medicating with their addictive behaviours. During sessions, individuals with an addiction begin to deal with issues related to their addiction.
- **Group therapy.** The group provides an opportunity for developing communication skills and offers an environment where individuals with an addiction learn how to be honest with themselves and others. The standard care in a treatment program is to combine group therapy with individual therapy.
- **Family therapy.** Family therapy helps all members of the family to recover from their potentially codependent roles.

- **12-step programs.** One of the most common types of peer support groups is a 12-step program, patterned after Alcoholics Anonymous. These programs are designed to keep individuals free of their addictions through honest acknowledgment of their shortcomings and through the mutual support of others who had similar experiences. There are 12-step programs for every addiction, including Narcotics Anonymous and Sex and Love Addicts Anonymous, as well as for families and others who have a relationship with the person who has the addiction.
- **Alternatives to 12-step programs.** Because 12-step programs adhere to a spiritual basis in the recovery process, some individuals for whom a spiritual approach is uncongenial have sought or started alternative groups. LifeRing Canada (2011) is one example of an alternative to a 12-step program. All meetings, materials, and anything associated with the program are non-secular as the philosophy of this program is that addiction and recovery should be placed in the hands of the individual who is an addict (LifeRing Canada, 2011).

DRUG DYNAMICS

Have you ever walked into a drugstore looking for some cough syrup or a pain reliever and become overwhelmed by the options available? Do you think they are all safe because they are available for you to purchase without a prescription or anyone's advice? Although there are literally tens of thousands of drugs at our disposal, choices among them should not be made lightly. All drugs are chemical substances that have the potential to alter the structure and function of our bodies. Quite simply, all drug use involves risks in addition to the intended benefits. You can minimize these risks by asking appropriate questions of health care providers and by becoming a critical consumer of all drugs. Your pharmacist is a good person to talk to. You should share your symptoms and be clear regarding which symptoms you wish to relieve. Questions you might ask relate to how often you can take the drug and does the drug interact with any other drugs you may be taking (e.g., caffeine, alcohol, a pain reliever, and so on).

Drugs work because they physically resemble the chemicals produced naturally within the body (see Figure 9.1). For example, many painkillers resemble the endorphins (literally "morphine within") manufactured in the body. Most bodily processes result from chemical reactions or changes in electrical charge. Because drugs possess an electrical charge and a chemical structure similar to chemicals that occur naturally in

FIGURE 9.1

How the Body Metabolizes Drugs

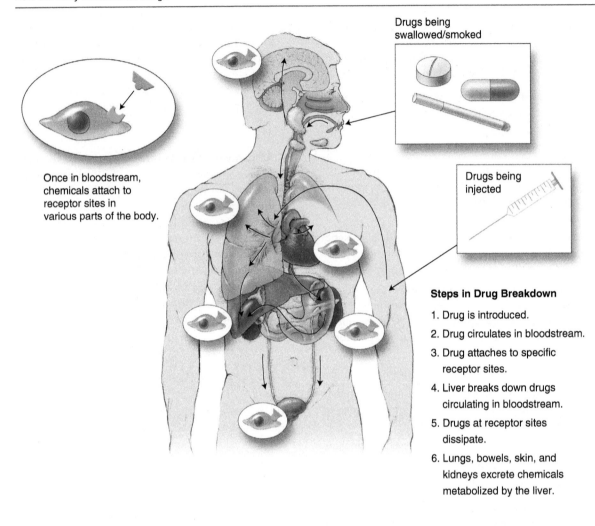

Once in bloodstream, chemicals attach to receptor sites in various parts of the body.

Drugs being swallowed/smoked

Drugs being injected

Steps in Drug Breakdown

1. Drug is introduced.
2. Drug circulates in bloodstream.
3. Drug attaches to specific receptor sites.
4. Liver breaks down drugs circulating in bloodstream.
5. Drugs at receptor sites dissipate.
6. Lungs, bowels, skin, and kidneys excrete chemicals metabolized by the liver.

the body, they can affect physiological and psychological functions in many different ways.

Drugs attach themselves to specific **receptor sites** in the body. Receptor sites are specialized proteins found in all body cells. Different cells and body tissue contain different receptors, so different drugs will have different effects. The size, shape, and electrical charge of the drug and the receptor determine how they will interact. Most drugs can attach at multiple receptor sites located throughout the body including the heart, blood vessels, lungs, liver, kidneys, brain, and gonads (testicles or ovaries). The physiology of drug activity and its effect on human behaviours is very complex.

Receptor sites Specialized cells to which drugs can attach themselves.

Psychoactive drugs Drugs that have the potential to alter mood or behaviours.

Prescription drugs Drugs that can be obtained only with a written prescription from a licensed physician.

TYPES OF DRUGS

Drugs are divided into six categories: prescription drugs, recreational drugs, over-the-counter (OTC) drugs, herbal preparations, illicit drugs, and commercial drugs. Each category includes drugs that stimulate the body, depress body functions, produce hallucinations, or have the potential to alter a person's mood or behaviours. When the drug alters a person's mood or behaviour it is called a **psychoactive drug**.

- **Prescription drugs** can be obtained only with a written prescription from a licensed physician or nurse practitioner. Common drugs prescribed in Canada include Tylenol with Codeine for pain relief, Lipitor for reducing cholesterol, and Pariet for stomach discomfort often related to anxiety (Canada.com, n.d.). In 2014, prescribed drug spending was approximately $28.8 billion, accounting for 85.0 percent of total drug spending ($33.9 billion) and 13.4 percent of total health expenditure (Canadian Institute of Health Information, 2015).

- **Recreational drugs** belong to a vague category, with boundaries dependent upon the definition of recreation. Generally, these drugs contain chemicals that people use to help them relax or socialize and thus are part of people's typical recreation. Alcohol, tobacco, and caffeine are common examples included in this category. These drugs are legal even though they are psychoactive. Others may place illegal drugs in this category too.

- **Over-the-counter (OTC) drugs** can be purchased without a physician's prescription. You need only look at your local grocery or drug store for examples of OTCs. Pain relievers such as Tylenol, Advil, and Aspirin are available over-the-counter. Another large section of OTCs includes various remedies aimed at relieving symptoms due to coughs and colds. Expenditures specifically on OTC products (which are not usually covered by health care) were equivalent to $141 per Canadian in 2011 (Canadian Institute of Health Information, 2012).

- **Herbal preparations** form another vague category of drugs that includes at least 750 substances such as herbal teas and other products of botanical origin believed to have medicinal or healthful properties. Vickers, Zollman, and Lee (2001) noted that herbal medicine uses whole plants (most often as an unpurified extract) or a combination of herbs, and diagnostic principles based on treating the "underlying causes" of the health issue presented. Examples for herbal preparations for osteoarthritis include the following (Vickers, Zollman, & Lee, 2001):

  - Turmeric (*Curcuma longa*) tincture 20 mL—For anti-inflammatory activity and to improve local circulation at affected joints

  - Devil's claw (*Harpogophytum procumbens*) tincture 30 mL—For anti-inflammatory activity and general well-being

  - Ginseng (*Panax* spp) tincture 10 mL—For weakness and exhaustion

  - White willow (*Salix alba*) tincture 20 mL—For anti-inflammatory activity

  - Licorice (*Glycyrrhiza glabra*) 5 mL—For anti-inflammatory activity and to improve palatability and absorption of herbal medicine

  - Oats (*Avena sativa*) 15 mL—To aid sleep and for general well-being

- **Illicit (illegal) drugs** are often considered the most notorious substances. Although laws governing their use, possession, cultivation, manufacture, and sale differ from country to country, use of illicit drugs is generally recognized as harmful. These drugs are psychoactive. Examples of illegal drugs include marijuana, cocaine, heroin, and many others. Because these drugs are not monitored or regulated, their potency and purity may vary.

- **Commercial preparations** are the most universally used yet least commonly recognized as products with a drug action. More than 1000 of these substances exist, including seemingly benign items such as perfumes, cosmetics, household cleansers, paints, glues, inks, dyes, gardening chemicals, pesticides, solvent glue, and industrial by-products.

Routes of Administration of Drugs

Routes of administration refer to the ways in which a drug is taken into the body. Common routes include oral ingestion, injection, inhalation, inunction, and suppository.

Oral ingestion is the most common method for taking drugs and includes tablets, capsules, and liquids that we swallow. Oral ingestion generally results in relatively slow absorption because the drug must pass through the stomach, where it is acted on by digestive juices, and then moves on to the small intestine before it enters the bloodstream. Alcohol is an exception since the majority of it is absorbed into the bloodstream without digestion.

Many oral preparations that can irritate the stomach are coated to keep them from being dissolved by corrosive stomach acids before they reach the intestine and, in this way, protect the stomach lining from irritation. When your stomach contains food, drug absorption is slower than when your stomach is empty. Some drugs should not be taken with certain foods because they inhibit the drug's action (discussed later). Other drugs are recommended to be taken with food to prevent stomach irritation.

Injection, another common method of taking a drug, involves the use of a hypodermic syringe. This method

Recreational drugs Drugs that people use to relax or socialize during their recreational time.

Over-the-counter (OTC) drugs Drugs that can be purchased without a physician's prescription.

Herbal preparations Substances of plant origin believed to have medicinal properties.

Illicit drugs Drugs whose use, possession, cultivation, manufacture, and/or sale are illegal.

Commercial preparations Commonly used chemical substances with a drug action, such as cosmetics, household cleaning products, and industrial by-products.

Routes of administration The manner in which a drug is taken into the body.

Oral ingestion Intake of drugs through the mouth.

Injection The introduction of drugs into the body via a hypodermic needle.

usually results in rapid absorption, the rapidity of which depends on the type of injection. **Intravenous injection**, or injection directly into a vein, puts the drug in its most concentrated form directly into the bloodstream. In this way, the effects of the drug will be felt within three minutes—this route is extremely effective, particularly in medical emergencies. However, there is risk of serious or even fatal reactions as a result of this effective and efficient method of drug administration. For example, when illicit drugs are injected, the risk of overdose is particularly high, since the administrator or user may not be able to effectively control the dose and, once injected, the effects cannot be slowed (Kerr et al., 2007). In addition, some serious diseases, such as hepatitis and HIV infection, can be transmitted through needle use. For these reasons, intravenous injection is also one of the most dangerous routes of administration. **Intramuscular injection** results in much slower absorption of the drug than by intravenous injection. This type of injection places the hypodermic needle into muscular tissue, usually in the buttocks or in the triceps on the back of the upper arm. Normally used to administer antibiotics and vaccinations, this route of administration ensures a slow and consistent dispersion of the drug into the body tissues. **Subcutaneous injection** puts the drug into the layer of fat directly beneath the skin. Its common medical uses are for administration of local anesthetics and for insulin replacement therapy. A drug injected subcutaneously will circulate even more slowly than an intramuscularly injected drug because it takes longer to be absorbed into the bloodstream.

Inhalation refers to the ingestion of drugs through the nostrils. This method transfers the drug rapidly into the bloodstream through the alveoli (air sacs) in the lungs. Some examples of inhalation include nasal sprays, and the inhalation of aerosol sprays, gases, or fumes from solvents. The drug effects are usually felt immediately after inhalation and do not last long because only small amounts can be absorbed and metabolized in the lungs. A risk with this type of drug administration, particularly when sprays,

gases, and solvents are inhaled, is that the amount of drug consumed is not known and the risk for overdose is great.

Inunction introduces drugs into the body through the skin. Common examples include the small adhesive patches used to alleviate motion sickness or nicotine patches used to assist individuals when they stop smoking (see Chapter 10). These patches slowly release their chemicals for a consistent dispersal of drug so that the drug's effects are long-lasting. Rubbing ointments and oils on skin is also another way to introduce drugs into the body.

Suppositories are drugs mixed with a waxy medium designed to melt at body temperature. Most suppositories are inserted into the anus past the rectal sphincter muscles. As the wax melts, the drug is released and absorbed through the rectal walls into the bloodstream. Since there are many blood vessels in this area of the body, the effects of the drug are usually felt within 15 minutes. Other suppositories are inserted in the vagina. These drugs usually contain antifungal agents to treat problems in the vagina itself as opposed to drugs meant to travel in the bloodstream to treat another health issue.

Although not involving a waxy substance to be dissolved, also in this category are alcohol enemas (butt chugging) and vodka tampons (slimming) (Boynton Health, 2016). As the name implies, an alcohol enema involves pouring alcohol directly into the anus—usually through a tube—for quick absorption into the bloodstream via the abundant vasculature of the rectum (CNN Health, 2012). Vodka (or another type of alcohol)-soaked tampons are inserted vaginally, and again because of the vascularity of the area, the alcohol is rapidly absorbed (Go Ask Alice, n.d.). More details on these two types of alcohol consumption are included in Chapter 10.

DRUG INTERACTIONS

Most people are not aware of the risks of taking several drugs simultaneously. In fact, often little thought is given to the various drugs taken, whether over-the-counter, prescription, or recreational. The most dangerous interactions are synergism, antagonism, inhibition, and intolerance. Other negative interactions can occur when certain drugs and nutrients are consumed together.

Synergism, also known as potentiation, is an interaction of two or more drugs in which the effects of the individual drugs are multiplied beyond what is normally expected. Synergism can be expressed

Intravenous injection The introduction of drugs directly using a hypodermic needle into a vein.

Intramuscular injection The introduction of drugs directly into a muscle using a hypodermic needle.

Subcutaneous injection The introduction of drugs into the layer of fat directly beneath the skin using a hypodermic needle.

Inhalation The introduction of drugs through the nostrils.

Inunction The introduction of drugs through the skin.

Suppositories Mixtures of drugs and a waxy medium where the drug is slowly released when the wax melts in the vascular regions of the anus or vagina.

Synergism An interaction of two or more drugs in which the effects of the individual drugs are magnified beyond what is expected of their individual contribution.

mathematically as 2 + 2 = 10. A synergistic interaction is most likely to occur when central nervous system depressants such as alcohol, opiates (morphine, heroin), antihistamines (cold remedies), sedative hypnotics (Quaaludes), minor tranquillizers (Valium, Librium, and Xanax), and barbiturates are combined. The worst possible combination is alcohol and barbiturates (sleeping preparations such as Seconal and phenobarbital) because the combination leads to a slowdown of the brain centres that normally control vital functions. Respiration, heart rate, and blood pressure can drop to the point of inducing coma or death.

Prescription drugs carry special labels warning their users of potential drug interactions. Many OTC preparations carry similar warning labels. Because the dangers associated with synergism are so great, you should always check for possible drug interactions before using a prescribed, herbal, or OTC drug. You should also consider synergistic actions when consuming recreational drugs with or without prescription and/or OTC drugs. Pharmacists, physicians, drug information centres, nurse practitioners, naturopathic doctors, or community drug education centres can answer your questions. Even if one of the drugs in question is an illegal substance, you should still try to determine the dangers involved in combining it with other drugs. Health-care professionals are legally bound to maintain confidentiality even when they know that a client is using illegal substances.

Antagonism, or opposition, although not usually as serious as synergism, can produce unwanted and unpleasant effects. In an antagonistic reaction, one drug blocks the action of the other at the receptor site. The "blocking" drug occupies the receptor site, preventing the second drug from attaching, and this alters its absorption and action. An example of this is when nonsteroidal anti-inflammatory drugs (NSAIDs) such as ibuprofen and Aspirin are taken at the same time as a thiazide diuretic, resulting in reduced antihypertensive effects of the diuretic (Pharmainfo.net, n.d.).

Inhibition is a type of interaction in which the effects of one drug are eliminated or reduced by the presence of another drug, again due to interaction at the receptor site. A common inhibitory reaction occurs between antacid tablets and Aspirin. Antacids inhibit the absorption of Aspirin, resulting in less effective pain relief. Other inhibitory reactions occur between alcohol and contraceptive pills and between antibiotics and contraceptive pills. Specifically, alcohol and antibiotics diminish the effectiveness of birth control pills in some women.

Intolerance occurs when drugs combine in the body, resulting in extremely uncomfortable reactions.

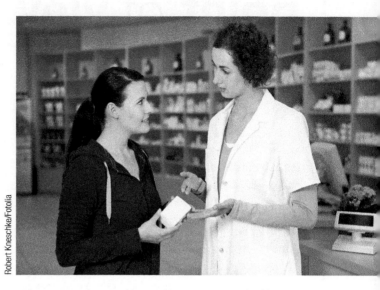

Whenever you take more than one drug at a time, you should consider how they will interact. For example, women who take oral contraceptives should strictly follow the dosage instructions and be aware that medicines such as penicillin can alter the contraceptive's effectiveness. Asking a pharmacist or other health-care practitioners is an effective way to learn about drug interactions.

The drug Antabuse, used to help individuals addicted to alcohol to give it up, works using this type of interaction. It binds liver enzymes (the chemicals the liver produces to break down alcohol), making it impossible for the body to metabolize alcohol. As a result, if the user of Antabuse drinks alcohol, he or she experiences nausea, vomiting, and, occasionally, fever.

Cross-tolerance occurs when a person develops a physiological tolerance to one drug and, as a result, a similar tolerance to other drugs with similar effects (Guzman, 2013). For example, cross-tolerance can develop between alcohol and barbiturates, two depressant drugs.

In addition to the various drug interactions noted above, there is the potential for drug nutrient interactions and drug–herbal preparation interactions. Drug–nutrient interactions are defined as physical, chemical, physiologic, or pathophysiologic relationships between a drug and a nutrient (Chan, 2013) and can cause serious health issues, particularly for geriatric patients. An example of a concerning drug herbal interaction is the combined intake of ginseng and caffeine where there is a synergistic stimulant effect (Kuhn, 2002).

Antagonism A type of interaction in which one drug blocks the action of another at the receptor site.

Inhibition A type of interaction in which the effects of one drug are eliminated or reduced by the presence of another drug at the receptor site.

Intolerance A type of interaction in which two or more drugs taken together produce extremely uncomfortable reactions.

Cross-tolerance The development of a tolerance to one drug that carries over to another similar drug.

point of view

FLU SHOT: Should you get one?

Each fall, as flu season approaches, you likely are aware of the many flu-shot clinics in your community, and potentially on your campus as well. Given the number of students living in your residence, as well as the number of students, faculty, and staff you are in contact with on a daily basis, should you be immunized? Before you make the decision as to whether or not you get a flu shot, you should learn more about it, including the risks and benefits.

Unlike other immunizations, such as the MMR (measles, mumps, and rubella) which boasts a near 100 percent success rate in preventing measles,

mumps, and rubella in children who receive two doses, the flu vaccination is less than 60 percent effective for healthy adults between the ages of 18 and 59 years. In fact, the efficacy rate of the flu shot fluctuates from year to year as each year a new vaccination is created to combat particular strains of the flu. Choosing which strains to include is complex and may not be on track; thus, a vaccination can be created for flus that may not be experienced that year and may miss coverage for what does become the most prevalent flu.

Are you in favour of the flu shot or against it?

IN FAVOUR

○ Of course I would get a flu shot—any reduction in the risk of missing school or work or potentially becoming seriously ill, even by only half, is worth my time and effort.

○ Of course I would get a flu shot—it reduces my risk of spreading the flu to people in the high risk category (under the age of 5, older adults, or people with compromised immune systems) who have a higher chance of dying or having permanent health effects if infected with the flu.

AGAINST

○ I don't get a flu shot—since I am not in the high risk category (under the age of 5, older adult [65+], or with a compromised immune system), I do not need it.

○ I don't get a flu shot—I would rather build my immune system the natural way, so I do not want one.

Sources: Based on Branswell, H. (2013). Doctor stirs debate over mandatory flu shots, *The Canadian Press*, Retrieved on May 9, 2013 from http://www.theglobeandmail.com/life/health-and-fitness/health/conditions/doctor-stirs-debate-over-mandatory-flu-shots/article10322395/. Gardam, M. & Lemieux, C. (2013). Mandatory influenza vaccination?

First we need a better vaccine CMAJ cmaj.122074; published ahead of print March 25, 2013. Weeks, C, If the flu shot is only 50-50, do we really need it? *The Globe & Mail*, Retrieved on May 9, 2013 from http://www.theglobeandmail.com/life/health-and-fitness/health/if-the-flu-shot-is-only-50-50-do-we-really-need-it/article7882154/.

PRESCRIPTION DRUGS

Even though prescription drugs are recommended (i.e., prescribed) under medical supervision, their misuse is one of the leading public health and safety issues in Canada (Canadian Centre on Substance Abuse [CCSA], 2013). In the March 27, 2013, press release for the comprehensive 10-year, pan-Canadian strategy, "First Do No Harm: Responding to Canada's Prescription Drug Crisis," Michel Perron, Chief

Executive Officer, CCSA and National Advisory Council Co-Chair, stated:

"Harms such as addiction, overdose, and death associated with certain prescription drugs—opioids, sedatives and tranquilizers, and stimulants—are a leading public health and safety concern in Canada that has now reached crisis proportions" (CCSA, 2013).

Complications and serious negative health consequences arising from the use and misuse of prescription drugs are common. For you to make appropriate decisions regarding your prescription drug use requires basic drug knowledge.

Types of Prescription Drugs

Antibiotics are drugs used to fight bacterial infection. Bacterial infections continue to be among the most common serious diseases in the world, with the vast majority cured by antibiotics. There are almost 100 different antibiotics available, dispensed by intramuscular or intravenous injection or in tablet or capsule form. Some, called broad-spectrum antibiotics, are designed to control diseases caused by a number of bacterial species. These medications may also kill off helpful bacteria in the body, thus triggering secondary infections. For example, some vaginal infections are related to long-term use of antibiotics. Further, it is believed that the misuse of antibiotics has led to an increase in drug-resistant bacteria. Thus, as resistance occurs, practitioners are advised to use discretion in prescribing.

Sedatives are central nervous system depressants that induce sleep and relieve anxiety. Used heavily in the 1950s and 1960s in the form of phenobarbital or Seconal, they gradually fell out of favour because of the risks involved, including a high potential for addiction. Detoxification can be life-threatening and must be medically supervised. In recent years, different types of sedatives, such as diazepam (Valium) and lorazepam (Ativan), with fewer side effects have been developed and, thus, are more commonly used today.

Tranquillizers are another form of central nervous system depressant. They are classified either as major or minor tranquillizers. The most powerful tranquillizers are used in the treatment of major psychiatric illnesses. When used appropriately, these strong sedatives are capable of reducing violent aggressiveness and self-destructive impulses. About 5 percent of Canadians aged 15 and older report using sleeping pills, and 5 percent report using tranquillizers (Turner, MacDonald, & Somerset, 2007). Women and older Canadians are more likely to report using these medications (The Annenburg Public Policy Center, 2005).

Antidepressants are powerful substances used to treat clinically diagnosed cases of depression. These drugs inhibit the release of certain neurotransmitters in the brain, thereby moderating the user's mood.

Amphetamines are stimulants prescribed less commonly now than in the past. Like other psychoactive drugs, they can be purchased legally and illegally. Amphetamines suppress appetite and elevate respiration, blood pressure, and pulse rate. These drugs are often prescribed to treat ADHD. Unfortunately, however, amphetamines are abused and used for recreation, particularity among teens and young adults. Tolerance to these powerful stimulants develops rapidly, and the user trying to cut down or quit may experience unpleasant **rebound effects**. These severe withdrawal symptoms, peculiar to stimulants, include depression, irritability, violent behaviours, headaches, nausea, and deep fatigue.

Analgesics are pain relievers that are available as prescription and OTC drugs. More details about how analgesics work is presented later in this text. A common prescription analgesic is OxyContin, or more recently Oxyneo. OxyContin is the trade name for the long-lasting form of the prescription opioid analgesic (pain reliever) oxycodone (Centre for Addiction and Mental Health, 2004). Oxycodone is also an ingredient in Percocet and Percodan, though OxyContin contains much higher doses—10 to 80 mg. OxyContin is specially formulated for slow release and, as such, is intended to provide relief from moderate to severe pain for up to 12 hours. Individuals prescribed OxyContin swallow one tablet twice daily. Although most users take this medication appropriately, they should be monitored closely because of their high risk of dependency (Centre for Addiction and Mental Health, 2004).

How is OxyContin abused? OxyContin is formulated to be swallowed whole to provide slow release into the bloodstream; however, when it is chewed or crushed, the slow release properties are destroyed (Centre for Addiction and Mental Health, 2004). Thus, when users chew or crush tablets, the oxycodone effects occur very rapidly, causing a high or euphoria described as similar to the high from heroin. So, a method of misuse that can lead to abuse is taking OxyContin in ways other than as prescribed.

Oxycodone is a potent opioid. When large amounts of oxycodone are released into the body all at once (whether chewed, snorted, or injected), there is a high risk of overdose and death, similar to a heroin overdose (Centre for Addiction and Mental Health, 2004). Symptoms of overdose include laboured or slow breathing, extreme somnolence progressing to coma, cardiac arrest, and death.

OxyContin users who inject the drug have the additional risks associated with sharing needles (e.g., hepatitis and HIV).

Addiction is also a problem—tolerance develops quickly, so the user requires larger and larger doses to achieve the desired effect (Centre for Addiction and Mental Health, 2004). Eventually, the drug is needed to simply prevent feeling sick. Withdrawal symptoms include

Antibiotics Prescription drugs designed to fight bacterial infection.

Sedatives Central nervous system depressants that induce sleep and relieve anxiety.

Tranquillizers Drugs taken to relax the body and relieve anxiety.

Antidepressants Drugs used to treat clinically diagnosed depression.

Amphetamines Drugs that suppress appetite and increase breathing rate, blood pressure, and heart rate.

Rebound effects Severe withdrawal effects, including depression, nausea, and violent behaviours.

Analgesics Pain relievers.

muscle aches, nausea, diarrhea, loss of appetite, restlessness, insomnia, runny nose, teary eyes, and sweating.

Use of Generic Drugs

Generic drugs are sold under a chemical name rather than a brand name. These alternatives to more expensive brand-name drugs contain the same active ingredients and should theoretically have the same main effect. There is, however, some controversy about the effectiveness of some generic drugs. Differences in minor ingredients can affect the way the drug is absorbed, which may cause discomfort or an allergic reaction in some users. If you experience any allergic reactions to a prescribed generic drug, tell your pharmacist or doctor, who can recommend an alternative drug. A list of medicines that can be interchanged has been approved in Canada. If your doctor or pharmacist fails to offer you the option of using a generic drug, you should ask if such a substitute exists and if it would be safe for you to use it.

OVER-THE-COUNTER (OTC) DRUGS

Over-the-counter (OTC) drugs are nonprescription drugs used in self-diagnosis and self-medication. Altogether, Canadians spend many millions of dollars yearly, around $141 per capita, on OTC preparations for relief of everything from runny noses to ingrown toenails (Canadian Institute for Health Information, 2012). Most OTC drugs are manufactured from a basic group of 1000 chemicals with combinations of as few as 2 and as many as 10 of these chemicals resulting in the many different types available today. Perhaps because of the common belief that OTC products are safe and effective, indiscriminate use, misuse, and abuse often occur. OTC drugs, like any other drugs, have the potential to produce dependency, tolerance, and addiction, as well as adverse toxic and other potentially negative reactions.

Generic drugs Drugs marketed by their chemical name rather than a brand name.

Prostaglandin inhibitors Drugs that inhibit the production and release of prostaglandins where prostaglandins are released by the body in response to pain.

Types of OTC Drugs

Analgesics

Analgesics are pain relievers. The earliest pain relievers were made of derivatives manufactured from the opium poppy. Today, pain relievers, ranging from Aspirin to dilaudid or morphine, are among the most commonly used drugs. In fact, most Canadians when surveyed said they had taken pain relievers in the past month (Single et al., 2000). Although pain relievers come in several forms, the most common are Aspirin, acetaminophen (Tylenol, Pamprin, Pandol), ibuprofen (Advil, Motrin, Nuprin), and ibuprofen-like drugs such as naproxen sodium (Aleve, Anaprox) and ketoprofen (Orudis).

Most pain relievers work at the receptor sites by interrupting pain signals. Some are categorized as nonsteroidal anti-inflammatory drugs (NSAIDs), also called **prostaglandin inhibitors**. Prostaglandins are chemicals that resemble hormones and are released by the body in response to pain. Scientists propose that the additional pain caused by the release of prostaglandins signals the body to begin the healing process. Prostaglandin inhibitors restrain the release of prostaglandins, thereby reducing the pain. Common NSAIDs include ibuprofen, naproxen sodium, and Aspirin.

Acetylsalicylic acid (ASA), commonly known as Aspirin, relieves pain by inhibiting the body's production of prostaglandins. It brings down fever by increasing the flow of blood to the skin's surface, which causes sweating and therefore cooling of the body. ASA is also commonly used to reduce the inflammation and swelling of arthritis. Furthermore, ASA's anticoagulant (interference with blood clotting) effects make it a useful daily medication for reducing the risk of heart attacks, but should be taken under the supervision of a primary care practitioner.

Acetaminophen is the active ingredient found in Tylenol and related medications, including muscle relaxants such as robaxacet. Like ASA, acetaminophen is an effective analgesic and antipyretic (fever-reducing) drug. It does not, however, provide relief from inflamed or swollen joints. The side effects associated with acetaminophen are generally minimal, though overdose can cause liver damage.

Most analgesics have side effects, the most common of which is drowsiness due to the depression of the central nervous system. It is important to read the label warnings. Some warnings caution specifically against driving or operating heavy machinery when using analgesics, and most state they should not be taken with alcohol. Specific to ASA, possible side effects include allergic reactions, ringing in the ears, stomach bleeding, and ulcers. Since research has linked ASA to the potentially fatal condition Reye's syndrome, children, teenagers, and young adults (up to age 25) who are at risk for developing this syndrome are recommended to use an alternative analgesic.

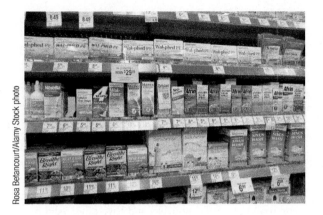

Read the labels of any drug you choose to take to relieve symptoms for your cough or cold to be sure that you chose the best product for your symptoms.

Cold, Cough, Allergy, and Asthma Relievers

Likely the most popular OTC drugs are those intended to provide relief of the symptoms of coughs, colds, allergies, and asthma that affect millions of people each year. The operative word in their titles is *reliever*. Most of these drugs are designed to alleviate or reduce some or all of the discomforting symptoms associated with upper-respiratory-tract maladies. Unfortunately, no drug exists to actually cure coughs, colds, allergies, or asthma. The drugs available provide temporary relief until the sufferer's immune system prevails. Aspirin or acetaminophen are often included in cold preparations. The basic types of OTC cold, cough, and allergy relievers are

- **Expectorants.** These drugs are formulated to loosen phlegm, allowing the user to cough and clear congested respiratory passages.

- **Antitussives.** These drugs are designed to calm or curtail the cough reflex. They are most effective when the cough is "dry," and does not produce phlegm (for which an expectorant is required).

- **Antihistamines.** These drugs are central nervous system depressants that dry runny noses, clear post-nasal drip and sinus congestion, and reduce tears.

- **Decongestants.** These drugs are designed to reduce nasal stuffiness due to colds.

- **Anticholinergics.** These drugs are often added to cold preparations to reduce nasal secretions and tears.

It is important for you to read the labels of cough, cold, allergy, and asthma relievers for a number of reasons. First, some cold compounds contain alcohol in concentrations that can exceed 40 percent, while others contain a lot of sugar. Equally important to consider are the various drugs included and the potential interactions likely to result. For example, many cough and cold medications contain expectorants or antitussives, which means conflicting actions could result in the body if you mix them (e.g., phlegm loosened to be coughed and cleared combined with a curtailed or reduced cough reflex), and you will receive little, if any, relief from your symptoms. The common cold is an interesting health issue to treat—there is a saying that it takes one week to get over a cold when medicated, and seven days when not. In other words, the cold bug has to work its way through the body. This does not mean that you should not take medication, but rather recognize that the medication you take will relieve the symptoms, not cure the cold.

Stimulants

Nonprescription stimulants are sometimes used by students in college or university in the last minute panic to complete assignments or in "all-nighter" study sessions. The active ingredient in most OTC

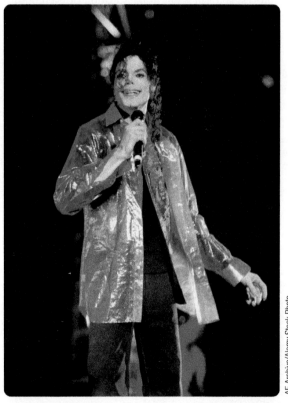

Abusing prescription drugs is no safer than abusing illicit drugs, as tragically demonstrated by the 2010 death of pop star Michael Jackson, whose death ultimately stemmed from his abuse of numerous prescription medications.

stimulants is caffeine. Although caffeine heightens wakefulness, increases alertness, and relieves fatigue, it also can result in increased nervousness, irritability, anxiety, and involuntary muscle twitches (see Chapter 10). Other drinks with similar properties, also mentioned in Chapter 10, are energy drinks; these too contain caffeine and other drugs and are used to provide energy when needed.

Sleeping Aids and Relaxants

These drugs are often used to induce the drowsy feelings that precede sleep. The principal ingredient is an antihistamine called pyrilamine maleate. Chronic reliance on sleeping aids can lead to addiction.

Dieting Aids

Some people use **laxatives** or **diuretics** ("water pills") to achieve weight loss. Since laxatives were designed to relieve constipation, their use to reduce body weight is considered drug misuse. There are health risks associated with the use of laxatives and diuretics. Frequent use of laxatives disrupts the body's natural elimination process and can result in constipation or even obstipation (inability to have a bowel movement). In addition to being inefficient in producing weight loss, laxatives deplete the body of needed fluids, salts, and minerals. Further, the user of laxatives gains the lost weight back upon drinking fluids, and may have created dangerous chemical imbalances with the elimination of potassium and sodium, which have important roles in maintaining electrolyte balance and supporting cardiac functioning. Depletion of these vital minerals can cause weakness, dizziness, fatigue, and sometimes death.

Laxatives Drugs used to soften stool and relieve constipation.

Diuretics Drugs that increase the excretion of urine from the body.

Inhalants Products sniffed or inhaled in order to produce highs.

Inhalants

Inhalants are chemicals that produce vapours. When inhaled, these chemicals or drugs cause hallucinations, as well as intoxicating and euphoric effects. Inhalants are not commonly recognized as drugs. They are legal to purchase, universally available, and have other valid purposes, but are potentially dangerous when used incorrectly. These drugs and the high that results from their use often appeal to those who cannot afford illicit substances.

Included in this category are organic solvents resulting from the distillation of petroleum products (e.g., rubber cement, model glue, paint thinner, lighter fluid, varnish, wax, spot removers, and gasoline). Most of these substances are sniffed by users. Because they are inhaled, the volatile chemicals in these products reach the bloodstream within seconds. This inhaled substance is not diluted or buffered by stomach acids or other body fluids and thus is more potent and dangerous than the same substance would be if swallowed. This characteristic, along with the fact that dosages are extremely difficult to control because everyone has unique lung and breathing capacities, makes inhalants particularly dangerous. An overdose of fumes can result in unconsciousness. If the user's oxygen intake is reduced during the inhaling process, death can result within five minutes. Further, accidental overdosing can occur from inadvertently mixing regular household chemicals; therefore, it is strongly advised to read all product labels.

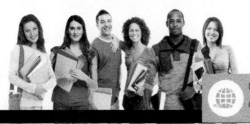

assess YOURSELF

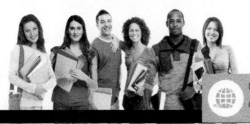
Go to MasteringHealth to complete this questionnaire with automatic scoring

TAKING CHARGE: Managing Drug Use and Potentially Addictive Behaviours

After reading this chapter, you should know that addictions produce devastating effects not only on the user, but also on the user's family and friends. Addictions usually, but not always, progress gradually, and it is difficult to know when a person crosses the line from habit to addiction. Keep in mind that drug use is problematic when it results in negative personal, social, financial, work- or study-related consequences. If you continue to use a drug despite the negative consequences you or others are experiencing as a result, chances are that you are addicted to it. Similarly, a particular behaviour that, when engaged in, results in negative consequences and symptoms of withdrawal when no longer engaged in is one that you are addicted to and treatment will be required to manage that behaviour in a more healthy way. Review (and complete) the questionnaires that follow to determine whether or not you may be addicted to alcohol or drugs.

The following three tests can be used to determine if you are addicted to alcohol (The CAGE Test and the AUDIT Test) or drugs (The Modified CAGE Test) (Babor et al., 1993). For the first two tests, you simply answer yes or no. Be honest as you review the questions.

The CAGE Test for Alcohol Addiction

1. Have you ever felt you should **C**ut down on your drinking?
2. Have you ever been **A**nnoyed when people have commented on your drinking?
3. Have you ever felt **G**uilty or badly about your drinking?
4. Have you ever had an **E**ye opener first thing in the morning to steady your nerves or get rid of a hangover?

Your Score

Score one point for each yes answer.

If you scored 1, there is an 80 percent chance you're addicted to alcohol.

If you scored 2, there is an 89 percent chance you're addicted to alcohol.

If you scored 3, there is a 99 percent chance you're addicted to alcohol.

If you scored 4, there is a 100 percent chance you're addicted to alcohol.

The Modified CAGE Test for All Addictions

Most self-test questionnaires apply to alcohol addiction, but can be easily adapted to any addiction.

1. Have you ever felt you should **C**ut down your use of drugs?
2. Have you ever been **A**nnoyed when people have commented on your use?
3. Have you ever felt **G**uilty or badly about your use?
4. Have you ever used drugs to **E**ase withdrawal symptoms, or to avoid feeling low after using?

Your Score

Score one point for each yes answer.

If you scored 1, there is an 80 percent chance you're addicted to a drug.

If you scored 2, there is an 89 percent chance you're addicted to a drug.

If you scored 3, there is a 99 percent chance you're addicted to a drug.

If you scored 4, there is a 100 percent chance you're addicted to a drug.

The AUDIT Test for Alcohol Addiction (Alcoholism)

To correctly answer some of these questions you need to know the definition of a drink. For this test one drink is:

One can of beer (12 oz or approx 330 mL of 5% alcohol), or

One glass of wine (5 oz or approx 140 mL of 12% alcohol), or

One shot of liquor (1.5 oz or approx 40 mL of 40% alcohol).

(continued)

1. How often do you have a drink containing alcohol?

   Never (score 0)
   Monthly or less (score 1)
   2–4 times a month (score 2)
   2–3 times a week (score 3)
   4 or more times a week (score 4)
2. How many alcoholic drinks do you have on a typical day when you are drinking?
   1 or 2 (0)
   3 or 4 (1)
   5 or 6 (2)
   7 to 9 (3)
   10 or more (4)
3. How often do you have six or more drinks on one occasion?
   Never (0)
   Less than monthly (1)
   Monthly (2)
   Weekly (3)
   Daily or almost daily (4)
4. How often during the past year have you found that you drank more or for a longer time than you intended?
   Never (0)
   Less than monthly (1)
   Monthly (2)
   Weekly (3)
   Daily or almost daily (4)
5. How often during the past year have you failed to do what was normally expected of you because of your drinking?
   Never (0)
   Less than monthly (1)
   Monthly (2)
   Weekly (3)
   Daily or almost daily (4)
6. How often during the past year have you had a drink in the morning to get yourself going after a heavy drinking session?
   Never (0)
   Less than monthly (1)
   Monthly (2)
   Weekly (3)
   Daily or almost daily (4)
7. How often during the past year have you felt guilty or remorseful after drinking?
   Never (0)
   Less than monthly (1)
   Monthly (2)
   Weekly (3)
   Daily or almost daily (4)
8. How often during the past year have you been unable to remember what happened the night before because of your drinking?
   Never (0)
   Less than monthly (1)
   Monthly (2)
   Weekly (3)
   Daily or almost daily (4)
9. Have you or anyone else been injured as a result of your drinking?
   No (0)
   Yes, but not in the past year (2)
   Yes, during the past year (4)
10. Has a relative, friend, doctor, or health-care worker been concerned about your drinking, or suggested that you cut down?
   No (0)
   Yes, but not in the past year (2)
   Yes, during the past year (4)

Your Score

If you scored 8–10 or more, you are probably addicted to alcohol.

It may seem like the AUDIT questionnaire is an easy test to fail. If you applied this test to other aspects of your life you will almost certainly come up as being addicted to something. For example, most people watch too much television or eat too much of their favourite food. But those are so-called "soft addictions" and the AUDIT questionnaire was not designed to assess them. It is extremely reliable when it comes to assessing alcohol addiction.

The AUDIT (Alcohol Use Disorders Identification Test) was developed by the World Health Organization (WHO). The test correctly classifies 95 percent of people into either alcoholics or non-alcoholics. It was tested on 2000 people before being published.

(The pdf format version of the AUDIT is available through the WHO website. Copyright © 1993 World Health Organization.)

Source: Reprint from *The Alcohol Use Disorders Identification Test*, 2nd ed., by Thomas F. Babor, John C. Higgins, John B. Saunders, Maristela G. Monteiro. © 2001.

Making Decisions for You

At one time or another you will use prescription or OTC drugs to restore or maintain your health. How can you be certain that you need a drug in the first place, that you are taking the right drug for you, and that your drug is not robbing you of vital nutrients or being rendered ineffective by other drugs you are taking or foods you are ingesting? You can only be sure by asking the right questions of the right people. Listed below are questions to pose to your physician, your pharmacist, or yourself before you take any drug.

1. What is your diagnosis?
2. Is your physician or pharmacist aware of all the other drugs you take, including prescription drugs (counting birth control pills), over-the-counter drugs, recreational drugs, and others?
3. Do you know the name of the drug you are taking? Is it the chemical name, a generic name, or a brand name? Are you able to take a generic version of the drug?
4. Are you certain of how often you should take the drug, for how long you should take it, and in what dosage?
5. Do you know when your drug should be taken in relation to food intake?
6. Do you know if you can drink alcohol while on your drug?
7. If taking oral contraceptives, do you know if the drug will influence the effectiveness of your oral contraceptive? Are you aware of reduced effectiveness when taken with some analgesics and alcohol? Do you protect yourself from pregnancy accordingly?
8. What are the known side effects of the drug? What should you do if you experience any of the side effects?
9. Can you stop taking your drug when you start feeling better, or should you continue to take the drug until the prescription is finished?
10. Do you know what you should do if you forget to take your drugs at the scheduled time?
11. Do you know what signs and symptoms signal that you are allergic to the drug?
12. Do you know how and where to store your drug?
13. Are there any drug–nutrient interactions that you should be aware of?
14. Are there any potential drug interactions that you should be aware of?
15. Are there any adverse consequences of long-term use of the medication?

Critical Thinking

You have a major term paper due in three days, and you just completed the reading for it. You are worried about how you will get it done, and realize you may have to pull an all-nighter. If you don't get at least a B, you will lose your academic scholarship and be forced to leave school. A friend tells you that last semester she consumed energy drinks to help her stay awake and to stimulate her thinking. She got an A– on the paper and experienced no side effects. She suggests you try them, too.

Using the DECIDE model described in Chapter 1, how will you keep yourself awake to finish your paper? Will you take an energy drink? What is the best approach for you to handle this situation?

DISCUSSION QUESTIONS

1. How does an addiction develop? Is it possible to gauge your drug use (quantity and frequency) and behaviours to prevent becoming addicted?

2. How does the set and setting influence a person's response to drugs and potentially addictive behaviours? What environmental factors influence the main effects and side-effects of psychoactive drugs?

3. How do analgesics work? Are they all equally effective and interchangeable for various maladies?

4. What general precautions should OTC drug users consider?

5. Create three health promotional 'items' regarding drug misuse and abuse aimed at primary, junior, or secondary school children. Think about what messages would have reached you at those particular age levels.

6. Design an interactive webpage that clearly describes drug use, misuse, and abuse relevant to students in your community.

APPLICATION EXERCISE

Reread the "Consider This . . ." scenario at the beginning of the chapter and answer the following questions.

1. Why is it drug misuse for Tracey to consume Laken's prescription?

2. Why is it drug misuse for Laken to not complete her prescription?

3. Do you think prescription drugs are often shared? Why or why not? What about OTCs?

MASTERINGHEALTH

Go to MasteringHealth for assignments, the eText, and the study Area with case studies, self-quizzing, and videos.

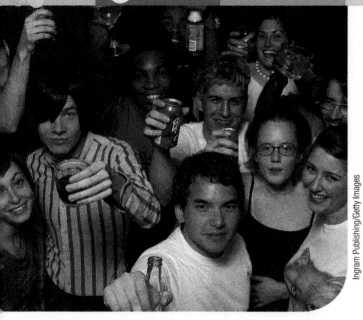

Ingram Publishing/Getty Images

CHAPTER 10

USING ALCOHOL AND CAFFEINE RESPONSIBLY AND REFRAINING FROM TOBACCO USE

◀️◉ CONSIDER THIS ...

Landyn, a second-year student, is celebrating the completion of first-term exams with her friends. Prior to going out to the bar, she and her friends are playing some drinking games. Considerable quantities of alcohol are consumed. Landyn and her friends call for a taxi to take them from home to the bar. While waiting, everyone gathers for a couple of shots. The drinking continues between periods of dancing—with Jägerbombs (an energy drink mixed with alcohol). When it is time to go home, Landyn and her friends are visibly drunk, incoherent, and having difficulty walking.

How typical is this scenario at your college or university? What risks are there for Landyn and her friends? What could they do differently to ensure their safety?

LEARNING OUTCOMES

- Describe the alcohol-use patterns of post-secondary students as well as the physiological and behavioural effects of alcohol consumption.

- Identify the short-term risks of binge drinking.

- Identify the social issues involved in tobacco use, including those surrounding smokeless tobacco.

- Explain the physiological short- and long-term effects of smoking.

- Compare the benefits and risks of caffeine consumption.

When you hear references to the dangers of drugs, what comes to mind? Usually the term *drugs* conjures images of derelict-looking individuals using cocaine, heroin, marijuana, LSD, PCP, or other illegal substances. Although people use the word *drugs* to refer to one set of dangerous substances, they often do not consider alcohol as a drug, primarily because its consumption is socially accepted and alcohol sales continue to boom in Canada. Similarly, tobacco and caffeine are seldom considered drugs, also likely because of their legality and acceptable use. Prescription and over-the-counter drugs are most often considered 'safe' for use with many people oblivious to the potential for drug interactions (see Chapter 9) and the consequences or risks of multiple drug use.

ALCOHOL: AN OVERVIEW

Most of us think of alcohol the way it is portrayed in ads or in the movies—a way of having fun while socializing and an important adjunct to a romantic dinner or a cozy evening in front of the fireplace. Moderate use of alcohol can be part of celebrations or special times without health risk. In fact, research shows that low levels of alcohol consumption may actually reduce some health risks. Still, alcohol is a drug that affects your physical and emotional behaviours. Further, the tragedies associated with alcohol receive far less attention than cocaine-related deaths, drug busts, and efforts to eradicate marijuana crops. Nevertheless, these tragedies are far more common—with potentially devastating effects on people of all ages.

In 2013, 80 percent of Canadians reported drinking alcohol in the past year, a rate similar to that reported in 2011 (78.0 percent) (Public Health Agency of Canada, 2016). There was, however, a decrease in past-year alcohol use among youth 15 to 24 years of age compared to 2004, from 82.9 to 70.0 percent in 2012. Similar to previous years higher percentage of males than females reported past-year alcohol use (82.7 percent versus 74.4 percent, respectively). (Health Canada, 2013)

According to Canada's Low Risk Drinking Guidelines (Canadian Centre on Substance Abuse, n.d.):

Low-risk drinking Guideline 1 (chronic)	People who drink within this guideline must drink "no more than 10 drinks a week for women, with no more than 2 drinks a day most days and 15 drinks a week for men, with no more than 3 drinks a day most days. Plan non-drinking days every week to avoid developing a habit."

Low-risk drinking Guideline 2 (acute)	Those who drink within this guideline do so by "drinking no more than 3 drinks (for women) or 4 drinks (for men) on any single occasion. Plan to drink in a safe environment. Stay within the weekly limits outlined" in Guideline 1.
Special Occasions	Reduce your risk of injury and harm by drinking no more than 3 drinks (for women) or 4 drinks (for men) on any single occasion. Plan to drink in a safe environment. Stay within the weekly limits outlined above.

Among people who consumed alcohol in the past 12 months, 18.6 percent exceeded Guideline 1 for chronic effects and 12.8 percent exceeded Guideline 2 for acute effects. A higher percentage of males than females drank in patterns that exceeded both guidelines. The chronic-risk guideline (1) was exceeded by 21.2 percent of male drinkers and 15.9 percent of female drinkers, while the acute-risk guideline (2) was exceeded by 15.8 percent of male drinkers and 9.7 percent of female drinkers. The guidelines were exceeded by youth aged 15 to 24 years at higher rates than among adults aged 25 years and older. One in four (24.4 percent) youth drinkers versus 17.6 percent of adult drinkers exceeded the guideline for chronic risk, while the acute-risk guideline was exceeded by 17.9 percent of youth drinkers and 11.9 percent of adult drinkers (Health Canada, 2013).

Another way to look at consumption of alcohol in Canada is through the term *heavy drinkers*. For this research, a heavy drinker was classified as men who consumed five or more drinks and women who consumed four or more drinks per occasion at least once per month over the past year (Statistics Canada, 2013). The latest Canadian data indicated the highest rates for heavy drinking for males was among those aged 20 to 34 (37.1 percent). For females, the highest rates were among those aged 18 to 19 and 20 to 34. In the 18 to 19 age group, 27.0 percent of females reported heavy drinking, and in the 20 to 34 age group, the rate was 23.7 percent. Clearly, males are more likely to drink than females, with both greater frequency and in greater quantity.

Although not directly associated with consumption because it does not include homemade wine and beer, alcohol sales can provide another indication of drinking patterns in Canada. Canadians purchase a considerable amount of alcohol each year. In the fiscal year ending March 31, 2014, Canada's beer and liquor sales were $20.5 billion. This was up 1.1 percent from the previous year. (Statistics Canada, 2014a). Although beer continues to be the alcoholic drink of choice for most Canadians in volume and dollar value sold, more consumers are turning to wine.

Reports of alcohol sales from 2014 indicated that when total sales were considered, per capita sales were highest in the Northwest Territories and Nunavut ($1344.7), and the lowest per capita sales were found in Prince Edward Island ($563.4) (Statistics Canada, 2014a).

Alcohol can both benefit and harm you. Most scientific evidence about the benefit as well as the harm comes from industrialized countries such as Canada, cultures where alcohol consumption is largely accepted and where dietary intake, low levels of physical activity, and high levels of sedentary behaviour lend themselves to numerous chronic diseases. Moderate alcohol consumption reduces, in certain age groups, the risk of coronary heart disease and ischemic stroke. Low-risk drinking guidelines, as mentioned above, suggest consuming no more than 15 standard drinks for men or 10 standard drinks for women per week (Canadian Centre on Substance Abuse, n.d.). Despite the potential for individual health benefits from light and infrequent consumption of alcohol, the harm associated with the misuse and abuse of alcohol still constitutes a major public health problem in developed and developing countries.

Almost 10 percent of drinkers reported some sort of harm to themselves in the past year as a result of their drinking (Health Canada, 2008). Of these, 3 percent report negative effects on friendships and social life and 5.4 percent report negative effects to their physical health. More alarming is that 32.7 percent of the respondents to the Canadian Addiction Survey reported being harmed the past year because of someone else's drinking (Health Canada, 2008). Of these, 10 percent indicated family or marriage difficulties, 22.1 percent reported being insulted or humiliated, 15.5 percent indicated serious arguments or quarrels, 15.8 percent reported verbal abuse, 10.8 percent were pushed or shoved, and 3.2 percent were physically assaulted. Alcohol is a significant factor in hospital admissions, road deaths, industrial accidents, accidental drowning, homicide, and suicide (World Health Organization, 2011). The World Health Organization (2011) estimates that alcohol results in 2.5 million deaths per year worldwide. In 2002 it was determined that 4258 deaths in Canada were related to alcohol abuse, this accounted for 1.9 percent of all deaths (Rehm et al., 2006), and that 82 014 Canadians were hospitalized due to alcohol misuse (Single et al., 2000). Total costs of alcohol abuse in 2002 (the latest data available), when measured in terms of health care, law enforcement, loss of productivity in the work place and home, and premature death or disability, were estimated at $14.6 billion or 36.6 percent of the total costs for substance abuse (also includes tobacco and illicit drugs) (Rehm et al., 2006).

Alcohol and the Post-Secondary Student

Alcohol is the most widely used, misused, and abused recreational drug in our society. It is also the most popular drug on campuses. According to the Canadian Addictions Survey, more than 90 percent of 18- to

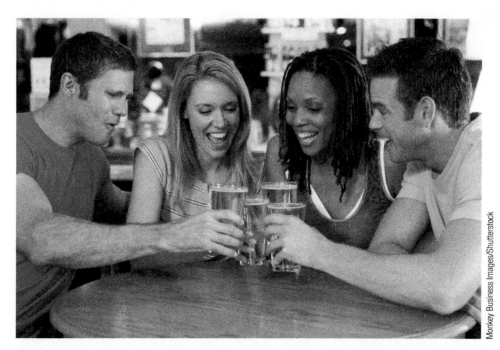

While alcohol has long been seen as a "social lubricant" by post-secondary students, alcohol abuse and associated behaviours continue to be serious problems on many campuses.

19-year-olds reported alcohol consumption in the past year (Health Canada, 2011).

University or college is a critical time to develop responsibility about your drinking. A number of social factors are involved in drinking at this stage of life and as part of the campus culture. There is little doubt that alcohol is a part of campus culture and tradition, with heavy drinking considered a problem on most Canadian campuses (Tamburri, 2012). Alcohol is often seen as a rite of passage and is used to relieve stress and to celebrate. Its ability to lower inhibitions makes it the "social lubricant" of choice for many students, giving them an easy way to initiate conversations, create friendships, and find a date and/or companion for the evening.

Students consistently report that their friends drink much more than they do (Lewis et al., 2011). These overestimations of peers' drinking behaviour are explained by two theories: pluralistic ignorance and false consensus. Pluralistic ignorance refers to when people think their behaviour differs from others even though it is the same, while false consensus refers to the tendency for people to overestimate others' behaviours in order to perceive themselves as the same as these others (Lewis et al., 2011). Further, actual alcohol consumption by post-secondary students is higher than self-reports. Such misinformation may promote or be used to excuse excessive drinking practices among post-secondary students when it could be used to create awareness and improve knowledge regarding drinking behaviours.

Binge drinking Drinking to become intoxicated; five drinks in one drinking occasion for men and four drinks for women.

Binge drinking on campuses continues to be an issue for a number of reasons. **Binge drinking** is defined as the consumption of five drinks in a row by men or four in a row by women on a single occasion (Flegal, MacDonald, & Hébert, 2011). The express purpose of binge drinking is to become intoxicated. Figure 10.1 illustrates the percentage of males and females in Canada according to age groups (Figure 10.1) who self-report binge drinking. Although these figures do not show data only from university and college age students, they provide context for heavy drinking in Canada. Clearly more men than women report binge drinking; and there is a greater rate of binge drinking in the territories.

Binge drinking is common—and expected—at pub crawls, keg parties, and the various events that are part of frosh week (Tamburri, 2012). In addition to the risk of alcohol poisoning and death, considerable property damage occurs to campuses and communities when students consume excessive quantities of alcohol. Examples from recent years highlight the severity of the binge drinking issues on Canadian campuses. Consider the two alcohol-related deaths at Queen's University in 2010, the St Patrick's Day binge drinking at Fanshawe College (London, Ontario) that led to a riot in 2011, the September 2012 alcohol poisoning death of a student at Acadia during frosh week (Tamburri, 2012), and the alcohol-related death of another Acadia student in May 2013 on a student-organized graduation trip. Until the drinking cultures of our Canadian campuses changes, you can expect tragedies like these to continue.

FIGURE 10.1

Heavy Drinking, by Age Group and Sex

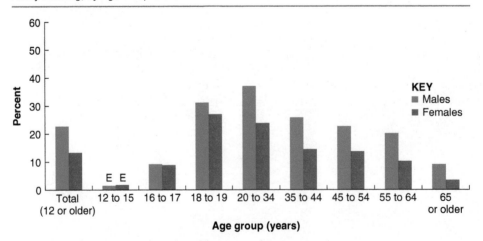

E use with caution (these data have a coefficient of variation from 16.6% to 33.3%)

Note: Heavy drinking refers to males who reported having 5 or more drinks, or women who reported having 4 or more drinks, on one occasion, at least once a month in the past year.

Source: Statistics Canada, Canadian Community Health Survey, Copyright © 2014. Reproduced and distributed on an "as is" basis with the permission of Statistics Canada.

Changing the drinking culture on your campus involves more than awareness campaigns (Tamburri, 2012). A concerted effort by administration, including student unions, faculty, staff, and the surrounding community, is required to create a safer environment where responsible drinking is promoted and expected. Policies and controls need to be put in place that allow for meaningful change in drinking practices on and off campus (Tamburri, 2012). Examples include restricting the volume of drinks sold (e.g., pitchers of beer, number of shots) after a certain time (midnight), reducing sales (e.g., reduced prices or special happy hour prices), restricting where alcohol can be consumed in residences, and so on. Further, stricter penalties for violations should be created—and applied when needed.

Although everyone is at risk for alcohol-related problems, including alcoholism, post-secondary students are particularly vulnerable for the following reasons:

- Alcohol exacerbates their already high risk for suicide, automobile accidents, and falls.

- Many university and college customs, norms, traditions, and mores encourage several dangerous practices and patterns of alcohol use, misuse, and abuse.

- Campuses are heavily targeted by advertising and promotions from the alcohol industry, including the employment of liquor representatives and distributors on most campuses.

- It is more common for post-secondary students than their peers to drink excessively in a variety of drinking games and other dangerous drinking practices.

- The strong need to be accepted by their peers means they are therefore heavily influenced by their peers.

Recently, there has been concern raised about two new ways of consuming alcohol—alcohol enemas or butt chugging and vodka tampons or slimming. As it sounds, an alcohol enema involves pouring alcohol directly into the anus—usually through a tube—for quick absorption into the bloodstream via the abundant vasculature of the rectum (CNN Health, 2012). One of the frightening consequences of this type of consumption of alcohol is the rapid, unaltered absorption. When alcohol passes through the stomach, it is acted upon by alcohol dehydrogenase that breaks down ethanol to make it less toxic for the body. This preliminary breakdown of alcohol does not happen when alcohol is absorbed through the anus, resulting in a more rapid and toxic rate of absorption (CNN Health, 2012). Further, once ingested, there is no possibility of reducing the amount consumed (as in, for instance, vomiting when too much alcohol is passed through the stomach).

Vodka- (or another type of alcohol) soaked tampons are inserted vaginally and, once again, because of the vascularity of the area, rapid absorption of alcohol takes place. Similar to butt chugging or alcohol enemas, there is risk for alcohol poisoning with the use of vodka (or any other alcohol-soaked tampon) as once the alcohol is in the bloodstream, there is no way to get it back, unlike when a person drinks too much, too quickly, and vomits (Go Ask Alice, n.d.).

Another 'drinking' concern related to students is 'drunkorexia'. The National Eating Disorder Association (NEDA, n.d.) defines drunkorexia as "replacing food consumption with excessive alcohol and/or using alcohol to induce vomiting as a method of purging and numbing feelings." It is estimated that this may affect as many as one in five college and university students (Mangat, 2011).

In an effort to prevent alcohol misuse and abuse, many universities and colleges institute policies aimed to address excessive consumption. You should also be made aware of where on your campus you can get help regarding yours or someone else's drinking problems. Most campuses offer individual and group counselling or can direct you to community resources. Considerable attention is directed toward the prevention of alcohol misuse and abuse. Some student organizations also promote responsible drinking and responsible party hosting as well as "safe" ride home options.

Rights versus Responsibilities

You likely recognize the dangers associated with alcohol consumption in general, yet are likely to deny that such things could happen to you. You, like others, likely think you are invincible, that it will not happen to you. You are aware of the relationship between alcohol and traffic accidents, spouse battering and child abuse, violent crimes, unprotected sexual activity, and family disruption, and you likely also believe that these tragedies happen to other people. Many students refuse to acknowledge that alcohol is a drug simply because they do not wish to see themselves as drug users. Is this true for you too? The society in which you live, particularly on campus, condones, approves, and often encourages the consumption of alcoholic beverages. You are also told from a number of sources how to drink responsibly, and yet the reality is that seldom do these words match what happens, particularly in the university or college environment, where excessive consumption of alcohol is most often the expectation, not the exception.

If you make the choice to drink, you should do so judiciously, with complete information about the potential risks and benefits. The physiological and psychological reactions of the human body to alcohol are strong. For this reason, you should approach the drug carefully and be well informed. To avoid the devastating effects of alcohol abuse, you must adhere to the same principles of prevention that apply to any potentially harmful substance. As previously noted, the Canadian Centre on Substance Abuse (n.d.) identified the following in the recently released low-risk drinking guidelines:

- no more than 15 standard drinks per week for men and 10 standard drinks per week for women

- no more than three drinks per day for men and two drinks per day for women

- several days per week with no alcohol consumption

- The fourth guideline suggests that we do NOT drink if you are/have:

   planning to drive

   taking any other drug, including prescription or over-the-counter drugs

   taking part in risky physical activities

   concurrent physical or mental health issues

   pregnant or trying to be

   responsible for the safety of others, young children or otherwise

   making an important decision

   dependent on alcohol

Other suggestions include setting limits for yourself, drinking slowly—no more than two drinks in three hours, alternate drinks with alcohol with non-alcoholic drinks, and finally to pay attention to your current health status, mood, and the amount you have eaten.

Ethyl alcohol (ethanol) A drug produced by fermentation and found in many beverages.

Fermentation The process whereby yeast organisms break down plant sugars to yield ethanol.

Distillation The process whereby mash is subjected to high temperatures to release alcohol vapours, which are then condensed and mixed with water to make the final product.

Proof A measure of the percentage of alcohol in a beverage.

THE PRODUCTION OF ALCOHOL

The intoxicating substance found in beer, wine, liquor, and liqueurs is **ethyl alcohol**, or **ethanol**. It is produced during a process called **fermentation**, whereby plant sugars are broken down by yeast organisms, yielding ethanol and carbon dioxide. Fermentation continues until the solution of plant sugars (called mash) reaches a concentration of 14 percent alcohol. At this point, the alcohol kills the yeast and halts the chemical reactions that produce it.

Manufacturers then add other ingredients that dilute the alcohol content of the beverage, such as in beer and wine. Other alcoholic beverages are produced through further processing called **distillation**, during which alcohol vapours are released from the mash at high temperatures. The vapours are then condensed and mixed with water to make the final product, such as in fortified wines and spirits.

The **proof** of an alcoholic drink is a measure of the percentage of alcohol in the beverage. The word *proof* comes from "gunpowder proof," a reference to the gunpowder test, whereby potential buyers tested the distiller's product by pouring it on gunpowder and attempting to light it. If the alcohol content was at least 50 percent, the gunpowder would burn; otherwise the water in the product would put out the flame. Thus, alcohol percentage is 50 percent of the given proof. For example, 80-proof whiskey or scotch is 40-percent alcohol by volume. In other words, the proof of an alcoholic drink provides an indication of its strength. Therefore, consuming the same amount (that is, volume) of lower-proof drinks will produce fewer alcohol effects than higher-proof drinks. Most spirits are 40 percent alcohol, wines are usually between 12 and 15 percent alcohol, ales are between 6 and 8 percent, and most other beers are between 2 and 6 percent.

PHYSIOLOGICAL AND BEHAVIOURAL EFFECTS OF ALCOHOL

Behavioural Effects

Behaviour changes caused by alcohol vary with the set and setting (see Chapter 9 for more details) for each individual. Alcohol may allow shy people to be less inhibited and more willing to talk to others. Consuming a drink or two may also cause a depressed person to feel even more depressed. In people

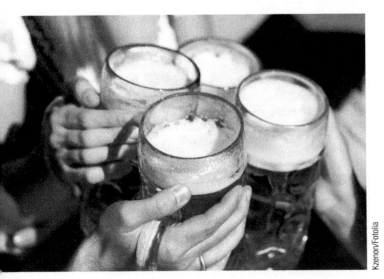

Kzenon/Fotolia

When drinking alcohol and monitoring your consumption, it is important to recognize what constitutes a drink as well as which drinks are more potent (i.e., have a higher alcohol content).

reluctant to share emotions, it may bring out violence and aggression. In many—if not most—cases, alcohol will do for the drinker what the drinker expects and wants it to do, making it possible for the user to blame his or her inappropriate behaviours on the alcohol. It is because of this expected effect, combined with reduced inhibitions, that a person who normally does not dance well 'tears a strip off the dance floor'. In other words, a person who normally inhibits his/her dancing behaviours may actually dance better after a drink or two, simply because his or her inhibitions have been reduced.

Blood alcohol concentration (BAC) is the ratio of alcohol to total blood volume. It is the factor used to measure the physiological and behavioural effects of alcohol. Despite individual differences, alcohol produces some general behavioural effects based on BAC (see Table 10.1). At a BAC of 0.02, a person feels slightly relaxed and his or her mood—whatever that may be—is generally enhanced. At a BAC of 0.05, relaxation increases, there is some motor impairment, and a willingness to talk becomes apparent. At a BAC of 0.08, the person feels elated and there is further motor impairment. At a BAC of 0.10, the depressant effects of alcohol become apparent, drowsiness sets in, and motor skills are further impaired, followed by a loss of judgment. Thus, if driving, the drinker may not be able to estimate distances or speed, and some lose the ability to make value-related decisions and may do things he or she would not do when sober. As BAC increases, the drinker experiences increased physiological and psychological effects. All these changes result in further deterioration of physical and mental functions.

People can acquire physiological and psychological tolerance to the effects of alcohol through regular use. The nervous system adapts over time, so greater quantities of alcohol are required to produce the same physiological and psychological effects. Furthermore, some people learn to modify their behaviours so that they appear to be sober even when their BAC is quite high. This ability is called **learned behavioural tolerance**. It should be pointed out though that this tolerance does not extend to BAC; in other words, although a person may appear 'sober', his or her BAC still reflects the amount of alcohol consumed and his or her reaction time as well as judgment are impaired as previously noted.

Absorption and Metabolism

Alcohol is rapidly absorbed into the bloodstream from the small intestine, and less rapidly from the stomach and colon. In proportion to its concentration

Blood alcohol concentration (BAC) The ratio of alcohol to total blood volume; the factor used to measure the physiological and behavioural effects of alcohol.

Learned behavioural tolerance The ability of drinkers to modify their behaviours so that they appear sober—or in control—even when they have high BAC levels.

TABLE 10.1

Psychological and Physiological Effects of Various Blood Alcohol Concentration Levels

Blood Alcohol Concentration (BAC)	Psychological and Physical Effects
Not Impaired	
<0.1%	Negligible.
Sometimes Impaired	
0.01%–0.04%	Slight muscle relaxation, mild euphoria, slight body warmth, increased sociability and talkativeness.
Usually Impaired	
0.05–0.07%	Lowered alertness, impaired judgment, lowered inhibitions, exaggerated behaviour, loss of muscle control.
Always Impaired	
0.08–0.14%	Slowed reaction time, poor muscle coordination, short-term memory loss, judgment impaired, inability to focus.
0.15–0.24%	Blurred vision, lack of motor skills, sedation, slowed reactions, difficulty standing and walking, passing out.
0.25–0.34%	Impaired consciousness, disorientation, loss of motor function, severely impaired or no reflexes, impaired circulation and respiration, uncontrolled urination, slurred speech, possible death.
0.35 and up	Unconsciousness, coma, extremely slow heartbeat and respiration, unresponsiveness, probable death.

in the bloodstream, alcohol decreases activity in parts of the brain and spinal cord. Your blood alcohol concentration depends on

- the amount consumed in a given time
- your size, sex, body build, and metabolism
- the type and amount of food in your stomach

Once alcohol has passed into the bloodstream, you cannot slow its absorption by eating or drinking. Mood also influences the rate of absorption, since emotions affect how long it takes for the contents of the stomach to empty into the intestine. Powerful moods, such as stress and anxiety, are likely to cause the stomach to "dump" its contents into the small intestine. That is why alcohol is absorbed much more rapidly when people are tense than when they are relaxed.

Consuming fruit sugar may shorten the duration of alcohol's effect by increasing the rate of elimination from the blood (that is, metabolism). In the average adult, the rate of metabolism is about 8.5 grams (that is, about two-thirds of a drink) of alcohol per hour. This rate varies dramatically among individuals, however, depending on the user's drinking history, physique, sex, liver size, and genetic factors (Addiction Research Foundation, n.d.).

Alcohol is metabolized in the liver, where it is converted by the enzyme alcohol dehydrogenase to acetaldehyde. It is then rapidly oxidized to acetate, converted to carbon dioxide and water, and eventually excreted from the body. Acetaldehyde is a toxic chemical that can cause immediate symptoms such as nausea and vomiting as well as long-term effects such as liver damage.

Like food, alcohol contains calories. Proteins and carbohydrates (starches and sugars) each contain 4 kilocalories per gram, while fat contains 9 kilocalories per gram (see Chapter 5). Alcohol, although similar in structure to carbohydrates, contains 7 kilocalories per gram. Alcohol is a source of energy—and therefore considered a food—however, it is not considered a nutrient because it is not essential to our body, nor does it perform any necessary function (Thompson, Manore, & Sheeska, 2007).

Your BAC depends on your weight and body fat, the water content in your body tissues, the concentration of alcohol in the beverage consumed, your rate of consumption, and the volume of alcohol consumed. Heavier people have larger body surfaces through which to diffuse alcohol; therefore, they have lower concentrations of alcohol in their blood than thin people after drinking the same amount. Alcohol does not diffuse as rapidly into body fat as into water; thus, assuming all other things are equal, alcohol concentration will be higher in a person with more body fat. Since women, on average have more body fat than men, they also have less water in their body tissues and as a result a higher BAC than a man of the same weight in response to drinking the same amount of alcohol (see Figure 10.2).

Women and Alcohol

Body fat is not the only contributor to the differences in alcohol's effects on men and women. Compared to men, women have half as much alcohol dehydrogenase, the enzyme that breaks down alcohol in the stomach before it has a chance to get to the bloodstream and the brain. Therefore, if a man and a woman drink the same amount of alcohol, the woman's BAC will be approximately 30 percent higher

FIGURE 10.2

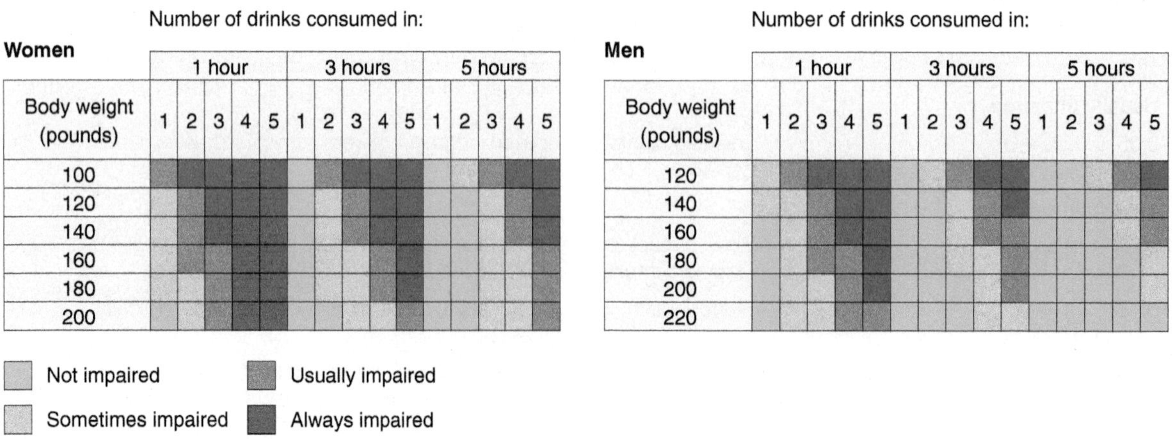

Approximate blood alcohol concentration (BAC) and the physiological and behavioural effects. Remember there are many variables that can affect BAC, so this is only an estimate of what your BAC would be.

than the man's, leaving her more vulnerable to the physiological and psychological effects. Figure 10.2 compares blood-alcohol levels by sex, weight, and consumption. Caution should be used when examining this table as there are many additional factors that may cause considerable variation in response to alcohol as previously noted. For this reason, you should always err on the side of caution when gauging your BAC.

Breathalyzer and Other Tests

The breathalyzer tests used by law enforcement officers are designed to determine BAC based on the amount of alcohol exhaled in the breath. Urinalysis yields a BAC based on the concentration of unmetabolized alcohol in the urine. Breath analysis, urinalysis, and blood tests are used to determine whether a driver is over the legal limit, with blood tests providing the most accurate measures.

Immediate Effects

Alcohol is a central nervous system (CNS) depressant. The primary action of ethanol is to reduce the frequency of nerve transmissions and impulses at synaptic junctions. This reduction of nerve transmissions causes a significant reduction in CNS functions, with resulting decreases in respiratory rate, pulse rate, and blood pressure. As CNS depression deepens, vital functions become noticeably reduced. In extreme cases, coma and death can result (see also Table 10.1).

Alcohol is a diuretic that increases urinary output. Although this effect might be expected to lead to automatic **dehydration** (loss of water), the body actually retains water, most of it in the muscles or in the cerebral tissues. This is because water is usually pulled out of the **cerebrospinal fluid** (fluid within the brain and spinal cord) instead, leading to what is known as mitochondrial dehydration at the cellular level within the nervous system. Mitochondria are miniature organs within cells responsible for specific functions. They rely heavily on fluid balance. When mitochondrial dehydration occurs from drinking, the mitochondria cannot carry out their normal functions, resulting in symptoms that include the "morning-after" headaches suffered by some drinkers.

Alcohol is also an irritant to the gastrointestinal system and can cause indigestion and heartburn if consumed on an empty stomach. Long-term use of alcohol causes repeated irritation that has been linked to cancers of the esophagus and stomach. In addition, people who engage in brief drinking sprees during which they consume unusually high amounts of alcohol put themselves at risk for irregular heartbeat or even total loss of heart rhythm, which can cause disruption in blood flow and possible damage to the heart muscle.

A **hangover** is sometimes experienced the morning after consuming alcohol. The symptoms of a hangover are familiar to those who drink: headache, upset stomach, anxiety, depression, thirst, and, in severe cases, an almost overwhelming desire to crawl back into bed. People who get hangovers often also stay up too late or engage in other behaviours likely to leave them feeling unwell the next day. The causes of hangovers are not well known, but the effects of congeners are suspected. **Congeners**, more prevalent in darker forms of alcohol (i.e., whiskey vs. vodka; red vs. white wine), are toxic forms of alcohol metabolized more slowly than ethanol. Your body metabolizes the congeners after the ethanol is gone from your system, and their toxic by-products are thought to contribute to the hangover. It is speculated that a hangover is actually a sign of withdrawal. It usually takes 12 hours to recover from a hangover. Bed rest, plenty of fluids, solid food, and a pain reliever may reduce the discomforts of a hangover; however, nothing but time can completely cure it.

Drug Interactions

When you use any drug (and alcohol is a drug), you need to be aware of the possible interactions with prescription drugs, over-the-counter drugs, or other drugs you are taking or considering taking. Table 10.2 summarizes possible interactions (see also Chapter 9).

Long-Term Effects

Effects on the Nervous System

Since alcohol is a CNS depressant, the nervous system is especially sensitive to it. Even people who drink moderately experience a decrease in brain size and weight accompanied by a slight loss of intellectual ability. The damage that results from alcohol use is localized primarily in the left side of the brain, which is responsible for written and spoken language, logic, and mathematical skills. The degree of shrinkage appears to be directly related to the amount of alcohol consumed. In terms of memory loss, the evidence suggests that having one drink every day is less likely to result in damage than saving up for a binge and consuming an excessive number of drinks at one time.

Dehydration Loss of fluids from body tissues.

Cerebrospinal fluid Fluid within and surrounding the brain and spinal cord tissues.

Hangover The physiological reaction to excessive drinking, including such symptoms as headache, upset stomach, anxiety, depression, diarrhea, and thirst.

Congeners Forms of alcohol metabolized more slowly than ethanol that produce toxic by-products.

TABLE 10.2

Drugs and Alcohol: Actions and Interactions

Drug Class/Name(s)	Effects with Alcohol
Anti-alcohol: Antabuse	Severe reactions to even small amounts: headache, nausea, blurred vision, convulsions, coma, possible death.
Antibiotics: Penicillin, Cyantin	Reduces therapeutic effectiveness of antibiotics.
Antidepressants: Elavil, Sinequan, Tofranil, Nardil	Increased central nervous system (CNS) depression, blood pressure changes. Combined use of alcohol and MAO inhibitors, a specific type of antidepressant, can trigger massive increases in blood pressure, even brain hemorrhage and death.
Antihistamines: Allerest, Dristan	Drowsiness and CNS depression. Impairs driving ability.
ASA: Aspirin, Anacin, Excedrin, Bayer	Irritates stomach lining. May cause gastrointestinal pain, bleeding.
Depressants: Valium, Ativan, Placidyl	Dangerous CNS depression, loss of coordination, coma. High risk of overdose and death.
Narcotics: Heroin, Codeine, Darvon	Serious CNS depression. Possible respiratory arrest and death.
Stimulants: Caffeine, Cocaine	Masks depressant action of alcohol. May increase blood pressure, physical tension.
Tylenol, Acetaminophen	Risk of liver damage, particularly with heavy alcohol consumption and maximum recommended doses of acetaminophen.

Source: Adapted by permission from *Drugs and Alcohol: Simple Facts about Alcohol and Drug Combinations* (Phoenix: DIN Publications, 1988), No. 121. http://www.doitnow.org/pdfs/121.pdf.

Cardiovascular Effects

The cardiovascular system may be affected by alcohol consumption in a number of ways. There is considerable evidence to suggest that moderate alcohol consumption reduces risk of heart attack, ischemic (clot-caused) stroke, peripheral vascular disease, sudden cardiac death, and death from all cardiovascular causes by 25 to 40 percent (Goldberg et al., 2001). The reason for this reduced risk for heart disease is primarily related to an improved blood lipid profile with higher levels of HDLs (see Chapter 12) and improvements in insulin sensitivity and other factors related to blood clotting (Booyse et al., 2007). Still, drinking is not recommended as a preventive measure against heart disease because the benefits do not outweigh the risks. For example, drinking too much alcohol contributes to high blood pressure and a slightly increased heart rate and cardiac output (Sheps, 2012). Further, alcohol contains calories and may relate to weight gain—another risk factor for high blood pressure (Sheps, 2012).

People who engage in brief drinking sprees, during which they consume unusually large amounts of alcohol, incur risks, including irregular heartbeats or total loss of heart rhythm (Abdelaziz, Kamalanathan, & John, 2011). This condition has been called "holiday heart syndrome" because it typically occurs around holidays such as Thanksgiving, Christmas, and New Year's Eve—occasions when drinkers are likely to overindulge. It can cause disruption in blood flow and possible damage to the heart muscle. Prolonged drinking can also lead to deterioration of the heart muscle, a condition called cardiomyopathy.

Liver Disease

One of the most common diseases related to alcohol abuse is **cirrhosis** of the liver (Figure 10.3). It is among the top 10 causes of death in Canada and the third largest contributor to the global burden of disease (Flegal, MacDonald, & Hébert, 2011). One result of heavy drinking is that the liver begins to store fat—a condition known as "fatty liver." If there is insufficient time between drinking episodes, this fat cannot be transported to storage sites and the fat-filled liver cells stop functioning. Continued drinking causes a further stage of liver deterioration called fibrosis, in which the damaged area of the liver develops fibrous scar tissue (National Institute on Alcohol Abuse and Alcoholism, 2010). Cell function can be partially restored at this stage with proper nutrition and abstinence from alcohol. However, if the person continues to drink, cirrhosis results—liver cells die and the damage is permanent (National Institute on Alcohol Abuse and Alcoholism, 2010). **Alcoholic hepatitis** is a serious condition

Cirrhosis The last stage of liver disease associated with chronic heavy use of alcohol, during which liver cells die and damage is permanent.

Alcoholic hepatitis Condition resulting from prolonged use of alcohol in which the liver is inflamed. It can result in death.

FIGURE 10.3

Comparison of a Healthy Liver with a Cirrhotic Liver

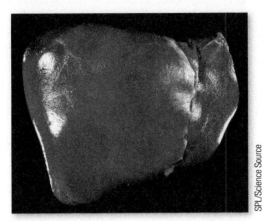

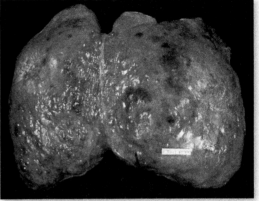

a A normal liver

b A liver with cirrhosis

In cirrhosis, healthy liver cells are replaced with scar tissue that interferes with the liver's ability to perform its many vital functions.

resulting from prolonged use of alcohol. A chronic inflammation of the liver develops, which may be fatal in itself or progress to cirrhosis.

Cancer and Other Effects

Heavy drinkers (more than five drinks per day, more than 12 times per year) are at higher risk for certain types of cancer, particularly those of the gastrointestinal tract. The repeated irritation caused by long-term use of alcohol has been linked to cancers of the esophagus, stomach, mouth, tongue, and liver (see also Chapter 12). It is unclear how alcohol exerts its carcinogenic effects, though it is thought that it inhibits the absorption of carcinogenic substances, permitting them to be taken to sensitive organs.

Evidence also suggests that alcohol impairs the body's ability to recognize and fight foreign bodies such as bacteria and viruses (National Institute on Alcohol Abuse and Alcoholism, 2010). Thus, individuals become more susceptible to colds and flus and less able to fight the abnormal cells that develop and may lead to cancer. It is worth noting that this reduced ability of the immune system occurs in chronic drinkers as well as in binge drinkers (National Institute on Alcohol Abuse and Alcoholism, 2010).

An irritant to the gastrointestinal system, alcohol may cause indigestion and heartburn if consumed on an empty stomach. It also damages the mucous membranes and leads to inflammation of the esophagus, chronic stomach irritation, problems with intestinal absorption, and chronic diarrhea. Excessive alcohol use is a major cause of chronic inflammation of the

pancreas, the organ that produces digestive enzymes and insulin. Chronic abuse of alcohol inhibits enzyme production, which further inhibits the absorption of nutrients (Wagnerberger, Kanuri, & Bergheim, 2012). Drinking alcohol can block the absorption of calcium, a nutrient that strengthens bones (Davis, 2013). This should be of particular concern to women because as women age their risk for osteoporosis (loss of bone mineral content and density) increases. Heavy consumption of alcohol worsens this condition.

Fetal Alcohol Spectrum Disorders

Alcohol consumed by the mother has potential harmful effects on fetal development dependent upon timing and amount of consumption. Alcohol consumed during the first trimester of pregnancy poses the greatest threat to organ development, while exposure during the last trimester, when the brain is developing rapidly, is most likely to affect CNS development.

A series of disorders collectively called **fetal alcohol spectrum disorder (FASD)** is caused by prenatal exposure to alcohol and leads to lifelong developmental and cognitive disabilities among Canadian children (Stade et al., 2006). FASD occurs when alcohol ingested by the mother passes through the placenta into the fetus's bloodstream. Because the fetus is so small, its BAC will be

Fetal alcohol spectrum disorder (FASD) A broad category of disorders relating to consumption of alcohol during pregnancy—includes fetal alcohol syndrome, fetal alcohol effects, partial fetal alcohol effects, alcohol-related neurodevelopmental disorders, and neurobehavioural disorder–alcohol exposed.

much higher than that of the mother. Thus, consumption of alcohol during pregnancy affects the fetus far more seriously than the mother.

FASD is the leading cause of developmental delay in Canada and North America, with an incidence estimated at 1 to 6 in 1000 live births (Stade et al., 2006). FASD includes the following disorders related to alcohol consumption during pregnancy: **fetal alcohol syndrome (FAS)**, **fetal alcohol effects (FAE)**, partial fetal alcohol effects, alcohol-related neurodevelopmental disorders, and neurobehavioural disorder-alcohol exposed. FAS is characterized by retarded growth prenatally and postnatally, facial anomalies, CNS dysfunction as noted by intellectual impairment, structural abnormalities, developmental delay, and complex behavioural problems (Stade et al., 2006). One-fifth of FAS children have difficulty sleeping and are hyperactive. Many have severe learning disabilities and are dyslexic. Congenital heart problems are more common than in normal babies, as are genitourinary problems. There is an increased incidence of spina bifida, hip dislocation, and delayed skeletal maturation. FAE is used to describe children with prenatal exposure to alcohol but only some FAS characteristics.

As there is no definitive information regarding a safe quantity of alcohol during pregnancy, women who are or wish to become pregnant should abstain from alcohol. Health professionals should reassure women who have consumed small amounts of alcohol occasionally during pregnancy that the risk is likely minimal. Pregnant women should also know that not drinking at any time during a pregnancy will benefit themselves and their babies.

In June 1992, the Standing Committee on Health and Welfare, Social Affairs, Seniors, and the Status of Women released its report *Fetal Alcohol Syndrome: A Preventable Tragedy*. Since then, Health Canada has worked with health-care professionals to identify and implement prevention strategies; produced pamphlets and videos on FAS; and, with the Association of Canadian Distillers and the Brewers' Association of Canada, sponsors a national information service resource centre providing links to support groups, prevention projects, and experts on FASD (1-800-559-4514).

Fetal alcohol syndrome (FAS) A disorder that may result in the fetus if a mother regularly consumes alcohol during pregnancy. Among its effects are mental retardation, small head, tremors, and abnormalities of the face, limbs, heart, and brain.

Fetal alcohol effects (FAE) A syndrome describing children with a history of prenatal alcohol exposure but without all the physical or behavioural symptoms of FAS. Among its symptoms are low birthweight, irritability, and possible permanent mental impairment.

Alcohol abuse (alcoholism) Excessive use of alcohol that interferes with work, school, or personal relationships or that entails violations of the law.

Drinking and Driving

The leading cause of death for all age groups from 15 to 24 years old (including university and college students) is accidents, including traffic accidents (Statistics Canada, 2012b). In 2011, there were 121 incidents of impaired driving causing death (Statistics Canada, 2011). Moreover, in 2010, MADD Canada estimated that approximately 1082 individuals were killed in accidents resulting from impaired driving due to alcohol consumption.

ALCOHOLISM

Alcohol use becomes **alcohol abuse** or **alcoholism** when there is excessive consumption or a level of consumption that interferes with work, school, or social and family relationships. Alcoholism is considered a disease and is one of many addictions or dependencies on substances or behaviours that have mood-altering consequences.

As noted previously, 8.8 percent of Canadians between the ages of 15 and 65 reported harm to self in the past year as a result of their drinking. Of the past-year drinkers, 6.2 percent indicated heavy drinking (five or more drinks for males and four or more drinks for women on a single occasion) at least once per week, with men between the ages of 20 and 35 years the most likely to report heavy drinking. Further, as previously noted, 18.7 percent of past-year drinkers exceeded the low-risk drinking guidelines (that is, consuming no more than 15 standard drinks for men or 10 standard drinks for women per week).

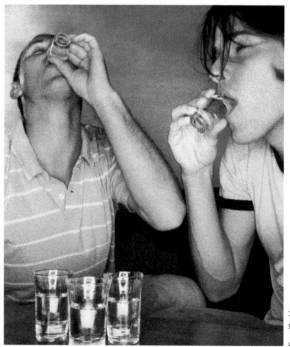

Deciding when and how much to drink is no simple matter. Irresponsible consumption of alcohol can easily result in negative consequences.

The most common areas affected by excessive drinking are physical health (5.4 percent), financial position (4.7 percent), and social health (3.0 percent). Almost one-third (32.7 percent) of Canadians say they have had problems from other people's drinking, such as being disturbed by loud parties (23.8 percent), being insulted or humiliated (22.1 percent), having a serious argument (15.5 percent), being physically abused (14.0 percent), and experiencing marital difficulties (10.0 percent). In 2010, it was estimated that about 299 838 individuals were injured in motor vehicle crashes. MADD Canada estimates that approximately 63 821 of these individuals were injured in impairment-related crashes (this equates to about 175 per day).

How, Why, Whom?

As with other addictions, tolerance, psychological dependence, and withdrawal symptoms must be present to qualify a person as addicted to alcohol. Addiction usually results from chronic use over a period of time that varies from person to person. People who have problems with alcohol, including irresponsible users, are not necessarily people addicted to it. The stereotype of the person on skid row (homeless, impoverished, and living on the streets) addicted to alcohol applies to only 5 percent of those affected. The remaining 95 percent of individuals addicted to alcohol live in some type of extended family unit. They can be found at all socioeconomic levels and in all professions, ethnic groups, geographic locations, and religions. You have a 1 in 10 chance or risk of becoming addicted to alcohol. Individuals addicted to alcohol tend to have a number of attitudes and behaviours in common. People who recognize in themselves any of these attitudes and behaviours discussed in the following paragraphs should seek professional help to determine whether alcohol has become a controlling factor in their lives (see also the Assess Yourself Questionnaires included at the end of Chapter 9).

Women are the fastest-growing component of the population becoming addicted to alcohol. They tend to become addicted at a later age and after fewer years of heavy drinking than men. Women at highest risk for alcohol-related problems are those living common law in their 20s or early 30s, or who have a husband or partner who drinks heavily.

The Causes of Alcoholism

Alcoholism is a disease with biological, psychological, and social/environmental components, but we do not know what role—or how much of a role—each of these components plays.

Biological and Family Factors

Research into the hereditary and environmental causes of alcoholism has found higher rates of alcoholism among family members. In fact, alcoholism is four to five times more common among the children of those who are addicted to alcohol than in the general population (Mental Health Canada, n.d.).

Individuals categorized with type 1 alcoholism have had at least one parent who was a problem drinker and grew up in an environment that encouraged heavy drinking. Their drinking is reinforced by family and social events that include heavy drinking. These individuals share certain personality characteristics—for instance, they avoid novelty and harmful situations and are concerned about the thoughts and feelings of others. Type 1 alcoholism accounts for about 75 percent of all cases and does not occur until after the age of 25 (Perkinson, 2011). Individuals classified with type 2 alcoholism are typically males under the age of 25 years (Perkinson, 2011). These men are the biological sons of fathers who, in addition to being alcoholics, have a history of violence and drug use. These men display the opposite characteristics of individuals considered type 1 alcoholics—they do not seek social approval, they lack inhibition, and they are prone to novelty-seeking behaviours (Goodwin & Gause, 1990).

Because the effects of heredity and environment are so difficult to separate, some researchers have chosen to examine this issue through twin and adoption studies. So far, these studies have produced inconclusive results. However, a slightly higher rate of similar drinking behaviours has been demonstrated among identical twins. Further, sons living away from their biological parents who are alcoholics tend to more closely resemble their biological parents in drinking behaviours than their adoptive or foster parents.

Social and Cultural Factors

There are numerous factors that can mitigate or exacerbate problems with alcohol. Many individuals begin to drink because of peer pressure—everyone else is doing it. The average age that Canadians start to drink is around 12 years of age, well before the legal age of drinking (Statistics Canada, 2012c). Others may begin drinking or continue to drink as a way to dull the pain of an acute loss or an emotional or social problem. For example, students may drink to escape the stress involved in university or college life; disappointment over unfulfilled expectations; difficulties in forming relationships; or the loss of the security of home, loved ones, and close friends. Unfortunately, the emotional discomfort that causes many people to turn to alcohol also ultimately causes them to become even more uncomfortable as the depressant effect of the drug begins to take its toll. Thus, the person who is already depressed may become even more depressed, antagonizing friends and other social supports until these supports turn away.

Family attitudes toward alcohol also influence the role alcohol may play in a person's life as well as whether or not a person will develop a drinking problem. It has been demonstrated that people raised in cultures in which drinking is a part of religious or of ceremonial activities or in which alcohol is a traditional part of the family meal are less prone to alcohol dependency. In contrast, in societies in which alcohol purchase is carefully controlled and drinking is regarded as a rite of passage to adulthood, such as that found in Canada, the tendency for abuse appears to be greater (Ray & Kisr, 1990).

Certain social factors have been linked with alcoholism as well. These include urbanization, the weakening of links to the extended family and a general loosening of kinship ties, increased mobility, and changing religious and philosophic values. Apparently, then, some combination of heredity and environment plays a decisive role in the development of alcoholism.

Recognizing Your Personal Risk

There is a strong relationship between age of initiation and future drinking problems (Foxcroft et al., 2013). Generally, individuals who start drinking by 14 years of age are at greater risk than those who start drinking later. Simple screening tools can be effective at identifying personal risk for alcohol-related problems, including dependence. If you respond 'yes' to two or more of the questions listed below, there is a 90 percent chance that you have an alcohol use disorder (George, 2007).

- Have you felt you needed to cut down on your drinking?
- Have you felt annoyed by criticism of your drinking?
- Have you felt guilty about your drinking?
- Have you felt you needed a drink first thing in the morning?

Effects of Alcoholism on the Family

It has been recognized that not only the person addicted to alcohol, but also his or her entire family and close friends, suffer. Although most research focuses on family effects during the late stages of alcoholism, the family unit actually begins to react early on as the person starts to show symptoms of addiction to alcohol.

Many families affected by alcoholism have no idea what normal family life is like. Family members unconsciously adapt to the behaviours of the person who is addicted to alcohol by adjusting their own behaviours in an attempt to maintain a level of normalcy within the home. To minimize their feelings about the addiction or out of love for him or her, family members take on various abnormal roles. These roles actually help keep the person drinking. Children in such dysfunctional families generally assume at least one of the following roles:

- Family hero: tries to divert attention from the problem by being really good, almost too good to be true
- Scapegoat: draws attention away from the family's primary problem through delinquency or misbehaviour
- Lost child: becomes passive and quietly withdraws from upsetting situations as well as family life
- Mascot: disrupts tense situations by providing comic relief

Life is a struggle for children in alcoholic homes. They have to deal with constant stress, anxiety, and embarrassment. Because the individual who is an alcoholic is often the centre of attention, the children's wants and needs are usually ignored. It is not uncommon for these children to be victims of violence, abuse, neglect, or incest. As previously noted, when such children grow up, they have a greater tendency to become alcoholics themselves than children from nonalcoholic families. A question that remains for these children, is it nature or nurture?

Over time, we have come to recognize the unique problems of adult children of individuals addicted to alcohol whose difficulties in life stem from a lack of parental nurturing during childhood. Among these problems are an inability to develop social attachments, a need to be in control of all emotions and situations, low self-esteem, and depression.

Not all individuals who grew up in alcoholic families have lifelong problems. Many of these people develop a resiliency in response to their family's problems and enter adulthood with positive strengths and valuable career-oriented skills, such as the ability to assume responsibility, strong organizational skills, and realistic expectations of their jobs and those of others.

Costs to Society

As previously noted, the alcohol industry in Canada registered sales of more than $20.3 billion in the fiscal year ending March 31, 2011, providing employment for more than 14 000 persons and generating significant revenue for provincial and federal governments. The average beverage sales per capita per year for Canadians was $712.40 (Statistics Canada, 2012a).

The benefits of alcohol sales to the economy should be considered alongside the consequences of alcohol abuse and addiction. Wider society suffers the consequences of individuals' alcohol abuse. The total alcohol sales in Canada is equivalent to about 2.7 percent of GDP and represents the most optimistic estimate of the cost of addiction to society. The actual number could be significantly higher. Of this amount, alcohol abuse accounts for approximately 40 percent (Single et al., 1996).

Women and Alcoholism

In the past, women have consumed less alcohol and had fewer alcohol-related problems than men. Now, a greater percentage of women, especially college- and university-aged women, are choosing to drink and many are drinking more heavily.

There are now almost as many women as men who become alcoholics. However, there appear to be differences between men and women when it comes to alcohol abuse:

1. Women attribute the onset of problem drinking to a specific life stress or traumatic event more frequently than men.

2. Women's alcoholism starts later and progresses more quickly than men's; this phenomenon is called "telescoping."

3. Women tend to be prescribed mood-altering drugs more often than men; women thus face the risks of drug interaction or cross-tolerance more often.

4. Men not addicted to alcohol tend to divorce their spouses who are addicted nine times more often than they do their spouses without an alcohol addiction; women addicted to alcohol are thus not as likely to have a family support system to aid them in their recovery.

5. Women addicted to alcohol do not tend to receive as much social support as men in their treatment and recovery.

6. Unmarried, divorced, or single-parent women tend to have significant economic problems that may make entry into a treatment program especially difficult (Kinney & Leaton, 1991).

RECOVERY

Most individuals addicted to alcohol who seek help have experienced a turning point or dramatic occurrence, such as a failed relationship, confrontation at work, or some other impactful experience. Regardless of the reasons for seeking help, it has finally been recognized that alcohol controls the person's life—this is a critical component of recovery. Prior to this point, denial of the problem prevents the individual from moving forward. The first step to recovery is to recognize there is a problem and to assume responsibility for personal actions.

The Family's Role

Family members of an individual addicted to alcohol sometimes take action before that person does. They may go to an organization or a treatment facility to seek help for themselves and the affected individual. An effective method of helping an individual addicted to alcohol confront the disease is a process called **intervention**. Essentially, an intervention is a planned confrontation with the person who is an alcoholic that involves several family members plus professional counsellors. The family members express their love and concern, telling the person who has the addiction that they will no longer refrain from acknowledging the problem and affirming their support for appropriate treatment. A family (and friend) intervention is often the turning point for a growing number of individuals addicted to alcohol.

Treatment Programs

Once a person has recognized and admitted to the problem there are many sources of support available. Depending on the severity of the addiction an individual may be able to overcome the addiction through the use of outpatient resources and services. This could include working with an addictions counselor and following a decision support framework. Such a framework provides a form of clinical counseling, decision aids and coaching, which can be used to overcome addiction (O'Connor, 2006). An example of this framework is the Ottawa Decision Support Framework (Figure 10.4).

There are hundreds of residential care facilities in Canada for the treatment of alcohol and drug addiction, funded by a mix of municipal, provincial, federal sources, and private donations. There are also outpatient, detox, walk-in, and crisis centres. Treatment is also available at private treatment centres costing several thousand dollars, but some insurance programs or employers will assume most of this expense. Treatment programs are based on various models and offered in many other languages in addition to French and English.

Intervention A planned confrontation with a person addicted to alcohol in which family members and/or friends express their concern about the drinking.

FIGURE 10.4

The Ottawa Decision Support Framework

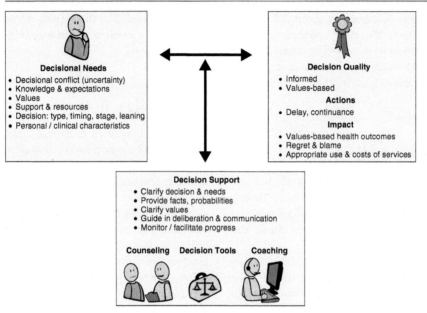

Source: AM O'Connor (2006). Ottawa Decision Support Framework to Address Decisional Conflict. Reproduced by permission of The Ottawa Hospital Research Institute. Retrieved from www.ohri.ca/decisionaid.

Individuals addicted to alcohol who quit drinking typically experience withdrawal symptoms, such as

- hyperexcitability
- confusion
- sleep disorders
- convulsions
- agitation
- tremors of the hands
- brief hallucinations
- depression
- headache
- seizures

In a small percentage of individuals, alcohol withdrawal results in a severe syndrome known as **delirium tremens (DTs)**. Delirium tremens is characterized by confusion, delusions, agitated behaviours, and hallucinations.

Withdrawal from alcohol is very difficult and medically risky—more so than for many other addictive substances or behaviours. Thus, for withdrawal from any long-term addiction to alcohol, medical supervision is usually necessary. Detoxification, the process by which individuals addicted to alcohol end their dependence, is commonly carried out in a medical facility where they can be monitored to prevent fatal withdrawal reactions. Withdrawal usually takes 7 to 21 days. Shortly after detoxification, treatment begins for psychological addiction. Most treatment facilities keep their patients from three to six weeks.

Family, Individual, and Group Therapy

Various individual and group therapies are also available. In family therapy, the person and family members gradually examine the psychological reasons underlying the addiction. In individual and group therapy, individuals addicted to alcohol learn positive coping skills for use in situations that have regularly resulted in them choosing to drink. On some campuses, the problems associated with alcohol abuse, primarily excessive drinking, are so great that student health centres are offering their own treatment and awareness programs.

Other Types of Treatment

Two other treatments are drug and aversion therapy. For drug therapy, disulfiram (trade name Antabuse) is the drug of choice for treating individuals addicted to alcohol. When taking this drug, if alcohol is consumed, it causes unpleasant intolerant effects such as headache, nausea, vomiting, drowsiness, and hangover. These symptoms discourage one from drinking. Aversion therapy is based on conditioning therapy. It

Delirium tremens (DTs) A state of confusion brought on by withdrawal from alcohol. Symptoms include hallucinations, anxiety, and trembling.

works on the premise that the sight, smell, and taste of alcohol will acquire aversive properties if repeatedly paired with a noxious stimulus. For a period of 10 days, the individual takes drugs that induce vomiting when combined with alcohol. These treatments work best in conjunction with counselling.

Alcoholics Anonymous (AA) is a private, non-profit, self-help organization founded in 1935. The organization, which relies on group support to help people stop drinking, has more than one million members, with branches all over the world. People attending their first AA meeting will find that last names are never used. Neither is anyone forced to speak. Members are taught to believe that their alcoholism is a lifetime problem. They share their stories with the group and are asked to place their faith, and control of the habit, in the hands of a "higher power." The road to recovery is taken one step at a time. AA offers specialized meetings for individuals who are homosexual, atheist, HIV-positive, and professionals. The psychosocial support from AA has been helpful for many to achieve long-term sobriety and reduces risk for alcohol-related suicide (George, 2007).

Alcoholics Anonymous also has auxiliary groups to help spouses or partners, friends, and children of individuals addicted to alcohol. Al-Anon is the group dedicated to helping adult relatives and friends of the person who is addicted understand the disease and learn how they can be part of the recovery process. The support gained from talking with others with similar problems is one of the greatest benefits derived from participation in Al-Anon. Many members learn how to exert greater control over their own lives. Some are able to rid themselves of the guilt they feel about their participation in their loved one's alcoholism.

Alateen, another AA-related organization, is designed to help adolescents live with a parent or parents who are alcoholics. Teens are taught that they are not at fault for their parents' problems with alcohol. They learn skills to develop their self-esteem so they can function better socially. Alateen also helps the children of people addicted to alcohol to overcome their guilt feelings.

Brief Interventions

It is worth noting that brief (i.e., less than five minutes) motivational interventions can also be effective in getting heavy drinkers to address their drinking habits when used in primary care, emergency department, and specialty care settings (George, 2007). Individuals who do not respond to these brief interventions require more intensive behavioural interventions as already discussed.

Relapse

Roughly 60 percent of individuals addicted to alcohol relapse (resume drinking) within the first three months of treatment. Why is the relapse rate so high? Treating an addiction requires more than getting the person who is addicted to stop using; it also requires getting the person to break a pattern of behaviours that has dominated his or her life—often for some time.

People seeking to regain a healthy lifestyle must not only confront their addiction, but also prevent relapse. Individuals with compulsive personalities need to learn to understand themselves and take control. Others need to view treatment as a long-term process that takes a lot of effort beyond attending a weekly self-help group meeting. In order to work, a recovery program must offer the individual addicted to alcohol ways to increase self-esteem and resume personal growth.

SMOKING

Health consequences of the tobacco epidemic in developed and developing countries are devastating. It was estimated in 1998 by the World Health Organization that by 2020, tobacco use would kill more people than any single disease, and that since the middle of the twentieth century tobacco products have killed more than 60 million people in developed countries alone. It is currently estimated that smoking is the single most preventable cause of death, killing five million people worldwide each year (World Health Organization, 2013). It is now estimated that if the current trends regarding smoking continue, that it will kill eight million people per year by 2030 (World Health Organization, 2013).

Canadians have been smoking less since 1966, when 54 percent of men and 28 percent of women were smokers. In 2014, 18.1 percent of Canadians 12 years of age and older, (approximately 5.4 million people), smoked either daily or occasionally (Statistics Canada, 2014b). This is a decrease from 2013 (19.3 percent) and is the lowest smoking rate reported since 2001. More men (21.4 percent) than women (14.8 percent) smoke. For males this was a decrease from 2012 and for females it was a decrease from 2013.

On a positive note and potentially related to the various efforts to reduce smoking in the population such as restricted smoking indoors and taxation as well as a decrease in social acceptance, fewer young people report occasional or daily smoking. In fact the the percentage of daily or occasional smokers was the lowest for

Alcoholics Anonymous (AA) An organization whose goal is to help individuals addicted to alcohol stop drinking; includes auxiliary branches such as Al-Anon and Alateen.

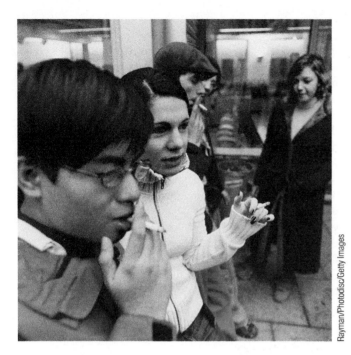

Is social smoking really that bad for me?
An occasional puff once in a while when you are out with friends doesn't hurt, right? Wrong! There is no "safe" amount of tobacco use—any smoking or smokeless tobacco has the potential for negative effects on your health. Further, even if you only smoke once or twice a week and consider yourself a social smoker, chances are you are on the road to dependence and a more frequent habit and addiction.

youths aged 12 to 17 (4.3 percent). In addition, 55 percent of Canadians aged 20 to 24 had never smoked, which is a significantly higher percentage than the 39 percent of 20 to 24 year olds who never smoked in 2001 (Statistics Canada, 2014b).

Despite the reduced rate of smoking in the population, it remains the number one preventable cause of death in Canada. Every year, smoking kills five times more Canadians than car accidents, murder, suicide, and alcohol abuse combined. The latest figures for deaths attributed specifically to tobacco suggested that almost 17 percent of all deaths were related to tobacco use, while acute-care hospital days attributable to tobacco were 10.3 percent of all hospital days (Rehm et al., 2006).

Tobacco and Its Effects

Tobacco is available in several forms. Cigarettes, cigars, and pipes are used for burning and inhaling tobacco. **Snuff** is a finely ground form of tobacco that can be inhaled, chewed, or placed against the gums. **Chewing tobacco**, also known as "smokeless tobacco," is placed between the gums and teeth for sucking or chewing.

The chemical stimulant nicotine is the major psychoactive substance in these products. In its natural form, **nicotine** is a colourless liquid that turns brown upon oxidation (exposure to oxygen). When tobacco leaves are burned in a cigarette, pipe, or cigar, nicotine is released and inhaled into the lungs. Sucking or chewing tobacco releases nicotine into the saliva, and is then absorbed through the mucous membranes in the mouth. The stimulant effects of nicotine are discussed later in this chapter. Smoking is the most common form of tobacco use. Smoking delivers a strong dose of nicotine to the user, along with an additional 5000 chemicals, 50 of which are known to cause cancer (Reid et al., 2012). Among these chemicals are various gases and vapours that carry particulate matter in concentrations that are 500 000 times as great as the most air-polluted cities in the world. Particulate matter condenses in the lungs to form a thick, brownish sludge called tar. **Tar** contains various carcinogenic (cancer-causing) agents such as benzopyrene and chemical irritants such as phenol. Phenol has the potential to combine with other chemicals to contribute to the development of lung cancer.

In healthy lungs, millions of tiny hairlike tissues called cilia sweep away foreign matter. Once the foreign material is swept up and collected by the cilia, it can be expelled from the lungs by coughing. Nicotine impairs the cleansing function of the cilia by paralyzing them for up to one hour following the smoking of a single cigarette. Tars and other solids in tobacco smoke are thus allowed to accumulate and irritate sensitive lung tissue.

Tar and nicotine are not the only harmful chemicals in cigarettes. In fact, tars account for only 8 percent of the components of tobacco smoke. The remaining 92 percent is made up of various gases, the most dangerous of which is **carbon monoxide**. In tobacco smoke, the concentration of carbon monoxide is 800 times higher than the level considered safe. In the human body, carbon monoxide reduces the oxygen-carrying capacity of the red blood cells by binding with the receptor sites for oxygen (Centre for Addiction and Mental Health, 2012). Smoking thus diminishes the capacity of the circulatory system to carry oxygen, causing oxygen deprivation in many body tissues. It is not a surprise then to discover that smokers, particularly heavy smokers, find physical tasks such as walking quickly or climbing the stairs result in them feeling 'winded' because they are not able to get sufficient oxygen to the working tissues. The heat from tobacco smoke, which can reach 880°C, is also harmful to the smoker. Inhaling hot gases and vapours

Snuff A powdered form of tobacco sniffed and absorbed through the mucous membranes in the nose or placed inside the cheek and sucked.

Chewing tobacco A type of tobacco placed in the mouth and then sucked or chewed.

Nicotine The stimulant chemical in tobacco products.

Tar A thick, brownish substance condensed from particulate matter in smoked tobacco.

Carbon monoxide A gas found in cigarette smoke that binds at oxygen receptor sites in the blood.

exposes sensitive mucous membranes to irritating chemicals that weaken the tissues and contribute to the development of cancers of the mouth, larynx, and throat.

Filtered cigarettes are designed to reduce levels of gases such as hydrogen cyanide and hydrocarbons, yet may actually deliver more hazardous carbon monoxide to the user than nonfiltered brands. Some smokers use low-tar and nicotine products (that is, mild, special, or "lite") thinking these are safer forms of cigarettes. True, they contain 10 percent less carbon monoxide and 8 percent less nicotine, but they contain the same level of the other harmful chemicals. However, since there is less nicotine, smokers tend to inhale more deeply and actually inhale more of the dangerous chemicals than they would if they smoked regular cigarettes.

Nicotine is a powerful central nervous system (CNS) stimulant that produces an aroused, alert mental state rapidly, since it enters the brain 10 seconds after inhalation (Health Canada, 2007). Nicotine also stimulates the adrenal glands, increasing the production of adrenaline. The physical effects of nicotine stimulation include increased heart and respiratory rate, constriction of blood vessels, and subsequent increased blood pressure because the heart must work harder to pump blood through the narrowed vessels (Health Canada, 2007). Because smoking increases the "stickiness" of the blood, there is an increased risk of developing blood clots when you smoke. This risk is further elevated when smoking is combined with use of oral contraceptives.

Nicotine decreases the stomach contractions that signal hunger. It also decreases blood sugar levels. These factors, along with decreased sensation in the taste buds, reduce appetite. For this reason, many smokers eat less and are typically thinner than nonsmokers. New smokers usually feel the effects of nicotine with their first puff. These symptoms, called **nicotine poisoning**, include dizziness; lightheadedness; rapid, erratic pulse; clammy skin; nausea; vomiting; and diarrhea (Health Canada, 2007). This effect is further enhanced in children, because of their physiologically and chemically immature bodies. These effects of nicotine poisoning cease when tolerance develops. Tolerance develops almost immediately in new users, perhaps after the second or third cigarette (Health Canada, 2007). In contrast, tolerance to most other drugs, such as alcohol, develops over a period of months or years.

Smoking—A Learned Behaviour

In most cases, becoming a smoker is a gradual process. It begins with forming a predisposition to smoking—that is, a perception that smoking is a normal behaviour accepted by your peer group, regardless of how it is perceived in society. Smoking usually starts with an experimental stage in which you smoke repeatedly but irregularly, followed by regular use, then addiction. The transition from first experimenting with smoking to daily use usually takes an average of two to three years.

About 85 percent of smokers start before age 16. New smokers do not expect to become addicted, believing instead that they will be able to quit whenever they want to. Only 10 percent of smokers begin after the age of 18. It seems probable that the level of knowledge and experience acquired by age 18 relates to the decision not to smoke.

Tobacco product promotions are intended to convey a positive brand image and convey as many "impressions" (exposures to the consumer) as possible in order to create and maintain the perception that tobacco use is desirable, socially acceptable, healthy, sexy, and more pervasive in society than it really is. These promotions are primarily directed at young people, particularly young women, partly because the tobacco companies know that most people make the decision as to whether or not to smoke by the age of 16. Another reason tobacco companies need to target new users is that when their product is used as recommended, it is likely to kill you.

Smokeless Tobacco

Smokeless tobacco is as addictive as cigarettes due to its nicotine content. Although there is nicotine in all tobacco products, smokeless tobacco contains more than cigarettes. An average-sized dip or chew held in your mouth for 30 minutes releases as much nicotine as smoking four cigarettes. Thus, a two-can-a-week snuff dipper gets as much nicotine as a one-and-a-half-pack-a-day smoker.

One of the major risks of chewing tobacco is **leukoplakia**, a condition characterized by leathery white patches inside the mouth produced by contact with irritants in tobacco juice. Smokeless tobacco also impairs the senses of taste and smell, often resulting in the user adding salt and sugar to food, which can contribute to high blood pressure and obesity. Some smokeless tobacco products contain high levels of sodium (salt), which also contributes to high blood pressure. In addition, dental problems are common among users: contact with tobacco juice causes receding gums, tooth decay, bad breath, and discoloured teeth. Damage to the teeth and jawbone can contribute to early loss of teeth. Users of all tobacco products may not be able to use the vitamins and other nutrients in food effectively. In some cases, vitamin supplements may be recommended by a physician.

Nicotine poisoning Symptoms experienced by new smokers including dizziness; diarrhea; lightheadedness; rapid, erratic pulse; clammy skin; nausea; and vomiting.

Leukoplakia A condition characterized by leathery white patches inside the mouth produced by contact with irritants in tobacco juice.

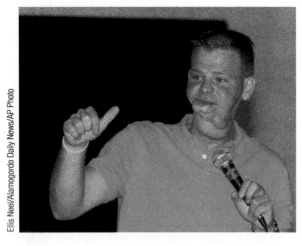

VonBehrens, a 27-year-old cancer survivor, talks about his experiences with chewing tobacco, cancer, doctors and disfiguring surgeries during an anti-tobacco presentation to middle school students. VonBehrens was 17 when he was diagnosed with oral cancer; his jaw, teeth, and part of his tongue were removed in surgeries to save his life.

Environmental Tobacco Smoke

As the population of nonsmokers rises, so does the demand for the right to breathe smoke-free air. As a result, smoking is banned in many public places, particularly those that are indoors. In recent years, further banning has occurred in parks, campuses, and in vehicles when a child under the age of 18 is in it.

Environmental tobacco smoke (ETS) is divided into two categories: mainstream smoke and secondhand smoke (also called sidestream smoke). **Mainstream smoke** refers to smoke drawn through tobacco while inhaling; **secondhand smoke** refers to smoke from the burning end of a cigarette and the smoke exhaled by a smoker. People who breathe smoke as a result of someone else's smoking are said to be involuntary or passive smokers.

Although involuntary smokers breathe less tobacco than active smokers, they still face risks from exposure to tobacco smoke. Secondhand smoke actually contains more carcinogenic substances than the smoke that a smoker inhales directly—about twice as much tar and nicotine, 5 times as much carbon monoxide, and 50 times as much ammonia or window cleaner (The Canadian Lung Association, 2012). Exposure to secondhand smoke increases risk of lung disease (by 25 percent), heart disease (by 10 percent), emphysema,

Environmental tobacco smoke (ETS) Smoke from tobacco products, including mainstream and sidestream smoke.

Mainstream smoke Smoke drawn from a cigarette, cigar, or pipe while inhaling.

Secondhand smoke Cigarette, pipe, or cigar smoke released into the air and inhaled by nonsmokers (as well as smokers).

Nicotine withdrawal Symptoms, including nausea, headaches, and irritability, experienced by individuals who cease using tobacco.

chronic bronchitis, asthma, and other diseases (The Canadian Lung Association, 2012).

Lung cancer and heart disease are not the only risks involuntary smokers face. Children exposed to secondhand smoke also have a greater chance of developing other respiratory problems, such as coughing, wheezing, asthma, and chest colds, along with a decrease in pulmonary performance. In fact, the greatest effects of secondhand smoke are seen in children under the age of five.

Cigarette, cigar, and pipe smoke in enclosed areas present other hazards to nonsmokers. The level of carbon monoxide from cigarette smoke contained in enclosed places is 4000 times higher than the standard recommended by the U.S. Environmental Protection Agency as a definition of clean air. An estimated 10 to 15 percent of nonsmokers are extremely sensitive (hypersensitive) to cigarette smoke. These people experience itchy eyes, difficulty breathing, painful headaches, nausea, and dizziness in response to minute amounts of smoke.

Efforts to reduce the hazards associated with passive smoking have been rolling along for years. As previously mentioned, smoking is illegal in most public places, including government buildings, restaurants, cafés, coffee shops, shopping malls, schools, and universities, as well as many public outdoor places. Hotels and motels, if not completely smoke-free, set aside rooms for nonsmokers, and car rental agencies designate certain vehicles for nonsmokers. Smoking has also been banned for some time on all domestic airline flights. Recently, some provinces have declared vehicles containing children under the age of 18 years to be smoke-free as well.

QUITTING

Quitting smoking is often a lengthy process involving several unsuccessful attempts before success is finally achieved. Even successful quitters have occasional slips, emphasizing the fact that quitting smoking is a dynamic process that may actually be never-ending. Various programs have been developed and there are various prescription and nonprescription drugs that can be used to assist you when you choose to quit.

Breaking the Nicotine Addiction

Nicotine addiction may be one of the toughest addictions to overcome given that most (80 percent) smokers have a cigarette every one to two hours (Health Canada, 2007). When smokers quit, **nicotine withdrawal** occurs; the symptoms of withdrawal include headaches, anxiety and irritability, restlessness and difficulty concentrating, nausea, vomiting, and intense cravings for tobacco (Health Canada, 2007). Smokers who attempt to quit may also experience fatigue and coughing, both indications that the body is attempting to remove the poisons accumulated from smoking (Health Canada, 2007). If you are a smoker and choose to quit, you have several options to manage the symptoms of your withdrawal.

Nicotine Replacement Products

Non-tobacco products that put nicotine in the bloodstream may help you to stop using tobacco. The two most common nicotine-replacement products are nicotine chewing gum and the nicotine patch, both available by prescription. One prescription chewing gum containing nicotine is called Nicorette. Nicorettes help with the withdrawal symptoms by reducing your nicotine consumption gradually over time. The gum delivers about as much nicotine as a cigarette, but because it is absorbed through the mucous membrane of the mouth, it does not produce the same rush as the nicotine that is inhaled from a cigarette. As a result, the individual who stopped his/her tobacco use does not experience withdrawal symptoms, and fewer cravings for nicotine are felt as the dosage is reduced until the person is completely weaned from the drug. There is some controversy surrounding the use of nicotine replacement gum. Opponents believe that it substitutes one addiction for another. Successful quitters counter that it is a valid way to help break a deadly habit without suffering the unpleasant withdrawal symptoms and cravings that often lead ex-smokers to resume smoking.

The nicotine patch, first marketed in 1991, is a popular method for those attempting to quit smoking. It is generally used in conjunction with a comprehensive smoking-behaviour cessation program. A small, thin patch is placed on the smoker's upper body to deliver a continuous flow of nicotine through the skin for 24 hours. This continuous flow of nicotine, like the regular chewing of Nicorette, reduces and potentially eliminates the withdrawal symptoms typically experienced. The patch is worn for 8 to 12 weeks under the guidance of a physician. During this time, the dose of nicotine in the patch is gradually reduced until the smoker is fully weaned from nicotine. Occasional side-effects include mild skin irritation, insomnia, dry mouth, and nervousness. The patch is relatively inexpensive compared to the price of a pack of cigarettes, and some insurance plans will pay for it.

Two other prescription drugs available to assist you when you choose to quit smoking are Zyban and Champix[r] (quit 4 life, n.d.). Zyban (Buproprion) is prescribed for two weeks at a time with most individuals requiring on average nine weeks of treatment. When taking Zyban, the previous enjoyment of smoking is lost, thus reducing the smoker's desire to smoke. Similar to Zyban, Champix[r] (Varenicline) works by preventing the enjoyment of smoking by blocking your brain's ability to take in nicotine. Further, Champix[r] enables the brain to produce dopamine, which reduces cravings for nicotine. It generally takes 12 weeks of Champix[r] for most individuals to successfully quit smoking. Both drugs have various potential side effects, some of which are similar to nicotine withdrawal. Individuals who take Zyban are recommended to not consume alcohol, as violent reactions have been noted after even one or two drinks in previous users (quit 4 life, n.d.). If you experience depression or suicidal thoughts when taking Champix[r], you are advised to discontinue use immediately (quit 4 life, n.d.).

Breaking the Habit

For many smokers, the road to quitting includes some type of antismoking therapy. Among the more common therapy techniques are aversion therapy, operant conditioning, and self-control therapy. Prospective quitters must decide which method or combination of methods will work best for them. Programs that combine several approaches have shown the most promise. It should be recognized that when people choose to quit smoking, they have a habit to break as well as an addiction. Smoking is often done at regular intervals during the day, and thus is a habit or lifestyle choice. Successful smoking cessation programs will also attempt to manage the 'habit' part of smoking too.

Benefits of Quitting

Many tissues damaged by smoking can repair themselves over time. As soon as smokers stop, their bodies begin the repair process. Within eight hours, carbon monoxide and oxygen levels return to normal, and "smoker's breath" disappears. Within a few days of quitting, the mucus clogging airways is broken up and eliminated. Circulation and the senses of taste and smell improve within weeks. Many ex-smokers who have successfully stopped smoking say they have more energy, sleep better, and feel more alert. By the end of one year, the risk for lung cancer and stroke decreases. Within two years, the risk for heart attack drops to almost the same levels as for non-smokers. At the end of 10 tobacco-free years, the ex-smoker can expect to live out his or her normal life span. Figure 10.5 shows the health benefits of quitting smoking.

FIGURE 10.5

When Smokers Quit

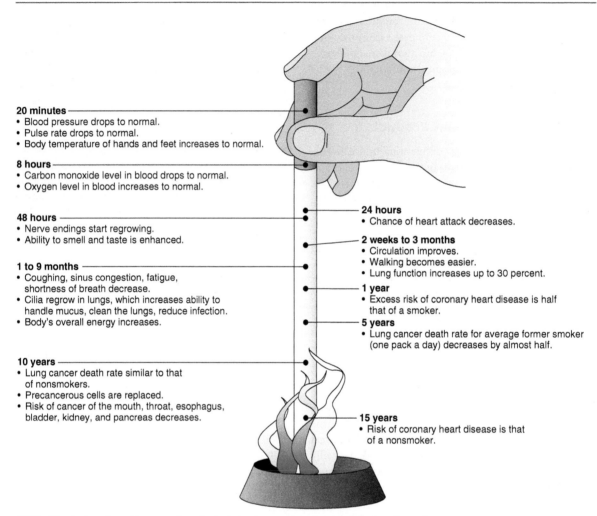

20 minutes
- Blood pressure drops to normal.
- Pulse rate drops to normal.
- Body temperature of hands and feet increases to normal.

8 hours
- Carbon monoxide level in blood drops to normal.
- Oxygen level in blood increases to normal.

48 hours
- Nerve endings start regrowing.
- Ability to smell and taste is enhanced.

1 to 9 months
- Coughing, sinus congestion, fatigue, shortness of breath decrease.
- Cilia regrow in lungs, which increases ability to handle mucus, clean the lungs, reduce infection.
- Body's overall energy increases.

10 years
- Lung cancer death rate similar to that of nonsmokers.
- Precancerous cells are replaced.
- Risk of cancer of the mouth, throat, esophagus, bladder, kidney, and pancreas decreases.

24 hours
- Chance of heart attack decreases.

2 weeks to 3 months
- Circulation improves.
- Walking becomes easier.
- Lung function increases up to 30 percent.

1 year
- Excess risk of coronary heart disease is half that of a smoker.

5 years
- Lung cancer death rate for average former smoker (one pack a day) decreases by almost half.

15 years
- Risk of coronary heart disease is that of a nonsmoker.

Within 20 minutes of smoking cessation, the body begins a series of changes that continues for years.

Source: From *Drugs and Society* by Glen R. Hanson, Peter J. Venturelli, Annette E. Fleckenstein. Copyright year 1998. Reprinted with permission of Jones and Bartlett Publishers.

CAFFEINE

Caffeine is the most popular and widely consumed drug in Canada with the average per person consumption estimated to be between 210 to 238 mg per day (Centre for Addiction and Mental Health, 2011). Almost half of Canadians drink coffee every day, and many others consume caffeine in some other form (tea, colas, chocolate), mainly for its well-known "wake-up" effect. Drinking coffee is legal and socially encouraged. Many people do not realize caffeine is a drug and it too is addictive. To most, coffee and other caffeine-containing products seem harmless. Though in most cases, the moderate consumption of caffeine is safe, you should be aware of the potential risks involved and clear on what is moderate consumption. **Caffeine** is a drug derived from the chemical family called **xanthines** (National Library of Medicine, 2013). Two related chemicals, theophylline and theobromine, are found in tea and chocolate, respectively. Xanthines are mild CNS stimulants that enhance mental alertness and reduce feelings of fatigue. Other stimulant effects of caffeine include increases in heart muscle contractions,

Caffeine A stimulant found in coffee, tea, chocolate, and some soft drinks.

Xanthines The chemical family of stimulants to which caffeine belongs.

Student
Health
TODAY

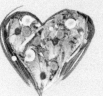

E-cigarettes: Risks and Concerns

Electronic cigarettes, also called e-cigarettes, are increasingly used worldwide, even though there is limited information on their health effects. Most e-cigarettes consist of a battery, a charger, an atomizer, and a cartridge containing nicotine and propylene glycol. When a smoker draws air through an e-cigarette, an airflow sensor activates the battery and heats the atomizer to vapourize the propylene glycol and nicotine. Upon inhalation, the aerosol vapour delivers a dose of nicotine into the lungs of the smoker, after which, residual aerosol is exhaled into the environment. Nothing is known, however, about the chemicals present in the aerosolized vapours emanating from e-cigarettes.

Although manufacturers claim that electronic cigarettes are a safe alternative to conventional cigarettes, the U.S. Food and Drug Administration (FDA) analyzed samples of two popular brands and found variable amounts of nicotine and traces of toxic chemicals, including known cancer-causing substances (carcinogens). These carcinogens included an ingredient used in antifreeze and formaldehyde, which was present in higher amounts when higher-voltage charges are used. Although e-cigarettes do not involve combustion and the vapour contains fewer toxic chemicals than tobacco smoke, e-cigarettes are a relatively new product and thus the long-term health effects of vaping are unknown.

In Canada, e-cigarettes containing nicotine are regulated as drugs/drug delivery devices under the Food and Drugs Act. Nicotine-containing e-cigarettes, with or without a health claim, require market authorization from Health Canada as new drugs before they can be imported, marketed, or sold. To date, no such product has received market approval; therefore, e-cigarettes containing any level of nicotine have not been approved for sale in Canada. In contrast, e-cigarettes that do not contain nicotine and do not make health claims are legal. Health Canada has issued public advisories against using e-cigarettes, as these products "may pose health risks and have not been fully evaluated for safety, quality, and efficacy." Several provinces have begun to develop policies for the sale, marketing, and use of both nicotine- and non-nicotine-containing e-cigarettes. At the municipal level, a growing number of jurisdictions are adopting by-laws or modifying their smoking policies to prohibit and/or restrict the use of e-cigarettes.

An increasing number of Canadians are trying e-cigarettes, particularly smokers and young Canadians. In 2013, 8.5 percent of all Canadians age 15 and older (approximately 2.5 million) reported trying an e-cigarette; 1.8 percent had used an e-cigarette in the past 30 days. Recent estimates from national surveys of Canadian adults suggest that between one-third and one-half of smokers had tried e-cigarettes. Studies of Quebec and Ontario high school students indicate even higher levels of use among youth smokers. In Ontario, 43 percent of youth who had used a tobacco product in the past 12 months reported ever using e-cigarettes. A larger study of high school students in Ontario and Alberta found that 35 percent of past-month smokers also reported using e-cigarettes in the past month. In Quebec, 90 percent of youth smokers reported ever using e-cigarettes, including 30 percent who reported use in the past 30 days. Young nonsmokers are also trying e-cigarettes. Among high school students in Ontario, 7 percent of never smokers reported ever using e-cigarettes, compared to 28 percent of youth nonsmokers in Quebec. In general, few nonsmokers reported use of e-cigarettes in the past month; several recent studies suggest that approximately 4 percent of nonsmoking youth reported past-month use of e-cigarettes.

Overall, there is evidence indicating the use of e-cigarettes in Canada is on the rise. However, much of the existing evidence relies upon non-representative surveys with limited geographic scope. The data collected using the 2013 Canadian Tobacco, Alcohol and Drugs Survey (CTADS) provides the first nationally representative, comprehensive examination of e-cigarette use in the Canadian population. Therefore, health professionals recommend those using e-cigarettes should proceed with caution and further research is needed to determine the long-term effects of e-cigarette use.

Sources: Based on the report from Czoli C. D., Reid J. L., Rynard V. L., & Hammond D. *E-cigarettes in Canada – Tobacco Use in Canada: Patterns and Trends*, 2015 Edition, Special Supplement. Waterloo, ON: Propel Centre for Population Health Impact, University of Waterloo. Retrieved from http://www.tobaccoreport.ca/2015/TobaccoUseinCanada_2015_EcigaretteSupplement.pdf.

oxygen consumption, metabolism, and urinary output. These effects are felt within 15 to 45 minutes of ingesting a product that contains caffeine.

Side effects of xanthines include wakefulness, insomnia, irregular heartbeat, dizziness, nausea, indigestion, and sometimes mild delirium. Some people also experience heartburn. As with other drugs, the user's psychological outlook and expectations or set (see also Chapter 9) will influence the effects. Different products contain different concentrations of caffeine. A 156-mL (5-ounce) cup of brewed coffee contains 65 to 115 milligrams. Caffeine concentrations vary with the brand and strength of the brew. Typically, the darker the coffee bean, the less caffeine it contains. This is because in the roasting process caffeine is lost, thus, the longer the coffee beans are roasted, the darker they become, resulting in more of a coffee flavour but less caffeine. Small chocolate bars (28 grams) contain up to 15 milligrams of caffeine and theobromine. Table 10.3 outlines the caffeine content of various products.

Caffeinism Caffeine intoxication brought on by excessive caffeine use; symptoms include chronic insomnia, irritability, anxiety, muscle twitches, and headaches.

Caffeine Addiction

As the effects of caffeine wear off, users may feel let down—mentally or physically depressed, tired, and weak. To counteract this, people commonly choose to drink another cup of coffee. Habitually engaging in this practice leads to tolerance and psychological dependency. Until the mid-1970s, caffeine was not medically recognized as addictive. Chronic caffeine use and its attendant behaviours were called "coffee nerves." This syndrome is now recognized as caffeine intoxication, or **caffeinism**. Symptoms of caffeinism include chronic insomnia, jitters, irritability, nervousness, anxiety, and involuntary muscle twitches. Withdrawing the caffeine may compound the effects and produce severe headaches. (Some physicians ask their patients to take a simple test for caffeine addiction—do not consume anything containing caffeine, if you get a severe headache within four hours, you are addicted and experiencing withdrawal symptoms.) Because caffeine meets the requirements for addiction—tolerance, psychological dependency, and withdrawal symptoms—it can be classified as addictive. Although you would have to drink 67 to 100 cups of coffee in a day to produce a fatal overdose of caffeine, you may experience sensory disturbances after consuming 10 cups of coffee within a 24-hour period. These symptoms include tinnitus (ringing in the ears), spots before the eyes,

TABLE 10.3
Caffeine Content of Various Products

Product	Size*	Caffeine†
Coffee		
Brewed	8 oz. (237 mL)	95–200 mg
Brewed, decaffeinated	8 oz. (237 mL)	2–12 mg
Espresso, restaurant-style	1 oz. (30 mL)	47–75 mg
Instant	8 oz. (237 mL)	27–173 mg
Tea		
Black tea, decaffeinated	8 oz. (237 mL)	0–12 mg
Green tea	8 oz. (237 mL)	24–45 mg
Black tea	8 oz. (237 mL)	14–70 mg
Soda Pop		
Coca-Cola	12 oz. (355 mL)	23–35 mg
Diet Coke	12 oz. (355 mL)	23–47 mg
Diet Pepsi	12 oz. (355 mL)	27–37 mg
Sweets		
Chocolate chips, semisweet	1 cup (168 grams)	104 mg
Dark chocolate-coated coffee beans	28 pieces	336 mg

*Sizes are listed in fluid ounces (oz.) and millilitres (mL).

†Caffeine is listed in milligrams (mg).

numbness in arms and legs, poor circulation, and visual hallucinations (Handwerk, 2009). Because 10 cups of coffee is not an extraordinary amount to drink in one day for some, caffeine use poses a health risk.

Energy Drinks

Because they contain caffeine, it makes sense to include a section on energy drinks in this chapter. Energy drinks are, in fact, one of the fastest growing components of the beverage industry (CTV Montreal News, 2013). The Centre for Addiction and Mental Health (2011) reported that the per capita consumption of energy drinks increased from 0.8 litres in 2001 to 1.1 litres in 2006. Energy drinks are powerful stimulants available in a variety of sizes and with various levels of caffeine, sugar, and calories (see Table 10.4 for details). Not included in Table 10.4 are the amount of other ingredients included in these beverages—other stimulant ingredients such as guarana, taurine, ginseng—and B vitamins (Sifferlin, 2013). If you recall the section in Chapter 9 on drug interactions, you might question the safety of these energy drinks—even though most contain only as much caffeine as a large cup of coffee—given the potential for synergistic reactions. Please also see the Point of View box on page 307 for a discussion of energy drinks mixed with alcohol.

Energy drinks are most often consumed for the 'rush of energy' promised, with many students making them a part of their daily consumption (CTV Montreal News, 2013). As you likely know, there have been several deaths reported linked to energy drink consumption, though autopsy results cannot specifically indicate the energy drink consumed, but rather can provide toxicology results that include levels of caffeine and other drugs found.

In addition to the risks and benefits of consumption (something you should consider for any decision you make that may impact your health), you might consider why it is that energy drinks have become 'essential' for many? Have they simply replaced cola consumption? Coffee consumption? Is there really a need to boost your energy to get your work done? Or would you be better off taking care of your overall health needs so that you can do what needs to be done without ingesting drugs to help you?

The Health Consequences of Long-Term Caffeine Use

Long-term caffeine use has been tentatively linked to a number of serious health problems, ranging from heart disease and cancer to mental dysfunction and birth defects. Further, high consumption (more than six cups of coffee per day) of unfiltered coffees such as French press and boiled/perked coffee are linked to elevated low-density-lipoprotein concentrations (van Dam, 2008). However, no strong evidence exists to suggest that moderate caffeine use (less than 300 milligrams daily—approximately three cups of coffee) produces harmful effects in healthy, nonpregnant people. In fact, there may be some benefit to frequent moderate consumption of coffee—whether decaffeinated or caffeinated—in terms of reducing risk for type 2 diabetes, though more research is warranted to better understand the mechanisms providing this benefit (Tunnicliffe et al., 2008). Coffee and other products containing caffeine also have potential benefits as ergogenic aids, facilitating athletic performances and potentially positively altering carbohydrate and fat metabolism during exercise (Graham et al., 2008; Tarnopolsky, 2008; Tunnicliffe et al., 2008).

It appears that caffeine does not cause long-term high blood pressure and is not linked to strokes, nor is there any evidence of a relationship between caffeine and heart disease. However, people who experience irregular heartbeat are cautioned against using caffeine because the resultant increase in heart rate might be life-threatening. Both decaffeinated and caffeinated coffee products contain ingredients that can irritate the stomach lining and be harmful to people with stomach ulcers. For years, caffeine consumption was linked with fibrocystic breast disease, a condition characterized by painful, noncancerous lumps in the breasts. Although these conclusions have been challenged, many clinicians advise patients with mammillary cysts to avoid or limit their caffeine use.

TABLE 10.4

Caffeine Content of a Variety of Energy Drinks

Ratings

In order of caffeine content, lowest to highest. Ties are in alphabetical order.

Product	Size (fl. oz.)	Cost ($)	Per serving Calories	Sugars (g.)	Caffeine (mg.)
5-hour Energy Decaf	1.9	2.00	4	0	6
FRS Healthy Energy	11.5	2.00	20	2	17
Archer Farms Energy Drink Juice Infused (Target)	12	1.80	80	19	55
Amp Energy	8	1.00	110	29	71
Bawls Guarana	10	2.00	120	32	71
Steaz Energy	8	1.33	90	23	72
Red Rain Energy Drink	8	.50	100	24	75
SK Street Kings 6 Hours of Energy	2.5	1.75	0	0	78
Rockstar Energy Drink Double Strength	8	1.00	140	31	80
Sambazon Organic Amazon Energy	8	1.17	90	21	81
Red Bull Energy Drink	8.4	1.75	110	27	83
Monster Energy	8	1.00	100	27	92
Xyience Xenergy	8	1.25	0	0	94
Nestlé Jamba	8.4	2.00	90	20	98
Venom Energy	8	1.00	120	27	110
Guru Energy Drink	8.4	2.50	100	25	118
Arizona Energy	8	1.00	100	26	129
Clif Shot Turbo Energy Gel	1.2*	1.00	110	12	133
Stacker 2 6-Hour Power	2	1.50	0	0	149
Starbucks Doubleshot	15	2.50	210	26	162
Full Throttle	8	2.50	220	58	210
Celsius Your Ultimate Fitness Partner	12	1.75	10	0	212
5-hour Energy	1.9	2.00	4	0	215
Monster X-presso	6.8	2.25	90	12	221
NOS High Performance Energy Drink	16	2.50	220	52	224
Rockstar Energy Shot	2.5	2.00	10	0	229
5-hour Energy Extra Strength	1.9	3.00	4	0	242

*Serving size is in gram weight, not volume.

Source: *Consumer Reports* magazine (December, 2012) The buzz on energy-drink caffeine: Caffeine levels per serving for the 27 products we checked ranged from 6 milligrams to 242 milligrams per serving. Retrieved May 10, 2013. Reprinted with permission.

point of view

ENERGY DRINKS AND ALCOHOL: Your Choice Drink?

In addition to energy drinks giving you wings to assist in your daily tasks, they are also often combined with alcohol to assist you in dancing or partying into the wee hours of the morning. Despite the combination of drugs with opposing effects (e.g., stimulants and depressants), Hsu (2012) suggests that the combination of energy drinks and alcohol has become a "staple drink for club-going young people in need of an energy fix as they party till the wee hours of the morning." Risks of this combination include a reduction in your body's natural ability to recognize that you have had enough to drink and to shut down, thus allowing you to drink more alcohol, which increases your risk of alcohol poisoning as well as various other potentially negative consequences associated with excess alcohol consumption (e.g., unprotected sex, unintentional sex, acts of aggression, and so on) (Hsu, 2012). Further, other risks associated with energy drinks are abnormal heart rhythms, difficulty sleeping, jitteriness, rapid pulse, and elevated blood pressure (Consumer Reports, 2012). Combined, there is the potential for tremors, irritability, and bursts of energy followed by exhaustion (Hsu, 2012).

What is your reaction to this combination? Are you willing to take the risk and combine energy drinks with alcohol in an attempt to dance or party longer? Or will you find a more natural way to keep the party/dancing going?

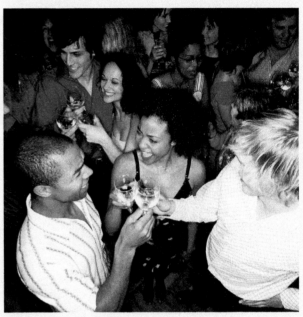

George Doyle/Stockbyte/Getty Images

assess YOURSELF

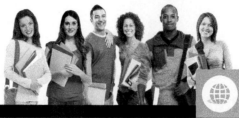

Go to MasteringHealth to complete this questionnaire with automatic scoring

TAKING CHARGE: Managing Your Alcohol and Tobacco Use

To better manage your alcohol and tobacco use, it is important to ask yourself questions regarding it. Honest reflection of your behaviours can help you to make better decisions regarding these recreational drugs.

Alcohol and Tobacco: Are Your Habits Placing You at Risk?

1 What's Your Risk of Alcohol Abuse?

Many college and university students engage in potentially dangerous drinking behaviours. Is your approach to drinking safe? Take the following quiz and reflect upon your responses and what they might indicate.

1. How often do you have a drink containing alcohol?

   Never (0)

   Monthly or less (1)

   2 to 4 times a month (2)

   2 to 3 times a week (3)

   4 or more times a week (4)

2. How many alcoholic drinks do you have on a typical occasion when you are drinking?

   1 or 2 (0)

   3 or 4 (1)

   5 or 6 (2)

   7 to 9 (3)

   10 or more (4)

3. How often do you have four or five drinks or more on one occasion?

   Never (0)

   Less than monthly (1)

   Monthly (2)

   Weekly (3)

   Daily or almost daily (4)

4. How often during the past year have you been unable to stop drinking once you started?

   Never (0)

   Less than monthly (1)

   Monthly (2)

   Weekly (3)

   Daily or almost daily (4)

5. How often during the past year have you failed to do what was normally expected from you because of drinking?

   Never (0)

   Less than monthly (1)

   Monthly (2)

   Weekly (3)

   Daily or almost daily (4)

6. How often during the past year have you needed a drink in the morning to get yourself going after a day or night of heavy drinking?

   Never (0)

   Less than monthly (1)

   Monthly (2)

   Weekly (3)

   Daily or almost daily (4)

7. How often during the past year have you had a feeling of guilt or remorse after drinking?

   Never (0)

   Less than monthly (1)

   Monthly (2)

   Weekly (3)

   Daily or almost daily (4)

8. How often during the past year have you been unable to remember what happened the night before because you had been drinking?

   Never (0)

   Less than monthly (1)

Monthly (2)

Weekly (3)

Daily or almost daily (4)

9. Have you or someone else been injured as a result of your drinking?

No (0)

Yes, but not in the past year (1)

Yes, during the past year (2)

10. Has a relative, friend, or a doctor or other health-care professional been concerned about your drinking or suggested you cut down?

No (0)

Yes, but not in the past year (1)

Yes, during the past year (2)

Interpreting Your Responses

Scores below 6: Congratulations! You are in control of your drinking behaviours and do a good job of consuming alcohol responsibly and in moderation.

Scores between 6 and 8: Your alcohol consumption is possibly risky. Take steps to change your drinking behaviour and make some positive changes for your health and safety.

Scores above 8: Your drinking patterns are putting you at high risk for illness, unsafe sexual situations, or alcohol-related injuries, and may even affect your academic performance.

Source: Abridged and adapted from National Institutes of Health, 1990. *Why Do You Smoke?* NIH Pub. No. 93-1822. U.S. Department of Health and Human Services.

This Assess Yourself activity gave you the chance to evaluate your alcohol consumption. If some of your answers surprised you or if you were unsure how to answer some of the questions, consider taking steps to change your behaviour.

Today, you can:

- Start a diary of your drinking habits. Keeping track of how much you drink—as well as how much money you spend on drinks and how you feel when you are drinking—will make you more aware of your true drinking habits.

- Spend some time thinking about the ways your family members use alcohol. Is there a family history of excessive use of alcohol or alcohol abuse? Did your family's alcohol consumption have any effect on you while you were growing up? Consider whether your current alcohol use is healthy, or whether it is likely to create problems for you in the future.

Within the next two weeks, you can:

- Make your first drink a glass of water or another nonalcoholic beverage the next time you go to a party. Intersperse alcoholic drinks with nonalcoholic beverages to pace your consumption.

- Challenge yourself and a few close friends to get together at least once a week for a nonalcoholic social occasion, such as a sports event or movie night.

- Commit yourself to limiting your alcohol intake at every social function you attend. Decide ahead of time whether you want to drink and, if so, what your limit will be; then stick to it.

- Cultivate friendships and explore activities that do not centre on alcohol. If your current group of friends drinks heavily, and it is becoming a problem for you, you may need to step back from the group for a while.

2 Why Do You Smoke?

Identifying why you smoke can help you develop a plan to quit. Answer the following questions and evaluate your reasons for smoking.

1. I smoke to keep from slowing down.

☐ Often ☐ Sometimes ☐ Never

2. I feel more comfortable with a cigarette in my hand.

☐ Often ☐ Sometimes ☐ Never

3. Smoking is pleasant and enjoyable.

☐ Often ☐ Sometimes ☐ Never

4. I light up a cigarette when something makes me angry.

☐ Often ☐ Sometimes ☐ Never

5. When I run out of cigarettes, it is almost unbearable until I get more.

☐ Often ☐ Sometimes ☐ Never

6. I smoke cigarettes automatically without even being aware of it.

☐ Often ☐ Sometimes ☐ Never

7. I reach for a cigarette when I need a lift.

☐ Often ☐ Sometimes ☐ Never

8. Smoking relaxes me in a stressful situation.

☐ Often ☐ Sometimes ☐ Never

(continued)

Interpreting Your Responses

Use your answers to identify some of the key reasons why you smoke, then use the tips presented in this chapter to develop a plan for quitting.

Regardless of your current level of use, if you smoke at all, now is the time to take steps toward stopping the habit.

Today, you can:

- Develop a plan to stop using tobacco. The first step is to identify why you want to quit. Write your reasons down and carry a copy of it with you. Every time you are tempted to smoke, go over your reasons for quitting.
- Think about the times and places you usually smoke. What could you do instead of smoking at those times? Make a list of positive tobacco alternatives.

Within the next two weeks, you can:

- Pick a day to stop smoking, review the information presented in Chapter 1 regarding behaviour change.
- Throw away all your cigarettes, lighters, and ashtrays.

By the end of the semester, you can:

- Focus on the positives. Now that you have stopped smoking, your mind and your body will feel better—recognize this positive change. Make a list of the good things about not smoking. Carry a copy with you, and look at it whenever you have the urge to smoke.
- Reward yourself for stopping. Go to a movie, go out to dinner, go for a walk, spend time in an outdoor place that gives you pleasure, or buy yourself a gift from the money you saved by not smoking.

Source: From *Why Do You Smoke?*, by National Institutes of Health, 2014.

DISCUSSION QUESTIONS

1. When it comes to drinking alcohol, how much is too much? How often is too often? How can you control your consumption of alcohol so that you do not drink too much or too often?

2. What factors may cause someone to progress from being a social drinker to becoming addicted to alcohol? What effect does alcoholism have on the family of the person who becomes addicted?

3. Describe your campus culture regarding alcohol. Create a video/commercial that portrays this culture and the risks associated with it.

4. Discuss the varied forms in which you can ingest tobacco. In each form, how do chemicals enter your system? What are the physiological effects of nicotine?

5. Discuss the risks of smokeless tobacco. Do you think that smokeless tobacco should be banned from all levels of sport? Why or why not?

6. People who smoke often claim they have the right to smoke in public places. From what you have learned about secondhand smoke, how would you argue against an individual's right to smoke in public?

7. Do you drink coffee or other beverages that contain caffeine? Do you limit your consumption of these beverages? Why or why not? Are you addicted to caffeine? How could you find out? What are the risks of caffeine addiction or excessive caffeine consumption?

8. Describe the health risks and potential benefits of caffeine consumption.

APPLICATION EXERCISE

Reread the "Consider This . . ." scenario at the beginning of the chapter and answer the following questions.

1. Considering the culture around alcohol in your community, how realistic is the situation described? How might it be different? How is it the same?

2. What are some of the typical outcomes after a night of excessive alcohol consumption such as this? Would the outcomes be different for a group of men than women? Why or why not?

3. Despite the known risks of mixing drugs such as those found in energy drinks plus alcohol, why has it become popular among young people? What are the risks?

4. Is it possible for students to enjoy the 'party' lifestyle of their post-secondary years without excessive alcohol consumption as is often currently experienced?

MASTERINGHEALTH

Go to MasteringHealth for assignments, the eText, and the study Area with case studies, self-quizzing, and videos.

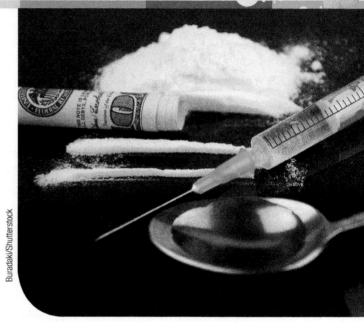

Buradaki/Shutterstock

CHAPTER 11

UNDERSTANDING ILLICIT DRUGS

LEARNING OUTCOMES

- Identify the most commonly used illicit drugs in Canada.
- Compare the risks of the various methods of using cocaine.
- Describe the physiological and psychological effects of marijuana and its potential to affect students' performance.
- Identify common designer drugs and the risks of their use.
- Discuss harm reduction practices in Canada.

◄◉ CONSIDER THIS . . .

Kwame is a student-athlete on the varsity football team. Overall, he is a dedicated student-athlete who likes to live life to the fullest and is willing to experience life outside the box. As a result, he infrequently smokes a little pot when he does not have a game on the next day or two. At the Vanier Cup one year, Kwame is randomly selected for drug testing. Although he did not smoke up the night before, Kwame tests positive for marijuana.

What would happen to a student-athlete in Kwame's situation at your university/college? What would happen to a student caught smoking pot? Is the treatment/reaction to these situations the same among students, faculty, administration, and the community? Why or why not? How does infrequent marijuana use influence an athlete's ability to train and/or compete? How does infrequent marijuana use influence a student's academic ability?

ILLICIT DRUGS

Illicit or illegal drug use continues to be a problem in our society today. Although you may not be a user yourself, you are influenced by illicit drug use in one way or another. It is important to understand how these drugs work and why people use them. In this chapter, we focus our attention on illicit drugs—drugs that are illegal to possess, produce, or sell.

On June 19, 1996, the Senate passed Bill C-8, the Controlled Drugs and Substances Act. The Act came into force on May 14, 1997. It replaced Canada's main laws on illicit drugs—the Narcotic Control Act and parts of the Food and Drugs Act. The Controlled Drugs and Substances Act significantly expanded the reach of Canada's drug laws and continued Canada's heavy reliance on a failed policy of criminal prohibition (Canadian Foundation for Drug Policy, 1997).

Illicit drug users come from all walks of life. Most illicit drug use occurs in places other than dilapidated crack houses, and few users fit the stereotype of the crazed junkie. The reasons people give for using illicit drugs vary from one situation to another and from one person to another. Age, sex, genetic background, culture, education, physiology, personality, life experiences, and expectations are factors that play a role in a person's choice to use illicit drugs.

The Canadian Tobacco, Alcohol and Drug Survey (CTADS) provides the most recent data on drug use in Canada (Statistics Canada, 2015). Illicit drug use varies with age, sex, province (Figure 11.1), marital status, education, and income. In 2013, 11 percent (3.1 million) of Canadians reported using at least one of the following drugs in past 12 months (cannabis, cocaine or crack, speed, ecstasy, hallucinogens, or heroin) (Statistics Canada, 2015). Fewer females (8 percent or 1.0 million) than males (14 percent or 2.0 million) reported using illicit drugs. Among youth aged 15 to 19 and young adults aged 20 to 24, 23 percent (473 000) and 27 percent (651 000) respectively, reported engaging in drug use.

In 2010, it was estimated that between 153 and 300 million people worldwide—or 3.4 to 6.6 percent of the population aged 15 to 64 years—used illicit drugs at least once in the past year (United Nations Office of Drugs and Crime, 2012). Of these, an estimated 12 percent or 15.5 to 38.6 million users were considered to be drug-dependent or with a drug-use disorder. Globally, 0.4 percent of deaths and 0.8 percent of "disability adjusted life years" (that is, the time a person lives with a physical or mental disability) were attributed to illicit drug use (World Health Organization, n.d.). In 2002 (the latest data available), between

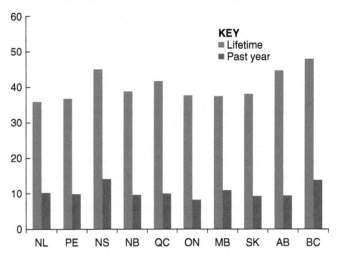

FIGURE 11.1

Percent of Canadians that Self-reported Lifetime and Past Year Use of All Illicit Drugs, According to Province

Source: Data from Health Canada, 2012, retrieved May 11, 2013, from www.hc-sc.gc.ca/hc-ps/drugs-drogues/stat/_2011/tables-tableaux-eng.php#t2.

1455 and 1695 deaths in Canada were attributed to illicit drug use and acute care hospital days were estimated to be 318 000 to 352 000 (Canadian Centre on Substance Abuse and the Centre for Addiction and Mental Health, 2002). The World Health Organization (n.d.) suggested that "illicit drugs account for the highest proportion of disease burden among low mortality, industrialized countries in the Americas, Eastern Mediterranean, and European regions [and that the] economic reliance on the drug trade, and drug dependence leaves many individuals open to exploitation by criminals and criminal organizations; threatening the health of men, women and children, the rule of law, and ultimately, the vitality and strength of all our communities." Canada collects data regarding self-reported harms with illicit drug use (Health Canada, 2012). In 2012, 2.0 percent of Canadians aged 15 years and older reported experiencing at least one harm in the past year due to their illicit drug use. The prevalence of reported harm due to their own drug use was four times higher among youth aged 15 to 24 years (5.5 percent) than adults aged 25 years and older (1.4 percent).

Why do Canadians choose to use illicit drugs? There is no clear answer. Economic despair, issues related to the family or community, a general sense of hopelessness, or a need to relieve boredom may be powerful engines leading to use. These factors, combined with increased availability and diversity of drugs, attitudes and beliefs that illicit drug use is common, and potentially liberal parental attitudes may explain the use of illicit drugs for some.

Social policy also affects drug use, although its effects are difficult to evaluate. Illicit drug use declined significantly during the first five years of Canada's Drug Strategy, when the focus was on the general public. It started rising again during Phase II, when the focus shifted to street youth and high-risk groups. The resurgence of drug use currently witnessed is led largely by mainstream youth, as noted, for example, by the average age of marijuana initiation in the 15- to 24-year-old age group at 15.6 years. Ultimately, health promotion messages aimed at the prevention of illicit drug use should be targeted toward our youth. According to the Canadian Centre on Substance Abuse (n.d.), all young people—dropouts and A+ students alike—are vulnerable to drug use and should be viewed as an at-risk population.

Anti-drug programs have been developed to deal with the problems of illegal drug use. For these programs to be successful, they need to take a multi-dimensional approach. The tendency in many of these programs has been to focus on only one aspect of drug use rather than the many interrelated factors that contribute to the individual's choice to use. For example, many programs consider the drugs themselves the culprits. Other programs at preventing illicit drug use oversimplify the reality of drug use by exhorting potential users to "just say no," ignoring the fact that drugs are an integral part of many people's social or cultural lives. The pressures to take drugs are often tremendous, and the reasons for using them complex. Thus, the treatment or programs to cease use must also be complex.

People who develop drug problems usually think they can control their use when they start. Initially, their drug use is viewed as a fun and controllable pastime. Peer influence is a strong motivator for drug use, especially among adolescents. Typically, teens and young adults believe that drug use in others is much greater than it really is. Some people use drugs to cope with feelings of worthlessness and despair, others to battle depression and anxiety. Some view drugs as the quick answer to life's difficulties. Still others take these drugs because they are bored or are hoping to find excitement through the drug use. The reasons for illicit drug use are varied and should be recognized as such. Since the majority of illegal drugs produce physiological and psychological dependence, the idea that a person can use these substances regularly without becoming addicted is not substantiated. To find out how much you might be controlled by drugs or by a drug user, complete the questionnaires in the Assess Yourself Questionnaire at the end of this chapter.

Cocaine A powerful stimulant drug with strong psychological effects.

Cocaine

Cocaine is a crystalline white alkaloid powder derived from the leaves of the South American coca shrub (not related to cocoa plants) (Centre for Addiction and Mental Health, 2006). These leaves have been chewed for thousands of years by people in Peru and Bolivia to lessen hunger and fatigue. Pure cocaine was isolated in 1860 by a German pharmacology graduate student. In the 1880s, the famous psychiatrist Sigmund Freud praised the powerful stimulant effects of cocaine as the treatment for a variety of illnesses, including depression, as well as for alcohol and opioid addiction. Cocaine use then increased and it was widely and legally available in Canada in medicine and soft drinks. With increased use, the risks of cocaine became clear, and, in 1911, Canada passed laws restricting its importation, manufacture, sale, and possession.

Cocaine is generally sold on the street as a hydrochloride salt—a fine, white crystalline powder known as "blow," "C," "coke," "crack," "flake," "freebase," "rock," or "snow," among other names (CAMH, 2006). Other street names include: all-American drug, aunt nora, barbs, dream, foo-foo dust, her, king's habit, Peruvian lady, tardust, witch, and zip (Cas Palmera, 2012). Street dealers often dilute it with inert (non-psychoactive) but similar-looking substances such as cornstarch, talcum powder, and sugar, or with active drugs such as procaine and benzocaine (used as local anesthetics), or other central nervous system stimulants such as amphetamines.

According to the most recent Canadian Alcohol and Drug Use Survey, lifetime cocaine use for 2011 was reported as 6.2 percent, while 0.9 percent indicated past year use (Health Canada, 2012). The highest rate of lifetime use of cocaine is reported in British Columbia at 9.1 percent and lowest in New Brunswick at 3.7 percent and Prince Edward Island at 3.8 percent.

Cocaine affects mood, judgment, and motor skill coordination. Cocaine has its most dramatic effects on vision, as it may cause a higher sensitivity to light, the perception of halos around bright objects, and difficulty focusing. Users have also reported blurred vision, glare problems, and hallucinations, particularly "snow lights"—weak flashes or movements of light in the peripheral field of vision, which tend to make drivers swerve toward or away from the lights. Some users have also reported auditory hallucinations (for example, ringing bells) and olfactory hallucinations (for example, the smell of smoke or gasoline).

Cocaine also heightens feelings such as irritability, excitability, and startle response. Users who were driving at the time reported that sudden sounds, such as horns or sirens, caused them severe anxiety coupled with rapid steering or braking reactions, even when the source of the sound was not in the immediate vicinity of their vehicles. Suspiciousness, distrust, and paranoia—other reactions to cocaine—have prompted users to flee in their cars or drive evasively. Further, users report attention lapses while driving, reckless driving, and ignoring relevant stimuli such as changes in traffic signals (Addiction Research Foundation, 1991).

Methods of Cocaine Use

Cocaine can be taken in several ways. The powdered form of the drug is "snorted" through the nose. Smoking (freebasing) and intravenous injections are more dangerous means of using cocaine. When cocaine is snorted, it can cause damage to the mucous membranes in the nose and sinusitis. Further, snorting cocaine can damage the user's sense of smell, and occasionally it creates a hole in the septum. Smoking, or "freebasing," cocaine can result in lung and liver damage. Freebasing is more popular than injecting cocaine because of the risk inherent with drug use with a needle, and, in particular, the risk of contracting diseases such as AIDS and hepatitis by sharing needles. A major risk of freebasing relates to the volatile mixes required and the risk of explosion; some users have been killed or seriously burned.

Many cocaine users still occasionally "shoot up." Injecting allows the user to introduce relatively large amounts of cocaine rapidly into the body. Within seconds, there is an incredible sense of euphoria. This intense high lasts only 15 to 20 minutes, and then the user heads into a "crash." To prevent the unpleasant effects of the crash, users often shoot up frequently. Regular injections into the veins can cause severe damage to them which may be why persistent users find

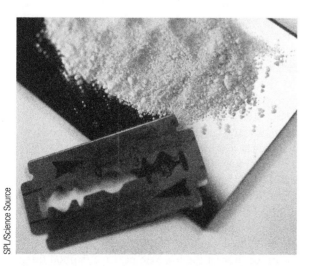

Although cocaine use has declined from its peak in the 1980s, it continues to be a commonly used and abused illicit drug today.

various places for injection including wrists, elbows, arms, ankles, neck, bottoms of feet—even the groin (Rhodes et al., 2006). Besides AIDS and hepatitis, users who inject themselves are at risk for skin infections, inflammation of the arteries, and infection of the lining of the heart.

Physical Effects of Cocaine

The effects of cocaine are felt rapidly and are dependent upon how it is taken. Snorted cocaine enters the bloodstream through the lungs in less than one minute and reaches the brain in about five minutes (Health Canada, 2009a). Cocaine that is smoked or injected reaches the brain a little more quickly. When cocaine binds at its receptor sites in the central nervous system, it produces intense pleasure due to the increased amount of dopamine in the brain (Health Canada, 2009a). The euphoria quickly abates and the desire to regain the pleasurable feelings makes the user want more and relates to the strong physiological and psychological dependence upon the drug.

Cocaine is an anesthetic and a central nervous system stimulant. In tiny doses, it can slow heart rate. In larger doses, the physical effects are dramatic: increased heart and breathing rate and blood pressure, loss of appetite, postponed physical and mental fatigue, convulsions, muscle twitching or exaggerated reflexes, irregular heartbeat, paranoid thinking, anxiety, even death due to overdose (Health Canada, 2009a). Other effects of cocaine include temporary relief of depression, decreased fatigue, talkativeness, increased alertness, and heightened self-confidence. Again, however, as the dose increases, users become irritable and apprehensive and their behaviours may turn paranoid or violent.

Cocaine-Affected Babies

Because cocaine easily crosses the placenta (as virtually all drugs do), the fetus is vulnerable when a pregnant woman uses the drug. The most threatening problem during pregnancy is the increased risk of a miscarriage and premature delivery (Health Canada, 2009a). Should the pregnant user reach full term, her baby is usually born with brain damage, heart defects, kidney problems, and malformed heads, arms, and fingers. These babies tend to show signs of withdrawal at birth, including irritability, jitteriness, and the inability to eat or sleep properly (Health Canada, 2009a). They seem unable to respond or relate to people the way normal babies do, and are difficult to console and comfort. Because it is so difficult for adults to interact with them, their social and emotional development is negatively affected. Cocaine is also transmitted through breast milk. The baby is then exposed to all the physical and mental effects of cocaine use (CAMH, n.d.a).

Freebase Cocaine

Freebase is a form of cocaine more powerful and costly than the powder or chip (crack) form. Street cocaine (cocaine hydrochloride) is converted to pure base by removing the hydrochloride salt and many of the "cutting agents." The end product, freebase, is smoked through a water pipe. Because freebase cocaine reaches the brain within seconds, it is more dangerous than cocaine that is snorted. It produces a quick, intense high that disappears quickly, leaving an intense craving for more. Freebasers typically increase the amount and frequency of the dose. They often become severely addicted and experience serious health problems and financial ruin (CAMH, 2006). Side effects of freebasing include weight loss, increased heart rate and blood pressure, depression, paranoia, and hallucinations. Freebase is an extremely dangerous drug and is responsible for a large number of cocaine-related hospital emergency-room visits and deaths.

Crack

Crack is the street name given to freebase cocaine processed from cocaine hydrochloride using ammonia or sodium bicarbonate (baking soda) and water, then heating the substance to remove the hydrochloride. Crack can also be processed with ether, but this is much riskier because ether is a flammable solvent. The mixture (90-percent-pure cocaine) is then dried. The soapy-looking substance that results can be broken up into "rocks" and smoked. These rocks are approximately five times as strong as cocaine. Crack gets its name from the popping noises it makes when burned. A crack user may quickly become addicted to the drug. Addiction is accelerated by the speed at which crack is absorbed through the lungs (it hits the brain within seconds after use) and by the intensity of the high.

Freebase The most powerful distillate of cocaine.

Crack A distillate of powdered cocaine that comes in small, hard "chips" or "rocks."

Amphetamines A large and varied group of synthetic agents that stimulate the central nervous system.

Methamphetamine (meth) A powerfully addictive drug that strongly activates certain areas of the brain and affects the central nervous system.

Amphetamines

Amphetamines include a large and varied group of synthetic agents that stimulate the central nervous system. Small doses of amphetamines act like adrenaline (a hormone that naturally stimulates the body) and improve alertness, lessen fatigue, and generally elevate mood (CAMH, 2004b). With repeated use, physiological and psychological dependence develops. Sleep patterns are affected (insomnia); heart rate, breathing rate, and blood pressure increase; restlessness, anxiety, appetite suppression, and vision problems are common. High doses over long time periods can produce hallucinations, delusions, and disorganized behaviours. Abusers become paranoid, fearing everything and everyone. Some become very aggressive or antisocial.

Amphetamines are sold under a variety of names. "Bennies" (amphetamine/Benzedrine), "dex" (dextroamphetamine/Dexedrine), and "meth" or "speed" (methamphetamine/Methedrine) are some of the most common. Other street terms for amphetamines are "cross tops," "crank," "uppers," "wake-ups," "lid poppers," "cartwheels," and "blackies." Amphetamines do have therapeutic uses in the treatment of attention deficit hyperactivity disorder in children (Ritalin, Cylert) and obesity (Pondimin).

Methamphetamine

An increasingly common form of amphetamine, **methamphetamine** (**meth**) is a potent, long-acting, addictive drug that strongly activates the brain's reward centre by producing a sense of euphoria (CAMH, 2005a) "Crystal meth" can cause brain damage, resulting in impaired motor skills and cognitive functions, psychosis, and increased risk for heart attack and stroke. Methamphetamine can be snorted, smoked, injected, or orally ingested. Street names for meth include: crank, crystal, crystal glass, Christina, Tina, cris, Cristy, chalk, chalk dust, ice, speed, geep, getter, getgo, go fast, trash, garbage, wash, white cross, white crunch, hanyak, hironpon, hiropon, hot ice, super ice, batu, kaksonjae, LA glass, LA ice, ice cream, quartz, chunky love cookies, cotton candy, dunk, gak, go-go juice, junk, no doze, pookie, rocket fuel, and scooby snax (Cas Palmera, 2010a). Depending on the method of use, the drug will affect the user in different ways. Users often experience tolerance immediately, making meth a highly addictive drug from the very first time it is used. When snorted, the effects can be felt in three to five minutes; if orally ingested, the user will experience effects within 15 to 20 minutes. The pleasurable effects of meth are typically an intense rush lasting only a few minutes when snorted or a high lasting over eight hours when smoked.

According to the most recent Canadian Alcohol and Drug Use Survey, lifetime methamphetamine/crystal meth use for 2011 for Canadian men and women between the ages of 15 to 64 years was reported as 0.6 percent, while no value is reported for past year use given the low value found (Health Canada, 2012). Again, because of the low rate of usage (a good thing really), provincial data is not reported for lifetime or past year use of methamphetamine/crystal meth.

Physical Effects of Methamphetamine

Smaller doses of methamphetamine produce increased physical activity, alertness, and a decreased appetite. However, the drug's effects quickly wear off, and the user seeks more. Long-term use of meth can cause severe dependence, psychosis, paranoia, aggression, weight loss, and stroke. Abusers often do not sleep or eat for days, as they continually inject up to 1 gram of the drug every two to three hours. A high state of irritability and agitation has been associated with violent behaviours among some users. A common symptom among users is the sensation of insects crawling under their skin; thus, these individuals may have scratches on their skin caused by their efforts to relieve the sensation. Use of meth is an increasingly serious problem. A possible contributing factor to the increasing rate of meth use is that it is relatively easy to make. Meth is produced by "cookers," using recipes that often include common OTC ingredients such as ephedrine and pseudoephedrine, found in cold and allergy medication, as well as lethal ingredients such as drain cleaner, battery acid, and others.

Ice is a potent form of methamphetamine created in Canada and imported primarily from Asia, particularly South Korea and Taiwan. When smoked, ice is odourless, and its effects can last for more than 12 hours. Like other methamphetamines, the "down" side of this drug is devastating. Prolonged use can cause fatal lung and kidney damage, as well as long-lasting psychological damage. In some instances, major psychological dysfunction can persist as long as two and a half years after last use.

Marijuana (Cannibis)

Although archaeological evidence documents the use of **marijuana** (also known as "grass," "weed," "pot," "dope," and "ganja," among other names [CAMH, 2005b]) as far back as 6000 years, the drug did not become popular in North America until the 1960s. Marijuana remains by far the most extensively used illicit drug, as previously reported, CTADS reported that the prevalence of past-year use of marijuana was three times higher among Canadian youth aged 15 to 24 compared to adults (24.4 percent vs. 8.0 percent) (Statistics Canada, 2015). Among youth aged 15 to 19, the rate of past-year marijuana use was 22.4 percent; the corresponding rate was 26.2 percent among young adults aged 20 to 24. Reasons postulated for the elevated levels of marijuana use in teens is that they do not think it is a drug (because it does not come in a pill form, nor is it injected), their access to it is relatively easy, and because of the decriminalization of medical marijuana (Hui, 2013).

Figures 11.2 and 11.3 show yearly and provincial lifetime and past year use, respectively. Highest rates of lifetime marijuana use are found in British Columbia, Nova Scotia, and Alberta, while highest past year use was found in Nova Scotia and British Columbia (Health Canada, 2012).

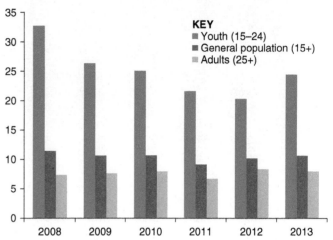

FIGURE 11.2

Percent of Canadians Who Self Reported Past Year Use of Marijuana

Source: Statistics Canada. (2015). Canadian Tobacco, Alcohol and Drugs Survey: Summary of results for 2013. Ottawa, ON: Author. Retrieved April 10, 2015, from http://healthycanadians.gc.ca/science-research-sciences-recherches/data-donnees/ctads-ectad/summary-sommaire-2013-eng.php.

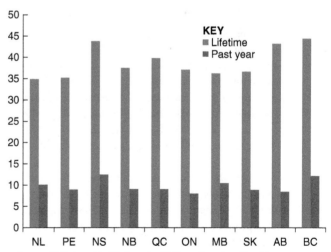

FIGURE 11.3

Percent of Canadians Who Self-Reported Lifetime and Past Year Use of Marijuana

Source: Data from Health Canada, 2012, retrieved on May 11, 2013 from www.hc-sc.gc.ca/hc-ps/drugs-drogues/stat/_2011/tables-tableaux-eng.php#t2.

Ice A potent, inexpensive stimulant with long-lasting effects.

Marijuana A psychoactive stimulant that intensifies reactions to environmental stimuli.

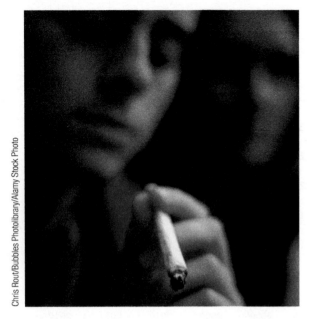

Many college or university students have a false perception of how much their peers use marijuana. In a recent survey, students estimated that 79.4 percent of their peers had used marijuana in the past month and that 11.3 percent used it daily. Reality is that only 14.2 percent used marijuana in the past month and only 1.9 percent used it daily.

Source: Data from the American College Health Association, American College Health Association—National College Health Assessment (ACHA_NCHA): Reference Group Data Report Fall 2010 (Baltimore: American College Health Association, 2011).

Physical Effects of Marijuana

Marijuana is derived from either the *cannabis sativa* or *cannabis indica* (hemp) plants. Today's top-grade cannabis produces reactions similar to hashish. **Tetrahydrocannabinol (THC)** is the psychoactive substance in marijuana and the key to determining how powerful a high the marijuana will produce. Two decades ago, marijuana ranged in potency from 1 to 5 percent THC, while today's crop averages 8 to 15 percent.

Hashish, a potent cannabis preparation derived mainly from the thick, sticky resin of the plant, contains high concentrations of THC. Hash oil, a substance produced by percolating a solvent such as ether through dried marijuana to extract the THC, is a tarry liquid that can contain up to 70 percent THC.

Marijuana can be brewed and drunk in tea or baked into quick breads or brownies. THC concentrations in such products are impossible to estimate. Most of the time, however, marijuana is rolled into cigarettes (joints) or packed firmly into a pipe. Some people smoke marijuana through water pipes called "bongs." Effects are generally felt within 10 to 30 minutes and wear off within three hours.

Tetrahydrocannabinol (THC) The chemical name for the active ingredient in marijuana.

Hashish The sticky resin of the cannabis plant, high in THC.

The most noticeable effect of THC is the dilation of the eyes' blood vessels, which produces the characteristic bloodshot eyes. Smokers of the drug also exhibit coughing, dry mouth and throat ("cotton mouth"), increased thirst and appetite, lowered blood pressure, and mild muscular weakness, primarily exhibited in drooping eyelids. Users who take a high dose in an unfamiliar or uncomfortable setting are more likely to experience anxiety and the paranoid belief that their companions are ridiculing or threatening them.

Effects of Chronic Marijuana Use

Potential long-term effects of heavy or regular marijuana use include:

- psychological dependence
- an increased risk of cancer because of the tar and other known cancer-causing agents in cannabis
- irritation to the respiratory system (in fact, smoking three to four joints per day has an effect similar to that of smoking 20 cigarettes)
- reduced motivation for work and study
- schizophrenia
- impaired attention, memory, and ability to process complex information
- suppression of the immune system
- blood pressure changes (CAMH, 2005b.)

Research suggests that pregnant women who smoke marijuana are at a higher risk for stillbirth or miscarriage and for delivering low-birthweight babies and babies with abnormalities of the nervous system. Babies born to women who use marijuana during pregnancy are five times more likely to have features similar to those exhibited by children with fetal alcohol spectrum disorders (see Chapter 10 for more details).

Debates concerning the effects of marijuana on the reproductive system have yet to be resolved. Studies conducted in the mid-1970s suggested that marijuana inhibited testosterone (and thus sperm) production in males and caused chromosomal breakage in ova and sperm. Subsequent research in these areas was inconclusive. The question of whether the high-level THC plants currently available will increase the risks associated with this drug is, as yet, unanswered.

Marijuana and Medicine

Although recognized as an addictive drug by the Canadian government, marijuana also has several medical purposes. Marijuana (particularly in the form of nabilone) helps to control side effects such

Chris Rout/Bubbles Photolibrary/Alamy Stock Photo

as the severe nausea and vomiting produced by chemotherapy, the chemical treatment for cancer. It also improves appetite and reduces or delays the loss of lean muscle mass associated with AIDS-wasting syndrome. Marijuana reduces the muscle pain and spasticity caused by diseases such as multiple sclerosis. It also temporarily relieves the eye pressure of glaucoma (a progressive disease characterized by increased fluid pressure in the eyeball).

Health Canada implemented the Marihuana Medical Access Regulations on July 30, 2001. These regulations clearly define the circumstances and the manner in which access to marijuana for medical purposes will be permitted with three main components:

- authorizations to possess dried marijuana
- licences to produce marijuana, which include Personal-Use Production Licences and Designated-Person Production Licences; and
- access to supply of marijuana seeds or dried marijuana.

Furthermore, storefront operations selling marijuana, commonly known as "dispensaries" and "compassion clubs," are not licensed by Health Canada and are illegal under the current law.

There are two categories for which you may be considered eligible for Medical Marijuana:

Category 1
Any symptom treated as part of compassionate end-of-life care,

OR

Symptoms related to specific medical conditions, namely:

Severe pain and/or persistent muscle spasms from multiple sclerosis

Severe pain and/or persistent muscle spasms from a spinal cord injury

Severe pain and/or persistent muscle spasms from a spinal cord disease

Severe pain, cachexia, anorexia, weight loss, and/or severe nausea from cancer

Severe pain, cachexia, anorexia, weight loss, and/or severe nausea from HIV/AIDS infection

Severe pain from severe forms of arthritis

Seizures from epilepsy

Category 2
A debilitating symptom that is associated with a medical condition or with the medical treatment of that condition, other than those described in Category 1 (Health Canada, 2013).

Marijuana and Driving

Marijuana use presents clear hazards for drivers of motor vehicles as well as for others on the road. The drug substantially reduces a driver's ability to react and to make quick decisions in a way comparable to that of drinking and driving (Canada Centre on Substance Abuse, 2011). Perceptual and other performance deficits resulting from marijuana use can persist for some time after the high subsides. Users who attempt to drive, fly, or operate heavy machinery often fail to recognize their impairment. In a report by Health Canada (2013), drivers aged 18 to 19 years were most likely to report driving after using cannabis (8.3 percent), followed by those aged 15 to 17 years (6.4 percent). Moreover, males were three times more likely than females to report that they drove after using cannabis.

Opiates

Opiates are among the oldest analgesics known. These drugs cause drowsiness, relieve pain, and induce euphoria. Also called **narcotics**, they are derived from the parent drug **opium**, a dark, resinous substance made from the milky juice of the opium poppy. Other opiates include morphine, codeine, heroin, and black tar heroin.

The word *narcotic* comes from the Greek word for "stupor" and is generally used to describe sleep-inducing substances. For many years, opiates were widely used by the medical community to relieve pain, induce sleep, curb nausea and vomiting, stop diarrhea, and sedate psychiatric patients. During the late nineteenth and early twentieth centuries, many patent medicines contained opiates. Suppliers advertised these concoctions as cures for everything from menstrual cramps to teething pains.

Among the opiates widely used by medical practitioners was **morphine**. First manufactured in the early nineteenth century, morphine was named after Morpheus, the Greek god of sleep, and is more powerful than opium. Street names for morphine include: duramorph, M, miss Emma, monkey, roxanol, and white stuff (Drug Guide, 2013). **Codeine**, a less powerful analgesic, is derived from morphine. The three most common street names for codeine are T-threes (Tylenol 3), syrup (Phenergan), and empi (Empirin with Codeine) (Drug Overdose, 2013).

All opiates are highly addictive. Growing concern

Narcotics Drugs that induce sleep and relieve pain; primarily the opiates.

Opium The parent drug of the opiates; made from the milky juice of the opium poppy.

Morphine A derivative of opium; sometimes used by medical practitioners to relieve pain.

Codeine A drug derived from morphine; used in cough syrups and some painkillers.

point of view

MEDICAL MARIJUANA: Too Legal or not Legal Enough?

There have been strong arguments both for and against the legalization of marijuana over the past few decades. Below are some of the major points from both sides of the issue.

ARGUMENTS FOR LEGALIZATION

Marijuana is a safe and effective treatment for certain complications of dozens of conditions, such as cancer, AIDS, multiple sclerosis, pain, migraines, glaucoma, and epilepsy.

Legalizing marijuana and taxing its sale would bring in revenue for the government.

The government could control the standardization of marijuana growth and production and promote more responsible cultivation methods.

ARGUMENTS AGAINST LEGALIZATION

It is not necessary to legalize marijuana for medical use because there are already approved drugs that are just as effective in treating the same conditions.

Marijuana use poses dangerous side effects including lung injury, immune system damage, and interference with fertility that make it inappropriate for medical use.

Marijuana is known to be addictive and may lead to use of harder drugs.

Where Do You Stand?

○ Do you think marijuana use in general should be legalized?

○ What criteria do you think should be used to determine the legality of a particular substance? Who should make those determinations?

○ What are your feelings on drug laws in general — do you think they should be more or less prohibitive? What sort of policies would you propose to protect individuals and their rights?

Sources: Based on Marijuana Policy Project, *State by State Medical Marijuana Laws: How to Remove the Threat of Arrest* (Washington, DC: 2008); Marijuana Policy Project, "Medical Marijuana Overview," 2009, www.mpp.org/library/research/medical-marijuana-overview.html; ProCon.org, "Medical Marijuana," 2009, http://medicalmarijuana.procon.org.

---

about addiction led to government controls of narcotic use. Subsequent legislation required physicians prescribing opiates to keep careful records. Physicians are still subject to audits of their prescriptions of these agents. Some opiates are still used today for medical purposes. Morphine is sometimes prescribed by doctors in hospital settings for relief of severe pain. Codeine is found in prescription cough syrups and in other painkillers, many of which are available as OTCs. Several prescription drugs, including Percodan, fentanyl, and Dilaudid, contain synthetic opiates. All opiate use is strictly regulated.

Physical Effects of Opiates

Opiates are powerful central nervous system depressants. In addition to relieving pain, these drugs lower heart rate, respiration, and blood pressure (Drug Guide, 2013). Side effects include weakness, dizziness, nausea,

Heroin A derivative of morphine, usually injected into the bloodstream.

vomiting, euphoria, decreased sex drive, visual disturbances, and lack of coordination. Of all the opiates, heroin is the most notorious. Because all opiate addiction follows a similar progression, only heroin will be described in the following paragraphs.

Heroin Addiction

Heroin and black tar heroin are powerful opiates. Heroin is a white powder derived from morphine. Black tar heroin is a sticky, dark brown, foul-smelling substance, also made from morphine. Street names for heroin include: smack, H, black tar, chiba or chiva, junk, brown sugar, skag, mud, dragon, dope, white, China white, white nurse, white lady, white horse, white girl, white boy, white stuff boy, he, black, black tar, black pearl, black stuff, black eagle, brown, brown crystal, brown tape, brown Rhine, Mexican brown, Mexican mud, Mexican horse, snow, snowball, scat, sack, skunk number 3, number 4, and number 8 (Cas Palmera, 2010b). Heroin is a depressant. It produces

Although it is the number one used illicit drug in Canada, many users, including students in university or college, do not know of the potential effects of their use on their ability to think. In one study of memory and impulsivity in regular marijuana users, all participants in the sample of more than 100 marijuana users between the ages of 18 to 44 years who had used at least two days a week in the past month and at least weekly in the past six months reported at least one marijuana-related problem (Day et al., 2013). The most frequent problems noted were "to procrastinate" and "to have a lower energy level" with these two factors combining and resulting in "lower productivity." Another study of marijuana users' functional brain activity performance highlighted the negative impact of chronic marijuana use (though not under the influence at the time of test) particularly related in the time to complete the task (Tropp Sneider et al., 2013). These two studies provide clear examples of how your school performance can be negatively impacted by your choice to use marijuana.

References

Day, A. M., Metrik, J., Spillane, N. S., & Kahler, C. W. (2013). Working memory and impulsivity predict marijuana-related problems among frequent users. *Drug Alcohol Dependance, 131*(0), 171–174.

Tropp Sneider, J., Gruber, S. A., Rogowska, J., Silveri, M. M., & Yurgelun-Todd, D. A. (2013). A preliminary study of functional brain activation among marijuana users during performance of a virtual maze task, *Journal of Addiction*, Volume 2013, Article ID 461029, 12 pages.

a dreamy, mentally slow feeling and drowsiness in the user. It also can cause drastic mood swings of euphoric highs followed by depressive lows. Heroin slows respiration and urinary output and constricts the pupils of the eyes (hence the image of the stereotypical drug user hiding his eyes behind a pair of dark sunglasses). Symptoms of tolerance and withdrawal can appear within three weeks of first use.

The most common route of administration for heroin addicts is "mainlining"—intravenous injection of powdered heroin mixed in a solution—though fear of HIV and hepatitis infection has resulted in some users avoiding needles. As noted later in this chapter, safe injection sites have been established to reduce risk. Many users describe the "rush" they feel when injecting themselves as intensely pleasurable, whereas others report unpredictable and unpleasant effects. The temporary nature of the rush contributes to the drug's high potential for addiction—many addicts shoot up four or five times a day. Mainlining causes veins to scar and, if this practice is frequent enough, the veins collapse. Once a vein has collapsed, it can no longer be used to inject heroin into the bloodstream. Those who are addicted to heroin, similar to other injection drug users, become expert at locating new veins to use: in the feet, the legs, and the temples. When they do not want their needle tracks (scars) to show, they inject themselves under the tongue, in the groin, or other places that are less visible to others.

According to the most recent Canadian Alcohol and Drug Use Survey, lifetime heroin use in 2011 for Canadian men and women between the ages of 15 to 64 years was reported as 0.5 percent, with no value reported for past year use given the low level reported (Health Canada, 2012). Again, because of the low rate of usage (a good thing really), provincial data is not reported for either lifetime or past year use of heroin.

Treatment for Heroin Addiction

Most programs designed to help individuals addicted to heroin have not been successful. The rate of relapse (tendency to return to previous behaviours) is high. Some individuals resume their drug use even after years of drug-free living because the craving for the euphoric feel from the drug is still so strong. It takes a great deal of discipline to seek alternative, non-drug euphoric feelings. Individuals addicted to heroin experience a distinct pattern of withdrawal. They begin to crave another dose four to six hours after their last dose. Symptoms of withdrawal include an intense desire for the drug, yawning, a runny nose, sweating, and crying. About 12 hours after the last dose, individuals addicted to heroin experience sleep disturbance, dilated pupils, loss of appetite, irritability, goosebumps, and muscle tremors. The most difficult time in the withdrawal process occurs 24 to 72 hours after last use. All the preceding symptoms continue along with nausea, abdominal cramps, restlessness, insomnia, vomiting, diarrhea, extreme anxiety, hot and cold flashes, elevated blood pressure, and rapid heartbeat and respiration. Once the peak of withdrawal has passed, these symptoms begin to subside. Still, the person recovering from the addiction has many hurdles to jump.

Methadone has been used since the 1960s to assist people addicted to synthetic opioids such as codeine, and opiates such as morphine and heroin (Canadian Public Health Association, n.d.). Methadone

Methadone A synthetic narcotic; used to block withdrawal symptoms as a treatment for people addicted to opiates.

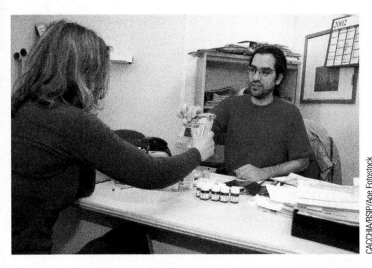

Methadone administered under the supervision of a clinic or pharmacy staff (as shown) allows many individuals addicted to heroin to lead somewhat normal lives.

CACCHIA/BSIP/Age Fotostock

is a synthetic narcotic that blocks the effects of opiate withdrawal and reduces cravings. It is chemically similar enough to opiates to control the tremors, chills, vomiting, diarrhea, and severe abdominal pains of withdrawal. The methadone dose is decreased over a period of time with the intent to wean the individual. In this way, methadone is made available on a daily basis to individuals addicted to opioids or opiates through specialized drug treatment clinics or prescribed by family physicians and dispensed by community pharmacists (Canadian Public Health Association, n.d.). In these settings, methadone is combined with juice so that the euphoric effect is not felt, nor is there interference in the capacity to think.

The use of methadone to treat opioid or opiate addiction is considered a hard reduction approach in that it assists those that are addicted to reduce or eliminate the harmful effect of their addiction (Canadian Public Health Association, n.d.). However, it is controversial because of its potential for addiction. Critics contend that the program merely substitutes one drug for another, with the addiction remaining. Proponents argue that people on methadone are less likely than those still using heroin to engage in criminal activities to support their addictions. For this reason, many methadone programs are government financed and available to clients free of charge or at reduced costs.

Psychedelics

Psychedelics are a group of drugs whose primary pharmacological effect is to alter feelings, perceptions, and thoughts in the user. The major receptor sites for most of these drugs are in the part of the brain responsible for interpreting outside stimuli before allowing these signals to travel to other parts of the brain. This area is called the **reticular formation** and is located in the brain stem at the upper end of the spinal cord. When a psychedelic drug is present at a reticular formation receptor site, messages become scrambled and the user may see wavy walls instead of straight ones or smell colours or hear tastes. This mixing of sensory messages is known as synesthesia.

In addition to synesthetic effects, users may recall events long buried in the subconscious mind or become less inhibited than when in a non-drug state. Some psychedelic drugs are erroneously labelled "hallucinogens." Hallucinogens are substances capable of creating auditory or visual **hallucinations**, or images that are perceived but not real. Not all psychedelic drugs are capable of producing hallucinations. The most widely recognized psychedelics are LSD, mescaline, psilocybin, and psilocin.

According to the most recent Canadian Alcohol and Drug Use Survey, lifetime hallucinogen use for 2011 for Canadian men and women between the ages of 15 to 64 years was reported as 10.4 percent and 0.6 percent for past year use (Health Canada, 2012). The highest rate of lifetime use of hallucinogens was reported in British Columbia at 15.3 percent, followed by Alberta at 14.8 percent, and lowest in New Brunswick at 8.1 percent and Ontario at 8.2 percent.

LSD

Of all the psychedelics, **lysergic acid diethylamide (LSD)** has the most notoriety. This chemical was first synthesized in the late 1930s by the Swiss chemist Albert Hoffman. It resulted from experiments aimed at deriving medically useful drugs from the ergot fungus found on rye and other cereal grains. Psychiatrists initially felt it could be beneficial to patients unable to remember and recognize suppressed traumas, and the drug was used for such purposes from 1950 through 1968. Known on the street as "acid," LSD continues to be widely available.

An odourless, tasteless, white crystalline powder, LSD is most frequently dissolved in water to make a solution that can then be used to manufacture the street forms of the drug: tablets, blotter acid, and "windowpane." What the LSD consumer usually buys is blotter acid—small squares of blotter-like paper that have been impregnated with the liquid. The blotter is swallowed or chewed briefly. LSD also comes in tiny thin squares of gelatin called "windowpane" and in tablets called "microdots," which are less than 3 millimetres across (it would take 10 or more of these to add up to the size of an ASA tablet). Street names for LSD include: acid,

Psychedelics Drugs that distort the processing of sensory information in the brain.

Reticular formation An area in the brain stem responsible for relaying messages to other areas in the brain.

Hallucination An image (auditory or visual) perceived but not real.

Lysergic acid diethylamide (LSD) Psychedelic drug causing sensory disruptions; also called "acid."

battery acid, blotter, boomers, California sunshine, cid, doses, dots, golden dragon, heavenly blue, loony toons, Lucy in the sky with diamonds, microdot, pane, purple heart, tab, window pane, yellow sunshine, and zen (Foundation for a Drug-Free World, 2013).

LSD is one of the most powerful drugs known, producing strong effects in doses as low as 20 micrograms (equivalent in size to the average-sized postage stamp). The potency of the typical dose of LSD currently ranges from 20 to 80 micrograms, compared to the 150 to 300 micrograms commonly used in the 1960s.

Despite its reputation for being primarily a psychedelic, LSD produces a large number of physical effects, including slightly increased heart rate, elevated blood pressure and temperature, goose flesh (roughened skin), increased reflex speeds, muscle tremors and twitches, perspiration, increased salivation, chills, headaches, and mild nausea. Since the drug also stimulates uterine muscle contractions, it can lead to premature labour and miscarriage in pregnant women. Research into the effects of long-term LSD use remains inconclusive. Similar to other illegally purchased drugs, LSD users are also exposed to the risks associated with the purchase of an impure product.

The psychological effects of LSD vary from person to person. The set and setting in which the drug is used are particularly strong influential factors with LSD. Euphoria is the common psychological state produced by the drug, but dysphoria (a sense of evil and foreboding) can also be experienced. The drug shortens attention span, causing the mind to wander. Thoughts may be interposed and juxtaposed as well. The user may thus be able to experience several different thoughts simultaneously. Synesthesia occurs occasionally. Users become introspective, and suppressed memories may surface, often taking on bizarre symbolism. Many more effects are possible, including, but not limited to, decreased aggressiveness and enhanced sensory experiences.

While there is no evidence of physiological dependence with LSD use, psychological dependence is likely. Many LSD users become depressed for one or two days following a trip and use the drug to relieve this depression. The result is a cycle of LSD use to relieve post-LSD depression, which often leads to psychological addiction.

Mescaline

Mescaline is one of hundreds of chemicals derived from the **peyote** cactus. Street names for mescaline include: anhalontum, beans, buttons, cactus, hikori, huatari, mesc, mescal, mescal buttons, moon, plants, seni, and wakowi (Drug Library, n.d.). This small, button-like cactus grows in the southwestern United States and parts of Latin America. Natives of these regions have long used the dried peyote buttons during religious ceremonies. In fact, members of the Native American Church (a religion practised by thousands of North American First Nations peoples) have been granted special permission to use the drug during ceremonies in some U.S. states.

Users normally swallow 10 to 12 dried peyote buttons. These buttons taste bitter and generally induce immediate nausea or vomiting. Long-time users claim that the nausea becomes less noticeable. Those who are able to keep the drug down begin to feel the effects within 30 to 90 minutes, when mescaline reaches maximum concentration in the brain. The effects may persist for up to 9 or 10 hours. Mescaline is a powerful hallucinogen. It is also a central nervous system stimulant.

Products sold on the street as mescaline are likely synthetic chemical relatives of the true drug. Street names of these products include DOM, STP, TMA, and MMDA. These drugs can be toxic in small quantities.

Psilocybin

Psilocybin and psilocin are the active chemicals in a group of mushrooms sometimes called "magic mushrooms." Street names for psilocybin include: magic, magic mushrooms, mushrooms, shrooms, mushies, fungus, fungus delight (Health Canada, 2009b). *Psilocybe* mushrooms, which grow throughout the world, can be cultivated from spores or can be harvested wild. These mushrooms, like others, can be eaten raw or cooked. They can be used to make a mushroom "tea" or mixed with fruit juice to make "fungus delight" (Health Canada, 2009b). Less often, they may be sniffed, snorted, or injected. Because many mushrooms resemble the psilocybe variety, people who use wild mushrooms for any purpose should be cautious as wild mushrooms can easily be misidentified, and mistakes can be fatal. Psilocybin is similar to LSD in its physical effects, which wear off in four to six hours. The exact chemical content is difficult to determine and varies in each mushroom; therefore, the effects can vary tremendously.

According to Health Canada (2009b), the short time effects of "magic mushrooms" include:

- anxiety, including panic attacks
- hallucinations and a loss of touch with reality
- distorted visual perceptions
- lightheadedness
- dilated pupils (causing blurred vision)
- nausea and vomiting
- dry mouth
- numbness, particularly facial numbness (paresthesia)

Mescaline A hallucinogenic drug derived from the peyote cactus.

Peyote A cactus with small "buttons" that, when ingested, produce hallucinogenic effects.

Psilocybin The active chemical found in psilocybe mushrooms that produces hallucinations.

- exaggerated reflexes
- sweating and increased body temperature followed by chills and shivering
- muscle weakness and twitching
- increased blood pressure and heart rate

In addition, a person could potentially experience:

- paranoia
- confusion and disorientation
- severe agitation
- loss of coordination
- loss of urinary control
- convulsions

After the effects of the mushrooms wear off, a user may feel very tired, depressed, and lethargic for a few days.

Deliriants

Delirium is an agitated mental state characterized by confusion and disorientation. Almost all psychoactive drugs will produce delirium at high doses, with **deliriants** producing this effect at relatively low (subtoxic) levels.

PCP

Phencyclidine (PCP) is one of the best-known deliriants. It is a synthetic substance that became a black-market drug in the early 1970s. PCP was originally developed as a "disassociative anesthetic," which means that patients given this drug could keep their eyes open, apparently remain conscious, and feel no pain during a medical procedure. Patients would afterward experience amnesia for the time the drug was in their system. Such a drug had obvious advantages as an anesthetic during surgery, but its unpredictability and drastic effects (post-operative delirium, confusion, and agitation) resulted in a discontinuation of its use, and it was withdrawn from the legal market.

On the illegal market, PCP is a white, crystalline powder that users often sprinkle onto marijuana cigarettes. It is dangerous and unpredictable regardless of how it is administered. Common street names for PCP are angel dust (for the crystalline powdered form), peace pill, horse tranquillizer, supergrass, boat, tic tac, zoom and shermans (for the tablet form).

Delirium An agitated mental state characterized by confusion and disorientation produced by psychoactive drugs.

Deliriant Any substance that produces delirium at relatively low doses, including PCP and some herbal substances.

Phencyclidine (PCP) A deliriant commonly called "angel dust."

Designer drug A synthetic analogue (creates effects similar to the drug it mimics) of an existing illicit drug.

The effects of PCP depend on the dosage. As little as five milligrams produces effects similar to strong central nervous system depressants. These effects include slurred speech, impaired coordination, reduced sensitivity to pain, and reduced heart and respiratory rates. Doses between 5 and 10 milligrams cause fever, salivation, nausea, vomiting, and total loss of sensitivity to pain. Doses greater than 10 milligrams result in a dramatic drop in blood pressure, coma, muscular rigidity, violent outbursts, and possible convulsions and death.

Psychologically, PCP may produce either euphoria or dysphoria. It is also known to produce hallucinations as well as delusions and overall delirium. Some users experience a prolonged state of "nothingness." The long-term effects of PCP use are unknown.

Designer Drugs

Designer drugs are structural analogues (drugs that produce similar effects) of more familiar illicit drugs. These illegal drugs are manufactured by underground chemists to mimic the psychoactive effects of controlled drugs. At present, at least three types of synthetic drugs are available on the illegal drug market: analogues of phencyclidine (PCP), fentanyl and meperidine (both synthetic narcotic analgesics), and amphetamine and methamphetamine, which have hallucinogenic and stimulant properties (National Institute on Drug Abuse, 1989).

Although PCP analogues have been identified in street samples of drugs, they are less frequently used today than other forms of designer drugs. Analogues of fentanyl are much more common; the pharmacological properties are similar to those of heroin or morphine. These analogues, known as "synthetic heroin" or "new heroin," can be addictive and carry the risk of overdose. Amphetamine and methamphetamine analogues are the most common forms of designer drugs on campuses today. These analogues often cause hallucinations and euphoria.

Ecstasy is one example of a designer drug; the chemical name for it is 3,4-methylenedioxymethamphetamine (MDMA) and the chemical structure is similar to that of amphetamine (a stimulant) and mescaline (a hallucinogen) (Health Canada, 2009b). According to the most recent Canadian Alcohol and Drug Use Survey, lifetime use of ecstasy in 2011 for Canadian men and women between the ages of 15 to 64 years was reported as 3.8 percent and 0.7 percent for past year use (Health Canada, 2009c). The highest rate of lifetime use of hallucinogens was reported in British Columbia at 5.1 percent and lowest in Prince Edward Island at 2.6 percent.

Ecstasy is usually sold in tablet, capsule, or powder forms. The tablets vary in shape, size, colour, and in the amount of ecstasy they contain—in fact, they may not even contain any ecstasy at all (Health Canada, 2009c)! Common names for ecstasy include: X, E, or XTC, Adam, beans, candy, dancing shoes, disco biscuits, doves, E-bomb, egg rolls, happy pill, hug drug, love drug, Malcolm (or Malcolm X), scooby snacks, smartees, sweets, skittles, thizz, vitamin E or vitamin X, and vowels (Cas Palmera, 2010c).

In small to moderate doses, ecstasy can produce feelings of energy, confidence, pleasure, well-being, increased sociability, and closeness to others. Larger doses do not enhance these desired effects. In fact, large doses of ecstasy are associated with grinding of teeth, jaw pain, sweating, increased blood pressure and heart rate, anxiety, panic attacks, blurred vision, nausea, vomiting, and convulsions (CAMH, n.d.a).

One risk of ecstasy use is hyperthermia (Health Canada, 2009c). This risk occurs because MDMA increases body temperature and, given that ecstasy is often used during raves where there is dancing in large crowds, there is considerable risk of overheating (Health Canada, 2009c). When the increase in body temperature is combined with an increase in blood pressure and heart rate, there is the possibility of kidney or heart failure, strokes, and seizures. Another risk related to excessive water consumption is if users drink excessive water to alleviate their increase in body temperature, which can lead to the salt levels in their blood decreasing dramatically, leading to confusion, convulsions and delirium, and then progress quickly to coma and death from the swelling of the brain (Health Canada, 2009c).

Bath salts are another example of a designer drug that has garnered significant attention recently; you might recall the highly publicized cannibal-like attack in Miami in the spring of 2012 and the link to the Maritimes (Visser, 2012). It is not exactly clear what drugs are included in bath salts, though they do contain synthetic chemicals similar to amphetamines (McMillen, 2013). Street names for bath salts include ivory wave, purple wave, vanilla sky, and bliss—they are nothing like the Epsom salts you might put in your bath (McMillen, 2013). Bath salts can be snorted, shooted, or mixed with food and drink, resulting in effects such as agitation, paranoia, hallucinations, chest pain, rapid heart rate, increased blood pressure, and suicidal thinking and behaviour (McMillen, 2013).

Steroids

Public awareness of **anabolic steroids** is often heightened by media stories about their use in amateur and professional athletes at World and Olympic class levels. Anabolic steroids are artificial forms of the male

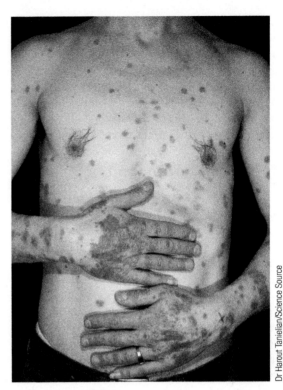

Steroid acne.

Dr Harout Tanielian/Science Source

hormone testosterone that promote muscle growth and strength. When used for medicinal purposes, the dose is one-tenth to one-hundredth of what is used illicitly (HealthLinkBC, 2013). Although these **ergogenic drugs**—that is, substances used to enhance athletic performance—are used primarily by young men to increase their strength, power, bulk (weight), and speed, as well as reduce body fat in efforts to improve their athletic performance, others not involved in athletics use steroids for the intimidation factor of increased muscle size or simply to improve their physique.

Most steroids are obtained through black-market sources. Steroids are available in two forms: injectable solution and pills (CAMH, n.d.b). Anabolic steroids produce a state of euphoria, diminished fatigue, and increased bulk and power in both sexes. These qualities give steroids an addictive quality. When users stop, they appear to undergo psychological withdrawal, partly caused by the disappearance of the physique they have become accustomed to. Steroids cause several adverse effects in men and women (HealthLinkBC, 2013). These drugs cause mood swings (aggression and violence, sometimes known as "roid rage"), acne, liver tumours, elevated cholesterol levels, hypertension, liver disease, heart attack or stroke, oily skin and acne, male-patterned hair loss, and skin infections. When steroids are used in children and youth, they may stop bone growth,

Anabolic steroids Artificial forms of the hormone testosterone that promote muscle growth and strength.

Ergogenic drug Substance that enhances athletic performance.

thus preventing the child from reaching his or her full adult height (HealthLinkBC, 2013). There is also a danger of HIV transmission through shared needles. In women, large doses of anabolic steroids trigger masculine changes, including lowered voice, increased facial and body hair, rough skin, enlarged clitoris, decreased breast size, and changes in or absence of menstruation (HealthLinkBC, 2013). When taken by healthy males, anabolic steroids shut down the body's production of testosterone, causing men's breasts to grow and testicles to shrink (HealthLinkBC, 2013).

A continued alarming trend is the use of other drugs to achieve the "performance-enhancing" effects of steroids. These steroid alternatives are sought in order to avoid the penalties (such as being banned from sports) for illicit use of anabolic steroids. Two common steroid alternatives are gamma hydroxybutyrate (GHB) and Clenbuterol. GHB is a deadly, illegal drug that is a primary ingredient in many of these "performance-enhancing" formulas. GHB does not produce a high. It does, however, cause headaches, nausea, vomiting, diarrhea, seizures and other central nervous system disorders, and possibly death. Another steroid alternative, Nandrolone, has turned up in drug tests, and yet another, Clenbuterol, has become an extremely popular item on the black market. Canada conducts around 2000 doping control tests per year on premier athletes. Most (70 percent) are random. Excluding body building, power lifting, and junior football (which have a 25 percent positive test result), there is about a 3 percent violation rate. For Olympic sports, the rate is 1 percent (Zilkowsky, 2001).

SOLUTIONS TO THE PROBLEM

Since 2004 and the first Canadian Addiction Survey, the self-report of lifetime and past year use of cannabis has decreased from 44.5 percent to 39.4 percent in lifetime use and from 14.1 percent to 9.1 percent in past year use (Health Canada, 2012). A similar decline in self-reported illicit drug use was found with a decrease in the past year use from 14.5 percent to 9.4 percent (Health Canada, 2012), but illicit drug use is still a cause for concern in our society today. It is generally agreed that a multimodal approach to drug education is best. Students should be taught about the use, misuse, and abuse of licit and illicit drugs. Factual information free from scare tactics must be presented; moralizing about drug use or nonuse is not effective in most cases. Critical to these teachings is expanding your decision-making and critical thinking skills so that

you can make the most appropriate decisions for you at various points in time of your life (see Chapter 1). Further, the realities of drug use and the potential short- and long-term consequences for that use should be presented. As mentioned previously, you are likely to assume that drug use among your peers is higher than it really is. Programs that teach you to control your drug use, as opposed to allowing your drug use to control you, are needed. Similarly, interventions should include content regarding the potential influence of set and setting. Reinforcing self-esteem along with decision-making skills should also be considered. It is not enough to urge you to "just say no"; alternatives to drug use should also be included as well as the opportunity to critically consider situations where you may feel pressured to use licit and illicit drugs.

All drug use/abuse prevention approaches have the potential to help a bit, but neither alone nor in combination do they offer a total solution to the problem. Drug use, misuse, and abuse have been a part of human behaviours for thousands of years, and are not likely to disappear in the near future. For this reason, you need to educate yourself and develop responsible thinking and actions necessary to avoid dangerous drug use and potential misuse and abuse or drug addiction.

Harm Reduction

A controversial form of harm reduction regarding illicit drug use is supervised injection sites. Controversy exists because drug users inject illicit drugs under the direct supervision of a nurse or other health-care provider. Proponents for this form of harm reduction note, in addition to access to immediate lifesaving attention should the drug user overdose, the drug user has access to clean needles, thus reducing risk for hepatitis, HIV, and other transmissible infections. InSite, operated by Vancouver Coastal Health and opened in 2003, is the first legal supervised injection site in North America (Vancouver Coastal Health, n.d.). They report a 35 percent decrease in overdose compared to a 9 percent decrease city-wide. In addition to providing 12 injection booths, InSite also supplies clean injection equipment such as syringes, cookers, filters, water, and tourniquets, as well as access to addiction counsellors, mental health workers, and peer staff who can connect clients to community resources for housing, addictions treatment, and other supportive services (Vancouver Coastal Health, n.d.). It is believed that the services provided by InSite may provide the first step of recovery for those addicted to illicit drugs. Recently Toronto has approved the opening of three supervised injection sites, based on the Vancouver model.

assess
YOURSELF

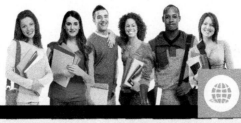

Go to MasteringHealth to complete this
questionnaire with automatic scoring.

TAKING CHARGE: Managing Drug Use Behaviour

After reading this chapter, you should be better informed regarding the most prevalently used illicit drugs in Canada. You should have enough information about each drug to assist you in a making an educated decision regarding whether or not you would want to use a particular drug in a particular situation. The following Assess Yourself questionnaire will help you to identify whether or not your drug use is controlling you. The questionnaire is followed by a series of questions that should help you decide whether or not to use an illicit drug. If you are honest in responding to each of these, you can learn about yourself and your drug use.

Recognizing a Drug Problem

Adult Version

These questions refer to the past 12 months.

		Circle Your Response
1. Have you used drugs other than those required for medical reasons?		Yes No
2. Have you abused prescription drugs?		Yes No
3. Do you abuse more than one drug at a time?		Yes No
4. Can you get through the week without using drugs?		Yes No
5. Are you always able to stop using drugs when you want to?		Yes No
6. Have you had "blackouts" or "flashbacks" as a result or drug use?		Yes No
7. Do you every feel bad or guilty about your drug use?		Yes No
8. Does your spouse (or parents) ever complain about your involvement with drugs?		Yes No
9. Has drug abuse created problems between you and your spouse or your parents?		Yes No
10. Have you lost friends because of your use of drugs?		Yes No
11. Have you neglected your family because of your use of drugs?		Yes No
12. Have you been in trouble at work (or school) because of drug abuse?		Yes No
13. Have you lost your job because of drug abuse?		Yes No
14. Have you gotten into fights when under the influence of drugs?		Yes No
15. Have you engaged in illegal activities in order to obtain drugs?		Yes No
16. Have you been arrested for possession of illegal drugs?		Yes No
17. Have you ever experienced withdrawal symptoms (felt sick) when you stopped taking drugs?		Yes No
18. Have you had medical problems as a result of your drug use (e.g., memory loss, hepatitis, convulsions, bleeding, and so on)?		Yes No
19. Have you gone to anyone for help for drug problem?		Yes No
20. Have you been involved in a treatment program specifically related to drug use?		Yes No

Source: Based on Substance Abuse Screening Instrument, The Drug Abuse Screening Test, www.drtepp.com/pdf/substance_abuse.pdf, Tepp, Alan.

(Continued)

Understanding Your Score

A "no" is scored 0, and a "yes" is scored 1, except for questions 4 and 5, which are reversed.

Total your score—your total reflects the severity of problems or consequences related to your drug abuse. An interpretation of your score should be based on the following guidelines:

0: No problem

1–5: Low level of problems related to drug abuse

6–10: Moderate level of problems related to drug abuse

11–15: Substantial level of problems related to drug abuse

16–20: Severe level of problems related to drug abuse

Interpretation of your score is most meaningful when considered within the context of the length of time that you have been using drugs, your age, your level of consumption, and other data collected as part of a more detailed assessment process.

The DAST questionnaire helps you to ask a broad range set of questions aimed at better understanding your use of drugs and your risk as a result. If you are concerned, you should seek an assessment/evaluation by a professional specifically trained and successfully experienced in dealing with drug addiction.

Disclaimer: Although these questions incorporate many of the common symptoms of drug addiction, the Drug Abuse Screening Test (DAST) is intended to be used for educational purposes only and should not be understood to constitute a diagnosis of drug addiction.

The following questions are provided to encourage you to further consider the decisions you make regarding your drug use.

- What other drugs (legal or illegal) are you currently using that could cause unwanted or unpleasant interactions?
- Do you know where the drug came from? Do you trust this source?
- Have you used this drug before? If so, how have you responded to it? If not, are you aware of how you might react?
- Should you have a negative reaction, do you know where you can go for help? Is there someone who can help you, if needed?
- Are you taking this drug to fit in?
- If you are caught using this drug, what will the personal and social consequences be? How will your family and friends feel about you? How will your future be affected if you are arrested and convicted?
- When pressured to use a drug, have you considered saying something like:
  - "Thanks, but I have a big test (game, meeting, something else) tomorrow morning."
  - "I already have a good buzz on right now, I don't need anything else."
  - "I don't know how _____ (the drug) will make me feel."
  - "I'm driving tonight, so I'm not using."
  - "I want to go for a run (or some other form of working out) in the morning."
  - "No thanks, I'm not interested."

Critical Thinking

You have a major exam tomorrow. In addition to your class notes, you have several chapters to review for it. You are worried about how you will get through it all, and think you may have to pull an all-nighter. If you don't get at least a B, you will lose your academic scholarship and be forced to leave school. A friend tells you that last semester she took a few lines of cocaine; it not only helped her stay awake, but also stimulated her thinking. She got an A– on her exam and experienced no side effects. She suggests you try it, too.

Using the DECIDE model described in Chapter 1, decide how you will keep yourself awake to study for your exam. What is the best approach for you to handle this situation?

DISCUSSION QUESTIONS

1. Describe the various methods of using cocaine. Which method is most effective? Why? Which method has the most health risks? Why?

2. Describe the various methods of using marijuana, both medicinally and non-medicinally. Which method is most effective? Why? Which method has the most health risks? Why?

3. Why is it difficult to determine the actual strength of marijuana?

4. Compare the physiological and psychological effects of marijuana and alcohol. Compare also the risks and benefits of their use.

5. What illicit drugs are you aware of on your campus? In your community? Why do you think these particular drugs are the 'drug of choice'?

6. Thinking about your particular campus, what kinds of drug education would be most effective? What drug(s) should be targeted? In what way?

7. What are the risks and benefits to harm reduction methods such as methadone clinics and supervised injection sites?

APPLICATION EXERCISE

Reread the "Consider This . . ." scenario at the beginning of the chapter and answer the following questions.

1. Do you think that university and college athletes should be tested for all illicit drugs? Why or why not? What about recreational drugs like tobacco, caffeine, and alcohol?

2. In what way(s) are university and college athletes held to a higher standard than other students regarding their attitudes and behaviours? Is this fair? Why or why not?

3. How would you feel about random illicit drug testing of students?

4. How might Kwame's academic and athletic performance be affected by his chronic marijuana use?

MASTERINGHEALTH

Go to MasteringHealth for assignments, the eText, and the study Area with case studies, self-quizzing, and videos.

focus on
Improving Your Sleep

Josh knew he was not ready for tomorrow's physics exam, but he went to his roommate's varsity basketball game anyway. By the time it was over and he started to study, it was past 11:00 p.m. To keep himself awake, he drank a can of Mountain Dew, an energy drink, and then a cup of instant coffee as he plowed through the text, his notes, and the online study guide. Just before 4:00 a.m., he fell into bed exhausted. Instead of drifting quickly to sleep, his mind kept racing. *Dynamics, inertia, action*, and *reaction* tumbled around with disjointed memories of all the stressful situations he had been through in the past few days—losing his cellphone, his girlfriend dumping him, the argument he had with his dad. He glanced at the clock; it said 5:30 a.m. The exam was in three hours.

Sound familiar? If you have ever tackled an exam or written a paper on too little sleep, you can probably predict what happened to Josh. He flunked.

In a recent survey, nearly 42 percent of students reported that they had only gotten enough sleep to feel rested in the morning less than two days during the past week (American College Health Association, 2011). Not surprisingly, nearly 61 percent of these students said they felt tired, dragged out, or sleepy during the day three to seven days of the week. Another study conducted by Canadian Association of College and University Student Services (2013) found that approximately 27 percent of Canadian post-secondary students have trouble sleeping largely due to stress and anxiety. It is not surprising then to think that today's students are sleep deprived, particularly given that they are going to bed an average of one to two hours later and sleeping 1 to 1.6 fewer hours than students of their parents' generation (Law, 2007). Between 15 and 30 percent of students report that they fall asleep in class on a regular basis, leading to an increased risk for low grades not to mention less enjoyment of their classes and overall educational experience (National Sleep Foundation, 2011).

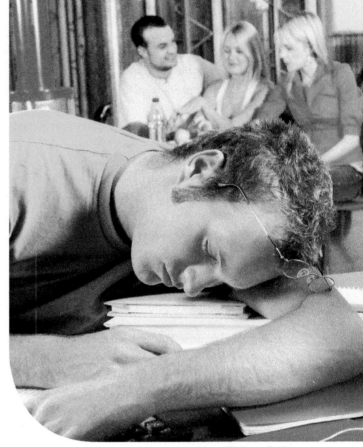

Vibe Images/Fotolia

One factor commonly implicated in reduced sleep time among college students is the internet and its 24-hour access to online games, social networking sites, videos, news, and more. Other things that might keep students awake include academic pressures, relationship problems, an underlying sleep disorder, chronic pain and other disease symptoms, anxiety or depression, the use of drugs (including alcohol), and stress from a variety of sources, including the stress of juggling finances, classes, and homework with a job or responsibilities at home.

These statistics are equally telling for working adults. A recent poll from the National Sleep Foundation (2008) found that 32 percent of working adults get a good night's sleep on only a few nights per month. A newer study examining sleep patterns among different ethnic groups found that sleep deficiencies were common among all groups (National Sleep Foundation, 2010). Specifically, individuals of African descent reported the least amount of sleep, while individuals of an Asian heritage reported the greatest amount of sleep. Regardless of ethnicity, when there are not enough hours in the day to get done what we think we need to, what typically gets shortchanged is sleep.

Because so many people are managing to function on campus and on the job with less sleep, you might think that sufficient sleep is not all that necessary or is not a component of your health that you need to pay attention to. The opposite is actually true; getting an adequate amount of sleep is much more important than most people realize. In this feature, we will examine the benefits of sleep and what happens when you do not sleep enough.

WHY DO YOU NEED TO SLEEP?

Sleep serves at least two biological purposes:

1. It conserves body energy. When you sleep, your core body temperature and the rate at which you burn calories drop. This leaves you with more energy to perform activities during your waking hours.

2. It restores you both physically and mentally. For example, certain reparative chemicals are released while you sleep. And there is some evidence, discussed shortly, that during sleep the brain is cleared of daily minutiae, learning is synthesized, and memories are consolidated.

Sleep Maintains Your Physical Health

Sleep has beneficial effects on most body systems. That is why, when you consistently do not get a good night's rest, your body does not function as well, and you become more vulnerable to a wide variety of health issues (Cappuccio et al., 2010). The following is a brief summary of the benefits of obtaining sufficient sleep:

- **Sleep maintains your immune system.** The common cold, strep throat, the flu, mononucleosis, cold sores, and a variety of other illnesses are more common when your immune system is depressed—which happens when you do not get enough sleep. Poor sleep quality, as well as shorter sleep duration, increases susceptibility to the common cold (Cohen et al., 2009). Another study reported that sleep disruption, particularly when circadian rhythms are disrupted repeatedly, results in an overall disruption of immune functioning (Bollinger et al., 2010).

- **Sleep reduces your risk for cardiovascular disease.** Research indicates that high blood pressure is more common in people who get fewer than seven hours of sleep a night (Cappuccio, Cooper Lanfranco, & Miller, 2011; Lanfranchi et al., 2010).

Interestingly, in this research both a short duration of sleep (less than six hours of sleep) and a long duration of sleep (greater than eight hours) were associated with greater risks of dying from heart disease. Two other studies found that poor sleep quality or reduced sleep time increased the prevalence of high levels in the blood of a substance called C-reactive protein (CRP), which is also a risk factor for heart disease (Okun, Coussons-Read, & Hall, 2009; Patel et al., 2009). Six or less hours of sleep also influences the risk of stroke (a blockage affecting a blood vessel in the brain—see Chapter 12) as noted in a study of more than 93 000 women (Chen et al., 2008).

- **Sleep contributes to a healthy metabolism.** Every moment of your life, your body's cells are participating in chemical reactions, many of which involve the breakdown of food and the synthesis of new compounds that the body needs. The sum of all these reactions is called *metabolism*. It is believed that sleep contributes to healthy metabolism and may be involved in maintaining a healthy body weight. While there is evidence that sleep deficiencies play a key role in increasing risk for type 2 diabetes and making diabetes harder to control, the link between sleep and obesity is far less clear (National Sleep Foundation, 2009; Nielson, Danielson, & Serensen, 2011). As noted, people are sleeping less today than they have in the past. Also as previously noted (see Chapter 6), the rate of overweight and obesity has increased in recent years. It is not illogical, then, to wonder if these two realities are related.

People who are overweight or obese tend to have more fat in their throats, tonsils, tongues, and supporting tissues, which increases their likelihood of a sleep disorder such as obstructive sleep apnea. Although excessive weight can lead to sleep disruption, is the reverse true as well? That is, does sleep deprivation lead to weight gain? Research suggests that two appetite-regulating hormones are affected by sleep deprivation: *ghrelin,* the "hungry hormone," which stimulates your appetite, and leptin, which signals you are full. Several studies showed to varying degrees that people who slept less than eight hours per night had lower levels of leptin, higher levels of ghrelin, and higher BMIs (Cappuccio et al., 2008; Hairston et al., 2010; Hasler, 2004; Nielsen et al., 2011; Spiegel et al., 2004).

Sleep Affects Your Ability to Function

If you routinely shortchange yourself on sleep, you could be sabotaging your grades (and any other intellectual work you do) and, if you drive while drowsy,

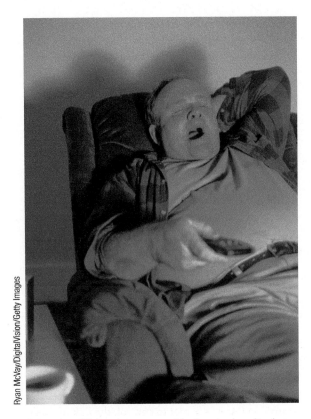

Ryan McVay/DigitalVision/Getty Images

Being overweight can increase your risk of certain sleep disorders.

endangering your life. The following section discusses how sleep—or lack thereof—affects your ability to function.

- **Sleep contributes to neurological functioning.** Restricting sleep can cause a wide range of neurological problems, including lapses of attention, slowed or poor memory, reduced cognitive ability, and a tendency for your thinking to get "stuck in a rut" (Banks & Dinges, 2007). Your ability not only to remember facts but also to integrate those facts, make meaningful generalizations about them, and consolidate what you have learned into lasting memories requires adequate sleep (Eichenbaum, 2007; Ellenbogen et al., 2009). In fact, students who pull all-nighters, as well as students who are short sleepers, have significantly lower overall grade-point averages compared to classmates who get adequate sleep (Thatcher, 2008).

- **Sleep improves motor tasks.** Sleep also has a restorative effect on motor function—that is, the ability to perform tasks such as shooting a basket, playing a musical instrument, or driving a car (Sheth, Janvelyan,

Circadian rhythm The 24-hour cycle by which you are accustomed to going to sleep, waking up, and performing habitual behaviours.

Hormone A "chemical messenger" released from one of the body's endocrine glands that travels in the bloodstream to another site where it helps to regulate body functions.

Sleep A readily reversible state of reduced responsiveness to, and interaction with, the environment.

Non-REM (NREM) sleep A period of restful sleep dominated by slow brain waves; during non-REM sleep, rapid eye movement is rare.

& Khan, 2008). It is one thing to mess up a Schubert sonata, it is another to fall asleep when you are driving! Some sleep researchers contend that a night without sleep impairs your motor skills and reaction time as much as if you were driving drunk (Tracy, 2008). As post-secondary students and working adults alike have become more sleep-deprived, the incidence of drowsy driving and so-called fall-asleep accidents has become a national concern.

Sleep Promotes Your Psychosocial Health

It is believed that certain brain regions, including the cerebral cortex (your "master mind"), can achieve some form of essential rest only during sleep (Bear, Connors, & Paradiso, 2007). So, if your roommate says you are grouchy after a few nights without enough sleep, do not take it too personally—your irritability is actually a sign of brain fatigue. In addition, you are more likely to feel stressed, worried, or sad when you are sleep-deprived. The relationship between sleep and stress is highly complex; stress can cause or contribute to sleep problems, and sleep problems can cause or increase your level of stress! The same is true of clinical psychiatric conditions such as depression and anxiety disorders. Reduced or poor quality sleep can trigger these disorders, but is also a common symptom resulting from them (Gregory et al., 2009; National Sleep Foundation, n.d.; Roth, 2004).

WHAT HAPPENS WHEN YOU SLEEP?

Each of us has an internal clock that subconsciously directs much of our daily activity. This 24-hour cycle by which you are accustomed to going to sleep, waking up, and performing habitual behaviours throughout your day is known as your **circadian rhythm**. Regulated in part by a tiny gland in your brain called the *pineal body,* it releases a **hormone** called *melatonin* that induces drowsiness.

You can fight the effects of melatonin for hours—even days!—especially if, like Josh in our opening story, you load up on caffeine. But like all human beings, and in fact all mammals, you will eventually succumb to **sleep**, which is clinically defined as a readily reversible state of reduced responsiveness to, and interaction with, the environment (Bear, Connors, & Paradiso, 2007). There are two primary sleep states: a state that is not characterized by rapid eye movement, called **non-REM (NREM) sleep**, and a state in which rapid eye

FIGURE 1

The Nightly Sleep Cycle

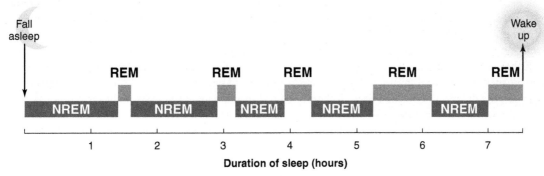

As the number of hours you sleep increases, your brain spends more and more time in REM sleep. Thus, sleeping for too few hours could deprive you of needed REM sleep.

movement does occur, called **REM sleep**. During the night, you slide through the stages of NREM sleep, then into REM, then back through NREM again, repeating one full cycle about once every 90 minutes (Bear, Connors, & Paradiso, 2007). Overall, you spend about 75 percent of each night in NREM sleep, and 25 percent in REM (Figure 1). As you age, you may sleep more lightly and spend less time in REM sleep.

Non-REM Sleep Is Restorative

During non-REM or "quiet" sleep, the body rests. Movement can occur, for instance, to shift your position in bed, but muscle tension is reduced. Your body temperature and your energy use drop during non-REM sleep; sensation is dulled; and your brain waves, heart rate, and breathing slow. In contrast, digestive processes speed up, and your body stores nutrients. During NREM sleep, you do not typically dream. Four distinct stages of NREM sleep have been distinguished by their characteristic progressive slowing of brain-wave patterns.

Stage 1. Your eyes may be open or closed, but essentially, you drift off. Stage 1 lasts only a few minutes, and is the lightest stage of sleep from which you are most easily awakened. This is the transition period between wakefulness and sleep in which the brain produces *theta waves,* which are slow brain waves. Many experience a sudden feeling of falling in this stage that can cause them to have a quick, jerky muscular reaction.

Stage 2. This stage is slightly deeper than Stage 1 and lasts from 5 to 15 minutes with even slower brain waves than in Stage 1. Your eyes are closed, eye and body movements gradually cease, and you disengage from your environment.

Stage 3. NREM sleep is also called *slow-wave sleep,* because during Stages 3 and 4, your brain generates slow brain waves known as *delta waves.* Your blood pressure drops, your heart rate and respiration slow considerably, and you enter deep sleep.

Stage 4. This is the deepest stage of sleep. Human growth hormone is released and signals your body to repair worn tissues. Speech and movement are rare during this stage, but can and do sometimes occur. For example, sleepwalking typically occurs during the first Stage 4 period of the night. You have probably heard that it is difficult to awaken a sleepwalker, and that is true of anyone in Stage 4 sleep.

During the deep phases of NREM sleep, your body repairs and regenerates tissue, builds bone and muscle, and promotes immune system health. If you do not reach or stay in deep NREM sleep for long periods, you may find that you tire more readily and have less resistance to disease.

REM Sleep Is Energizing

Dreaming takes place primarily during REM sleep. During REM, your brain-wave activity increases to be almost indistinguishable from that of someone who is wide awake, and your brain's energy use is higher than that of a person who is performing a difficult math problem (Bear, Connors, & Paradiso, 2007)! Your muscles are paralyzed during REM sleep—you may dream that you are rock climbing, but your body is incapable of movement with the exceptions of your heart and respiratory muscles, which allow you to breathe, and the tiny

REM sleep A period of sleep characterized by brain-wave activity similar to that seen in wakefulness; rapid eye movement and dreaming occur during REM sleep.

muscles of your eyes, which move your eyes rapidly as if you were following the scenario of your dream. This rapid eye movement gives REM sleep its name.

During REM sleep, your brain processes the experiences you have had and consolidates the information you have learned during the day. Some research suggests that if you are deprived of REM sleep, you may lose information or skills learned in the previous 24 to 48 hours. Other research suggests that REM sleep has little effect on memory (Genzel et al., 2009). As the night progresses, the duration of NREM sleep declines and you spend more and more time in REM. That is why a longer sleep is important to ensure that you get as much REM sleep as you need.

HOW MUCH SLEEP DO YOU NEED?

Given the importance of adequate sleep, especially REM sleep, you are probably asking yourself how much sleep you really need. Unfortunately, there is no magic number. Sleep needs vary from person to person, and your gender, health status, and lifestyle will also affect how much sleep your body requires.

Sleep Need Includes Baseline Plus Debt

The short answer to how much sleep you need is about seven to eight hours. This recommendation is given as the standard for "average" sleep time and is supported by a variety of studies over many years (Cappuccio et al., 2010; Sabanayagam & Shanker, 2010). Support for this recommendation comes from research that has shown that adults who sleep seven to eight hours a night have a lower risk of mortality than those who get fewer than seven or more than eight hours of sleep (Cappuccio et al., 2010; Cappuccio et al., 2010). Still, sleep is not a "one size fits all" proposition. Individual variations occur according to age (infants, children, and adolescents need more sleep), gender (women need more sleep), and many other factors. Because of individual differences, researchers cannot determine exactly how much sleep everyone needs. A good idea is to pay attention to how you feel after different amounts of sleep, and aim for the duration that feels best for you (National Sleep Foundation, 2011). Further, when sorting

Sleep debt The difference between the number of hours of sleep an individual needed in a given time period and the number of hours he or she actually slept.

Sleep inertia A state characterized by cognitive impairment, grogginess, and disorientation that is experienced upon rising from short sleep or an overly long nap.

out your sleep needs, you should consider two aspects: your body's physiological need plus your current **sleep debt**. Sleep debt refers to the total number of hours of missed sleep you carry around with you, either because you got up before your body was fully rested or because your sleep was interrupted. For example, if last week you managed just five hours of sleep a night Monday through Thursday and then get seven to eight hours a night Friday through Sunday, you will have an unresolved sleep debt of 8 to 12 hours. That means you need *more than* eight hours a night for the next several nights to "catch up."

The good news is that it is believed that you *can* catch up on lost sleep if you go about it sensibly. Getting five hours of sleep a night all semester long, then sleeping 48 hours the first weekend you are home on break will not restore your functioning, and will likely disrupt your circadian rhythm. Instead, whittle away at that sleep debt by sleeping nine hours a night throughout your break—then start the new term resolved to sleep seven to eight hours a night.

Do Naps Count?

Although naps cannot entirely cancel out a significant sleep debt, they can help to improve your mood, alertness, and performance (National Sleep Foundation, 2011). It is best to nap in the early to mid-afternoon, when the pineal body in your brain releases a small amount of melatonin and your body experiences a natural dip in its circadian rhythm. Try to avoid napping in the late afternoon, as it could interfere with your ability to fall asleep that night. It is best to keep your naps short (about 20 minutes), because a nap of more than 30 minutes can leave you in a state of **sleep inertia**, which is characterized by cognitive impairment, grogginess, and a disoriented feeling.

HOW CAN YOU GET A GOOD NIGHT'S SLEEP?

The following tips can help you get a longer and more restful night's sleep.

- **Let there be light.** Throughout the day, stay in sync with your circadian rhythm by spending time in the sunlight. If you live in an area where the sun seldom shines for weeks at a time, invest in special light-emitting diode (LED) lighting designed to mimic the sun's rays. Exposure to natural light outdoors is most beneficial, but opening the shades indoors and, on overcast days, turning on room lights can also help keep you alert.

- **Stay active.** Make sure you get plenty of physical activity during the day. Resist the temptation to postpone your physical activity until you are sleeping better. Start gently, but start now, because regular physical activity might help you maintain regular sleep habits.

- **Sleep tight.** Do not let a pancake pillow, scratchy or pilled sheets, or a threadbare blanket keep you from sleeping soundly. If your mattress is uncomfortable and you cannot replace it, try putting a foam mattress overlay on top of it.

- **Create a sleep "cave."** As bedtime approaches, keep your bedroom quiet, cool, and dark. Start by turning off your computer and cellphone. If you live in an apartment or dorm where there is noise outside or in the halls, wear ear plugs or get an electronic device that produces "white noise" such as the sound of gentle rain. Turn down the thermostat or, on hot nights, run a quiet electric fan. Install room-darkening shades or curtains or wear an eye mask if necessary to block out any light from the street.

- **Condition yourself into better sleep.** Go to bed and get up at the same time each day. Establish a bedtime ritual that signals to your body that it is time for sleep. For instance, sit by your bed and listen to a quiet song, meditate, write in a journal, take a warm bath or shower, or read something that lets you quietly wind down.

- **Make your bedroom a mental escape.** Do not stew about things you cannot fix right now. Clear your mind of worries and frustrations. Focus on listening to your body unwind.

- **Breathe.** Do it deeply, as soon as your head hits the pillow. Inhale through your nose slowly, filling your lungs completely, then exhale slowly through slightly pursed lips. Feel your stomach and diaphragm rising and falling. Repeat several times (see also Chapter 3 for stress relaxation techniques). In addition to giving your body the oxygen it needs, deep breathing can also decrease anxiety and tension that sometimes make it difficult to fall asleep.

- **Do not toss and turn.** If you are not asleep after 20 minutes, get up. Turn on a low light, and read something relaxing, not stimulating, or listen to some gentle music. Once you feel sleepy, go back to bed.

- **Get rid of technology in the bedroom.** Make a rule: No TV, texting, or chatting online after a certain time. If you cannot sleep, do not surf the net or check out your Facebook page. Sit quietly, focus on your breathing and relaxation, and try to recapture that drowsy, sleepy feeling.

To Prevent Sleep Problems, Avoid These Behaviours

Maybe you are already doing most of the actions suggested, and you still cannot sleep. If so, perhaps it is time to learn what *not* to do:

- Do not nap in the late afternoon or evening, and when you nap, make sure it is less than 30 minutes.

- Do not engage in strenuous physical activity within several hours of bedtime. Physical activity speeds up your metabolism and may make it harder to fall asleep.

- Do not read, study, watch TV, use your laptop, talk on the phone, eat, or smoke in bed. In fact, do not smoke at all—besides increasing your risk for cancer, heart disease, respiratory diseases, and others, smoking disturbs your sleep.

- Do not try to sleep if you are really hungry or really full. Allow at least three hours between your evening meal and bedtime, and if you feel hungry before bed, have a light snack.

- Do not drink coffee, energy drinks, or anything else that contains caffeine within several hours of bedtime. Once you consume caffeine, a stimulant (see also Chapter 10), it takes your body about six hours to clear just *half* of it from your system (National Sleep Foundation, 2011).

- Do not drink alcohol within several hours of bedtime. Although initially it may make you drowsy, it interferes with your natural sleep stages and can cause you to awaken in the middle of the night, unable to get back to sleep.

- Do not drink large amounts of any liquid before bed, to prevent having to get up in the night to use the bathroom.

- Do not take sleeping pills or nighttime pain medications unless they have been prescribed by your health-care provider. Casual use of over-the-counter sleeping aids can interfere with your brain's natural progression through the healthy stages of sleep. You may also experience "payback" later when you try to stop using the drug and your sleep challenges return, at a level worse than they were before you started using the medication.

- Do not get triggered. Remember the earlier advice about turning off your cellphone as you begin to prepare for bed? One reason is to avoid those late-night phone calls that can end up in arguments, disappointments, and other emotional stressors. If something—or someone—does trigger you shortly before bed, journal about it briefly, then promise yourself that you will make time the next day to explore your feelings more deeply.

WHAT IF YOU ARE NOT SLEEPING WELL?

If you are not sleeping well, you are not alone. Sleeplessness seems to have hit epidemic levels, causing millions of people to have difficulty performing everyday activities (Centers for Disease Control and Prevention, 2012). The data presented in Table 1 indicates the reasons that others reported for not being able to sleep. If you are following the advice in this chapter and you still are not sleeping well, then it is time to see your health-care provider. Although sleep disorders are relatively common in the general population, fewer than 5 percent of post-secondary students are diagnosed and in treatment for sleep disorders (American College Health Association, 2011). If you seek medical attention for your difficulties sleeping, you will probably be asked to keep a sleep diary such as the one in Figure 2, and you may be referred to a sleep disorders centre for an overnight stay. This type of evaluation is known as a clinical **sleep study**. While you are asleep in the sleep centre, sensors and electrodes record

TABLE 1

Self-Reported Sleep-Related Difficulties Among Adults 20 Years Old and Older

Difficulty	Percentage of Adults
Concentrating on things	23.2%
Remembering things	18.2%
Working on hobbies	13.3%
Driving or taking public transportation	11.3%
Taking care of financial affairs	10.5%
Performing employed or volunteer work	8.6%

Source: Centers for Disease Control and Prevention, "Insufficient Sleep is a Public Health Epidemic," Accessed October 5, 2011, www.cdc.gov/features/dsSleep/.

Sleep study A clinical assessment of sleep in which the patient is monitored while spending the night in a sleep disorders centre.

FIGURE 2

Sample Sleep Diary

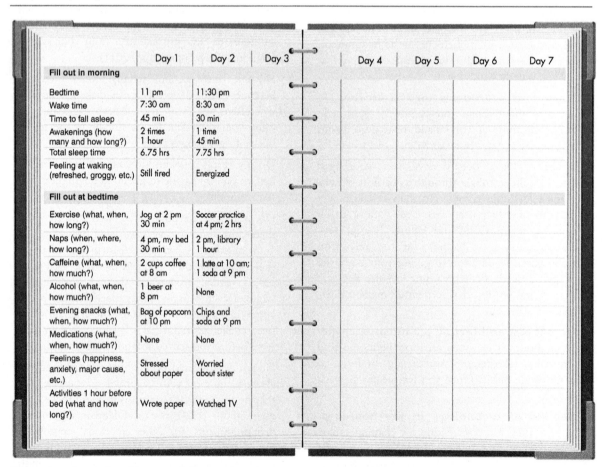

	Day 1	Day 2	Day 3	Day 4	Day 5	Day 6	Day 7
Fill out in morning							
Bedtime	11 pm	11:30 pm					
Wake time	7:30 am	8:30 am					
Time to fall asleep	45 min	30 min					
Awakenings (how many and how long?)	2 times 1 hour	1 time 45 min					
Total sleep time	6.75 hrs	7.75 hrs					
Feeling at waking (refreshed, groggy, etc.)	Still tired	Energized					
Fill out at bedtime							
Exercise (what, when, how long?)	Jog at 2 pm 30 min	Soccer practice at 4 pm; 2 hrs					
Naps (when, where, how long?)	4 pm, my bed 30 min	2 pm, library 1 hour					
Caffeine (what, when, how much?)	2 cups coffee at 8 am	1 latte at 10 am; 1 soda at 9 pm					
Alcohol (what, when, how much?)	1 beer at 8 pm	None					
Evening snacks (what, when, how much?)	Bag of popcorn at 10 pm	Chips and soda at 9 pm					
Medications (what, when, how much?)	None	None					
Feelings (happiness, anxiety, major cause, etc.)	Stressed about paper	Worried about sister					
Activities 1 hour before bed (what and how long?)	Wrote paper	Watched TV					

Using a sleep diary such as this one can help you and your health-care provider discover any behavioural factors that might be contributing to your sleep problem.

data that will be reviewed by a sleep specialist who will help your primary health-care provider determine the precise nature of your sleep problem.

There are more than 80 specific sleep disorders (American Academy of Sleep Medicine, 2008). The most common disorders in adults are insomnia, sleep apnea, and restless legs syndrome. Other common sleep disorders include narcolepsy and a group of disorders called parasomnias.

Insomnia

Insomnia—difficulty in falling asleep, frequent arousals during sleep, or early morning awakening—is the most common sleep complaint. Annual polls reveal that more than 50 percent of people experience insomnia at least a few nights a week (National Sleep Foundation, 2009). About 10 to 15 percent of people report that they have chronic insomnia, that is, insomnia that persists longer than a month, including about 3 percent of post-secondary students who require treatment for their insomnia (American College Health Association, 2011). Insomnia is more common among women than men, and its prevalence increases with age.

Symptoms of insomnia include difficulty falling asleep, waking up frequently during the night, difficulty returning to sleep, waking up too early in the morning, a sleep that was not refreshing, daytime sleepiness, and irritability. Sometimes, insomnia is related to stress and worry. In other cases, it may be related to disruptions to the body's circadian rhythms, which may occur with travel across time zones, shift work, and other major schedule changes. Insomnia can also occur as a side effect from taking certain medications. Left untreated, insomnia can be associated with increased illness or morbidity.

Treatment for Insomnia

Because of the close connection between behaviours and insomnia, cognitive behavioral therapy is often part of any treatment for insomnia. A cognitive behavioural therapist assists a patient in identifying thought and behavioural patterns that contribute to the inability to fall asleep. Once these patterns are recognized, the patient practises new habits that produce positive change. In some cases of insomnia, *hypnotic* or *sedative* medications may be prescribed. These drugs induce sleep, and some may help relieve anxiety. However, some have undesirable side effects ranging from daytime sleepiness and hallucinations to sleepwalking and other strange nighttime behaviours. Some can actually promote anxiety or depression. Many sedatives are also addictive and can lead to tolerance and dependence. Antidepressants are also commonly prescribed

for insomnia. Relaxation techniques, including yoga and meditation (see also Chapter 3), can be especially helpful in preparing the body to sleep. Physical activity, done early in the day, can also be helpful in reducing stress and promoting deeper sleep.

Sleep Apnea

Sleep apnea is a disorder in which breathing is briefly and repeatedly interrupted during sleep (National Sleep Foundation, 2011). *Apnea* refers to a breathing pause that lasts at least 10 seconds. During that time, the chest may rise and fall, but little or no air may be exchanged, or the person may actually not breathe until the brain triggers a gasping inhalation. Sleep apnea affects about 1 in every 15 people (Sleep Disorders Guide, n.d.).

There are two major types of sleep apnea: central and obstructive. *Central sleep apnea* occurs when the brain fails to tell the respiratory muscles to initiate breathing. Consumption of alcohol, certain illegal drugs, and certain medications can contribute to this condition. *Obstructive sleep apnea (OSA)*, which is the more common form, occurs when air cannot move in and out of a person's nose or mouth, even though the body tries to breathe.

Typically, OSA occurs when a person's throat muscles and tongue relax during sleep and block the airways (National Sleep Foundation, 2011). People who are overweight or obese often have more tissue that flaps or sags, which puts them at higher risk for sleep apnea. People with OSA are prone to heavy snoring, snorting, and gasping. These sounds occur because, as oxygen saturation levels in the blood fall, the body's autonomic nervous system is stimulated to trigger inhalation, often via a sudden gasp of breath. This response can wake the person, interrupting deep sleep, and causing the person to wake up in the morning feeling tired and unwell. More serious risks of OSA include high blood pressure, irregular heartbeats, heart attack, and stroke. Apnea-associated sleeplessness can be a factor in an increased risk of type 2 diabetes, immune system deficiencies, and a host of other problems.

Restless Legs Syndrome

Restless legs syndrome (RLS) is a neurological disorder characterized by unpleasant sensations in the legs when at rest combined with an uncontrollable urge to move in an effort to relieve these feelings. These sensa-

Insomnia A disorder characterized by difficulty in falling asleep quickly, frequent arousals during sleep, or early morning awakening.

Sleep apnea A disorder in which breathing is briefly and repeatedly interrupted during sleep.

Restless legs syndrome (RLS) A neurological disorder characterized by an overwhelming urge to move the legs when they are at rest.

tions range in severity from uncomfortable to irritating to painful. In general, the symptoms are more pronounced in the evening or at night. Lying down or trying to relax activates the symptoms, so people with RLS often have difficulty falling and staying asleep. Some researchers estimate that RLS affects as many as 10 percent of the population, with a wide range in symptom severity (National Institute of Neurological Disorders and Stroke, 2011).

The cause of RLS is unknown; however, there is growing support for some form of genetic predisposition (National Institute of Neurological Disorders and Stroke, 2011). In other cases, RLS appears to be related to other conditions such as kidney failure, diabetes, and peripheral neuropathy. Pregnancy or hormonal changes can worsen symptoms. If there is an underlying condition, treatment of that condition may provide relief. Other treatment options include use of prescribed medication, decreasing tobacco and alcohol use, and applying heat to the legs. For some people, practising relaxation techniques or performing stretching exercises can help alleviate symptoms.

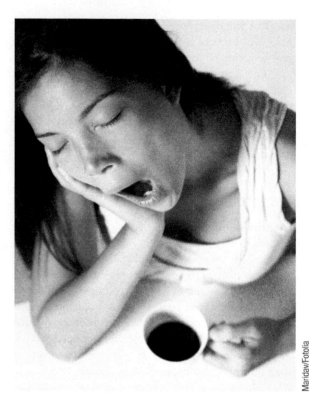

Because sleep is vital for daily functioning and well-being, disorders that prevent you from getting sufficient quality sleep can leave you feeling stressed and overall run down.

Narcolepsy

Narcolepsy is excessive, intrusive sleepiness. The person affected can fall asleep quite suddenly—in class, at work, driving, or in any other situation. Narcolepsy affects men and women in equal numbers. The condition is apparently due to a dramatic reduction in the number of nerve cells containing a substance called hypocretin in the brains of narcoleptics (American Academy of Sleep Medicine, 2006). Hypocretin plays a role in sleep regulation. There appears to be a genetic basis for the disorder.

Narcolepsy Excessive, intrusive sleepiness.

assess YOURSELF

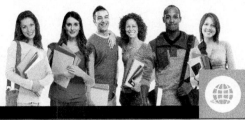

Go to MasteringHealth to complete this questionnaire with automatic scoring

TAKING CHARGE: Managing Your Sleep

Do you need a jolt of caffeine to get you jump-started in the morning? Do you find it hard to stay awake in class? Have you ever nodded off behind the wheel? These are all signs of inadequate or poor quality sleep. Complete the questionnaire below and reflect upon how well you are sleeping.

Are You Sleeping Well?

Read each statement below, then circle True or False according to whether or not it applies to you in your current school term.

1. I sometimes doze off in my morning classes.
   True   False

2. I sometimes doze off in my last class of the day.
   True   False

3. I go through most of the day feeling tired.
   True   False

4. I feel drowsy when I am a passenger in a bus or car.
   True   False

5. I often fall asleep while reading or studying.
   True   False

6. I often fall asleep at the computer or watching TV.
   True   False

7. It usually takes me a long time to fall asleep.
   True   False

8. My roommate (or partner) tells me I snore.
   True   False

9. I wake up frequently throughout the night.
   True   False

10. I have fallen asleep while driving.
    True   False

If you answer True more than once, you may be sleep deprived. Try the strategies in this chapter and those that follow for getting more or better quality sleep, and if you still experience sleepiness, see your health-care provider:

- Evaluate your behaviours and identify things you are doing that get in the way of a good night's sleep. Develop a plan. What can you do differently starting today?

- Write a list of personal Dos and Don'ts. For instance: Do turn off your cellphone after 11:00 p.m. Do not drink anything with caffeine after 5:00 p.m. (assuming a sleep time of 11 p.m.).

- Keep a sleep diary. Note not only how many hours of sleep you get each night, but also how you feel and how you function the next day.

- Arrange your room to promote restful sleep. Remember the "cave": Keep it quiet, cool, and dark, and replace any uncomfortable bedding.

- Visit your campus health centre and ask for more information about getting a good night's sleep.

- Establish a regular sleep schedule. Get in the habit of going to bed and waking up at the same time, even on weekends.

- Create a ritual, such as stretching, meditation, reading something light, or listening to music, that you follow each night to help your body ease from the activity of the day into restful sleep.

- If you are still having difficulty sleeping and feel you might have a sleep disorder or an underlying health problem disrupting your sleep, contact your health-care provider.

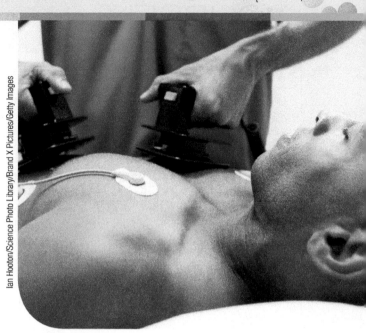

Ian Hooton/Science Photo Library/Brand X Pictures/Getty Images

CHAPTER 12
REDUCING RISK FOR CARDIOVASCULAR DISEASE AND CANCER

LEARNING OUTCOMES

- Explain the incidence, prevalence, outcomes, and impacts of cardiovascular disease in Canada.

- Describe the anatomy and physiology of the heart and the circulatory system.

- Identify the various types of heart disease and the risk factors for developing them.

- Identify the various types of cancer and the risk factors for developing them.

- Describe the suspected causes of cancer, including those factors that are controllable and uncontrollable.

- Explain the importance of lifestyle choices in preventing heart disease and cancer.

◄◉ CONSIDER THIS . . .

Kassandra is an avid sunbather. She thinks the glow of a tan makes her look healthy and attractive. In fact, when she cannot get the tan she desires from the sun, she spends time in a tanning bed. This year, she decided to get a jump on her tan and is studying for her final exams outside under the sun every minute she can. In her efforts to get tanned as quickly as possible, she has decided to not wear sunscreen.

How many others like Kassandra do you know? What is the risk of suntanning—under the sun or in tanning beds? What will it take to change the attitude that a suntan makes a person look healthy and attractive? What can a person do to reduce his or her risk of developing skin cancer? What do you know about sunscreen and how and when to apply it?

Heart disease and cancer continue to be the two leading causes of death in Canada. Together, they account for 50.1 percent of all deaths in Canada (Statistics Canada, 2012). In the past, heart disease was the leading cause of death, deemed responsible for at least 47 percent of all deaths. Cancer surpassed heart disease as the leading cause of mortality (that is, death rate) in 1993 for men and in 1998 for women (Milan, 2011). Not surprisingly, the actions you take today have a significant impact on reducing your risk for these diseases now and in the future. In other words, you can reduce your risk for heart disease and cancer by making certain lifestyle choices—at the very least, you can postpone the onset of these diseases. Postpone, rather than prevent, at times may be the more appropriate term, given that mortality is eventually a reality and there will be a cause for your death.

CARDIOVASCULAR DISEASES

Cardiovascular disease (CVD), a class of diseases of the heart and blood vessels, is the leading cause of death worldwide (World Health Organization, 2013). Approximately 30 percent of all deaths worldwide are a result of cardiovascular disease and the number of people expected to die from heart disease or stroke will reach 23.3 million by 2030 (World Health Organization, 2013). In Canada, CVD (heart disease—20. 7 percent; stroke—5.9 percent) accounted for more than 26.6 percent of all deaths (Statistics Canada, 2012). The mortality rate has decreased from 370.5 to 138.6 per 100 000 males and from 295.1 to 126.1 per 100 000 females between 1981 and 2007 (Milan, 2011).

How do medical professionals account for this decline? Why has there been a greater decline in men than women? There are no simple answers. Advances in medical techniques, earlier and better diagnostic procedures and treatments (better for men than women), better emergency medical assistance programs, and training of people in cardiopulmonary resuscitation (CPR) have greatly aided individuals with CVD. As noted later, women's signs and symptoms for heart attack are not as obvious as men's. Refinements in surgical techniques and improvements in heart transplants and artificial heart devices have enabled men and women to live longer lives. Despite these medical advances in treatment of CVD, the onus remains on the individual for prevention, since most premature deaths from CVD could be prevented by avoiding tobacco products; eating well and reducing obesity; increasing activity; and preventing high blood pressure, diabetes, and elevated blood lipids (World Health Organization, 2013). More specifically, you can reduce your risk for CVD by controlling high blood pressure and reducing your dietary intake of saturated fats and cholesterol. By maintaining your weight, decreasing your sodium intake, engaging in regular physical activity, and changing your lifestyle to reduce your stress response, you can lower your blood pressure. You can also monitor the levels of fat and cholesterol in your blood and adjust your dietary intake to prevent your arteries from becoming clogged. Understanding how your cardiovascular system works will help you to understand your risks for CVDs and what can be done to reduce these risks.

UNDERSTANDING YOUR CARDIOVASCULAR SYSTEM

The **cardiovascular system** refers specifically to the network of elastic tubes through which blood flows as it carries oxygen and nutrients to all parts of the body. It includes the heart, lungs, arteries, arterioles (small arteries), and capillaries (minute blood vessels). It also includes venules (small veins) and veins, the blood vessels through which blood flows as it returns to the heart and lungs (Heart and Stroke Foundation, 2009).

Under normal circumstances, the human body contains approximately six litres of blood. This blood transports nutrients, oxygen, waste products, hormones, and enzymes throughout the body. It also regulates body temperature, cellular water levels, and acidity levels of body components, and aids in bodily defence against toxins and harmful microorganisms (Heart and Stroke Foundation, 2009). An adequate blood supply is essential to health and well-being.

How does the heart ensure that blood is constantly recirculated to body parts? The four chambers of the heart work together to deliver oxygenated blood where it is needed and to remove carbon dioxide (see Figure 12.1).

The two upper chambers of the heart, called **atria**, or auricles, are large collecting chambers that receive blood from the rest of the body. The two lower chambers, known as **ventricles**, pump the blood out again. Small valves regulate the steady, rhythmic flow of blood

Cardiovascular diseases (CVD) Diseases of the heart and blood vessels.

Cardiovascular system A complex system comprising the heart and blood vessels that transports nutrients, oxygen, hormones, and enzymes throughout the body, and regulates temperature, the water levels of cells, and the acidity levels of body components.

Atria The two upper chambers of the heart, which receive blood.

Ventricles The two lower chambers of the heart, which pump blood through the vessels.

FIGURE 12.1

Anatomy of the Heart

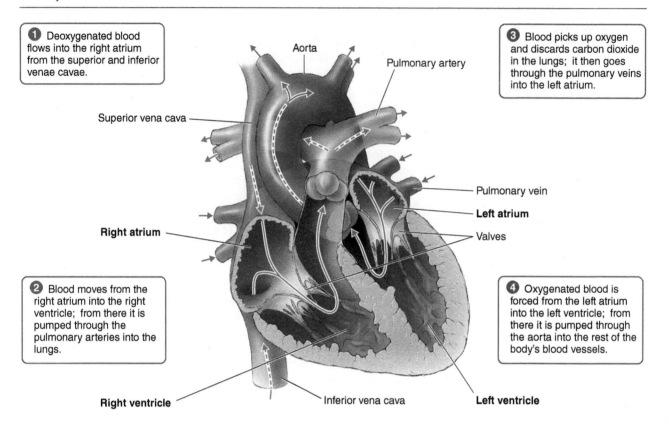

1 Deoxygenated blood flows into the right atrium from the superior and inferior venae cavae.

3 Blood picks up oxygen and discards carbon dioxide in the lungs; it then goes through the pulmonary veins into the left atrium.

Aorta

Pulmonary artery

Superior vena cava

Pulmonary vein

Left atrium

Right atrium

Valves

2 Blood moves from the right atrium into the right ventricle; from there it is pumped through the pulmonary arteries into the lungs.

4 Oxygenated blood is forced from the left atrium into the left ventricle; from there it is pumped through the aorta into the rest of the body's blood vessels.

Right ventricle

Inferior vena cava

Left ventricle

between chambers and prevent inappropriate backwash. The tricuspid valve, located between the right atrium and the right ventricle, the pulmonary (pulmonic) valve, between the right ventricle and the pulmonary artery, the mitral (bicuspid) valve, between the left atrium and left ventricle, and the aortic valve, between the left ventricle and the aorta, allow blood to flow in only one direction (Heart and Stroke Foundation, 2009).

Heart activity depends on a complex interaction of biochemical, physiological, and neurological signals (Heart and Stroke Foundation, 2009). The following is a simplified version of the steps involved:

1. Deoxygenated blood enters the right atrium after circulating through the body.

2. From the right atrium, blood moves to the right ventricle and is pumped through the pulmonary artery to the lungs, where it receives oxygen.

3. Oxygenated blood from the lungs then returns to the left atrium of the heart.

4. Blood from the left atrium is forced into the left ventricle.

5. The left ventricle pumps blood through the aorta to the body.

Different types of blood vessels are required for different parts of this process. **Arteries** carry blood away from the heart. Pulmonary arteries carry deoxygenated blood to the lungs, where they pick up oxygen and drop off carbon dioxide. As they branch off from the heart, the arteries divide into smaller blood vessels called **arterioles**, and then into even smaller blood vessels called capillaries.

Capillaries have thin walls that permit the exchange of oxygen, carbon dioxide, nutrients, and waste products with body cells. Carbon dioxide and waste products are transported to the lungs and kidneys through **veins** and venules (small veins).

For the heart to function properly, the four chambers must beat in an organized manner. This is governed by an electrical impulse that directs the heart muscle to move when the impulse moves across it, resulting in a sequential contraction of the four chambers. This signal starts in a small bundle of highly specialized cells, the **sinoatrial node (SA node)**, located in the right atrium. The SA node serves as a form of natural

Arteries Vessels that carry blood away from the heart.

Arterioles Small arteries.

Capillaries Minute blood vessels that branch out from the arterioles through which the exchange of oxygen, carbon dioxide, nutrients, and waste products happens.

Veins Vessels that carry blood back to the heart.

Sinoatrial node (SA node) Node serving as a form of natural pacemaker for the heart.

pacemaker for the heart (Heart and Stroke Foundation, 2009). People with damaged or nonfunctional natural pacemaker activity have a mechanical pacemaker inserted to ensure the smooth passage of blood through the sequential phases of the heartbeat.

At rest, the average adult heart beats 60 to 80 times per minute (Heart and Stroke Foundation, 2009). A woman's resting heart rate tends to be slightly higher than a man's. A person's heart with a higher level of cardiorespiratory fitness beats about 50 to 60 times per minute (see Chapter 4). To supply the working muscles with the nutrients they need, the heart beats harder when engaged in physical activity. When the mind and body experience severe stress, the heart may beat over 200 times per minute, particularly in an individual who is overweight and/or with a low level of physical fitness. A healthy heart functions more efficiently and is better able to accommodate various stresses upon it than a less healthy one.

TYPES OF CARDIOVASCULAR DISEASES

Although most of us associate CVD with heart attacks (or myocardial infarction), there are a number of different types. The four most common forms are:

- atherosclerosis (characterized by deposits of plaque in the inner lining of the arteries)

- coronary heart disease (a result of atherosclerotic plaque building up in the arteries such that coronary artery blood flow is reduced; when the blood flow is severely restricted or blocked, a heart attack results; when the blood flow is reduced [approximately 75 percent], but not blocked, chest pain [angina pectoris] often occurs)

- stroke (cerebrovascular accident that occurs as a result of reduced blood supply to the brain)

- hypertension (chronic high blood pressure)

Other less common forms of CVD include irregular heartbeat (arrhythmia), congestive heart failure, and congenital and rheumatic heart disease.

Irrespective of lifestyle behaviours, some individuals are at a greater risk than others for CVD (Heart and Stroke Foundation, 2009). Generally, risk increases with age; men are at a greater risk than women, and individuals of African, South Asian, and First Nations descent are at greater risk than other ethnicities. Others are at risk because of their lifestyle choices. These will be discussed later in this chapter.

Atherosclerosis

Atherosclerosis is a type of arteriosclerosis. **Arteriosclerosis** is a general term for the narrowing or "hardening" of the arteries. The end result of arteriosclerosis is reduced blood flow to vital organs. Atherosclerosis is characterized by deposits of fatty substances, cholesterol, cellular waste products, calcium, and fibrin (a clotting material in the blood) in the inner lining of an artery. The resulting build-up is referred to as atherosclerotic **plaque** (Heart and Stroke Foundation, 2011). Plaque may partially or totally block the blood's flow through an artery. When plaque develops, two things can happen: (1) bleeding (hemorrhage) into the plaque or (2) formation of a blood clot (thrombus) on the plaque's surface. If either of these occurs and an artery is blocked, the chances of a heart attack or stroke increase (see Figure 12.2) (Heart and Stroke Foundation, 2011).

Atherosclerosis does not occur suddenly. It is believed, in fact, that atherosclerotic plaque begins to form in the womb and worsens as the years pass (Mayo Clinic, 2012). As such, atherosclerosis is not an all-or-nothing disease but occurs in varying degrees. Further, there are lifestyle choices individuals make in regard to physical activity and dietary intake that significantly influence the amount of plaque that develops and remains in the arteries (Heart and Stroke Foundation, 2011). If the arteries are occluded (blocked with plaque) to about 75 percent in the heart, angina pectoris (chest pain) results. When the arteries are 90 to 95 percent occluded and a blood clot attempts to travel through them, a myocardial infarction (heart attack) or ischemic stroke (if the blood clot is in occluded arteries in the brain) occurs.

The process of plaque build-up begins when the protective inner lining of the artery (endothelium) becomes damaged, allowing fat, cholesterol, and other substances in the blood to affix to the arterial walls, eventually obstructing blood flow. The three major causes of such damage are (1) dramatic fluctuations in blood pressure, (2) elevated levels of cholesterol, triglycerides, and glucose in the blood, and (3) cigarette smoking. Viral infections may also be contributing factors. Cigarette smoke aggravates and speeds up the development of atherosclerosis, particularly in the coronary arteries, the aorta, and the arteries of the legs because of the damage caused to the inner arterial walls (Heart and Stroke Foundation, 2011).

Atherosclerosis A type of arteriosclerosis characterized by plaque deposits in the inner lining of arteries.

Arteriosclerosis Refers to narrowing and hardening of the arteries.

Plaque Combination of fatty substances, cholesterol, cellular waste products, calcium, and fibrin.

Coronary Heart Disease

Coronary heart disease (CHD), also called coronary artery

FIGURE 12.2

Atherosclerosis and Coronary Heart Disease

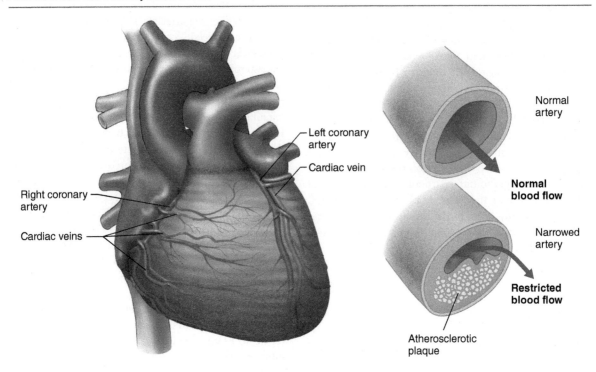

disease, is the major disease of the cardiovascular system. It is the result of atherosclerotic plaque accumulation such that a blockage occurs in one or more of the coronary arteries and blood flow is impeded. As previously mentioned, chest pain or angina pectoris results when the blockage in the cardiac arteries is equivalent to 75 percent or more while complete blockage results in a heart attack.

A **heart attack**, or **myocardial infarction**, involves a blockage of the normal blood supply to an area of the heart. This condition is often brought on by a **coronary thrombosis**, or blood clot in the coronary artery. When blood does not flow readily, there is a corresponding decrease in oxygen transportation. The symptoms of a heart attack vary from mild to severe and from specific to nonspecific. Women, in particular, experience less severe and less specific symptoms. The Heart and Stroke Foundation (2013) identifies the following as the most common symptoms:

Heart attack (myocardial infarction) A blood clot that prevents blood from flowing through the heart.

Coronary thrombosis A blood clot in a coronary artery.

Collateral circulation Following the complete occlusion of a coronary artery, rerouting of needed blood through unused or underused blood vessels.

- chest discomfort (uncomfortable chest pressure, squeezing, fullness or pain, burning or heaviness)

- discomfort in other areas of the upper body (neck, jaw, shoulder, arms, back)
- shortness of breath
- sweating
- nausea
- lightheadedness*

As previously noted, many women do not experience the common signs and symptoms as previously listed. For women, their symptoms of heart disease are vaguer and include unusual fatigue, shortness of breath, and sleep disturbances.

If the heart blockage is minor, the otherwise healthy heart will adapt over time by using small unused or underused blood vessels to reroute the needed blood and oxygen. This system, known as **collateral circulation**, is a form of self-preservation that allows a damaged heart muscle to heal itself. When heart blockage is more severe, the body is unable to adapt on its own and outside lifesaving support is critical. Chances of surviving a heart attack are greatest when you seek treatment immediately—thousands of Canadians die each year because they did not receive timely medical intervention (Heart and Stroke Foundation, 2013). Of those Canadians who initially survive their heart attack, 12 percent

*Based on "Signs of heart attack, cardiac arrest and sudden arrhythmia death syndrome (SADS)", http://www.heartandstroke.com/site/c.iklQLcMWJtE/ b.3483917/k.AA64/Heart_disease__Signs_of_heart_attack_cardiac_arrest_SADS.htm, published by Heart and Stroke Foundation of Canada.

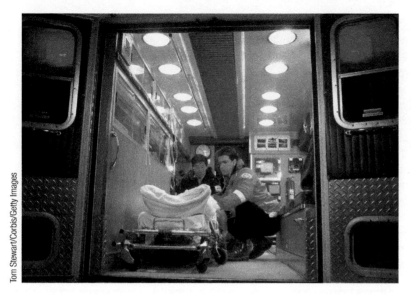

Because thousands of heart attack victims die within the first few hours, immediate attention is vital to the patient's survival.

Stroke

Like the heart muscle, brain cells must have a continuous and adequate supply of oxygen in order to survive. A **stroke** (also called a cerebrovascular accident) occurs when the blood supply to the brain is cut off. Strokes can be caused by a **thrombus** (blood clot), an **embolus** (a wandering clot), or an **aneurysm** (a weakening in a blood vessel that causes it to bulge and, in severe cases, burst).

When a stroke occurs—that is, the restriction or complete blockage of blood flow in the brain—brain cells die. Consequences of a stroke vary depending upon where the blood flow was restricted and for how long. They include speech impairment, memory loss, and loss of motor control. Although some strokes affect parts of the brain that regulate heart and lung function and result in death within minutes, others are mild and result in temporary dizziness or slight weakness or numbness. Mild strokes are called **transient ischemic attacks** and often indicate an impending major stroke. The key to surviving a stroke is to obtain medical treatment within 24 hours of the first symptom (Centers for Disease Control and Prevention, 2013). Although almost three-quarters of Canadians recognize at least one warning sign of stroke, only half would call 9-1-1 if they or someone they knew was experiencing the warning sign (Heart and Stroke Foundation, n.d.). According to the Heart and Stroke Foundation of Canada (2013) stroke can be treated. The Heart and Stroke foundation of Canada has developed the FAST tool for identifying warning signs of a stroke:

- **F**ace—is it drooping?
- **A**rms—can you raise them?
- **S**peech—is it slurred or jumbled?
- **T**ime—to call 9-1-1 right away.

If you experience any of these symptoms, call 9-1-1 or your local emergency

will die within 30 days. Long-term survival after 30 days reaches 91 to 93 percent (Canadian Institute for Health Information, 2003).

As a result of atherosclerosis and other circulatory impairments, the heart's oxygen supply is often reduced, a condition known as ischemia. Individuals with **ischemia** often suffer from varying degrees of **angina pectoris** or chest pains. Many of these individuals experience short episodes of angina when they exert themselves physically. Symptoms of angina range from a slight feeling of indigestion to a feeling that the heart is being crushed. Generally, the more serious the oxygen deprivation, the more severe the pain.

Currently, several methods of treating angina are available. In mild cases, rest is critical. The most common treatments for more severe cases involve using drugs that affect (1) the supply of blood to the heart muscle or (2) the heart's demand for oxygen. Pain and discomfort are often relieved with nitroglycerin, a drug used to relax (dilate) veins, thereby reducing the amount of blood returning to the heart and lessening its workload. Patients whose angina is caused by spasms of the coronary arteries are often given drugs called calcium channel blockers. Since excessive calcium and potassium are among the suspected causes of these spasms, calcium channel blockers are used to prevent calcium atoms from passing through coronary arteries and causing heart contractions. They also appear to reduce blood pressure and to slow heart rates. **Beta blockers** are another major type of drug used to treat angina. The chemical action of beta blockers serves to control potential overactivity of the heart muscle.

Ischemia Insufficient blood flow relative to the demand of the tissue, which results in a decrease in oxygen.

Angina pectoris Severe chest pain occurring as a result of reduced oxygen flow to the heart.

Beta blockers A type of drug used to treat angina; controls potential overactivity of the heart muscle.

Stroke Results when the blood supply to the brain is severely reduced or cut off.

Thrombus Blood clot.

Embolus Blood clot forced through the circulatory system.

Aneurysm A weakened blood vessel that may bulge under pressure and, in severe cases, burst.

Transient ischemic attacks Mild form of stroke; often an indicator of impending major stroke.

number immediately. If a person is diagnosed with a stroke caused by a blood clot, doctors can administer a clot-busting drug available only at a hospital, and only within a few crucial hours after symptoms begin. That is why it is very important to be able to recognize the five warning signs of stroke and *immediately* call 9-1-1 or your local emergency number.

If you are with someone who suddenly, and without plausible reason, experiences any or all of the symptoms described above, give them the 60-second test, also called FAST:

- Ask the person to smile. Does his or her **FACE** droop on one side?

- Ask the person to raise both **ARMS.** Does one arm sag?

- Ask the person to repeat a simple sentence like, "It's sunny today." Is his or her **SPEECH** slurred or unusual?

If the answer to any of the above is yes, it's **TIME** to call 9-1-1, even if the symptoms seem to lessen or disappear altogether.

Less common symptoms of stroke are loss of consciousness or reduced consciousness, including fainting, confusion, convulsions, or coma, and sudden nausea, fever, and vomiting coming on within seconds or minutes (Carolinas Medical Center Northeast, 2011; Centers for Disease Control and Prevention, 2013; Stanford School of Medicine, 2011; Women's Heart Foundation, 2007).

Hypertension

Hypertension or chronic high blood pressure is unique because it is a CVD itself, and a risk factor for CHD and stroke. When blood pressure is chronically elevated, the workload on the heart is greater, which may damage the heart's ability to pump blood effectively throughout the body and result in heart muscle damage (Heart and Stroke Foundation, 2012). High blood pressure may also damage the interior walls of the arteries, which facilitates atherosclerotic plaque accumulation (Heart and Stroke Foundation, 2012).

Sustained high blood pressure, or **hypertension**, that cannot be attributed to any specific cause is known as **essential hypertension**. Approximately 90 percent of all cases of high blood pressure fit this category. **Secondary hypertension** refers to high blood pressure caused by specific factors, such as kidney disease, obesity, or tumours of the adrenal glands.

Blood pressure is measured by two numbers, for example, 110/80 mm Hg, stated as "110 over 80 millimetres of mercury." The top number, **systolic blood pressure**, refers to the pressure of blood in the arteries when the heart muscle contracts, sending blood to the rest of the body. The bottom number, **diastolic blood pressure**, refers to the pressure of blood on the arteries when the heart muscle relaxes, as blood is reentering the heart chambers. Normal blood pressure varies depending on age, weight, and physical condition, and high blood pressure is usually diagnosed when systolic pressure is 140 or above (see Table 12.1). When only systolic pressure is high, the

---

Hypertension Chronic high blood pressure; 140/80 mmHg or greater.

Essential hypertension Hypertension as a result of unknown causes.

Secondary hypertension Hypertension as a result of another condition such as kidney disease, obesity, or tumours of the adrenal glands.

Systolic blood pressure The upper number in the blood pressure fraction, refers to the pressure on the walls of the arteries when the heart contracts.

Diastolic blood pressure The lower number in the blood pressure fraction, refers to pressure on the walls of the arteries during the relaxation phase of heart activity.

TABLE 12.1
Blood Pressure Classifications

Classification	Systolic Reading (mmHg)		Diastolic Reading (mmHg)
Normal	Less than 120	and	Less than 80
Prehypertension	120–139	or	80–89
Hypertension			
Stage 1	140–159	or	90–99
Stage 2	Greater than or equal to 160	or	Greater than or equal to 100
Hypertensive crisis	Greater than or equal to 180	or	Greater than or equal to 110

Source: The American Heart Association, "Understanding blood pressure readings," 2015, http://www.heart.org/HEARTORG/ Conditions/HighBloodPressure/HighBloodPressure/Understanding -Blood-Pressure-Readings_UCM_301764_Article.jsp.

condition is known as isolated systolic hypertension (ISH), the most common form of high blood pressure in older adults.

Systolic blood pressure tends to increase with age, whereas diastolic blood pressure typically increases until age 55 and then declines. Men under the age of 45 are at nearly twice the risk of becoming hypertensive as their female counterparts and have an increased risk of dying of vascular disease within 10 years of a stroke (Rutten-Jacobs et al., 2015). Women tend to have higher rates of hypertension after age 65 (Mozaffarian et al., 2015). More and more people (over 30 percent of the population) are considered to be **prehypertensive**, meaning that their blood pressure is above normal, but not yet in the hypertensive range. These individuals have a significantly greater risk of becoming hypertensive (Centers for Disease Control and Prevention, 2015).

New guidelines for the management/treatment of high blood pressure among those with a history of diabetes, heart disease, or stroke are available. In general, guidelines for treating and managing high blood pressure provide information about maintaining lower blood pressure levels, recommending certain types of medications, and optimal times to begin medicating. People 65 and over are usually put on meds when their blood pressure is 150 over 90 mmHg or higher; those under 60 years of age are recommended to take medications at 140 over 90 mmHg or higher, especially if they have kidney disease or diabetes. At current rates, more and more people will begin heart medications at a younger age (James et al., 2014; Rosendorf et al., 2015).

Arrhythmia, Congestive Heart Failure, and Congenital and Rheumatic Heart Disease

Arrhythmia refers to an irregular heartbeat. It may be suspected, for instance, when a person complains of a racing heart in the absence of physical activity or anxiety; *tachycardia* is the medical term for an abnormally fast heartbeat. On the other end of the continuum is *bradycardia*, or abnormally slow heartbeat. When a heart goes into **fibrillation**, it exhibits a sporadic, quivering pattern of beating resulting in extreme inefficiency in moving blood through the cardiovascular system. If untreated, this condition can be fatal. Not all arrhythmias are life-threatening. Excessive caffeine or nicotine consumption can trigger arrhythmia. For the most part, in the absence of other symptoms, arrhythmias are not serious. However, severe cases may require drug therapy or an external electrical stimulus to prevent further, more serious complications.

Congestive heart failure occurs when the heart muscle is damaged or overworked and lacks the strength to continue the blood circulating process. Individuals afflicted with rheumatic fever, pneumonia, or other cardiovascular problems in the past often have weakened heart muscles. In addition, the walls of the heart and the blood vessels can be damaged from previous radiation or chemotherapy treatments for cancer. These weakened muscles respond poorly when stressed; blood flow out of the heart is diminished, and the return flow of blood through the veins begins to back up, causing congestion in the tissues. This pooling of blood causes enlargement of the heart and decreases the amount of blood that can be circulated. Blood begins to accumulate in other body areas, such as in the vessels in the legs and ankles or the lungs, causing swelling or difficulty in breathing. If untreated, congestive heart failure results in death. Most cases respond well to diuretics (water pills) for relief of fluid accumulation, digitalis, a drug that increases the pumping action of the heart, and a vasodilator that expands blood vessels and decreases resistance, allowing blood to flow more easily, thus reducing the workload on the heart.

Approximately 1 percent of children are born with some form of **congenital heart disease**, when the heart or blood vessels near the heart do not develop normally before birth (Heart and Stroke Foundation, 2012). These diseases range from slight murmurs or reverses in blood flow within the heart, caused by valve irregularities,

prehypertensive Blood pressure is above normal, but not yet in the hypertensive range.

Arrhythmia An irregularity in heartbeat.

Fibrillation A sporadic, quivering pattern of heartbeat resulting in inefficient moving of the blood.

Congestive heart failure Occurs when the heart muscle is damaged or overworked and lacks the strength to maintain blood circulation.

Congenital heart disease Heart disease present at birth.

which some children outgrow, to serious complications in heart function that can only be corrected with surgery. The underlying causes of congenital heart diseases are unknown but believed to be related to hereditary factors; maternal diseases, such as German measles (rubella), occurring during fetal development; or drug or alcohol intake by the mother during pregnancy (Heart and Stroke Foundation, 2012). Due to advances in pediatric cardiology, the prognosis for children with congenital heart defects is better now than ever before with more than 90 percent of infants born with congenital heart disease living to adulthood (Heart and Stroke Foundation, 2012).

Rheumatic heart disease is attributed to rheumatic fever, an inflammatory disease caused by an unresolved streptococcal infection of the throat ("strep throat") that may affect many connective tissues of the body, especially those of the heart, the joints, the brain, or the skin. In a small number of cases, the streptococcal infection can lead to an immune response in which antibodies attack the heart as well as the bacteria.

CONTROLLING YOUR RISKS FOR CARDIOVASCULAR DISEASES

The four primary risk factors for CVD are high blood pressure (hypertension), high blood fats (hyperlipidemia), smoking, and physical inactivity. Secondary risk factors include stress, obesity, and diabetes. These primary and secondary risk factors are mostly under your control. There are other risk factors, such as age, sex, ethnicity, and hereditary factors, that you cannot control.

Knowledge of the factors that contribute to CVD and how to make lifestyle changes that reduce your risk may motivate you to make the necessary health-promoting lifestyle changes. Common lifestyle changes that can decrease your risk include:

- **quitting smoking**, or not starting,
- **reducing your blood pressure** through changes in your dietary intake (primarily through reducing intake of sodium) and by regular physical activity
- **reducing your cholesterol** through changes in your dietary intake (primarily reducing cholesterol and fat consumption) and by being more physically active
- **being physically active**, specifically including cardiorespiratory physical activities

Rheumatic heart disease A heart disease caused by unresolved streptococcal infection of the throat.

- **maintaining your ideal weight** through healthy eating and regular physical activity
- consuming alcohol in moderation
- taking low-dose aspirin
- treating hypertension with drugs

These risks have an elevated impact when combined. For example, if you have high blood pressure, high cholesterol, a family history of heart disease, and smoke cigarettes, you run a much greater risk of having a heart attack or other CVD than someone with only one risk. To assess your personal risks for heart disease, see the Assess Yourself questionnaire at the end of the chapter.

Risks You Can Control

High Blood Pressure

As mentioned previously, high blood pressure (hypertension) is a unique risk factor for CHD because it is also a CVD itself. It is considered the leading risk for stroke and a major factor for heart disease (Heart and Stroke Foundation, 2013). In general, the higher your blood pressure, the greater your risk for CHD. High blood pressure is known as the "silent killer," because it usually has no symptoms. The latest data available from Statistics Canada, from 2011, indicate that 17.6 percent of the population 12 years of age or older have been diagnosed with high blood pressure by a health professional (Statistics Canada, 2013). Overall, with all age groups combined, slightly more women than men have been diagnosed with high blood pressure: 17.7 versus 17.4 percent. Very few 12- to 19-year-olds (0.6 percent) or 20- to 34-year-olds (2.4 percent) have high blood pressure. In the 35- to 44-year-old age group, 7.3 percent have high blood pressure. Rates more than triple in the 45- to 64-year-old age group, with 23.6 percent having high blood pressure. In the older age groups, over the age of 65 years, 49.5 percent have been diagnosed with high blood pressure. After the age of 65, more females than males have high blood pressure (51.7 versus 46.9 percent). Individuals of African and South Asian descent are not only three times more likely to become hypertensive than the general population, but they are also more likely to develop the problem at younger ages (Heart and Stroke Foundation, 2008).

If your blood pressure exceeds 140 over 90, you should make lifestyle changes to lower it (engage in regular physical activity, eat healthily—including reducing your sodium intake—manage your stress, and attain a healthy body weight). Regular aerobic exercise normally lowers blood pressure by 5 to 15 mmHg (Scott, 2007). Controlling your sodium intake can also reduce your risk since it contributes to approximately 17 000 cases of stroke and heart disease in Canada each year (Heart and Stroke Foundation, 2008). Even though the average Canadian consumes more than 3100 mg of sodium per day, the adequate daily intake has been set at between 1200 and 1500 mg each day (Heart and Stroke Foundation, 2008). Since the majority of the sodium we consume comes from processed foods, reducing consumption of them assists in lowering your intake (see also Chapter 5). If these lifestyle changes do not reduce your blood pressure to more normal values, you may need to take medication. Similarly, if your blood pressure is high normal you should adjust your lifestyle in an attempt to lower your blood pressure to what is considered normal (less than 120 over less than 80 mmHg).

Blood Fat and Cholesterol Levels

Since your body actually produces all the cholesterol that it needs, anything you consume alters your blood levels. Cholesterol is only consumed from foods of animal origin. If your dietary intake is high in saturated fats, your LDL cholesterol levels will rise. This sends the body's blood-clotting system into high gear, increasing the viscosity of the blood in just a few hours, which in turn increases your risk for heart attack or stroke. A fatty diet also elevates the amount of cholesterol in the blood, contributing to atherosclerosis. Foods particularly high in saturated fat include coconut oil, palm kernel oil, butter, cream, whole milk, and fatty cuts of beef. Regular physical activity, reducing saturated and trans fat intake, and increasing monounsaturated fat and omega-3 fat intakes can benefit your blood lipid profile and reduce risk for heart disease (see Chapter 5 for more details). As shown in Table 12.2, healthy levels of total cholesterol are less than 5.2 millimoles per litre

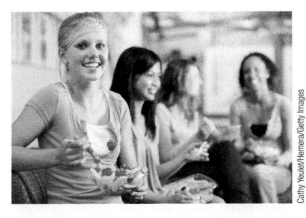

Controlling the amount and type of fat you eat is one thing you can do to lower your risk for heart disease.

TABLE 12.2

Healthy Values for Blood Cholesterol and Triglycerides

Type of Cholesterol	Healthy Concentration
Total cholesterol	6 to 19 yrs: < 4.5 mmol/L
	20 to 79 yrs: < 5.2 mmol/L
HDL* cholesterol	males: > 1.0 mmol/L
	females: > 1.3 mmol/L
LDL† cholesterol	< 3.5 mmol/L
Ratio of total cholesterol to HDL cholesterol	< 5.0
Triglycerides	< 1.7 mmol/L

*HDL = high density lipoproteins
†LDL = low density lipoproteins

Sources: Based on: Genest J, McPherson R, & Frohlich J. (2009). 2009 Canadian Cancer Society/Canadian Guidelines for the diagnosis and treatment of dyslipidemia and prevention of cardiovascular disease in the adult—2009 recommendations. *Canadian Journal of Cardiology.* 10:567–79.
Statistics Canada. (2010). Heart health and cholesterol levels of Canadians, 2007 to 2009, retrieved on June 14, 2013 from www .statcan.gc.ca/pub/82-625-x/2010001/article/11136-eng.htm.

(mmol/L) or 200 milligrams per decilitre (mg/dL) for individuals between 20 and 79 years of age (Genest, McPherson, & Frohlich, 2009). Values greater than 5.2 mmol/L (or 240 mg/dL) indicate an elevated risk for heart disease (Barrow, 1992). Values between 200 and 240 mg/dL are considered moderate risk.

Although risk values are established for total cholesterol, it is the individual components that you should be concerned about. **Low-density lipoproteins (LDLs)** are often referred to as "bad" cholesterol because they tend to build up or accumulate on artery walls. In contrast, **high-density lipoproteins (HDLs)**, or "good" cholesterol, remove cholesterol from artery walls, thus serving as a protector. In theory, if LDL levels get too high (see Table 12.2) or HDL levels too low (see Table 12.2)—largely because of too much saturated fat in the diet, lack of physical activity, high stress, or genetic predisposition—cholesterol will accumulate on the arterial walls and lead to CVD. The goal then is to manage the ratio of HDL to total cholesterol by lowering LDLs, raising HDLs, or both. Regular physical activity and a healthy dietary intake low in saturated and trans fat (see also Chapter 5 for more details) continue to be the best method for maintaining healthy levels of LDLs, HDLs, and total cholesterol.

Low-density lipoproteins (LDLs) A combination of protein, triglycerides, and cholesterol in the blood that accumulate on arterial walls.

High-density lipoproteins (HDLs) A combination of protein, triglycerides, and cholesterol in the blood that facilitate the transport of LDLs to the liver for metabolism and elimination from the body.

Triglycerides, the type of fat we normally consume, are also manufactured by our bodies. As people get older, fatter, or both, their triglyceride and cholesterol levels tend to rise. According to Statistics Canada (2010), a triglyceride level greater than or equal to 1.7 mmol/L increases risk for CVD.

Cigarette Smoking

The link between cigarette smoking and heart disease has been firmly established—smoking is considered responsible for more than half of all deaths due to CVD (Health Canada, 1997). Further, the risk for heart disease increases with the number of years smoked and the amount smoked per day—even with as few as five cigarettes smoked per day. Smokers who have a heart attack are four times more likely to die suddenly (within one hour) than nonsmokers. Evidence also indicates that chronic exposure to environmental tobacco smoke (passive smoking or secondhand smoke) also increases risk of heart disease (Canadian Institute of Health Information, 2003). If the effects of smoking are combined with other risk factors, the danger is greater than the sum of the added effects.

Cigarette smoking increases the risk of heart disease in several ways. First, the drug nicotine, a central nervous system stimulant, increases heart rate, heart output, blood pressure, and oxygen use by heart muscles. In other words, nicotine causes the heart to work harder with each cigarette smoked. Second, the carbon monoxide in cigarette smoke displaces oxygen in heart tissue, resulting in the heart being forced to work harder to get enough oxygen to the working tissues. Third, nicotine can lead to irregular heart rates (arrhythmias) that can result in sudden death. Fourth, cigarette smoke damages the lining of the arteries, allowing plaque to accumulate more easily. This additional accumulation constricts the vessels, increasing blood pressure and forcing the heart to work harder. In other words the negative effects of cigarette smoking occur at multiple levels and in many negative ways.

Physical Inactivity

Inactivity is another primary risk factor for CVD. The good news is that you do not have to be an exercise fanatic to reduce your risk for CVD. Even moderate levels of moderate-intensity physical activity are beneficial if done regularly and on a long-term basis. Such activities include walking for pleasure, gardening, housework, and dancing. See also Chapter 4 for other physical activity suggestions.

Engaging in physical activity on a regular basis reduces risk for heart disease in a number of

---

Triglycerides The most common form of fat in the body; consumed and manufactured in the body.

---

ways. Physical activity of a sufficient intensity (that is moderate intensity or greater) strengthens the heart, improves circulation, and improves your blood profile by increasing HDLs. Because of the increases in HDL, there is a reduced level of atherosclerotic plaque accumulation. Physical activity also plays an important role in reducing hypertension, maintaining body weight, and managing and preventing the stress response. In other words, physical activity may be one of the most important behaviours to engage in to reduce your risk for heart disease.

Obesity

Obesity also can increase risk for CVD. A body with excessive fat causes strain to the heart in its efforts to push blood through the many kilometres of capillaries that supply each kilogram of fat with needed nutrients. As such, people who are overweight or obese and sedentary are more likely to develop heart disease and stroke even if they have no other risk factors. Moreover, evidence indicates that where fat accumulates or is distributed on the body may affect a person's risk for CVD. Specifically, if excess fat accumulates around your upper body and waist (apple-shaped), you are at a greater risk than if your excess fat accumulates around your hips and thighs (pear-shaped). A waist girth greater than 102 centimetres for men and 88 centimetres for women significantly relates to elevated triglyceride levels, low HDL concentrations, and hypertension (Reeder et al., 1997).

Diabetes

Individuals with diabetes, particularly those who have taken insulin for a number of years (i.e., individuals with type 1 diabetes), have an increased risk for CVD. In fact, heart disease is the leading cause of death among individuals with diabetes. Because people who are obese have a higher risk for diabetes, distinguishing between the effects of the two conditions is difficult. Individuals with diabetes also tend to have elevated blood fat levels, increased atherosclerosis, and a tendency toward deterioration of small blood vessels, particularly in the eyes and extremities. Through a prescribed regimen of eating well, being physically active regularly, and taking medication (when necessary), individuals with diabetes can control much of their increased risk for heart disease.

Individual Response to Stress

Some people react to stress on a daily basis. These stress reactions occur because of or in reaction to normal, usual daily activities. These daily reactions may relate to higher levels of blood pressure in an unrested state (Health Canada, 1997). These people experience alarm and resistance so strongly that, when under stress, their bodies produce large amounts of stress chemicals, which in turn lead to tremendous strain for the cardiovascular system. These people are called "hot reactors." Although their blood pressure may be normal when they are not under stress—for example, in a doctor's office—it increases dramatically in response to even small amounts of everyday tension. "Cold reactors" are those who are able to experience stress without harmful cardiovascular responses. Cold reactors may internalize stress, but their self-talk and perceptions about the stressful events lead them to a nonresponse state in which their cardiovascular system remains virtually unaffected. Other research investigating the relationship of personality to heart disease suggests that personality plays a role in effective coping of the stress response. See Chapter 3 for tips on managing your stress response.

Risks You Cannot Control

There are some risk factors for CVD that you cannot prevent or control (Heart and Stroke Foundation, 2009). These include

- Heredity: Having a family history of heart disease increases your risk significantly.

- Age: Eighty percent of all fatal heart attacks occur in people over the age of 65. The risk for CVD increases with age for both sexes.

- Sex: Men are at a greater risk for CVD until older age. Women under 35 years of age generally have a fairly low risk for CVD. (For a more detailed discussion, see the next section.)

- Ethnicity: First Nations and Inuit people as well as individuals of African and South Asian descent are at greater risk for heart disease and stroke partly because they are more likely to have high blood pressure and diabetes.

WOMEN AND CARDIOVASCULAR DISEASE

Many more women die from heart disease and stroke than from breast cancer. Currently, two in three women have one or more of the major risk factors for heart disease (Heart and Stroke Foundation, 2009). While men have more heart attacks and have them earlier in life, women have a much lower chance of survival. Part of the reason, as previously mentioned, relates to the signs and symptoms of heart disease, which tend to be less apparent in women. Although we understand the mechanisms that cause heart disease in men and women, their experiences in the health-care system, their reactions to life-threatening diseases, and a host of other technological and environmental factors may play a role in their survival rates.

Risk Factors for Heart Disease in Women

Premenopausal women are unlikely to have a heart attack unless they also have diabetes, high blood pressure, kidney disease, or a genetic predisposition to high cholesterol levels. Family history, oral contraceptive use, and smoking also increase the risk for heart disease in premenopausal women. Once her estrogen production drops with menopause, a woman's chance of developing heart disease rises rapidly. In fact, a 60-year-old woman has the same heart attack risk as a 50-year-old man, and by her late 70s, a woman has the same heart attack risk as a man her age.

Cholesterol is another factor to consider in women's increased risk for heart disease as they age. Although women aged 25 and over tend to have lower cholesterol levels than men of the same age, when they reach 45 years things change. Most men's cholesterol levels become more stable, while LDL and total cholesterol levels in women rise, with the gap widening after the age of 55. It has been suggested for men that for every 1-percent drop in cholesterol, there is a 2-percent decrease in CVD risk. If this holds true for women, prevention efforts focusing on dietary interventions and physical activity may significantly help postmenopausal women reduce their risk for CVD.

When data from seven cycles of the National Population Health Survey were examined in a longitudinal research study, results indicated that women's risk of heart disease was significantly elevated if she also had depression—even after adjusting for other risk factors (for example, marital status, income, high blood pressure, diabetes, BMI, smoking, leisure-time physical activity, alcohol consumption, and use of hormone replacement therapy) (Gilmour, 2008). This same relationship was not found in men.

Recognizing Heart Disease in Women

Women often do not display the same recognizable symptoms of heart disease as men. The first sign of heart disease in men is generally a myocardial infarction. In women, the first sign is usually uncomplicated angina pectoris. Because chest discomfort rather than pain is the common manifestation of angina in women, and because angina has a much more favourable prognosis in women than in men, many physicians ignore the condition in their female patients or treat it too casually.

A heart attack also causes different symptoms in women than in men. In men, a heart attack usually manifests itself as crushing chest pain radiating to the shoulders, arms, neck, jaw, or back, as well as dizziness, paleness, difficulty breathing, sweating, nausea, vomiting, or anxiety (Heart and Stroke Foundation, 2009). In women, a heart attack results in much vaguer symptoms such as pain in the neck, jaw, or arms; heaviness in the shoulders, back, or the pit of the stomach; and feeling out of breath, tired, sweating, nausea, or vomiting (Heart and Stroke Foundation, 2009). If these symptoms are experienced for two minutes or longer, it is critical to seek help immediately (call 9-1-1) or get to the nearest hospital that offers emergency cardiac care.

Three reasons why signs of heart disease in women may be overlooked have been postulated: (1) physicians may be sex-biased in their delivery of health care, tending to concentrate on women's reproductive organs rather than on their whole body; (2) physicians tend to view heart disease in men as a more severe problem because they traditionally have a higher incidence of the disease; and (3) women decline major procedures more often than men. Other explanations for diagnostic and therapeutic difficulties encountered by women with heart disease include:

- Delay in diagnosing a possible heart attack, due to the complexity of interpreting chest pain in women because symptoms of heart attack are vague and much different than in men.

- Typically less aggressive treatment of women who have had a heart attack.

- Their older age, on average, and frequency of other health problems.

- Women's coronary arteries are often smaller than men's, making surgical or diagnostic procedures more difficult technically.

- Their increased incidence of post-infarction angina or heart failure (National Heart, Lung, & Blood Institute, 1995).

NEW WEAPONS AGAINST HEART DISEASE

The victim of a heart attack today has a variety of options not available a generation ago. Medications can strengthen heartbeat, control arrhythmias, remove fluids in cases of congestive heart failure, and relieve pain. Automated External Defibrillators (AEDs) exist in more public locations; there is even a legislation to support the installation of these devices. Further, bypass surgery and angioplasty have become relatively commonplace procedures in hospitals throughout the nation.

Techniques of Diagnosing Heart Disease

Several techniques can be used to diagnose heart disease, including electrocardiogram, angiography, and positron emission tomography scans. An **electrocardiogram** (ECG or EKG) is a record of the electrical activity of the heart measured during a stress test. Patients walk or run on treadmills while their hearts' functions are monitored. Another method of testing for heart disease is **angiography** (often referred to as "cardiac catheterization"), in which a needle-thin tube called a catheter is threaded through blocked heart arteries, a dye is injected, and an X-ray is taken to discover which areas are blocked. A more recent and even more effective method of measuring heart activity is **positron emission tomography**, also called a **PET scan**, which produces three-dimensional images of the heart as blood flows through it. During a PET scan, a patient receives an intravenous injection of a radioactive tracer. As the tracer decays, it emits positrons that are picked up by the scanner and transformed by a computer into colour images of the heart.

Other tests include the following:

- Radionuclide imaging (includes such tests as thallium test, multinucleated gated angiography scan, and acute infarct scintigraphy). In these procedures, substances called radionuclides are injected into the bloodstream. Computer-generated pictures can then show them in the heart. These tests can show how well the heart muscle is supplied with blood, how well the heart's chambers are functioning, and which part of the heart has been damaged.

Electrocardiogram A record of the electrical activity of the heart measured during a stress test.

Angiography A technique for examining blockages in heart arteries. A catheter is inserted into the arteries, a dye injected, and an X-ray taken to find the blocked areas.

Positron emission tomography (PET scan) Method for measuring heart activity by injecting a patient with a radioactive tracer scanned electronically to produce a three-dimensional image of the heart and arteries.

- Magnetic resonance imaging (MRI). This test uses powerful magnets to look inside the body. Computer-generated pictures can show the heart muscle, identify damage from a heart attack, diagnose certain congenital heart defects, and evaluate disease of larger blood vessels such as the aorta.

- Ultrafast computed tomography (CT). This is an especially fast form of X-ray of the heart designed to evaluate bypass grafts, diagnose ventricular function, and measure calcium deposits.

- Digital cardiac angiography. This modified form of computer-aided imaging records pictures of the heart and its blood vessels.

Angioplasty versus Bypass Surgery

During the 1980s, **coronary bypass surgery** seemed to be the ultimate technique for treating patients who had coronary blockages or suffered heart attacks. In coronary bypass surgery, a blood vessel taken from another site in the patient's body (usually the saphenous vein in the leg or the internal mammary artery) is implanted to transport blood by bypassing blocked arteries. The effectiveness of bypass operations, particularly for elderly people, has been questioned, particularly with less invasive treatment options now available.

A procedure called **angioplasty** (also called balloon angioplasty) has fewer risks and is believed by many to be more effective than bypass surgery in selected cardiovascular cases. This procedure is similar to angiography. A needle-thin catheter is threaded through blocked heart arteries. The catheter has a balloon at the tip, which is inflated to flatten fatty deposits against the artery walls, allowing blood to flow more freely. Angioplasty patients are generally awake but sedated during the procedure and spend only one or two days in the hospital after treatment. Most people can return to work within five days. Only about 1 percent of all angioplasty patients die during or soon after the procedure. Risks of this procedure include spontaneous collapse of the vessel worked on in 3 to 7 percent of cases, and in about 30 percent of all angioplasty operations, the treated arteries become clogged again within six months. Some patients may undergo the procedure as many as three times within a five-year period. Some surgeons argue that given angioplasty's high rate of recurrence, bypass may still be a more effective method of treatment.

Drug treatments may also be effective in prolonging life, but it is critical that doctors prescribe an aggressive drug treatment program and more important that patients comply. Among the most effective treatments are beta blockers and calcium channel blockers, used to reduce high blood pressure and treat other symptoms. Cholesterol-lowering medications are also effective.

Low-dose Aspirin (80 milligrams daily or every other day) is beneficial to heart patients because of its blood-thinning properties. It should be pointed out that higher doses do not provide additional protection. Aspirin is even recommended as a preventive strategy for individuals without current heart disease symptoms. However, given the additional risks from emergency surgery or accidental bleeding, ASA should not be taken, unless under the direction of a primary care practitioner.

Thrombolysis

Whenever a heart attack occurs, prompt action is the key factor in the patient's eventual prognosis. When a coronary artery gets blocked, the heart muscle does not die immediately, but time determines how much damage occurs. If a victim gets to an emergency room and is diagnosed fast enough (within two hours), a form of reperfusion therapy called **thrombolysis** can sometimes be performed. Thrombolysis involves injecting an agent such as tissue plasminogen activator (TPA) to dissolve the clot and restore some blood flow, thereby reducing the amount of tissue that dies from ischemia. These drugs must be used within one to three hours of a heart attack for best results, and once again, the importance of calling 9-1-1 when the symptoms of a heart attack are first noticed cannot be overemphasized.

CANCER INCIDENCE AND MORTALITY

Across Canada it is estimated that 196 900 (Figure 12.3) new cases of cancer will be diagnosed and 78 000 deaths from cancer will occur in 2015 (Canadian Cancer Society's Steering Committee on Cancer Statistics, 2015). In general, cancer rates increase with age and are more common in males than females. However, cancer incidence rates are slowly declining over time in males and slowly increasing in females. Over the course of their lifetime males have a greater chance (44.7 percent) then females (41.5 percent) of developing cancer. It is projected that males have a 29 percent lifetime probability (approximately a 1 in 3.5 chance) of dying from cancer and females have a 24 percent

Coronary bypass surgery A surgical technique in which one or more blood vessels are implanted to bypass one or more clogged coronary arteries.

Angioplasty A technique in which a catheter with a balloon at the tip is inserted into a clogged artery; the balloon is inflated to flatten fatty deposits against artery walls, allowing blood to flow more freely.

Thrombolysis Injection of an agent to dissolve clots and restore some blood flow, thereby reducing the amount of tissue that dies from ischemia.

FIGURE 12.3

Geographic Distribution of Estimated New Cancer Cases and Age-Standardized Incident Rates (ASIR) by Province and Territory, Both Sexes, Canada, 2015

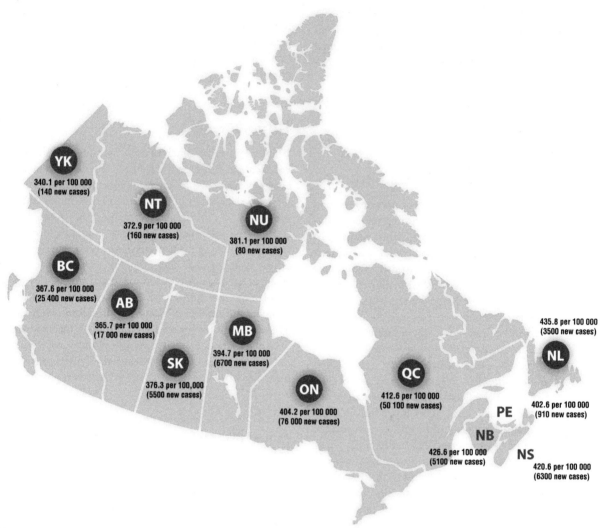

Source: Canadian Cancer Society's Steering Committee on Cancer Statistics. (2015). Canadian cancer statistics 2015. Toronto, ON: Canadian Cancer Society.

lifetime probability (approximately a 1 in 4.1 chance) of dying from cancer. The greater number of new cases of cancer is primarily due to an aging population with 89 percent of all cancers being diagnosed in Canadians over the age of 50, while 43 percent will occur in Canadians 70 years of age and older.

Among Canadians the leading cancers are prostate cancer for males (24 000 expected new cases annually) and breast cancer for females (25 000 expected new cases annually) (Figure 12.4) (Canadian Cancer Society's Steering Committee on Cancer Statistics, 2015). Lung, colorectal, breast, and prostate cancers account for approximately 50 percent of all cancer deaths combined in each sex. Lung cancer continues to be the leading cause of cancer death for both sexes.

Not everyone is equally at risk for all types of cancers. Cancer incidence and mortality vary greatly by age, sex, ethnicity, and socioeconomic status. Because cancer risk is strongly associated with lifestyle and behaviours, differences in ethnic and cultural groups can provide clues to factors involved in its development. Culturally influenced values and belief systems can also affect whether or not a person seeks care, participates in screenings, or follows recommended treatment options. For example, some cultures may only believe in naturalistic treatment options. In Canada, cancer incidence and mortality are highest in Atlantic Canada and Quebec and lowest in British Columbia (Canadian Cancer Society's Steering Committee on Cancer Statistics, 2015).

FIGURE 12.4

Percent Distribution of Estimated New Cancer Cases, by Sex, Canada, 2015

Males 100 500 New cases		Females 96 400 New cases	
Prostate	23.9%	Breast	25.9%
Colorectal	13.9%	Lung	13.5%
Lung	13.5%	Colorectal	11.5%
Bladder	6.1%	Body of uterus	6.5%
Non-Hodgkin lymphoma	4.5%	Thyroid	5.0%
Kidney	3.9%	Non-Hodgkin lymphoma	3.8%
Melanoma	3.6%	Melanoma	3.2%
Leukemia	3.5%	Ovary	2.9%
Oral	2.9%	Leukemia	2.8%
Pancreas	2.4%	Pancreas	2.5%
Stomach	2.1%	Kidney	2.4%
Brain/CNS	1.7%	Bladder	2.1%
Esophagus	1.7%	Cervix	1.5%
Liver	1.7%	Oral	1.5%
Multiple myeloma	1.5%	Brain/CNS	1.3%
Thyroid	1.4%	Stomach	1.3%
Testis	1.0%	Multiple myeloma	1.2%
Larynx	0.9%	Liver	0.6%
Hodgkin lymphoma	0.5%	Esophagus	0.5%
Breast	0.2%	Hodgkin lymphoma	0.5%
All other cancers	9.0%	Larynx	0.2%
		All other cancers	9.3%

CNS = central nervous system

Source: Canadian Cancer Society's Steering Committee on Cancer Statistics. (2015). Canadian cancer statistics 2015. Toronto, ON: Canadian Cancer Society. Retrieved from https://www.cancer.ca/~/media/cancer.ca/CW/cancer%20information/cancer%20101/Canadian%20cancer%20statistics/Canadian-Cancer-Statistics-2015-EN.pdf.

What Is Cancer?

Cancer is the name given to a large group of diseases characterized by the uncontrolled growth and spread of abnormal cells. It may be hard to understand how normal, healthy cells become cancerous, but if you think of a cell as a small computer, programmed to operate in a particular fashion, the process may become clearer. Under normal conditions, healthy cells are protected by the immune system as they perform their daily functions of growing, replicating, and repairing body organs. When something interrupts normal cell programming, uncontrolled growth and abnormal cellular development result in a new growth of tissue. This new tissue serves no physiological function and is called a **neoplasm**. When this neoplasmic mass forms a clump of cells it is known as a **tumour**.

Not all tumours are **malignant** (cancerous); in fact, most are **benign** (non-cancerous). Benign tumours are generally harmless unless they grow to obstruct or crowd out normal tissues or organs. A benign tumour of the brain, for instance, is life-threatening when it grows and causes blood restriction resulting in a stroke. The only way to determine whether a given tumour or mass is benign or malignant is through **biopsy**, or microscopic examination of cell development.

Benign and malignant tumours differ in several key ways. Benign tumours are generally composed of ordinary-looking cells enclosed in a fibrous shell or capsule that prevents their spreading to other body areas. Malignant tumours are usually not enclosed in a protective capsule and can therefore spread to other organs. This process, known

Cancer A large group of diseases characterized by the uncontrolled growth and spread of abnormal cells.

Neoplasm A new growth of tissue that serves no physiologic function, resulting from uncontrolled, abnormal cellular development.

Tumour A neoplasmic mass that grows more rapidly than surrounding tissues.

Malignant Very dangerous or harmful; refers to a cancerous tumour.

Benign Harmless; refers to a non-cancerous tumour.

Biopsy Microscopic examination of tissue to determine if a cancer is present.

FIGURE 12.5

Metastasis

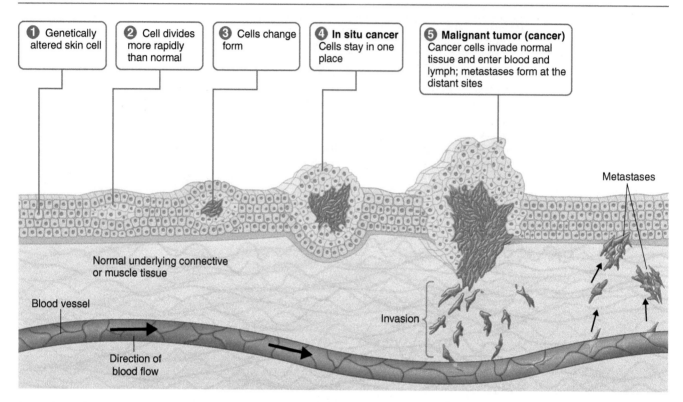

① Genetically altered skin cell

② Cell divides more rapidly than normal

③ Cells change form

④ In situ cancer Cells stay in one place

⑤ Malignant tumor (cancer) Cancer cells invade normal tissue and enter blood and lymph; metastases form at the distant sites

Metastases

Normal underlying connective or muscle tissue

Blood vessel

Invasion

Direction of blood flow

A mutation to the genetic material of a skin cell triggers abnormal cell division and changes cell formation, resulting in a cancerous tumour. If the tumour remains localized, it is considered in situ cancer. If the tumour spreads, it is considered a metastatic cancer.

as **metastasis**, makes some forms of cancer particularly aggressive in their ability to overcome bodily defences. (See Figure 12.5.) By the time they are diagnosed, malignant tumours have frequently metastasized throughout the body, reducing the likelihood that the cancer will be successfully treated. Unlike benign tumours, which merely expand to take over a given space, malignant cells invade surrounding tissue, emitting clawlike protrusions that disrupt chemical processes within healthy cells. More specifically, malignant cells disturb the ribonucleic acid (RNA) and deoxyribonucleic acid (DNA) within the normal cells. Tampering with these substances that control cellular metabolism and reproduction produces mutant cells that differ in form, quality, and function from normal cells.

What Causes Cancer?

After decades of research, most cancer epidemiologists believe that the majority of cancers are preventable and can be avoided by healthier choices in lifestyle and environment (Peto, 2001). In fact, the "Policy and Action for Cancer

Metastasis Process by which cancer spreads from one area to different areas of the body.

Prevention—Food, Nutrition, and Physical Activity: A Global Perspective," by the World Cancer Research Fund in conjunction with the American Institute for Cancer Research, clearly stated that two-thirds of all cancers could be prevented based on lifestyle changes (World Cancer Research Fund/American Institute for Cancer Research [WCRF-AICR], 2009). One-third could be prevented by not using tobacco and another one-third could be prevented by being physically active and eating well. Many specific causes of cancer are well documented; the most prevalent are smoking, obesity, and a few organic viruses. Most research supports the idea that cancer is caused by external (chemicals, radiation, viruses, and lifestyle) and internal (hormones, immune conditions, and inherited mutations) factors. These causal factors may act together or in sequence to promote cancer development. We do not know why some people have malignant cells in their body and never develop cancer, while others take 10 years or more to develop the disease and still others seem to rapidly develop and die from cancer. Many factors are believed to cause cancer, and a combination of these factors can dramatically increase one's risk of the disease.

One theory proposes that cancer results from spontaneous errors during cell reproduction. Perhaps cells that are overworked or aged are more likely to break down, causing genetic errors that result in mutant cells. Another theory suggests that cancer is caused by some external agent or agents that enter a normal cell and initiate the cancerous process. Numerous environmental factors, such as radiation, chemicals, hormonal drugs, immunosuppressant drugs (drugs that suppress the normal activity of the immune system), and other toxins are considered possible **carcinogens** (cancer-causing agents); perhaps the most common carcinogen is the tar found in cigarettes. The greater the dose or exposure to environmental hazards, the greater your risk. Thus, when you are forced to work, live, and pass through areas that have high levels of environmental toxins, you may also be at greater risk of cancer.

A third theory came out of research on certain viruses believed to cause tumours in animals. This research led to the discovery of **oncogenes**, suspected cancer-causing genes present on chromosomes. Although oncogenes are typically dormant, scientists theorize that certain conditions, such as age, stress, and exposure to carcinogens, viruses, and radiation may activate these oncogenes. Once activated, they begin to grow and reproduce in an out-of-control manner. Scientists are uncertain whether only people who develop cancer have oncogenes or whether we all have **proto-oncogenes**, genes that can become oncogenes under certain conditions. Many **oncologists** (physicians who specialize in the treatment of malignancies) believe that the oncogene theory may lead to a greater understanding of how individual cells function and bring us closer to developing an effective treatment for cancer.

Risks for Cancer

Lifestyle

Anyone can develop cancer; however, most cases affect adults beginning in middle age. In fact, nearly 80 percent of cancers are diagnosed at age 55 and over. Cancer researchers refer to one's cancer risk when they assess risk factors. *Lifetime risk* (absolute risk) refers to the probability that an individual, over the course of a lifetime, will develop cancer or die from it. As noted previously, 45 percent of men and 40 percent of women have a lifetime risk of developing cancer.

Relative risk is a measure of the strength of the relationship between risk factors and a particular cancer. Basically, relative risk compares your risk if you engage in certain known risk behaviours with that of someone who does not engage in the same behaviours. For example, if you smoke, you have a 20-fold relative risk of developing lung cancer compared to a nonsmoker. In other words, the chances of getting lung cancer are about 20 times greater in a smoker than in a nonsmoker (American Cancer Society, 2005).

Over the years, researchers have found that certain behaviours result in a higher incidence of cancer. In particular, smoking, a dietary intake high in total calories, fat, sodium, preservatives, and so on, engaging in little or no physical activity, living a predominantly sedentary lifestyle, being obese, consumption of alcohol, stress, and other lifestyle factors seem to play a role. Further confirming this theory is that colon and rectal cancer occur more frequently among persons with a high-fat, low-fibre dietary intake, in those who do not eat enough vegetables and fruits, and in those who are physically inactive.

Keep in mind that a high relative risk does not imply cause and effect, and has a direct relationship to absolute risk. It merely indicates the likelihood of a particular risk factor being related to a particular outcome. In other words, you can modify your lifestyle behaviours and reduce your risk.

Smoking

Of all the potential risk factors for cancer, smoking is among the greatest; it is the leading cause of preventable death in the world today. In developing countries, smoking is responsible for 80 to 90 percent of all deaths from lung cancer (World Health Organization, 2008). In Canada, tobacco is responsible for nearly one in five deaths annually. Recent declines in smoking, such that now fewer than one in five Canadians over the age of 12 years reported smoking occasionally or on a daily basis (Statistics Canada, 2012), have likely had a direct effect on the overall decrease in lung cancer rates. Still, lung cancer remains the leading cause of cancer death in men and women.

Researchers once believed that cigarettes caused only cancers of the lung, pancreas, bladder, and kidney, and (synergistically with alcohol) the larynx, mouth, pharynx, and esophagus. However, recent evidence indicates that several other types of cancer are also related to tobacco use. Most notably, cancers of the stomach, liver, and cervix are directly related to long-term smoking.

Obesity

It is difficult to sort through the volumes of evidence about the role of nutrients, obesity, sedentary lifestyle, low levels of physical activity, and related variables in the development of cancer. That said, cancer is more common among people who are obese, and risk increases as level of obesity increases. A study of

Carcinogens Cancer-causing agents.

Oncogenes Suspected cancer-causing genes present on chromosomes.

Proto-oncogenes Genes that can become oncogenes under certain conditions.

Oncologists Physicians who specialize in the treatment of malignancies.

more than 900 000 adults indicates a significant relationship between a high body mass index (BMI) and death rates for cancers such as those of the esophagus, colon, rectum, liver, kidney, and pancreas (Calle et al., 2003). Women with a high BMI have a higher mortality rate from breast, uterine, cervical, and ovarian cancers; men with a high BMI have higher death rates from prostate and stomach cancers. In this study, 34 percent of all cancer deaths were attributable to overweight and obesity. Other findings relevant to the obesity–cancer link are as follows:

- The relative risk of breast cancer in postmenopausal women is 50 percent higher for women who are obese.

- The relative risk of colon cancer in men is 40 percent higher for men who are obese.

- The relative risks of gallbladder and endometrial cancer are five times higher in individuals who are obese compared to those at a healthy weight.

Biologic Factors

Some early cancer theorists believed that we inherit a genetic predisposition toward certain forms of cancer (Knudson, 1986; Krontirus, 1983). Cancers of the breast, stomach, colon, prostate, uterus, ovaries, and lungs appear to have a heredity link. Specifically, a woman has a much higher risk of developing breast cancer if her mother, sisters, or daughters (i.e., primary relatives) had the disease, particularly if they had it at a young age. Hodgkin's disease and certain leukemias also show familial patterns. Whether these familial patterns are attributable to genetic susceptibility or to the fact that people in the same families experience similar environmental risks remains uncertain.

Sex also affects the likelihood of developing certain forms of cancer. For example, breast cancer occurs primarily among females, although men occasionally get breast cancer. Just over 25 percent of all cancer diagnoses among women are attributed to breast cancer; conversely, 0.2 percent of cancer diagnoses among men are attributed to breast cancer (Canadian Cancer Statistics, 2015). Obviously, factors other than heredity and familial relationships affect which sex develops a particular cancer. In the 1950s and 1960s, for example, women rarely contracted lung cancer. But with increases in the number of women who smoked and the length of time they smoked, lung cancer became a leading cause of cancer deaths for Canadian women in the 1980s. Although sex plays a role in certain cases, other variables, such as lifestyle, may be more significant in other cases.

Occupation and Environment Factors

Various occupational hazards are known to cause cancer when exposure levels are high or exposure is prolonged. Overall, however, workplace hazards account for only a small percentage of all cancers. One of the most common occupational carcinogens is asbestos, a fibrous substance once widely used in the construction, insulation, and automobile industries. Nickel, chromate, and chemicals such as benzene, arsenic, and vinyl chloride have been shown to be carcinogens for humans. Also, people who routinely work with certain dyes and radioactive substances may have increased risks for cancer. Working with coal tars, as in the mining profession, or working near inhalants, as in the auto-painting business, is also hazardous. Those who work with herbicides and pesticides also appear to be at higher risk, although the evidence is inconclusive to date for low-dose exposures.

Because people are sometimes forced to work near hazardous substances, it is imperative that worksites enact policies and procedures designed to minimize or eliminate toxic exposure.

Ionizing radiation—radiation from X-rays, radon, cosmic rays, and ultraviolet radiation (primarily UV-B radiation)—is the only form of radiation linked to cancer. (See the section on skin cancer.)

While reports about cancer-case clusters in communities around nuclear power facilities have raised public concerns, studies show that clusters do not occur more often near nuclear power plants than they do by chance in wider geographical areas (Canadian Nuclear Safety Commission, 2013).

Social and Psychological Factors

Although orthodox medical personnel are skeptical of overly simplistic prevention centres that focus on humour and laughter as the way to prevent cancer, we cannot rule out the possibility that negative emotional states contribute to disease development. People who are lonely, depressed, and lack social support are more susceptible to cancer than their mentally and emotionally healthy counterparts (see also Chapter 2). Similarly, people under chronic stress and those with poor nutrition or sleep habits develop cancer at a slightly higher rate than the general population. Experts believe that severe depression or prolonged stress may reduce the activity of the body's immune system, thereby wearing down bodily resistance to cancer.

Chemicals in Foods

Among the food additives suspected of causing cancer is sodium nitrate, a chemical used to preserve and give colour to red meat. Research indicates that the actual carcinogen is not sodium nitrate but nitrosamines, substances formed when the body digests sodium nitrates. Sodium nitrate has not been banned, primarily because it kills the bacterium *Clostridium botulinum,* which is

point of view

GO GREEN AGAINST CANCER

You may think it is someone else's responsibility to ensure the environment is free from carcinogens. Although there may be merit in that thinking, it is prudent for YOU to make more decisions that are 'environmentally friendly' not only for your personal health, but also for the health of future generations, including your children and grandchildren. In fact, there are many things you can do to help reduce the number of carcinogens in the environment and to limit your exposure to those that are there. The following are just a few ideas:

1. Leave your car at home. Use your bicycle, your feet, or some other way (skateboard, inline skates, scooter, and so on) instead of driving. This will reduce your daily carbon emissions and your risk for cancer by increasing your level of physical activity. If you cannot use active transportation all the way, use it for part of your trip. When you drive, park as soon as you are in the parking lot rather than circling for the closest spot to the entrance.

2. Choose organic foods when possible. Conventional produce is often sprayed with chemicals and pesticides. When you eat these chemicals, your risk for cancer can be elevated. Further, the spraying of chemicals contributes to air and water pollution (see Chapter 14).

3. When shopping for home furnishings, explore ecofriendly furniture, upholstery, and home textiles. Many furnishings are manufactured with toxic chemicals that are released into the air. Purchasing this kind of furniture can reduce indoor air quality and increase your risk for cancer. Select products that have not been treated with stain-resistant chemicals and look for ecofriendly flooring, carpets, and other products. Such ecofriendly products include bamboo, recycled glass or metal tiles, cork, and flooring made from reclaimed wood products.

4. Use "green" paper. By purchasing ecofriendly paper products that are bleach free, we reduce the amount of dioxins released into the atmosphere. Dioxins are carcinogenic, and fewer of them in the atmosphere will reduce everyone's risk for cancer. Consider your use of paper: reduce your consumption—think twice before printing, reuse what you can, and recycle everything possible.

5. Buy ecofriendly personal hygiene products. When purchasing personal hygiene products or cosmetics, select items that are environmentally responsible. Consider avoiding products containing the following chemicals, all of which are suspected or confirmed carcinogens:
   - diethanolamine (DEA)
   - formaldehyde (commonly found in eye shadows)
   - phthalates
   - parabens

6. Avoid dry cleaning when possible. Conventional dry cleaning uses a chemical called perchloroethylene (PERC), an agent known to increase the risk for cancer and harm the environment. If dry cleaning is unavoidable, explore dry cleaners using ecofriendly alternatives such as "wet cleaning," which includes biodegradable soaps or silicone-based solvents and special machinery used to reduce shrinkage.

---

the cause of the highly virulent food-borne disease botulism. It should also be noted that the bacteria found in the human intestinal tract may contain more nitrates than a person could ever take in when eating cured meats or other nitrate-containing food products. Nonetheless, concern about the carcinogenic properties of nitrates has led to the introduction of meats that are nitrate-free or contain reduced nitrates.

There is also concern about the possible harm caused by pesticide and herbicide residues. While some of these chemicals cause cancer at high doses in experimental animals, the very low concentrations found in some foods are well within government-established safety levels. Continued research regarding pesticide and herbicide use is essential for maximum food safety and the continuous monitoring of agricultural practices is necessary to ensure a safe food supply. It is important to find a balance between chemical use and the production of quality food products. Policies protecting consumer health and ensuring continued improvement in food production through development of alternative, low-chemical pest and herbicide control and reduced environmental pollution should be the goal of prevention efforts.

Infectious Diseases

Estimates hold that 16.1 percent of new cancers worldwide are attributable to infections (World Health

Organization, 2012). Infections are thought to influence cancer development in several ways, most commonly through chronic inflammation, suppression of the immune system, or chronic stimulation.

HBV, HCV, and Liver Cancer

Viruses such as hepatitis B (HBV) and C (HCV) are believed to stimulate cancer cells in the liver because they are chronic diseases that cause inflammation of liver tissue. This may prime the liver for cancer or make it more hospitable for cancer development. Global increases in HBV and HCV rates and concurrent increases in liver cancer rates provide evidence of such an association.

HPV and Cervical Cancer

Nearly 100 percent of women with cervical cancer have evidence of human papilloma virus (HPV) infection, believed to be a major cause of cervical and oropharyngeal cancer. HPV is a group of more than 100 different types of viruses, 40 of which are transmitted through sexual activity (Canadian Cancer Society, 2013a). In fact, it is estimated that at least 75 percent of sexually active men and women in Canada will have at least one HPV infection in their lifetime. HPV types 16 and 18 are responsible for 70 percent of all cervical cancers, while HPV types 6 and 11 are responsible for 90 percent of genital warts (Canadian Cancer Society, 2013a). A vaccine that protects against these HPV types is available for young and older women (up to age 40) and young men in Canada and should be viewed as a complement to cervical cancer screening (that is, the Pap test), not a replacement (see Chapter 9 for more details).

Medical Factors

Some medical treatments increase a person's risk for cancer. One example is the use of estrogen replacement therapy for postmenopausal women because of the potential increased risk of uterine cancer. Ironically, chemotherapy, which is used to treat cancer, may also increase risk for other forms of cancer.

TYPES OF CANCER

As noted previously, the term *cancer* refers to hundreds of different diseases. Four broad classifications are made according to the type of tissue from which the cancer arises.

- **Carcinomas**—Epithelial tissues (tissues covering body surfaces and lining most body cavities) are the most common sites for cancers. Carcinoma of the breast, lung, intestines, skin, and mouth are examples. These cancers affect the outer layer of the skin and mouth as well as the mucous membranes. They metastasize through the circulatory or lymphatic system initially and form solid tumours.

- **Sarcomas**—Sarcomas occur in the mesodermal, or middle, layers of tissue—for example, in bones, muscles, and general connective tissue. They metastasize primarily via the blood in the early stages. These cancers are less common but generally more virulent than carcinomas. They also form solid tumours.

- **Lymphomas**—Lymphomas develop in the lymphatic system—the infection-fighting regions of the body—and metastasize through the lymph system. Hodgkin's disease is one type of lymphoma. Lymphomas also form solid tumours.

- **Leukemia**—Cancer of the blood-forming parts of the body, particularly the bone marrow and spleen, is called leukemia. A non-solid tumour, leukemia is characterized by an abnormal increase in the number of white blood cells.

The seriousness and general prognosis of a particular cancer are determined through careful diagnosis by trained oncologists. Once laboratory results and clinical observations have been made, cancers are rated by level and stage of development. Those diagnosed as "carcinoma in situ" are localized and are often curable. Cancers given higher level or stage ratings have spread farther and are less likely to be cured.

Lung Cancer

Symptoms of lung cancer include a persistent cough, blood-streaked sputum, chest pain, and recurrent attacks of pneumonia or bronchitis. Treatment depends on the type and stage of the cancer. Surgery, radiation therapy, and chemotherapy are treatment options. If the cancer is localized, surgery is usually the treatment of choice. If the cancer has spread, surgery is used in combination with radiation and chemotherapy. Despite advances in medical technology, survival rates for lung cancer have improved only slightly in recent years. Just 17 percent of people with lung cancer live five or more years after diagnosis (Canadian Cancer Society's Steering Committee on Cancer Statistics, 2015).

Prevention

People who smoke cigarettes, especially those who smoked for more than 20 years, and people exposed to certain industrial substances such as arsenic and asbestos or to radiation from occupational, medical, or environmental sources, are at the highest risk for lung cancer (Center for Disease Control and Prevention, 2013). Exposure to secondhand cigarette smoke increases the risk for nonsmokers. Some researchers have theorized that as many as 90 percent of all lung cancers could be prevented if people did not smoke. Quitting smoking—or not starting—are the best measures you can take to prevent lung cancer. Any time is a good time to quit smoking, with health improvements noted almost immediately (see Chapter 10 for more details).

Breast Cancer

About one in nine women will develop breast cancer at some time in their lives and 1 in 27 will die as a result of it (National Cancer Institute of Canada, n.d.). Although this oft-repeated ratio has frightened many women, it represents a woman's lifetime risk. Thus, not until the age of 80 does a woman's risk of breast cancer rise to one in nine. Risks at earlier ages include:

- Age 50: 1 in 50
- Age 60: 1 in 24
- Age 70: 1 in 14

Breast cancer incidence among women has risen steadily over the past three decades—although the rate of increase is declining somewhat—whereas mortality rates for breast cancer have declined slightly since 1986 and particularly since 1990. This pattern of divergent trends is consistent with benefits achieved through screening programs and improved treatments (National Cancer Institute of Canada, n.d.).

Breast cancer can and does occur in men too. About 1 percent of all estimated breast cancer cases will occur in men (National Cancer Institute of Canada, n.d.). Men and women share the same risk factors for breast cancer and the same warning signs (Brinton et al., 2003). Potential signs of breast cancer include persistent breast changes such as a lump, thickening, swelling, dimpling, skin irritation, distortion, retraction or scaliness of the nipple, nipple discharge, pain, or tenderness. Risk factors for breast cancer vary considerably, as identified by the Public Health Agency of Canada, 2012:

- Age—80 percent of the cases of breast cancer occur in women over 50 years of age.
- Family history of breast cancer, especially in a mother, sister, or daughter diagnosed before menopause, or if a mutation on the BRCA1 or BRCA2 genes is present.
- Previous breast disorders with biopsies showing abnormal cells.

- No full-term pregnancies or having a full-term first pregnancy after age 30.
- High-density breast tissue.
- In post-menopausal women: obesity and physical inactivity.
- Beginning to menstruate at an early age.
- Later than average menopause.
- Taking hormone replacement therapy (estrogen plus progestin) for more than five years.
- Alcohol, as well as the use of oral contraceptives, may be associated with a slight increase in breast cancer risk.
- The effects of smoking and never breastfeeding are currently under study.

Although risk factors are useful tools, they do not always adequately predict individual susceptibility. Due to increased awareness, better diagnostic techniques, and improved treatments, individuals with breast cancer have a better chance of surviving today. A key factor in survival rests with individual recognition of early symptoms (Brinton et al., 2003).

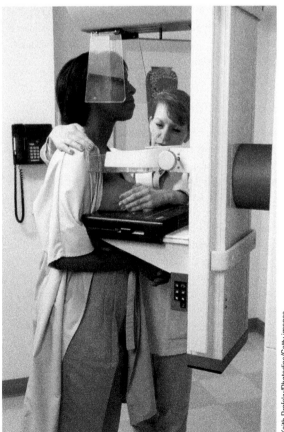

Mammography and other early detection techniques greatly increase a woman's chance of surviving breast cancer.

Prevention

Engaging in a regularly physically active lifestyle is related to a reduction in the risk for breast cancers. In one study of more than 1000 women aged 40 or younger (545 with breast cancer, 545 without), physical activity patterns were examined. The women who averaged four hours of physical activity per week since menstruating had a 58 percent lower risk. Researchers speculated that physical activity may protect women by altering the production of the ovarian hormones estrogen and progesterone during menstrual cycles (Bernstein et al., 1994).

Mammography offers the best hope for early detection of breast cancer. Although breast cancer screening with mammography and clinical breast exam could reduce mortality by nearly one-third in most women aged 50 to 69 years if they were regularly screened, only 34 percent participate in organized screening in Canada (Canadian Cancer Society/National Cancer Institute of Canada, 2006). All women, regardless of age, should become familiar with their breasts, how they feel, and what is normal for them. Despite the controversy over the cost-effectiveness and usefulness of a mammogram before the age of 40, many health professionals recommend that if you have any of the risk factors listed previously, are prone to fibrous breasts, and are worried about your condition, a mammogram may be warranted. Moreover, screening for women over the age of 50 is provincially funded. Consult with your physician if you are in doubt, as it is generally best to be a proactive health consumer.

Know Your Breasts

Early detection involves knowing and understanding what your breasts should look and feel like even if you are having regular screening tests. Many women and men discover their own breast cancer through changes in the look and feel of their breasts.

Breast tissue covers an area larger than just the breast. It extends up to the collarbone and from the armpit across to the breastbone in the centre of the chest. The breasts sit on the chest muscles that cover the ribs.

According to the Canadian Cancer Society (2008a), you should become familiar with your breast tissue by looking at and feeling your breasts (see Figure 12.6). In the past, experts suggested that this should be done by following a particular method every month. This is now no longer considered necessary. There is not a right or wrong way to check your breasts, as long as you get to know all of your breast tissue—up to your collarbone, under your armpits and including your nipples—well enough to notice changes.

It may be normal for your breasts to be lumpy or tender before your period (Canadian Cancer Society, 2008a). Breast tissue changes with age, too. Understanding what

FIGURE 12.6

Know Your Breasts

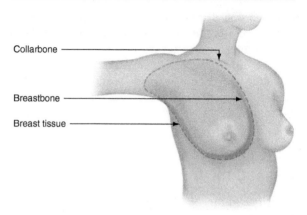

Collarbone

Breastbone

Breast tissue

Your breast tissue extends up to your collarbone and under your armpits, as well as your breast itself.

is normal for you will help you recognize changes and know what to report to your doctor.

What to Look For

Remember, lumps in the breast are very common, especially in women just before your period (Canadian Cancer Society, 2008a). Most lumps are not breast cancer. Most often breast cancer is first noticed as a painless lump in your breast or armpit. You or your partner may discover the lump, or your doctor may find it during a routine physical exam or screening mammogram.

Other signs might include:

- lump or swelling in the armpit
- changes in breast size or shape
- dimpling or puckering of the skin—thickening and dimpling skin is sometimes called orange peel
- redness, swelling, and increased warmth in the affected breast
- inverted nipple—nipple turns inwards
- crusting or scaling on the nipple

Often, these symptoms are not caused by cancer (Canadian Cancer Society, 2008a). Other health problems can cause them. Testing, via mammography, is necessary to make a diagnosis.

Treatment

Today, people with breast cancer (similar to any other type of cancer) have many treatment options. Fortunately, there are services available to help you get the best information, even if you live in a fairly remote area of the country. Often, cancer support groups can give you invaluable information and advice. Treatments range from the simple lumpectomy to radical mastectomy to various combinations of radiation or chemotherapy. Remember that it is always a good idea to seek more than one opinion before making a decision.

Colorectal Cancers

Although colorectal cancers are the second leading cause of cancer deaths in men and women, many people are unaware of potential risk factors and warning signs associated with colorectal cancers. Bleeding from the rectum, blood in the stool, and changes in bowel habits are the major warning signals. People over the age of 40, with a family history of colorectal cancer, a personal or family history of polyps (benign growths) in the colon or rectum, or inflammatory bowel problems such as colitis have an increased risk of being diagnosed with colorectal cancer. Canadian and international researchers have discovered four new genes related to colorectal cancer (Canadian Cancer Society, 2008b). This adds to the previous six already identified, and together these genes indicate an up to six-fold increase in lifetime risk of developing colorectal cancer. Further, a dietary intake high in fats or low in fibre may also increase risk (Canadian Cancer Society, 2013b).

Because colorectal cancer tends to spread slowly, the prognosis is quite good if it is caught in the early stages. As such, it is a common procedure in most provinces to screen for it in individuals over the age of 50 years using a technique called a colonoscopy. Treatment often consists of radiation or surgery. Chemotherapy, although not used extensively in the past, is a possibility today. A permanent colostomy, the creation of an abdominal opening for the elimination of body wastes, is seldom required for people with colorectal cancer (Canadian Cancer Society, 2013b).

Prostate Cancer

Cancer of the prostate continues to be the most frequently occurring cancer for men. It is the third leading cause of cancer deaths in males. In 2015, it is estimated that 24 000 Canadian men will be diagnosed with prostate cancer and about 4100 will die of the disease (Canadian Cancer Society's Steering Committee on Cancer Statistics, 2015). Beginning in 1994, the incidence of prostate cancer began to decline after increasing rapidly for several years. It was noted in 2008 that mortality rates due to prostate cancer continued to decline (Canadian Cancer Society's Steering Committee on Cancer Statistics, 2015).

Most signs and symptoms of prostate cancer are nonspecific—that is, they mimic the signs of infection

or enlarged prostate. Symptoms include weak or interrupted urine flow or difficulty starting or stopping the urine flow; the need to urinate frequently; pain or difficulty in urinating; blood in the urine; and pain in the lower back, pelvis, or upper thighs. Many males mistake these symptoms for other nonspecific conditions, such as infections, and delay treatment.

Fortunately, even with so many generalized symptoms, most prostate cancers are detected while they are still localized and have not progressed. Men with prostate cancer have an average five-year survival rate of 95 percent (Canadian Cancer Society's Steering Committee on Cancer Statistics, 2012). Prostate cancer is most frequently diagnosed in men between the ages of 60 and 69 years with deaths occurring most frequently in those over the age of 80 years (Canadian Cancer Society's Steering Committee on Cancer Statistics, 2012).

Skin Cancer

Skin cancer may be one of the most underrated of all cancers, particularly among young people. Although it is true that most people do not die of the common, highly curable basal or squamous cell skin cancers, many people do not know that another, highly virulent, form of skin cancer known as **malignant melanoma** has become a major killer. Estimates for 2015 indicated that 6800 Canadians will be diagnosed with melanoma (3700 men, 3100 women), with 1150 deaths expected (Canadian Cancer Society's Steering Committee on Cancer Statistics, 2015). Yet many people do not protect themselves from the sun whether on a beach tanning, on a golf course golfing, enjoying lunch outside, or doing other activities outdoors. Many often look for the 'glow' that is believed to come from a tan, and yet the perception that health and a well-tanned body go together could not be farther from the truth.

Symptoms

Many people do not have any idea what to look for when considering skin cancer. See the photographs included in this chapter for examples. Any unusual skin condition, especially a change in the size or colour of a mole or other darkly pigmented growth or spot, should be considered suspect. Scaliness, oozing, bleeding, the appearance of a bump or nodule, the spread of pigment beyond the border, change in sensation, itchiness, tenderness, and pain are all warning signs of the basal and squamous cell skin cancers. However, melanoma symptoms are slightly different. Often there is a sudden or progressive

Malignant melanoma A virulent cancer of the melanin (pigment-producing portion) of the skin.

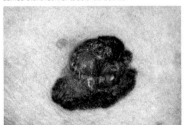 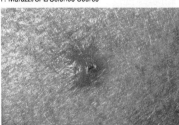 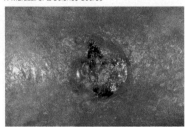

Prevention of skin cancer includes keeping a careful watch for any new pigmented growths and for changes to any moles. Melanoma symptoms, as shown in the left photo, include scalloped edges, asymmetrical shapes, discolouration, and an increase in size. Basal cell carcinoma and squamous cell carcinoma (middle and right photos) should be brought to your physician's attention but are not as deadly as melanoma.

change in a mole's appearance from a small, mole-like growth to a large, ulcerated, and easily-prone-to-bleeding growth. A simple ABCDE rule outlines the warning signals of melanoma:

- **A** is for *asymmetry*. One half of the mole does not match the other half.
- **B** is for *border irregularity*. The edges are ragged, notched, or blurred.
- **C** is for *colour*. The pigmentation is not uniform.
- **D** is for *diameter* greater than 6 millimetres.
- **E** is for *evolving*. The skin condition evolves/changes over time.

Any one of these symptoms should cause you to visit a physician.

Testicular Cancer

Testicular cancer is currently one of the most common types found in young adult men. Men between the ages of 17 and 34 years are at greatest risk. There has been a steady increase in diagnoses over the past several years in this age group. It was estimated that 1050 new cases of testicular cancer would be found in 2015 (Canadian Cancer Society's Steering Committee on Cancer Statistics, 2015).

FIGURE 12.7

Testicular Self-Exam

Follow the instructions in the diagram carefully and examine your testes immediately after your next hot bath or shower. Heat causes the testicles to descend and the scrotal skin to relax, making it easier to find unusual lumps.

Examine each testicle by placing the index and middle fingers of both hands on the underside of the testicle and the thumbs on the top. Gently roll the testicle between your thumb and fingers, feeling for small lumps.

Changes or anything abnormal will appear at the front or side of your testicle. Did you find any unusual lumps? Are there any unusual signs of any kind? Are there any markings or lumps at any site?

Keep in mind that not all lumps are a sign of testicular cancer. Unusual lumps at any location, however, should be checked by a physician. Early detection greatly increases your chances of a complete cure. Repeat the examination every month and record your findings.

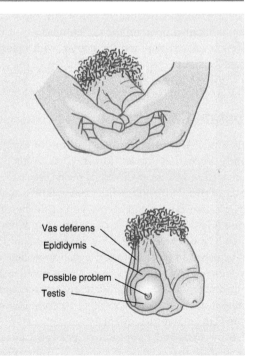

Although the exact cause of testicular cancer is unknown, several possible risk factors have been identified. Men with undescended testicles appear to be at greatest risk. In addition, some studies indicate that there may be a genetic influence. In general, testicular tumours are first noticed as a painless enlargement of the testis or as an apparent thickening in testicular tissue. Because this enlargement is often painless, it is extremely important that all men, particularly those between the ages of 17 and 34 years, practise regular testicular self-examination (see Figure 12.7). If a suspicious lump or thickening is found, medical follow-up should be sought immediately.

Ovarian Cancer

It was expected that 2800 new cases of ovarian cancer would be diagnosed in 2015, with 1750 women succumbing to the disease (Canadian Cancer Society's Steering Committee on Cancer Statistics, 2015). Ovarian cancer is often silent, showing no obvious signs or symptoms until late in its development. The most common sign is enlargement of the abdomen (or a feeling of bloating) in women over the age of 40 years. Other symptoms include vague digestive disturbances, such as gas and stomach aches, that persist without explanation (American Cancer Society, 1994).

The risk for ovarian cancer increases with age, with the highest rates found in women in their 60s. Women who never had children are twice as likely to develop ovarian cancer as those who have. The main risk factor appears to be exposure to the reproductive hormone estrogen. Women who have multiple pregnancies or use oral contraceptives, which inhibit estrogen, are at lower risk. In addition, having one or more primary relatives (mother, sisters, grandmothers) who had the disease increases individual risk. With the exception of Japan, the highest incidence rates are reported in industrialized countries (Canadian Cancer Society, 2013c).

Prevention

One study indicated that dietary intake may play a role in ovarian cancer (Risch et al., 1994). Researchers found that when comparing 450 Canadian women newly diagnosed with ovarian cancer with 564 demographically similar, healthy women, the women without ovarian cancer had a dietary intake lower in saturated fat. A recent systematic review also found that women consuming animal and dairy fat had an increased risk for ovarian cancer (Crane et al., 2014). Such results, particularly when combined with cardiovascular risks and other health risks, may provide yet another reason to reduce your overall intake of saturated fats.

The best way to protect yourself from ovarian cancer is with annual, thorough pelvic examinations. **Pap tests**, part of a pelvic exam, although useful in detecting cervical cancer, do not reveal ovarian cancer. Women over the age of 40 should have a cancer-related checkup every 3 years. If you have any of the symptoms of ovarian cancer and they persist, see your doctor.

Uterine Cancer

Most cervical and endometrial (that is, uterine) cancers develop in the body of the uterus, usually in the endometrium (lining). In 2015, 6300 new cases of cancer were expected to be diagnosed in the body of the uterus, leading to 1050 deaths (Canadian Cancer Society's Steering Committee on Cancer Statistics, 2015). The rest of uterine cancers develop in the cervix, located at the base of the uterus. The overall incidence of early-stage uterine cancer—that is, cervical cancer—has decreased at least 50 percent since 1977, but 1500 new cases were still estimated to be diagnosed in 2015 (Canadian Cancer Society's Steering Committee on Cancer Statistics, 2015). Further, invasive, later-stage forms of the disease appear to be decreasing, and mortality rates from cervical cancer have declined by at least 60 percent since 1977 with 380 deaths projected for 2015 (Canadian Cancer Society's Steering Committee on Cancer Statistics, 2015). Much of this apparent trend may be due to more effective regular screenings of younger women using the Pap test, a procedure in which cells taken from the cervical region are examined for abnormal cellular activity. Although these tests are very effective for detecting early-stage cervical cancer, they are less effective for detecting cancers of the uterine lining and not at all effective for detecting cancers of the fallopian tubes or ovaries (American Cancer Society, 1994).

Risk factors for cervical cancer include early age of first vaginal intercourse, multiple sex partners, cigarette smoking, use of oral contraceptives for 10 or more years, and sexually transmitted infections such as the herpes virus and HPV (the cause of genital warts) (Canadian Cancer Society, 2012). Risk factors for endometrial cancer include hormone factors, estrogen therapy, oral contraceptive use, total number of menstrual cycles (age), pregnancy, obesity, use of tamoxifen, ovarian tumours, polycystic ovarian syndrome, IUD use, poor diet and exercise choices, diabetes, family history, and history of breast or ovarian cancer (American Cancer Society, 2013). Early warning signs of uterine cancer include bleeding outside the normal menstrual period or after menopause; heavy menstrual

Pap test A procedure in which cells taken from the cervical region are examined for abnormal cellular activity.

bleeding during menopause; bleeding during vaginal intercourse; persistent unusual vaginal discharge that is foul smelling, pus-like, and blood-tinged; and pelvic pain or pressure (American Cancer Society, 2013).

Leukemia

Leukemia is a cancer of the blood-forming tissues that starts in the blood stem cells in the bone marrow, which leads to proliferation of millions of immature white blood cells (Canadian Cancer Society, 2013d). These abnormal cells crowd out normal white blood cells (which fight infection), platelets (which control hemorrhaging), and red blood cells (which prevent anemia). The signs and symptoms of leukemia are many, including fatigue, malaise, loss of appetite, paleness, weight loss, fever, anemia, shortness of breath, palpitations, weakness, dizziness, easy and widespread bruising, repeated and frequent infections, frequent or severe nosebleeds, bleeding gums, vomiting, headache, sore throat, night sweats, bone or joint pain, enlarged lymph nodes, abdominal discomfort, vision problems, sores in the eyes, and swollen testicles (Canadian Cancer Society, 2013d). In children, these symptoms can appear suddenly.

Leukemia can be acute or chronic in nature and can strike both sexes and all age groups. Chronic leukemia can develop over several months and have few symptoms. Although many people believe that leukemia is a childhood disease, leukemia strikes more adults than children (Canadian Cancer Society's Steering Committee on Cancer Statistics, 2012). Estimates for 2015 were that 6200 new cases of leukemia would be diagnosed (3500 in men, 2700 in women) (Canadian Cancer Society's Steering Committee on Cancer Statistics, 2015). Further, 2700 deaths were expected in 2015 from leukemia even though the survival rate of patients with acute lymphocytic leukemia has been increasing since the 1970s.

Oral Cancer

Cancer may develop in any part of the oral cavity. Most often it is found on the lips, the lining of the cheeks, the gums, and the floor of the mouth. The tongue, the pharynx, and the tonsils are other common sites. Recent estimates (from 2015) were that there would be 4400 new cases (2900 in men, 1450 in women) of oral cancer diagnosed in Canada with 1200 deaths forecasted (Canadian Cancer Society's Steering Committee on Cancer

Magnetic resonance imaging (MRI) A device that uses magnetic fields, radio waves, and computers to generate an image of internal tissues of the body for diagnostic purposes without the use of radiation.

Computerized axial tomography (CAT scan) A machine that uses radiation to view internal organs not normally visible on X-rays.

Statistics, 2015). Tobacco use—smoking, chewing, or dipping—is the most common risk factor for oral cancer.

FACING CANCER

As previously mentioned, 44 percent of men and 41 percent of women are likely to develop cancer in their lifetime, with at least one in four Canadians dying as a result. Many factors have contributed to the rise in cancer mortality—one being simply longer life expectancies—but the increase in the incidence of lung cancer is probably the most important reason. Recent advances in diagnosis and treatment have reduced much of the fear and mystery that surround cancer. Further, research continues with various studies, including a large, population-based prospective study in Alberta, called The Tomorrow Project (Alberta Cancer Foundation, 2013).

Detecting Cancer

The earlier a person is diagnosed with cancer, the better his or her prospect for survival. Various high-tech diagnostic techniques exist to detect cancer. New high-technology diagnostic imaging techniques have replaced exploratory surgery for some cancer patients. **Magnetic resonance imaging (MRI)** is one example of such technology. In MRI, a huge electromagnet is used to detect hidden tumours by mapping the vibrations of the various atoms in the body on a computer screen. **Computerized axial tomography scanning (CAT scan)** uses X-rays to examine parts of the body. In both of these painless, noninvasive procedures, cross-section pictures can show a tumour's shape and location more accurately than conventional X-rays.

These medical techniques, along with regular self-examinations and checkups, play an important role in the early detection and secondary prevention of cancer. Familiarize yourself with the Seven Warning Signals of cancer, as shown in Figure 12.8. If you notice any of these signs, and they do not appear to be related to anything else, you should see a doctor immediately. Make sure that appropriate diagnostic tests are completed whenever any warning signs appear. Also make a realistic assessment of your individual risk factors and try to avoid those you have control over.

New Hope in Cancer Treatments

Although cancer treatments have changed dramatically over the last 25 to 30 years, surgery, in which

FIGURE 12.8

Cancer's Seven Warning Signs

Cancer's Seven Warning Signals

1 Changes in bowel or bladder habits.

2 A sore that does not heal.

3 Unusual bleeding or discharge.

4 Thickening or lump in breast or elsewhere.

5 Indigestion or difficulty in swallowing.

6 Obvious change in a wart or mole.

7 Nagging cough or hoarseness.

If you have a warning signal, see your doctor.

the tumour and surrounding tissue are removed, is still most common. Today's surgeons tend to remove less surrounding tissue than previously and to combine surgery with either **radiotherapy** (the use of radiation) or **chemotherapy** (the use of drugs) to kill cancerous cells.

Radiation works by destroying malignant cells or stopping cell growth. It is most effective in treating localized cancer masses. In the process of destroying malignant cells, radiotherapy also destroys healthy cells.

When cancer has spread throughout the body, it is necessary to use some form of chemotherapy. Similar to radiation therapy, chemotherapy attacks and kills cancerous and healthy cells. Ongoing research will result in new, less toxic drugs more effective at attacking cancerous cells only.

Whether used alone or in combination, radiotherapy and chemotherapy have possible side effects, including extreme nausea, nutritional deficiencies, hair loss, and general fatigue. Long-term damage to the cardiovascular system and many other systems of the body can be significant. It is important that you discuss these matters fully with your doctor.

Psychosocial and behavioural research has become increasingly important as health professionals seek answers to questions concerning complex lifestyle factors that appear to influence risks for cancer, as well as the survivability of patients with particular psychological and mental health profiles. Also, health-care practitioners have become more aware of the psychological needs of patients and families and have begun to tailor treatment programs to meet the diverse needs of different people. In particular, individuals with cancer indicate higher levels of satisfaction and obtain better health outcomes when they are able to discuss their experience with health professionals (Bender et al., 2008). Research by Bender et al. (2008) indicates that women with breast cancer have many questions about the pain they will experience as a result of their treatment and of the cancer itself. Thus, it would be helpful for patients to be linked with support groups and fellow survivors so they can share and learn from each other's experiences.

Life after Cancer

Heightened public awareness and an improved prognosis for people with cancer has made the cancer experience less threatening and isolating than it once was. Assistance for individuals with cancer is more readily available than ever before. Cancer support groups, cancer information workshops, and medical consultation are just a few of the forms of assistance now offered in many communities. Increasing efforts in cancer research, improvements in diagnostic equipment, and advances in treatment provide hope for the future.

Radiotherapy The use of radiation to kill cancerous cells.

Chemotherapy The use of drugs to kill cancerous cells.

assess YOURSELF

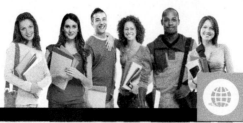

Go to MasteringHealth to complete this questionnaire with automatic scoring.

TAKING CHARGE: Managing Your Risk for Chronic Diseases

Although you may find it easy to read through a chapter like this and learn what you should be doing to keep yourself healthy, you are not really likely to think about what it takes to prevent serious illness like cancer or heart disease—partly because you are not likely to think it could happen to you. Relationships, financial worries, grades, time for fun, and other issues often take precedence over your long-term commitments to wellness.

You, similar to your classmates, have a unique level of risk for various diseases. Some of these risks you can take action to change, while others are risks that you need to manage as best you can as you plan a lifelong strategy for overall risk reduction. Complete the following questionnaire to gauge your risk and your understanding of the risks you may uniquely possess.

Understanding Your Risk for CVD

Respond to each of the following, then total your points in each section. The higher your score, the greater your risk. If you answer "don't know" for any question, talk to your parents or other family members as soon as possible to find out if you have any of these risks.

Part I: Assess Your Family Risk for CVD

1. Do any of your primary relatives (mother, father, grandparents, siblings) have a history of heart disease or stroke?

    Yes ___ (1 point) No___ (0 points) Don't Know ___

2. Do any of your primary relatives (mother, father, grandparents, siblings) have diabetes?

    Yes ___ (1 point) No___ (0 points) Don't Know ___

3. Do any of your primary relatives (mother, father, grandparents, siblings) have high blood pressure?

    Yes ___ (1 point) No___ (0 points) Don't Know ___

4. Do any of your primary relatives (mother, father, grandparents, siblings) have a history of high cholesterol?

    Yes ___ (1 point) No___ (0 points) Don't Know ___

5. Would you say that your family consumed a high-fat diet (lots of red meat, dairy, butter/margarine) during your time spent at home?

    Yes ___ (1 point) No___ (0 points) Don't Know ___

    Total ___

Part II: Assess Your Lifestyle Risk for CVD

1. Is your total cholesterol level higher than it should be?

    Yes ___ (1 point) No___ (0 points) Don't Know ___

2. Do you have high blood pressure?

    Yes ___ (1 point) No___ (0 points) Don't Know ___

3. Have you been diagnosed as prediabetic or diabetic?

    Yes ___ (1 point) No___ (0 points) Don't Know ___

4. Do you smoke?

    Yes ___ (1 point) No___ (0 points) Don't Know ___

5. Would you describe your life as being highly stressful?

    Yes ___ (1 point) No___ (0 points) Don't Know ___

    Total ___

Part III: Assess Your Additional Risks for CVD

1. How would you best describe your current weight?

    a. Lower than what it should be for my height and weight (0 points)

    a. About what it should be for my height and weight (1 point)

    c. Higher than it should be for my height and weight (1 point)

2. How would you describe the level of physical activity that you get each day?

    a. Less than what I should be doing each day (1 point)

b. About what I should be doing each day (0 points)

c. More than what I should be doing each day (0 points)

3. How would you describe your dietary intake?

   a. Eating only the recommended number of calories per day (0 points)

   b. Eating less than the recommended number of calories per day (0 points)

   c. Eating more than the recommended number of calories per day (1 point)

4. Which of the following best describes your typical dietary intake?

   a. I eat from the major food groups, trying hard to get the recommended amount of vegetables and fruits. (0 points)

   b. I eat too much red meat and consume too much saturated fat from meats and dairy products each day. (1 point)

   c. Whenever possible, I try to substitute olive oil or canola oil for other forms of dietary fat. (0 points)

5. Which of the following best describes you?

   a. I watch my sodium intake and try to reduce stress in my life. (0 points)

   b. I have a history of Chlamydia infection. (1 point)

   c. I try to eat 5 to 10 milligrams of soluble fibre each day and to substitute a soy product for an animal product in my diet at least once each week. (0 points)

Total ___

Source: Powers scott. k; Dodd stephen l; Noland; Virginia j., Total fitness and Wellness, 4th Ed., © 2006, pp. 277-278. Reprinted and Electronically reproduced by permission of Pearson Education, Inc., Upper saddle River, New Jersey.

Making Decisions for You, Right Now

List the five things that matter to you most right now. Is appearance part of your list? Is being able to get through a day without feeling tired or unusually fatigued important? Are you motivated to change your health behaviours and take action to reduce your risk for heart disease and cancer by engaging in more physical activity, reducing stress, and eating well? Was there anything about this chapter that made you think you should make a change now? Why is this important? What actions do you plan to take?

The following suggestions are things you might do to learn about your risks and make changes to reduce them:

- Determine your hereditary risks. If they are high, outline the steps that you can take to reduce your overall risk, focusing on lifestyle and the factors you can control.

- Learn about the normal CVD risk changes that occur with age. Take the steps needed to minimize these risks. Recognize that managing these risks will help you to feel better in your day-to-day life.

- If you smoke, quit. It will be easier to quit now than in five or ten years.

- If you do not smoke, do not start.

- Avoid secondhand smoke as much as possible.

- If you chew, dip, or use snuff, quit.

- Find out your cholesterol levels, including HDL and LDL levels.

- Reduce saturated and trans fat in your diet and take steps to reduce your triglyceride and cholesterol levels.

- Get out and do some physical activity. Every day. Even a relaxing walk every day is effective at reducing risk. Nobody says you have to run until you drop. Take it easy, but keep it up.

- Control your blood pressure. Monitor it regularly and see your doctor if you have high blood pressure.

- Manage your weight. You will feel better and be able to move more efficiently and effectively when you manage your weight. Obesity is a significant risk factor for CVD, diabetes, and cancer.

- Manage your stress.

- Avoid excessive sunlight particularly during the peak sunlight hours. When in the sun, wear sunscreen that contains at least SPF 15.

- Do not use tanning beds.

- Avoid excessive alcohol consumption.

- Monitor estrogen use—in the form of oral contraceptives or hormone replacement therapy, for instance—carefully.

- Avoid occupational exposures to carcinogens. Exposure to several different industrial agents (nickel, chromate, asbestos, vinyl chloride, and so on) increases risk for various cancers.

- Eat your vegetables and fruits. Eat at least seven or eight servings of fruits and vegetables every day to reduce your risk for lung, colon, pancreatic, stomach, bladder, esophageal, mouth, and throat cancer.

- Be happy; take care of your spiritual self.

(continued)

Critical Thinking

You have been good friends with one of your 30-something neighbours for some time. Recently, after spending a good deal of time working on a community project together, you start to date. After a few terrific dates, during which you really hit it off socially, you find out that your friend had cancer two years ago, and that there is a 50-percent chance it will return within five years. You really enjoy spending time with this person and may in fact be in love with him/her, but wonder what to do. What if you commit yourself to this relationship and the cancer returns? You want to have children, but are concerned about what would happen if your partner died of cancer while your children are young. On the other hand, there is a 50-percent chance that the cancer will not return.

Using the DECIDE model described in Chapter 1, decide whether or not you would continue the relationship. Does it make any difference to you whether the person who survived cancer is male or female? Explain why or why not.

DISCUSSION QUESTIONS

1. List the different types of cardiovascular diseases. Compare and contrast their symptoms, risk factors, prevention, and treatment.
2. Discuss why age is such an important factor in women's risk for CVD. What can be done to lower women's risks in later life?
3. Describe the role of healthy eating in preventing CVD.
4. Describe the unique role of physical activity in preventing and treating CVD.
5. What is cancer? What is the difference between a benign and a malignant tumour?
6. Describe the general risks for developing cancer. Which of these factors relate to you? What can you do to reduce this risk?
7. Why are breast and testicular self-exams important?
8. What symptoms signal that you have cancer instead of a minor illness? How soon should you seek treatment for any of the seven warning signs?

APPLICATION EXERCISE

Reread the "Consider This ... " scenario at the beginning of the chapter and answer the following questions.

1. Consider Kassandra's case in the chapter opener. Why do you think so many young Canadians deny their risk for skin cancer?
2. As a friend of Kassandra's, what advice might you give her?
3. Think about close friends or people in your family who also are at risk for developing skin cancer or any other form of cancer. What could you do to help them become aware of their risks without preaching to them about their lifestyle choices and turning them off?
4. What kinds of community efforts are needed to change the perceptions that a "healthy glow" results from suntanning?

MASTERINGHEALTH

Go to MasteringHealth for assignments, the eText, and the study Area with case studies, self-quizzing, and videos.

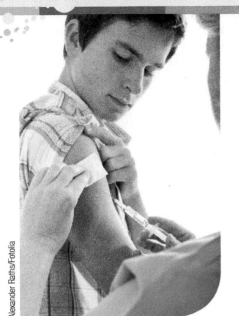

Alexander Raths/Fotolia

CHAPTER 13

CONTROLLING RISK FOR INFECTIOUS AND NONINFECTIOUS CONDITIONS

◄●) CONSIDER THIS . . .

Chandra and Michael have been seeing each other for a year. Their relationship is sexually active. Both had been sexually active prior to this relationship. Chandra is concerned and goes to the Health Unit for a sexual health checkup. She learns she has a sexually transmitted infection (STI). She can tell Michael herself, the Health Unit staff can arrange a confidential meeting and tell Michael for her, or she can ask her family doctor to talk with Michael. She is afraid of Michael's reaction and does not know if she is the carrier or became infected by Michael.

What do you think Chandra should do? What would you do? Why is Chandra worried about Michael's reaction? Is that a normal response? Why or why not? How would you react if your partner told you he or she had an STI?

LEARNING OUTCOMES

- Identify the risk factors for infectious diseases, including those you can and cannot control.

- Explain how the immune system works, as well as the role of vaccinations in fighting disease.

- Discuss the various sexually transmitted infections, including HIV, their means of transmission, and actions that prevent their spread.

- Identify common chronic diseases, including neurological disorders, sex disorders, diseases of the digestive system, and the varied musculoskeletal diseases.

Every moment of every day you are in contact with microscopic organisms that have the ability to make you sick. These disease-causing agents, or **pathogens**, are found in the air you breathe, in the foods you eat, and on nearly every person or object that you come into contact with. Most deaths from infectious diseases—almost 90 percent—are caused by only a handful of diseases. And most of these diseases have plagued humankind throughout history, often ravaging populations more effectively than wars (World Health Organization, 1999). There is fossil evidence that infections, cancer, heart disease, and a host of other ailments afflicted the earliest human beings. At times, infectious diseases wiped out whole groups of people through **epidemics** such as the Black Death or bubonic plague, which killed up to one-third of the population of Europe in the 1300s. A pandemic, or global epidemic, of influenza killed more than 20 million people in 1918, while strains of tuberculosis and cholera continue to cause premature death throughout the world.

In spite of our best efforts to eradicate them, these diseases continue to be a challenge around the world. The news is not all bad; even though we are bombarded by potential pathogenic threats, our immune systems are remarkably adept at protecting us. Endogenous microorganisms are those that live in peaceful coexistence with their human host most of the time. For people in good health, and whose immune systems are functioning well, endogenous organisms are usually harmless; however, in those with a compromised immune system or currently ill, these normally harmless pathogenic organisms can cause serious health problems.

Exogenous microorganisms are organisms that do not normally inhabit the body. When they do, they are apt to produce an infection or illness. The more easily these pathogens gain a foothold in the body and sustain themselves, the more **virulent** or aggressive the organism, the higher the probability that it will overcome your body defences and cause disease. However, if your immune system is strong and your internal capacity to ward off disease is substantial, you should be able to fight even the most virulent attacker. Just because you come in contact with a cold or flu virus does not mean that you will get sick. Just because your hands are teeming with bacteria does not mean that you will get a bacterial infection. Several factors influence your susceptibility to these diseases.

Infectious diseases in Canada are controlled through ongoing vigilance by public health networks operating at local, regional, provincial, and national levels. Clean food and water, immunizations, and an excellent health-care system have maintained Canadians' health. Eating well and engaging in regular physical activity are also factors in overall good health that help us as individuals combat infectious diseases. Nutritional status has been found to have an effect on resistance to infectious diseases in some population groups including infants, young children, and the elderly. Nutritional status can also affect the course of an infectious disease, as has been shown with individuals who are HIV-positive (Fields-Gardner & Campa, 2010). Regular physical activity of moderate or greater intensity boosts the efficacy of the immune system functioning (as noted in Chapter 4). Passive immunity is a natural occurring type of immunity that can also protect against the contraction of infectious diseases. This form of immunity occurs when a mothers' antibodies are transferred to the fetus through the placenta. It can also be induced artificially when high levels of antibodies specific are transferred to non-immune persons through blood.

INFECTIOUS DISEASE RISK FACTORS

While at one time it was believed that most diseases were caused by a single factor, it is now recognized that most diseases are **multifactorial**, or caused by the interaction of several factors from inside and outside the person (Figure 13.1). For a disease to occur,

Pathogen A disease-causing agent.

Epidemic Disease outbreak that affects many people in a community or region at the same time.

Virulent Strong enough to overcome host resistance and cause disease.

Multifactorial disease Disease caused by interactions of several factors.

FIGURE 13.1

Epidemiological Triad of Disease

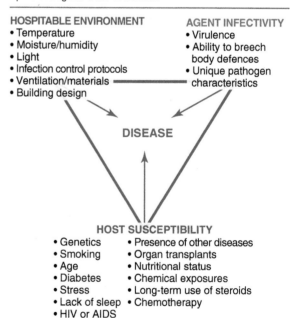

For a disease to occur, the agent, host, and environment must be conducive to overcoming the body's elaborate defence systems.

the host must be susceptible, which means that his or her immune system must be in a weakened or compromised condition; an agent capable of transmitting a disease must be present; and the environment must be hospitable to the pathogen in terms of temperature, light, moisture, and other requirements. Other factors also increase or decrease levels of susceptibility.

Risk Factors You Cannot Control

Uncontrollable risk factors (also known as nonmodifiable risk factors) are those factors that you may have little or no control over and increase your susceptibility to a disease. Some of the most common uncontrollable risk factors are discussed below.

Heredity

Perhaps the single greatest factor influencing your longevity is your parents' longevity. Being born into a family in which heart disease, cancer, or other illnesses are prevalent increases your risk. Some people with a close relative who has diabetes develop diabetes themselves even though they do what they can to reduce their risk by managing their weight, engaging in regular physical activity, and eating a diet that follows the guidelines identified in Eating Well with Canada's Food Guide. Some diseases are a result of chromosomal inheritance. **Sickle cell anemia**, an inherited blood disease that primarily affects individuals of African descent, is often transmitted to the fetus when both parents carry the sickle cell trait. It remains unclear whether hereditary diseases are a result of chromosomal abnormalities or deficiencies in immune system functioning.

Aging

After the age of 40, we become more vulnerable to chronic diseases. Similarly, as we age, our immune systems respond less efficiently to invading organisms, increasing our risk for infection and illness. The same flu that produces an afternoon of nausea and diarrhea in a younger person may cause days of illness or even death in an older person. The very young, as well as those with a compromised immune system, are also at risk for many diseases, particularly if not vaccinated against them.

Environmental Conditions

Unsanitary conditions and the presence of drugs, chemicals, and hazardous pollutants and wastes in our food and water have a significant effect on our immune systems. The weakening of **immunological competence**—the body's ability to defend itself against pathogens—in such situations has been well documented (Shulman, Phair, & Sommers, 1992).

Risk Factors You Can Control

You have some control over many risk factors for disease. Too much stress, an inadequate dietary intake, low levels of physical activity, high levels of sedentary behaviour, lack of sleep, misuse or abuse of legal and illegal drugs, poor personal hygiene, high-risk behaviours, and other variables significantly increase your risk for a number of diseases. Factors you can control—at least partly—through lifestyle choices include vigour of immune response; pre-existing level of immunity; pre-existing disease; use of substances such as cigarettes, chew, dip, alcohol, and drugs; and psychological factors such as stress, depression, and anxiety (Nelson, Williams, & Graham, 2001).

THE PATHOGENS: ROUTES OF INVASION

Pathogens enter the body in several ways. They may be transmitted by direct contact between infected persons, such as during sexual activity, kissing, or touching, or by indirect contact, such as by touching an object an infected person has contacted. Your hands are probably the greatest source of transmission. You can also **autoinoculate** yourself, or transmit a pathogen from one part of your body to another. For example, you might touch a sore on your lip teeming with viral herpes and then transmit the virus to your eye when you scratch your itchy eyelid.

Pathogens are also transmitted by airborne contact, either through inhaling the droplet spray from a sneeze or through breathing air that carries a particular pathogen. You may become the victim of foodborne infection if you eat something contaminated by microorganisms. The *E. coli* bacteria and other virulent pathogens are responsible for a variety of diseases that pose significant threats to humans. Examples of these are found in Table 13.1.

Your "best friend" may be the source of animal-borne pathogens. Dogs—as well as cats, livestock, and wild animals—can spread numerous diseases through their bites, feces, or by carrying infected insects into your living areas. For example, ticks in some regions carry Lyme disease. Water-borne diseases are transmitted directly from drinking water and indirectly from foods washed or sprayed with water containing their pathogens. These pathogens can also invade your body if

Sickle cell anemia Genetic disease resulting from chromosomal abnormalities commonly found among individuals of African descent.

Immunological competence Ability of the immune system to defend the body from pathogens.

Autoinoculation Transmission of a pathogen from one part of your body to another.

TABLE 13.1

Emerging Diseases: Challenges to Public Health

Over the past few decades, more than 30 diseases have been identified in humans. More than two-thirds of these diseases are known to have originated from animals—both wild and domestic species.

Disease/Cause Agent	Description
Avian influenza [Type A (H5N1)]	Previously thought to infect only birds (to whom it can be deadly), avian influenza first jumped to humans in 1997 in Hong Kong. Initial symptoms include fever, cough, and chills; most influenza infections cause only self-limited illness that does not require hospitalization. Symptoms after infection with the H5N1 strain can be severe in all age groups.
Ebola virus	A deadly disease concentrated in portions of Africa, Ebola can be transferred only by direct contact with infected blood, organs, secretions, semen, or contaminated needles. Transmission is enhanced by unsanitary, overcrowded conditions and poor preventive practices. No treatment or vaccine is available and 50 to 90 percent of those contracting the disease die.
Dengue fever	More than 200 000 cases of dengue fever occurred in Latin America alone during 1994, of which 5000 were dengue hemorrhagic fever (DHF), a severe form of the disease that causes high mortality. The type of mosquito that carries the disease is establishing new habitats in the Americas and parts of Africa and Asia. Over the past 40 or so years, the number of cases has increased at least 20-fold.
E. coli bacteria	Illness caused by the *Escherichia coli* bacteria as a result of eating unwashed or poorly washed vegetables and undercooked meat.
Flesh-eating strep	A rare disease caused by a strain of Group A streptococcus bacterium that produces materials that dissolve tissue. Early diagnosis and treatment with antibiotics stops the disease.
Cholera	A bacterial disease affecting the intestinal tract of individuals who eat or drink food or water contaminated by fecal waste of an infected person. In 1992, a new strain of cholera was detected in the Bay of Bengal and spread to 10 other countries.
Tuberculosis	A pulmonary disease once thought to be almost eliminated from North America. Depressed social conditions and improper use of antibiotics have revived this airborne disease, which is particularly threatening to people with weakened immune systems. Strict adherence to drug therapy for several months can cure the disease.
West Nile virus	A flavivirus commonly found in Africa, West Asia, and the Middle East that can infect mosquitoes, birds, horses, humans, and some other mammals. Increasingly common in North America, most people experience only a mild case, characterized by flu-like symptoms that last for a few days. However, more extreme forms of this disease can cause encephalitis (inflammation of the brain) and meningitis (inflammation of the membrane around the brain and spinal cord), which can prove to be fatal.
Malaria*	A life-threatening disease caused by parasites that are transmitted to people through the bites of infected female *Anopheles* mosquitoes.
Zika virus	A disease caused by a virus transmitted primarily by *Aedes* mosquitoes. People with zika virus disease can have symptoms including mild fever, skin rash, conjunctivitis, muscle and joint pain, malaise, or headaches. These symptoms normally last for two to seven days.

*World Health Organization. (2016). Emerging Diseases. Retrieved from www.who.int/topics/emerging_diseases/en/.

you wade or swim in contaminated streams, lakes, rivers, and reservoirs.

Bacteria

Bacteria are single-celled organisms. There are three major types of bacteria: cocci, bacilli, and spirilla. Bacteria may be viewed under a standard light microscope. Although there are several thousand species of bacteria, only approximately 100 cause diseases in humans. In many cases, it is not the bacteria themselves that cause disease but rather the poisonous substances, called **toxins**, that they produce. Some of these toxins are extremely powerful. Bacterial infections can take many forms, with the following being the most common.

Staphylococcal Infections

One of the most common forms of bacterial infection is the staph infection. **Staphylococci** are normally present on our skin at all times and seldom cause

Bacteria Single-celled organisms that can cause diseases in humans.

Toxins Poisonous substances produced by certain microorganisms that cause various diseases.

Staphylococci Found normally on our skin, only cause infection when there is a break in the skin.

problems. But when there is a cut or break in the **epidermis**, or outer layer of the skin, staphylococci may enter and cause a localized infection. If you have ever had acne, boils, styes (infections of the eyelids), or infected cuts, you probably had a staph infection.

At least one staph-caused disorder, **toxic shock syndrome**, is potentially fatal. Media reports in the early 1980s indicated that this disorder was exclusive to menstruating women, particularly those who used high-absorbency tampons for extended periods of time. Although tampons are strongly implicated, the actual mechanisms that produce this disease remain uncertain. Even though most cases of toxic shock syndrome occurred in menstruating women, the disease was first reported in 1978 in a group of children and continues to be reported in men, children, and nonmenstruating women. Most cases not related to menstruation occur in individuals recovering from wounds, surgery, and similar incidents.

To reduce the likelihood of contracting toxic shock syndrome, women should take the following precautions:

- avoid superabsorbent tampons except during the heaviest menstrual flow;
- change tampons frequently, at least every four hours;
- use pads at night instead of tampons.

Go to the closest emergency department or seek immediate medical attention if you have any of the following symptoms during menstruation: high fever, headache, vomiting, diarrhea and the chills, stomach pains, or shock-like symptoms such as faintness, rapid pulse, pallour (which can be caused by a drop in blood pressure), or a sunburn-like rash, particularly on fingers and toes.

Streptococcal Infections

Another common form of bacterial infection is caused by microorganisms called **streptococci**. A "strep throat" (severe sore throat characterized by white or yellow pustules at the back of the throat) is the typical streptococcal problem. Scarlet fever (characterized by acute fever, sore throat, and rash) and rheumatic fever (said to "lick the joints and bite the heart") are serious streptococcal infections.

Pneumonia

Pneumonia at one point (during the early 1900s) was one of the leading causes of death in North America and across the world. This disease is characterized by chronic cough, chest pain, chills, high fever, fluid accumulation, and eventual respiratory failure. One of the most common forms of pneumonia is caused by bacterial infection and responds readily to antibiotic treatment. Other forms are caused by the presence of viruses, chemicals, or other substances in the lungs. In these types of pneumonia, treatment may be more difficult.

Tuberculosis

One of the leading fatal diseases in Europe and North America in the early 1900s, **tuberculosis (TB)** is largely controlled through antibiotics, which must be taken for at least six to nine months. The exact drugs and length of treatment depend on your age, overall health, possible drug resistance, the form of TB (latent or active), and the infection's location in the body. While the mortality rate for TB worldwide has decreased by 41 percent since 1990, and even though it is treatable with antibiotics, it continues to be the top infectious disease killer worldwide. In 2014, 9.6 million people fell ill with TB and 1.5 million died from the disease (World Health Organization, 2015).

Several factors contribute to the resurgence of TB, including the phasing-out of surveillance and control programs, the emergence of multiple-antibiotic-resistant TB (MAR-TB), large-scale migration, social and natural disasters, and infection with the human immunodeficiency virus (HIV). The risk of developing clinical TB in tuberculin-positive individuals is very high in HIV-seropositive patients (Public Health Agency of Canada, 1996). For most Canadians, the risk of developing TB is low, although there are approximately 1600 new cases reported each year (Health Canada, 2012). Immunization has been used as a TB prevention strategy and control mechanism in Canada. In addition, public health programs use a combination of practices that include implementing standards and guidelines to manage disease.

Tuberculosis is caused by bacterial infiltration of the respiratory system. It is transmitted by breathing infected air from an infected person's coughing or sneezing. Many people infected with TB are contagious without actually showing symptoms themselves. Symptoms include persistent coughing, weight loss, fever, and coughing up blood. The average healthy person is not at high risk; however, those who may be fighting other diseases, such as some of the HIV-related diseases, may be at increased risk. Moreover, the burden of TB in the Aboriginal population is much greater than in the overall Canadian

Epidermis The outermost layer of the skin.

Toxic shock syndrome A potentially life-threatening bacterial infection most common in menstruating women.

Streptococci A bacteria that can cause strep throat or scarlet fever.

Pneumonia Disease of the lungs, usually caused by bacteria.

Tuberculosis (TB) A disease caused by bacterial infiltration of the respiratory system.

population. Factors contributing to these high rates include environmental factors and issues related to access healthcare.

The Mantoux tuberculin skin test (TST) or the TB blood test can usually detect TB. If you do have it, you can usually be treated and made noncontagious within two weeks and cured within six months.

Periodontal Diseases

Diseases of the tissues that surround the teeth including the gums, bones, and periodontal ligaments are called **periodontal diseases** (Health Canada, 2010). Gingivitis is a reversible gum disease that affects 32 percent of Canadian adults. Pocket depth is measured as an indicator of health of the teeth; 16 percent of Canadians have moderate disease and another 4 percent have severe disease. Loss of attachment is the third indicator of the health of the teeth and is directly related to age. Six percent of Canadians have severe loss of attachment (Health Canada, 2010). Improper home tooth care, including lack of flossing and poor brushing habits, and the failure to obtain regular professional dental care lead to increased bacterial growth, caries (tooth decay), and gum infections. If left untreated, permanent tooth loss may result. Further, untreated periodontal disease increases the risk for several systemic diseases, including coronary heart disease and type 2 diabetes.

Viruses

Viruses are extremely small pathogens, approximately 1/500 the size of bacteria. Because of their tiny size, they are visible only under an electron microscope and were therefore not identified until the twentieth century. At present, more than 150 viruses are known to cause diseases in humans.

A virus consists of a protein structure that contains either ribonucleic acid (RNA) or deoxyribonucleic acid (DNA). It is incapable of carrying out the normal cell functions of respiration and metabolism. It cannot reproduce on its own and exists only in a parasitic relationship with the cell it invades.

Treatment of viral diseases is difficult because many viruses can withstand heat, formaldehyde, and large doses of radiation with little effect on their structure. In addition, some viruses may have **incubation**

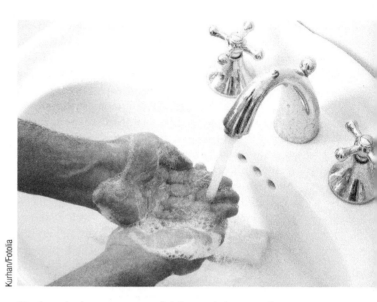

Kurhan/Fotolia

Hands can be the greatest source of viral transmission, so wash them thoroughly and often to prevent catching or transmitting the common cold.

periods (the length of time required to develop fully and cause symptoms in their hosts) measured in years rather than hours or days. Termed **slow-acting viruses**, these viruses infect the host and remain in a semidormant state for years, causing a slowly developing illness. HIV is an example of a slow-acting virus.

Drug treatment for viral infections is limited. Drugs powerful enough to kill viruses tend to kill the host cells too, although some drugs are available that block stages in viral reproduction without damaging the host cells. You have another form of virus protection within your body. When exposed to certain viruses, the body begins to produce a protein substance known as **interferon**. Interferon does not destroy the invading virus but sets up a protective mechanism to aid healthy cells in their struggle against the invaders. Although interferon research is promising, it should be noted that not all viruses stimulate interferon production.

The Common Cold

Caused by any number of viruses (some experts claim there may be more than 100 different viruses responsible for the common cold), colds are **endemic** among people throughout the world. Current research indicates that otherwise healthy people carry cold viruses in their noses and throats most of the time. These viruses are held in check until the host's resistance is lowered. In the true sense of the word, it is possible to "catch" a cold—from the airborne droplets of another person's sneeze or from skin-to-skin or mucous membrane contact—though recent studies indicate that your hands may be the greatest source of cold and other viral transmission.

Periodontal diseases Diseases of the tissue around the teeth.

Viruses Minute parasitic microbes that cause disease.

Incubation period The time between exposure to a disease and the appearance of the symptoms.

Slow-acting viruses Viruses with long incubation periods, causing slowly progressive symptoms.

Interferon A protein substance produced by the body that aids the immune system by protecting healthy cells.

Endemic Continued prevalence of a specific infection or disease in a specific population or area.

Although numerous ideas exist concerning how to prevent or cure the common cold, including taking megadoses of vitamin C, little hard evidence supports them. The best rule of thumb for preventing the common cold is to keep your resistance level high. Eating well (see Chapter 5), getting adequate rest (see Focus on Sleep), managing your stress (see Chapter 3), and engaging in regular physical activity (see Chapter 4) is your best approach to fighting off possible infection. Also, limit contact with people with newly developed colds since colds appear to be most contagious during the first 24 hours. Once you contract a cold, bed rest, plenty of fluids, and a pain reliever are the tried-and-true remedies for adults. Continue to eat well and be physically active at a light or moderate intensity. Keep in mind that children should not be given Aspirin for colds or the flu because of the possibility of Reye's syndrome. Several over-the-counter preparations are available to alleviate various cold symptoms (see also Chapter 9).

Influenza

In otherwise healthy people—that is, people without a compromised immune system—**influenza**, or flu, is usually not serious. Symptoms include aches and pains, nausea, diarrhea, fever, and cold-like ailments that generally pass quickly. However, in combination with other disorders, or among the elderly (people over 65), those with respiratory or heart disease, or the very young (children under the age of five), the flu can be very serious—even deadly.

Three major varieties of flu virus have been discovered to date, with many different strains existing within each variety. The "A" form of the virus is generally the most virulent, followed by the "B" and "C" varieties. If you contract one form of influenza you may develop immunity to it, but you may not necessarily be immune to other forms of it. There is little that can be done to treat individuals with the flu once it has become established. Similar to when you contract a cold, bed rest is recommended, as well as drinking plenty of fluids and trying to eat well. Physical activity should be limited or restricted until your fever has passed.

Some vaccines have proven effective for preventing certain strains of flu virus, but are totally ineffective against others. Flu vaccination is recommended for those with a compromised immune system, including adults and children with chronic pulmonary disorders, people of any age who are residents of nursing homes, people 65 years of age or over, and people with diabetes and other metabolic diseases—as well as people who work or volunteer in health services. It is also recommended for people who may come in contact with those with a compromised immune system. In other words, you may be recommended to have a flu shot simply because you may spread the flu to someone who may not be able to battle it well. In many jurisdictions, vaccination for these most vulnerable groups is provided free of charge. Vaccination for people not in essential health services is also recommended, but the person may have to pay the fee of $10 or $15. Because flu shots take anywhere from two to three weeks to become effective, you should get these shots in the fall, before the flu season begins.

Infectious Mononucleosis

This affliction of college- and university-aged people is often jokingly referred to as the "kissing disease." The symptoms of mononucleosis, or "mono," include sore throat, fever, headache, nausea, chills, abdominal discomfort, and a pervasive weakness or tiredness in the initial stages (Public Health Agency of Canada, 2011a). As the disease progresses, lymph nodes may continue to enlarge, and jaundice, spleen enlargement, aching joints, and body rashes may develop.

Theories on the transmission and treatment of mononucleosis are highly controversial. Caused by the Epstein-Barr virus, mononucleosis is readily detected through a monospot test, a blood test that measures the percentage of specific forms of white blood cells. Because many viruses are spread by transmission of body fluids, people once believed that young people passed the disease on when kissing. Although this is still considered a possible route of transmission, mononucleosis is not believed to be highly contagious. In fact, it does not appear to be easily contracted through normal, everyday personal contact. Multiple cases among family members are rare, as are cases between intimate partners.

Infectious mononucleosis usually lasts one to four weeks with protracted illness lasting one year occurring in some (Public Health Agency of Canada, 2011a). Treatment of mononucleosis is often a lengthy process that involves bed rest, a healthy dietary intake that follows Eating Well with Canada's Food Guide, and medications to control the symptoms of the disease. Gradually, the body develops a form of immunity to the disease and the person gets well again.

Hepatitis

One of the most highly publicized viral diseases is **hepatitis**. In response to an increased incidence of hepatitis in Canada, various educational programs were successfully implemented to reduce further outbreaks. In 2011 an estimated 220 697 to 245 987 Canadians were living with hepatitis C. That is the equivalent of six to seven people out of every 1000

Influenza A common viral disease of the respiratory tract.

Hepatitis A virally caused disease in which the liver becomes inflamed, resulting in fever, headache, and jaundice.

Canadians (Trubnikov, Yan, & Archibald, 2011). Most cases occur in males over the age of 30 years, though in recent years the gender gap is decreasing with a greater number of younger females being diagnosed. Most hepatitis C carriers are asymptomatic with 50 percent becoming chronic carriers. The incubation period for hepatitis C is 14 to 168 days. The rates of hepatitis B have also decreased in Canada in all age groups though it continues to be three times more prevalent in Aboriginal peoples (Public Health Agency of Canada, 2011b). Hepatitis B has an incubation period of 45 to 180 days with less than 10 percent of children and 50 percent of adults being symptomatic. Less than 10 percent of adults and more than 90 percent of perinatal and children infected become chronic carriers of the virus. Hepatitis A has a 15 to 45-day incubation period. Similar to hepatitis B, hepatitis A is symptomatic in less than 10 percent of children and in 50 percent of adults. There are no chronic carriers of the hepatitis A virus.

Hepatitis is generally defined as a virally caused inflammation of the liver, characterized by symptoms such as fever, headache, nausea, loss of appetite, skin rashes, pain in the upper right abdomen, dark yellow (with a brownish tinge) urine, and the possibility of jaundice. In fact, hepatitis is often "the disease your friends diagnose" because of the yellowing of the whites of the eyes and the skin.

Treatment of all the forms of viral hepatitis is somewhat limited. A healthy dietary intake, bed rest, and antibiotics to combat bacterial infections that can cause additional problems are recommended. Vaccines for hepatitis are available through a series of injections, although cost may be prohibitive for some. Many provinces are beginning to require vaccinations against hepatitis B for health-care workers and others who may be exposed to blood-borne pathogens. Vaccination for hepatitis is also recommended when travelling outside Canada and the United States to Africa, Asia, and Central and South America.

Mumps

Until 1969, mumps was a common viral disorder among children, with an average of 30 000 cases per year. That year, a vaccine became available and the number of reported cases decreased by 99 percent from 34 000 cases per year in the 1950s to fewer than 400 per year in the 1990s (Public Health Agency of Canada, 2012b). Rates in Canada in 2011 (the latest data available) are 0.82 per 100 000 (Public Health Agency of Canada, 2012b). Rates are highest in the 20- to 24-year-old category at 2.75 per 100 000 (Public Health Agency of Canada, 2012b). Since 2001 there have been two mumps outbreaks in Canada. Approximately one-half of all mumps infections are not apparent because they produce only minor symptoms. In fact, 20 percent have no symptoms at all (Public Health Agency of Canada, 2012b). Typically, there is an incubation period of 16 to 18 days, followed by symptoms caused by the lodging of the virus in the glands of the neck. The most common symptom is the swelling of the parotid (salivary) glands. One of the greatest dangers associated with mumps is the potential for sterility in men (20 to 30 percent of post-pubertal cases) who contract the disease in young adulthood, and although rare, women can also become infertile as a result of the inflammation (5 percent of post-pubertal cases) (Public Health Agency of Canada, 2012b).

Chicken Pox

Caused by the varicella-zoster virus, which also causes shingles (see below), chicken pox produces the characteristic symptoms of fever and tiredness 13 to 17 days after exposure, followed by skin eruptions that itch, blister, and produce a clear fluid. The virus is present in these blisters for approximately one week. Symptoms are generally mild, and immunity to subsequent infection appears to be lifelong. Although a chicken pox vaccine for children aged 12 months and older has been available in Canada since 2000, not all get vaccinated and a small percentage of those who do still develop chicken pox. It is believed that after the initial infection, the virus goes into permanent hibernation and, for most people, there are no further complications. For a small segment of the population, however, the zoster virus may become reactivated. Blisters will develop, usually on only one side of the body, and stop abruptly at the midline. Cases in which the disease, known as shingles, covers both sides of the body are far more serious. This disease is estimated to affect 15 to 28 percent of Canadians at some point in their lifetime (BC Centre for Disease Control, 2012). More cases of shingles have been reported in recent years, particularly in individuals over the age of 65 years.

Measles

Measles is the most contagious disease known to humans. Prior to the development of a vaccination in 1980, measles killed 2.6 million people each year (World Health Organization, 2015c). The disease remains one of the leading causes of death among young children globally, despite the availability of a safe and effective vaccine. Approximately 114 900 people died from measles in 2014—mostly children under the age of five (World Health Organization, 2015c). Since 1997, there have been no indigenous cases of measles reported—although imported cases do occur at a rate of about 11 per year (Public Health

Agency of Canada, 2013c). The **measles** virus may ultimately be responsible for more child deaths than any other single microbe, due to complications from pneumonia, diarrhea, and malnutrition. Technically referred to as rubeola, measles is a viral disorder that often affects young children. The incubation period for measles is about 10 days, though a 7 to 18 day range is normal with symptoms appearing about 14 days after exposure; these include an itchy rash and a high fever. The individual with measles is usually infectious from four days before the rash appears until 4 days after the rash appears (Public Health Agency of Canada, 2013c).

Rubella (or **German measles**) is a milder viral infection believed to be transmitted by inhalation, after which the virus multiplies in the upper respiratory tract and passes into the bloodstream. German measles causes a rash, especially on the upper extremities. It is not generally a serious health threat and usually runs its course in three to four days. The major exceptions to this rule are newborns and pregnant women. Rubella can damage a fetus, particularly during the first trimester, creating a condition known as congenital rubella, in which the infant may be born blind, deaf, cognitively impaired, or with heart defects. Immunization has greatly reduced the incidence of measles and German measles. Infections in children not immunized against measles can lead to fever-induced problems such as rheumatic heart disease, kidney damage, and neurological disorders.

YOUR BODY'S DEFENCES: KEEPING YOU WELL

Physical and Chemical Defences

Perhaps our single most critical early defence system is the skin. Layered to provide an intricate web of barriers, the skin allows few pathogens to enter. **Enzymes**, complex proteins manufactured by the body that appear in body secretions such as sweat, provide additional protection, destroying microorganisms on skin surfaces by producing inhospitable pH levels. Normal body pH is 7.0, but enzymatic or biochemical changes can cause the body chemistry to become more acidic (pH of less than 7.0), or more alkaline (pH of more than 7.0). In either case, microorganisms that flourish at a selected pH will be weakened or destroyed as these changes occur. A third protection is our frequent slight elevations in body temperature, which also create an inhospitable environment for many pathogens. Further, only when there are cracks or breaks, such as cuts in the skin, can pathogens gain easy access to the body.

The linings of the body provide protection against pathogens. Mucous membranes in the respiratory tract and other linings of the body trap and engulf invading organisms. Cilia, hairlike projections in the lungs and respiratory tract, sweep unwanted invaders toward body openings, where they are expelled. Tears, nasal secretions, ear wax, and other secretions found at body entrances contain enzymes designed to destroy or neutralize invading pathogens. Finally, any invading organism that manages to breach these initial lines of defence faces a formidable specialized network of defences from the immune system.

The Immune System: Your Body Fights Back

Immunity is the condition of being able to resist a particular disease by counteracting the substance that produces the disease. Any substance capable of triggering an immune response is called an **antigen**. An antigen can be a virus, a bacterium, a fungus, a parasite, or a tissue or cell from another individual. When invaded by an antigen, the body responds by forming substances called antibodies. **Antibodies** belong to a mass of large molecules known as immunoglobulins, a group of nine chemically distinct protein substances, each of which plays a role in neutralizing, setting up for destruction, or actually destroying antigens. Once an antigen breaches the body's initial defences, the body begins a careful process of antigen analysis. It considers the size and shape of the invader, verifies that the antigen is not part of the body itself, and then begins to produce a specific antibody to destroy or weaken the antigen. This process, which is much more complex than described here, is part of a system called humoral immune responses. Humoral immunity is the body's major defence against bacteria and bacterial toxins.

Cell-mediated immunity is characterized by the formation of a population of lymphocytes that can attack and destroy the foreign invader. These lymphocytes constitute the body's main defence against viruses, fungi, parasites, and some bacteria. Key players in this immune response are specialized groups of white blood cells known as macrophages (a type of phagocytic, or cell-eating, cell) and lymphocytes, other white blood cells in the blood, lymph nodes, bone marrow, and certain glands.

Two forms of lymphocytes in particular, the B-lymphocytes (B-cells) and T-lymphocytes (T-cells), are

Measles A viral disease that produces symptoms including an itchy rash and a high fever.

Rubella (German measles) A milder form of measles that causes a rash and mild fever in children and may cause damage to a fetus or a newborn baby.

Enzymes Organic substances that cause bodily changes and destruction of microorganisms.

Antigen Substance capable of triggering an immune response.

Antibodies Substances produced by the body to destroy or weaken specific antigens.

involved in the immune response. There are different types of B-cells, named according to the area of the body in which they develop. Most are manufactured in the soft tissue of the hollow shafts of the long bones. T-cells, in contrast, develop and multiply in the thymus, a multi-lobed organ that lies behind the breastbone. T-cells assist your immune system in several ways. Regulatory T-cells help direct the activities of the immune system and assist other cells, particularly B-cells, to produce antibodies. Dubbed "helper Ts," these cells are essential for activating B-cells, other T-cells, and macrophages. Another form of T-cell, known as the "killer Ts" or "cytotoxic Ts," directly attacks infected or malignant cells. Killer Ts enable the body to rid itself of cells infected by viruses or transformed by cancer; they are also responsible for the rejection of tissue and organ grafts. The third type of T-cells, "suppressor Ts," turns off or suppresses the activity of B-cells, killer Ts, and macrophages. Suppressor Ts circulate in the bloodstream and lymphatic system, neutralizing or destroying antigens, enhancing the effects of the immune response, and helping to return the activated immune system to normal levels. After a successful attack on a pathogen, some of the attacker T- and B-cells are preserved as memory T- and B-cells, enabling the body to quickly recognize and respond to subsequent attacks by the same kind of organism at a later time. Thus, macrophages, T- and B-cells, and antibodies are the key factors in mounting an immune response.

Once you have survived certain infectious diseases, you become immune to them, meaning that in all probability you will not develop those particular diseases again. When the disease-causing microorganism next attacks you, your memory T- and B-cells are quickly activated to come to your defence. Immunization works on the same principle. Vaccines containing an attenuated (weakened) or killed version of the disease-causing microorganism or an antigen similar to but not as dangerous as the disease antigen are administered to stimulate the immune system to produce antibodies to build immunity from the disease.

Autoimmune Diseases

Although white blood cells and the antigen–antibody response generally work in our favour, the body sometimes makes a mistake and targets its own tissue as the enemy, builds up antibodies against that tissue, and attempts to destroy it. This is known as autoimmune disease (auto means "self"). Common examples of this type of disease are rheumatoid arthritis, lupus erythematosus, and myasthenia gravis.

In some cases, the antigen–antibody response completely fails to function. The

Vaccination Inoculation with killed or weakened pathogens or similar, less dangerous antigens in order to prevent or lessen the effects of some disease.

result is a form of immune deficiency syndrome. Perhaps the most dramatic case of this syndrome was the "bubble boy," who died in 1984 after living his short life inside a sealed-off environment designed to protect him from all antigens.

Fever

If an infection is localized, pus formation, redness, swelling, and irritation often occur. These symptoms indicate a systemic response against the invading organisms. Another indication is the development of a fever, or a rise in body temperature above the norm of 37°C. Fever is frequently caused by toxins secreted by pathogens that interfere with the control of body temperature. Although this elevated temperature is often harmful to the body, it is also believed to act as a form of protection. A one- or two-degree elevation in temperature creates an environment that destroys some types of disease-causing organisms. Also, as body temperature rises, the body is stimulated to produce more white blood cells, which also destroy more invaders.

Pain

Although pain is not usually thought of as a defence mechanism, it plays a valuable role in the body's response to invasion. Pain is generally a response to injury. Pain may be either direct, caused by the stimulation of nerve endings in an affected area, or referred, meaning it is present in one place while the source is elsewhere. An example of referred pain is the pain in the arm or jaw often experienced by someone having a heart attack. Regardless of the cause of pain, most pain responses are accompanied by inflammation. Pain tends to be the earliest sign that an injury occurred and often causes the person to slow down or stop the activity, thereby protecting against further damage. Because it is often one of the first warnings of disease, persistent pain should not be overlooked, ignored, or masked with short-term pain relievers.

Vaccines: Bolstering Your Immunity

The body's natural defence mechanisms are our strongest allies in the battle against disease from birth until death. There are periods in our life, however, when either invading organisms are too strong or our natural immunity is too weak to protect us from catching a particular disease. It is at such times that we need outside assistance in developing immunity to an invading organism. Such assistance can be provided through **vaccination**. Vaccines are given orally or

TABLE 13.2

Recommended Childhood Immunization Schedule

Age	Immunization Against
2 months	Diphtheria, pertussis, tetanus, poliomyelitis, *haemophilus influenzae* b,* pneumococcal conjugate vaccine, meningococcal C conjugate vaccine
4 months	Diphtheria, pertussis, tetanus, poliomyelitis, *haemophilus influenzae* b, pneumococcal conjugate vaccine,** meningococcal C conjugate vaccine
6 months	Diphtheria, pertussis, tetanus, poliomyelitis,[†] *haemophilus influenzae* b, pneumococcal conjugate vaccine
12 months	Measles, mumps, rubella,[††] varicella,[‡] pneumococcal conjugate vaccine
18 months	Diphtheria, pertussis, tetanus, poliomyelitis, *haemophilus influenzae* b
4–6 years	Diphtheria, pertussis, tetanus, poliomyelitis
9–13 years	Hepatitis B[‡‡]
14–16 years	Diphtheria, tetanus, poliomyelitis, meningococcal C conjugate vaccine[§]

Notes:

Haemophilus influenzae b requires a series of immunizations. The exact number and timing of each may vary with the brand of vaccine used.

**Recommended schedule, number of doses, and subsequent use of pneumococcal vaccine depends on the age of the child when vaccination is begun.

[†]If oral polio virus vaccine is used exclusively in a series of immunizations, this dose may be omitted.

[††]A second dose of MMR vaccine is recommended for children and youth. It may be administered any time after a minimum one-month waiting period; provincial schedules differ.

[‡]Children aged 12 months to 12 years should receive one dose of varicella vaccine. Individuals aged 13 years or older should receive two doses at least 28 days apart.

[‡‡]Hepatitis B requires a series of immunizations. In some jurisdictions, they may be administered at a younger age.

[§]Recommended schedule and number of doses of meningococcal vaccine depends on the age of the child.

Source: © All Rights Reserved. *Canadian Immunization Guide,* 7th Edition. Public Health Agency of Canada, 2013. Reproduced with permission from the Minister of Health, 2014.

by injection, and this form of artificial immunity is termed *acquired immunity*, in contrast to *natural (passive) immunity*, which a mother passes to her fetus via their shared blood supply.

Today, depending on the virulence of the organism, vaccines containing live, weakened, or dead organisms are given to people for a variety of diseases. In some instances, if a person is already weakened by other diseases, vaccination may provoke an actual case of the disease. This happened with the smallpox vaccinations administered routinely in the 1960s. It was believed that the risk of contracting smallpox from the vaccine was actually greater than the chance of contracting the disease in an environment where it had essentially been eradicated. For this reason, routine smallpox inoculations were eliminated in the late 1960s. See Tables 13.2, 13.3, and 13.4 for the current recommendations in Canada for vaccines for children and adults.

TABLE 13.3

Adult Immunization Schedule—Routinely for All

Vaccine	Dosing Schedule (no record or unclear history of immunization)	Booster Schedule (primary series completed)
Tetanus and diphtheria given as Td; and pertussis given as Tdap	Doses 1 and 2, 4–8 weeks apart and dose 3 at 6–12 months later; one of the doses should be given as Tdap for pertussis protection	Td every 10 years; 1 dose should be given as Tdap if not previously given in adulthood
Measles, mumps and rubella given as MMR	1 dose for adults born in or after 1970 without a history of measles or those individuals without evidence of immunity to rubella or mumps; second dose for selected groups	Not routinely required
Varicella	Doses 1 and 2, at least 4 weeks apart for susceptible adults (no history of natural disease or seronegativity)	Not currently recommended

Source: © All Rights Reserved. *Canadian Immunization Guide,* 7th Edition. Public Health Agency of Canada, 2013. Reproduced with permission from the Minister of Health, 2014.

TABLE 13.4

Adult Immunization Schedule—Specific Risk Situations

Vaccine or Toxoid	Indication	Schedule
Influenza	Adults 65 years; Adults 65 years at high risk of influenza-related complications, their household contacts, health-care workers, and all those wishing to be protected against influenza.	Every autumn, using current recommended vaccine formulation
Pneumococcal polysaccharide	Adults 65 years; Adults 65 who have conditions putting them at increased risk of pneumococcal disease.	1 dose
Hepatitis A	Occupational risk, life-style, travel and living in areas lacking adequate sanitation. Outbreak control, post-exposure immunoprophylaxis. Patients with chronic liver disease.	2 doses 6–12 months apart
Hepatitis B	Occupational risk, life-style, post-exposure immunoprophylaxis. Patients with chronic liver disease.	3 doses at 0, 1, and 6 months
Bacille Calmette-Guérin (BCG)	Rarely used. Consider for high-risk exposure in selected cases.	1 dose
Cholera	High-risk exposure in travellers to endemic area(s).	1 oral dose of live attenuated vaccine; 2 doses at least 1 week apart but not greater than 6 weeks of oral inactivated vaccine
Japanese encephalitis	Travel to endemic area(s) or other exposure risk.	3 doses at days 0, 7, and 30
Poliomyelitis	Travel to endemic area(s) or other risk group.	Primary series doses 1 and 2, 4–8 weeks apart and dose 3 at 6–12 months later; 1 booster dose if 10 years since primary series
Meningococcal conjugate	Young adults	1 dose
Meningococcal polysaccharide	High-risk exposure groups	1 dose
Rabies, pre-exposure use	Occupational or high-risk travellers	3 doses at days 0, 7, and 21
Typhoid	High-risk travellers to endemic area(s) or other high-risk exposure	Parenteral capsular polysaccharide 1 dose; live attenuated 3–4 oral doses depending on preparation
Yellow fever	Travel to endemic area(s) or if required for foreign travel	1 dose with booster every 10 years if required
Smallpox	Laboratory staff working with vaccinia or other orthopoxviruses	1 dose

Source: © All Rights Reserved. *Canadian Immunization Guide,* 7th Edition. Public Health Agency of Canada, 2013. Reproduced with permission from the Minister of Health, 2014.

SEXUALLY TRANSMITTED INFECTIONS

There are more than 20 types of **sexually transmitted infections** (STIs, formerly called STDs, or sexually transmitted diseases). These infections were once referred to as venereal diseases—this newer classification is believed to be broader in scope and reflective of the numbers and types of communicable infections, which are sometimes asymptomatic (Health Canada, n.d.a). In Canada, the incidence of STIs is rising, particularly among young people—with the majority of new infections attributed to those between the ages of 15 and 24 years (Wong & Sutherland, 2002). Young people today generally become sexually active earlier and marry later—as a result, they have, on average, a greater number of partners, which increases their risk of acquiring an STI. Further, with the increase in the number of divorces, people are once again more likely to have multiple

Sexually transmitted infections (STIs) Infectious diseases transmitted via vaginal, anal, and oral sexual contact.

point of view

TO IMMUNIZE OR NOT TO IMMUNIZE:
Are Vaccinations Safe? Are Vaccinations Necessary?

You likely remember little about your early immunizations and had little to say about whether or not you would get them as your parents made that decision for you. Now that you are older and there is more information available about vaccinations, you are in a position to make that decision for your children when you have them. Further, you may need to make decisions regarding immunizations when you travel outside the country. It is important when you make the decision to immunize or not that you are well-informed of the risks and benefits.

Immunizations against widespread infectious diseases are one of the greatest public health success stories of all time—so successful, in fact, that most people have never seen or heard of anyone having the diseases that once wiped out entire populations. Today, fear of the old "killer" diseases has waned, and people raise questions as to whether they really need or want to get vaccinated. Add in the costs of vaccines and a growing distrust of health care, the government, and drug companies, and it is no wonder that there is growing anti-vaccine sentiment in some segments of the population.

How serious a problem is this? In some communities, such as Ashland, Oregon, up to 25 percent of kindergartners' parents opted their children out of at least one vaccine in 2010. In other U.S. school districts and counties, these rates are even higher, and a general trend of avoiding vaccinations is growing, in spite of clear evidence that this is risky business. Similar avoidance of vaccinations is happening in Canada.

Undervaccination rates are particularly high in non-Latino, college-educated white families with incomes above $75 000 a year. Religious tenets, fear of vaccine safety, and worry about vaccine overload are among some of the more common reasons for parents' refusal to vaccinate their children. Others object to mandatory vaccinations because they consider them to be a government intrusion into their individual rights.

The vaccine concerns receiving the most attention include fear that the measles, mumps, rubella (MMR) vaccine can lead to autism; fear that the hepatitis B vaccine is related to multiple sclerosis (MS); and fear that the combined tetanus, diphtheria, pertussis (Tdap) vaccine can cause sudden infant death syndrome (SIDS). Are these concerns valid? Research is ongoing, but the Centers for Disease Control and Prevention (CDC) has found no clear evidence that the MMR vaccine causes autism, that hepatitis B shots are the culprit behind MS, or that the Tdap vaccine leads to SIDS. Furthermore, the research that these fears were based upon has since been retracted as the results had been falsified. Virtually all medical and public health organizations support vaccinations, pointing to stringent safety controls in the manufacturing and testing of vaccines, as well as ongoing safety monitoring, the long history of vaccines in wiping out killer diseases across the globe, and the fact that risks from the diseases themselves are almost always much greater than any risks associated with a vaccine. If large numbers of people were to avoid vaccinations, old killers would be likely to reemerge, and those people who were already sick or weak from other conditions would be extremely vulnerable.

The reasons for vaccination far outweigh any arguments against. That said, it is important to note that, despite extensive testing, no vaccine is completely safe and effective and that there are often risks from temporary, minor side effects from any given vaccine. Local rashes and reactions at injection sites, low-grade fever, discomfort, and even allergic reactions can occur. Major risks from getting vaccinations are extremely rare and studies supporting the antivaccine rhetoric are unsubstantiated.

Vaccine pharmacovigilance, the science and activities relating to the detection, assessment, understanding, prevention, and communication of adverse events following immunization or of any other vaccine- or immunization-related issues, is monitored by the Public Health Agency of Canada. The Canadian Adverse Events Following Immunization Surveillance System is a Federal/Provincial/Territorial monitoring system with the following objectives:

1. to continuously monitor the safety of marketed vaccines in Canada;
2. to identify increases in the frequency or severity of previously identified vaccine-related reactions;

(continued)

3. to identify previously unknown adverse events following immunization that could possibly be related to vaccine;

4. to identify areas that require further investigation and/or research; and

5. to provide timely information on adverse effects following immunization reporting profiles for vaccines marketed in Canada that can help inform immunization-related decisions.

Although the government is responsible for ensuring that our vaccinations are safe and effective, it still remains up to you to make the best decisions for you and for those you are responsible for.

Sources: Based on Centers for Disease Control and Prevention, "Concerns about Autism," 2011, www.cdc.gov/vaccinesafety/Concerns/Autism/Index.html; Centers for Disease Control and Prevention, "Vaccine Adverse Event Reporting System," 2011, www.cdc.gov/vaccinesafety/Activities/VAERS.html; Centers for Disease Control and Prevention, "Vaccine Safety," 2011, www.cdc.gov/vaccinesafety/index.html; Centers for Disease Control and Prevention, "Vaccine Safety: Concerns about Autism," Modified January 2010, www.cdc.gov/vaccinesafety/Concerns/Autism/Index.html; Public Health Agency of Canada, (2012a) Vaccine Safety, retrieved on June 15, 2013 from www.phac-aspc.gc.ca/im/vs-sv/; Slade B. et al. (2009). "Postlicensure Safety Surveillance for Quadrivalent Human Papillomavirus Recombinant Vaccine," *Journal of the American Medical Association* 302, no. 7: 750–57.

sexual partners during their life and increase their risk of developing an STI.

In many, the early symptoms of an STI are not serious. They range from mild discomfort to annoying itching or discharge. (See Figure 13.2 for signs that may indicate an STI.) Left untreated, however, some STIs have grave consequences, such as sterility, blindness, central nervous system destruction, disfigurement, and even death. Infants born to mothers with STIs are at risk of a variety of health problems.

Similar to other communicable diseases, much of the pain, suffering, and anguish associated with STIs could be eliminated or substantially reduced through education, responsible action, and prompt treatment when symptoms first occur. Overcoming the tendency to pass moral judgments on those who contract an STI would certainly lower the barriers to treatment. Similarly, being prepared to deal with the pressure to engage in sexual activity, as well as the responsibility required when choosing to be sexually active.

Possible Causes: Why Me?

STIs affect men and women of all socioeconomic levels, ages, ethnicities, and regions of the world. Several reasons have been proposed to explain the present high rates of STIs. The first relates to the moral and social stigma associated with them. Shame and embarrassment often keep infected people from seeking treatment. Unfortunately, these people usually continue to be sexually active, thereby infecting others. People uncomfortable with discussing sexual issues may also be less likely to use, or to ask their partners to use, condoms as a means of protection against STIs.

Another reason proposed for the STI epidemic is the current casual attitude about sex—particularly on most campuses. There seems to be an attitude that everyone is 'doing it' and you should be 'doing it' too. Bombarded by media hype that glamorizes sex and the ease of being sexually active, many people engage in sexual activity without considering the physical, emotional, or spiritual consequences or being responsible for their actions. Others are pressured into sexual relationships they do not really want. Generally, the more sexual partners a person has, the greater the risk for contracting an STI. Evaluate your beliefs and attitudes about STIs by taking the Assess Yourself self-assessment in the Focus on STIs section.

FIGURE 13.2

Signs and Symptoms of STIs

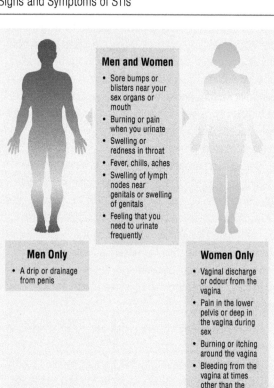

Men and Women
- Sore bumps or blisters near your sex organs or mouth
- Burning or pain when you urinate
- Swelling or redness in throat
- Fever, chills, aches
- Swelling of lymph nodes near genitals or swelling of genitals
- Feeling that you need to urinate frequently

Men Only
- A drip or drainage from penis

Women Only
- Vaginal discharge or odour from the vagina
- Pain in the lower pelvis or deep in the vagina during sex
- Burning or itching around the vagina
- Bleeding from the vagina at times other than the regular menstrual periods

Ignorance about the infections themselves and an inability to recognize actual symptoms or to acknowledge that a person may be asymptomatic yet still have an infection are also factors behind the current rise in STIs. A person infected but asymptomatic may unknowingly spread an STI to an unsuspecting and unprotected partner, who may then ignore or misinterpret symptoms that appear. By the time either partner seeks medical help, he or she may have infected several others.

Modes of Transmission

STIs are generally spread through some form of sexual contact. Vaginal and anal intercourse, oral–genital contact, and hand–genital contact are (in decreasing order of likelihood) the most common modes of transmission. More rarely, pathogens for STIs are transmitted from mouth to mouth or, even more infrequently, through contact with fluids from body sores. While each STI is a different infection caused by a different pathogen, all STI pathogens prefer dark, moist places, especially the mucous membranes lining the reproductive organs. The majority of these organisms are susceptible to light, excess heat, cold, and dryness, and many die quickly on exposure to air. (The toilet seat is not a likely breeding ground for most bacterial or viral STIs.) Although most STIs are passed on by sexual contact, other kinds of close contact, such as sleeping on the sheets used by someone who has pubic lice or using his or her towel, may also result in transmission from one person to another. One method of preventing the spread of STIs is to use a condom during any sexual activity, including vaginal, anal, and oral sex as well as during hand–genital contact. To fully protect yourself, follow these basic rules:

- Decide ahead of time that you will only have sex using a condom. Make sure you have one with you.
- Never reuse a condom.
- Use only latex condoms.
- Store condoms in a cool, dry place—not in the glove compartment of your car or in your wallet.
- If a condom appears brittle or sticky, do not use it.
- Put the condom on (correctly) before any sexual activity, including oral sex and hand–genital contact.
- Apply a water-based lubricant containing spermicide to the condom for additional protection.
- If the condom breaks, tears, or becomes dislodged, wash the genitals thoroughly with soap and water, apply a spermicide, and put on another condom before additional contact. It takes only a fraction of a second to become infected with disease-laden body fluids or to infect someone else.
- Hold the condom in place during withdrawal to make sure it does not come off.

Like other communicable diseases, STIs have both pathogen-specific incubation periods and periods of time during which transmission is most likely, called periods of communicability.

Although there are more than 20 types of STIs, only those most likely to pose a risk for you are discussed.

Chlamydia

Genital **chlamydia** (*Chlamydia trachomatis*) first became nationally reportable in 1990 and emerged as the most prevalent bacterial STI in Canada. Preventable and treatable, infection rates for genital chlamydia remains high in Canada—in 2012, the chlamydia rate was 298.7 per 100 000 (383.5 per 100 000 among females and) 212.0 per 100 000 among males) (Public Health Agency of Canada, 2015a). These rates continue to rise. The increase is partly due to more and better screening. In both males and females, the rates of chlamydia were highest in those aged 20 to 24 years, primarily because young people are not protecting themselves and others from this STI (see Table 13.5).

The name of the infection is derived from the Greek verb *chlamys*, meaning "to cloak," because, unlike most bacteria, chlamydia can live and grow only inside other cells. Although many people classify chlamydia as either nonspecific or nongonococcal urethritis (NGU), a person may have NGU without having the organism for chlamydia. In more than half of the cases of NGU (infections of the urethra and surrounding tissues not caused by gonococcal bacteria), *Chlamydia trachomatis*, the bacterial organism that causes chlamydia, is present. For this reason, the two disease terms tend to be used interchangeably, even though NGU may be caused by other organisms.

According to Health Canada (2006), those infected with chlamydia through oral sex generally have few symptoms. Symptoms of anal infection include:

- Rectal pain
- Bleeding
- Discharge

Symptoms from vaginal sex, when apparent, are relatively (within women and men) similar and include the following for women:

- A vaginal discharge
- A burning sensation when urinating
- Pain in the lower abdomen, sometimes with fever and chills

Chlamydia Bacterially caused STI of the urogenital tract.

TABLE 13.5
Screening for STIs

Screening to detect asymptomatic STIs is divided into three categories:

Case Finding: A patient-based strategy in individuals with an increased likelihood of one or more STIs—for example, sexual contacts with someone who has gonorrhea

Focused Screening: A group-based strategy in subpopulations with high STI prevalence rates—for example, street youth, core groups, adolescents, and those with a history of STI

General Screening: A population-based strategy in certain members of the general public who are not considered to be at increased risk for STI but in whom serious consequences might occur if infected—for example, syphilis and HIV testing in pregnancy

	Case Finding	Focused Screening	General Screening
Procedures			
Sexual history	x	x	x
Physical examination			
External genital	x	x	x
Internal genital	Adults, adolescents	Adults, adolescents	—
Targeted extragenital	x	x	x
Laboratory tests			
Chlamydia trachomatis	x	x	—
Treponema pallidum	x	x	x
Pap smear	Adults, adolescents	Adults, adolescents	—
Hepatitis B (HBV)	Optional	Optional	x
HIV	x	x	x

Source: © All Rights Reserved. Canada Communicable Disease Report—Supplement—Vol.21S4. Public Health Agency of Canada, 1995. Reproduced with permission from the Minister of Health, 2014.

- Pain during sex
- Vaginal bleeding between periods or after intercourse

Symptoms for men include:

- A discharge from the penis
- A burning sensation when urinating
- Burning or itching at the opening of the penis
- Pain and/or swelling in the testicles

Unfortunately, many individuals with chlamydia have no symptoms and therefore do not seek help until the infection has done secondary damage (Health Canada, 2006). Females are especially likely to be asymptomatic, with more than 70 percent of carriers unaware they have the infection until secondary damage occurs (Health Canada, 2006).

The secondary damage resulting from chlamydia is serious for males and females. Males suffer damage to the prostate gland, seminal vesicles, and bulbourethral glands, as well as arthritis-like symptoms and damage to the blood vessels and heart. In females, secondary damage from chlamydia includes inflammation that damages the cervix or fallopian tubes, causing sterility and damage to the inner pelvic structure and leading to pelvic inflammatory disease (PID, see next section). If an infected woman becomes pregnant, she has a high risk for miscarriages and stillbirths. Chlamydia may also be responsible for one type of **conjunctivitis**, an eye infection that affects not only adults but also infants, who contract the disease from an infected mother during delivery. Untreated conjunctivitis can cause blindness.

Chlamydia can be controlled through responsible sexual behaviours and familiarity with the early symptoms of the disease. If detected early enough, chlamydia is easily treatable with antibiotics such as tetracycline, doxycycline, or erythromycin. In most cases, treatment is successfully completed in two to three weeks.

Pelvic Inflammatory Disease (PID)

Pelvic inflammatory disease (PID) is actually not one disease but a term used to describe a number of infections of the uterus, fallopian tubes, and ovaries.

Conjunctivitis Serious inflammation of the eye caused by any number of pathogens or irritants; can be caused by STIs such as chlamydia.

Pelvic inflammatory disease (PID) Includes various infections of the female reproductive tract.

Although PID is often the result of an untreated STI, especially chlamydia or gonorrhea, it is not actually an STI. Nonsexual causes of PID are also common, including excessive vaginal douching, cigarette smoking, and substance abuse. PID is not a notifiable disease in Canada; thus, estimating prevalence is difficult. That said, it is estimated that there are 100 000 cases of symptomatic PID each year in Canada (Public Health Agency of Canada, 2013b). It is further estimated that 10 to 15 percent of women of a reproductive age experience at least one PID (Public Health Agency of Canada, 2013b).

Symptoms may include acute inflammation of the pelvic cavity, severe pain in the lower abdomen, menstrual irregularities, fever, nausea, and painful intercourse (Public Health Agency of Canada, 2013b). The major consequences of untreated PID are infertility, ectopic pregnancy, chronic pelvic pain, and recurrent upper genital infections. Risk factors include young age at first sexual intercourse, multiple sexual partners, and high frequency of sexual intercourse. Regular gynecological examinations and early treatment for STI symptoms reduce risk.

Gonorrhea

Gonorrhea continues to exist in Canada, though it has declined more than tenfold since 1980. In 2012, the rate of Gonorrhea was 36.2 per 100 000; rates were higher in males than females (41.4 vs. 31.0 per 100 000, Public Health Agency of Canada, 2015b). Females between the ages of 15 and 24 years and males between the ages of 20 and 29 years accounted for the highest rates of gonorrhea. Although there has been an overall decline since 1980, the lowest rates for gonorrhea were in the mid-1990s; current rates are stagnant (Public Health Agency of Canada, 2011d).

Currently, the majority of endemic gonococcal infections is thought to reside within core groups: a small subset of the population whose members frequently acquire new sexual partners. The highest rates of infection are found in the territories, with 1603.3 per 100 000 in Nunavut, 552.5 per 100 000 in the Northwest Territories, followed by Saskatchewan (84.9 per 100 000) and Manitoba (83.6 per 100 000) (Public Health Agency of Canada, 2011d). More research needs to be conducted to assess and describe core groups within a Canadian context; appropriate prevention and control strategies, aimed at reducing or ideally eliminating indigenous gonococcal infections, can then be implemented.

Caused by the bacterial pathogen *Neisseria gonorrhoea*, gonorrhea primarily infects the linings of the urethra, genital tract, pharynx, and rectum. It may be spread to the eyes or other body regions via the hands or body fluids.

In males, a typical symptom is a white milky discharge from the penis accompanied by painful, burning urination two to nine days after contact. The pain is usually severe enough to send most men to their physician for treatment. Only about 20 percent of all males with gonorrhea are asymptomatic.

In females, the situation is the opposite. Only about 20 percent of all females experience any form of discharge, and few develop a burning sensation upon urinating until much later in the infection (if ever). The organism can remain in the woman's vagina, cervix, uterus, or fallopian tubes for long periods with no apparent symptoms other than an occasional slight fever. Thus, a woman can be unaware that she has been infected and that she may be infecting her sexual partners.

Upon diagnosis, an antibiotic regimen using penicillin, tetracycline, spectiomycin, ceftriaxone, or other drugs is begun. A penicillin-resistant form of gonorrhea may require a particularly strong combination of antibiotics. Treatment is generally completely effective within a short period of time if the disease is detected early.

If the disease goes undetected in a woman, it can spread throughout the genital–urinary tract to the fallopian tubes and ovaries, causing sterility—or, at the very least, severe inflammation and pelvic inflammatory disease symptoms. If an infected woman becomes pregnant, the disease can cause conjunctivitis in her infant. In the past, to prevent this, physicians and midwives routinely administered silver nitrate or penicillin preparations to the eyes of newborn babies. Currently, an antibiotic ointment or drops are used, not only to prevent the spread of STIs but also to prevent other eye infections that might result because of bacteria.

Untreated gonorrhea in the male can spread to the prostate, testicles, urinary tract, kidney, and bladder. Blockage of the vasa deferentia due to scar tissue formation can cause sterility. In some cases, the penis develops a painful curvature during erection.

Syphilis

Syphilis, the other well-known STI, is also caused by a bacterial organism, the spirochete known as *Treponema pallidum*. Because it is extremely delicate and dies quickly on exposure to air, dryness, or cold, the organism is generally transferred only through direct sexual contact. Typically, this means contact between sexual organs during intercourse, but in rare instances the organism enters the body through a break in the skin, through deep kissing in which body fluids are exchanged, or through some other transmission of body fluids.

Gonorrhea Second most common STI in Canada; if untreated, can cause sterility.

Syphilis An STI caused by a bacterial infection, cured with antibiotics, spread through direct sexual contact.

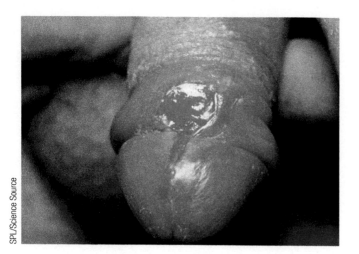

A chancre on the site of the initial infection is a symptom of primary syphilis.

With the arrival of HIV in the 1980s, syphilis took on new importance. It increases sexual transmission of HIV by six- to sevenfold, and neurosyphilis in HIV-infected patients is particularly difficult to treat. Early detection and treatment of STIs can have a major impact on the sexual transmission of HIV2-9. Because of this synergy, syphilis control can have a significant impact on the HIV epidemic in Canada (Health Canada, 1999).

Syphilis is called the "great imitator" because its symptoms resemble those of several other diseases. Only an astute physician who has reason to suspect the presence of the disease will order the appropriate tests for a diagnosis. Unlike most of the other STIs, syphilis generally progresses through several distinct stages.

Primary Syphilis

The first stage of syphilis, particularly for males, is often characterized by the development of a sore known as a **chancre** (pronounced "shank-er"), located most frequently at the site of the initial infection. This chancre is usually about the size of a dime and is painless, but it oozes bacteria, ready to spread to an unsuspecting partner. Usually the chancre appears between three and four weeks after contact.

In males, the site of the chancre tends to be the penis or scrotum because this is where the organism first made entry into the body. But, if the infection was contracted through oral sex, the sore can appear in the mouth, throat, or other "first contact" area. In females, the site of infection is often internal, on the vaginal wall or high on the cervix. Because the chancre is not readily apparent, the likelihood of detection is not great. In males and females, the chancre will completely disappear in three to six weeks.

Chancre Sore often found at the site of syphilis infection.

Secondary Syphilis

From a month to a year after the chancre disappears, secondary symptoms may appear, including a rash or white patches on the skin or on the mucous membranes of the mouth, throat, or genitals. Hair loss can occur, lymph nodes can become enlarged, and the individual infected might run a slight fever or develop a headache. In rare cases, sores develop around the mouth or genitals. As during the active chancre phase, these sores contain infectious bacteria, and contact with them can spread the disease. In some people, symptoms follow a textbook pattern; in others, there are no symptoms at all. In a few cases, there may be arthritic pain in the joints. Because symptoms vary so much and because the symptoms that do appear are so far removed from previous sexual experience that the individual infected seldom connects the two, the infection often goes undetected even at this second stage. Symptoms may persist for a few weeks or months and then disappear; thus, many individuals do not realize they have syphilis.

Latent Syphilis

The syphilis spirochetes begin to invade body organs after the secondary stage. There may be periodic reappearance of previous symptoms, including the presence of infectious lesions, for between two and four years after the secondary period. After this period, the infection is rarely transmitted to others, except during pregnancy, when it can be passed on to the fetus. The child will then be born with congenital syphilis, which can cause death or severe birth defects such as blindness, deafness, or disfigurement. Because in most cases the fetus does not become infected until after the first trimester, treatment of the mother during this period will usually prevent infection of the fetus.

In some instances, a child born to an infected mother will show no apparent signs of the disease at birth but within several weeks will develop body rashes, a runny nose, and symptoms of paralysis. Congenital syphilis is usually detected before it progresses much further. But sometimes the child's immune system will ward off the invading organism, and further symptoms may not surface until the teenage years.

In addition to causing congenital syphilis, latent syphilis, if untreated, will continue to progress, infecting more and more organs until the infection reaches its final stage, late syphilis.

Late Syphilis

Most of the horror stories concerning syphilis involve the late stages of the infection. Years after syphilis has entered the body and progressed through the various organs, its net effects become clearly evident. Late-stage syphilis symptoms include heart damage, central nervous system damage, blindness, deafness, paralysis, premature senility, and, ultimately, insanity.

Treatment for Syphilis

Treatment for syphilis is similar to that for gonorrhea. Because the organism is bacterial, it is treated with antibiotics, usually penicillin, penicillin G benzathine, or doxycycline. Although typically diagnosed through a swab of the area, blood tests are administered to determine the exact nature of the invading organism, and the doses of antibiotics are much stronger than those taken by the typical gonorrhea patient. The major obstacle to treatment is misdiagnosis of this "imitator" disease.

Pubic Lice

Often called "crabs," **pubic lice** are more annoying than dangerous. Pubic lice are small parasites usually transmitted during sexual contact. Pubic lice prefer the dark, moist regions of the body and, during vaginal and anal sex, move easily from partner to partner. Pubic lice are typically between 1.1 and 1.8 mm in length and attach most often to hair in the pubic region, though they can attach to the coarse hair of the body, such as eyebrows, eyelashes, underarm hair, mustache, or beard (MedicineNet.com, n.d.). Although sexual contact is the most common mode of transmission, it is possible to become infected with pubic lice from close personal contact with towels, linens, or clothing from an infected person. It is not likely that pubic lice can be transmitted from toilet seats given that the nits or larvae require a warm human body to survive (MedicineNet.com, n.d.).

Venereal Warts

Venereal warts (also known as genital warts or condylomas) are caused by a small group of viruses known as human papilloma viruses (HPVs). A person becomes infected when an HPV penetrates the skin and mucous membranes of the genitals or anus through sexual contact. The virus appears to be relatively easy to catch. The typical incubation period is from six to eight weeks. Many people have no apparent symptoms, particularly if the warts are located inside the reproductive tract. Others may develop a series of itchy bumps on the genitals, which range in size from a small pinhead to large cauliflower-like growths that can obstruct normal urinary or reproductive activity. On dry skin (such as on the shaft of the penis), the warts are commonly small, hard,

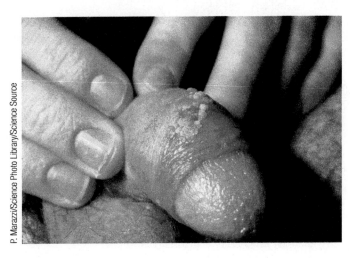

Genital warts are caused by the human papilloma virus and can be full blown or flat.

and yellowish-grey, resembling warts that appear on other parts of the body. Venereal warts are of two different types: (1) full-blown genital warts noticeable as tiny bumps or growths, and (2) the much more prevalent flat warts not usually visible to the naked eye.

Risks of Venereal Warts

Many venereal warts will eventually disappear without treatment. Others will grow and generate unsightly flaps of irregular flesh on the external genitalia. The greatest threat from venereal warts may be in the apparent relationship between them and a tendency for dysplasia, or changes in cells that may lead to a precancerous condition, usually on the cervix. Exactly how HPV infection leads to cervical or oropharyngeal cancer is uncertain. What is known is that within five years of infection, 30 percent of all HPV cases progress to the precancerous stage. Of those cases that become precancerous and are left untreated, 70 percent will eventually result in cancer. As mentioned previously in Chapter 12, a vaccination is now available for young women and men to protect them from the HPV. In addition, venereal warts can pose a threat to a pregnant woman's unborn fetus if the fetus is exposed to the virus during birth. Caesarean deliveries may be considered in serious cases.

Treatment for Venereal Warts

Treatment for venereal warts may take several forms:

1. Warts are painted with a medication called podophyllin during a visit to the doctor's office. The podophyllin is washed off

Pubic lice Parasites that most often cling to pubic hair; also called "crabs."

Venereal warts Warts that appear in the genital area or the anus; caused by the human papilloma viruses (HPVs).

Student

Health
TODAY

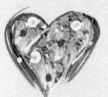

HPV Vaccines

Most sexually active people will contract some form of human papillomavirus (HPV) at some time in their lives, though they may never even know it. There are about 40 types of sexually transmitted HPV, most of which cause no symptoms and go away on their own. Low-risk types can cause genital warts, but some high-risk types can cause cervical cancer in women and other less common genital cancers—such as cancers of the anus, vagina, and vulva (area around the opening of the vagina). It was estimated by the Canadian Cancer Society (2012) in their annual report that there would be 1350 new cases and 390 women would die as a result of cervical cancer. There are currently two HPV vaccines (Cervarix™ or Gardasil®) that can help prevent women from becoming infected with HPV and subsequently developing cervical cancer.

- HPV vaccines are recommended for 9- to 13-year-old girls. It is also recommended for girls and women aged 13 through 26 who have not yet been vaccinated or completed the vaccine series. Ideally, females should get a vaccine before they become sexually active. Females who are sexually active may get less benefit from it, because they may have already gotten an HPV type targeted by the vaccines. However, they would still get protection from those types they have not yet contracted.
- One of the HPV vaccines, Gardasil®, is also licensed, safe, and effective for males aged 9 through 26 years (see Health Canada's recommendations that follow). Boys and young men may choose to get this vaccine to prevent genital warts.
- The vaccines (Cervarix™ or Gardasil®) have been widely tested in girls and women ages 9 through 45 years.
- Because the HPV vaccine is relatively new, some first-year college or university students who are eligible for vaccination have not yet received it. If you are one of these individuals, you should speak to your doctor about it.
- Both Cervarix™ and Gardasil® are very effective against high-risk HPV types 16 and 18, which cause 70 percent of cervical cancer cases. Although both vaccines are made with very small parts of the human papillomavirus, they cannot cause infection with HPV. Both vaccines are given as shots with three doses required for complete immunity.
- It should be pointed out that only Gardasil® protects against low-risk HPV types 6 and 11. These HPV types cause 90 percent of cases of genital warts in females and males, so Gardasil is approved for use with males as well as females.
- Neither Cervarix™ nor Gardasil® protect against all types of HPV, so they cannot prevent all cases of cervical cancer. About 30 percent of cervical cancers will not be prevented by the vaccines, so it is still important for sexually active women to continue screening for cervical cancer (through regular Pap tests). Also, the vaccines do not prevent other sexually transmitted infections (STIs), so it is still important for sexually active persons to protect themselves from other STIs.
- Based on an extensive review of the 2007 recommendations made by the National Advisory Committee on Immunizations, Health Canada (2012) has authorized use of HPV4 and HPV2 (Cervarix™ or Gardasil®) in the following ways:

1. HPV vaccine (Cervarix™ or Gardasil®) is recommended for females between 9 and 13 years of age
2. HPV vaccine (Cervarix™ or Gardasil®) is recommended for females between 14 and 26 years of age
3. HPV vaccine (Cervarix™ or Gardasil®) is recommended for females between 14 and 26 years of age who have had previous Pap abnormalities, including cervical cancer and EGW
4. HPV vaccine (Cervarix™ or Gardasil®) may be administered to females over 26 years of age (up to age 45 years)
5. HPV vaccine (HPV2 or HPV4) is not recommended in females under the age of 9 years
6. HPV4 (Gardasil®) is recommended in males between 9 and 26 years of age for the prevention of anal intraepithelial neoplasia (AIN) grades 1, 2, and 3, anal cancer, and anogenital warts

Sources: Based on Dawar, M., Harris, T., & McNeil, S. (prepared report, report approved by NACI). Canada Communicable Disease Report January 2012, Volume 38. An update on Human Papillomavirus (HPV) Vaccines, retrieved on May 6, 2013 from www.phac-aspc.gc.ca/publicat/ccdr-rmtc/12vol38/acs-dcc-1/assets/pdf/acs-dcc-1-eng.pdf. Centers for Disease Control and Prevention, "Vaccines and Preventable Diseases: HPV Vaccine— Questions & Answers," Reviewed April 2011, www.cdc.gov/vaccines/vpd-vac/hpv/vac-faqs.htm; American Cancer Society, 2009, "Human Papillomavirus (HPV), Cancer and HPV Vaccines—Frequently Asked Questions," Revised October 2009, www.cancer.org/Cancer/CancerCauses/OtherCarcinogens/InfectiousAgents/HPV/HumanPapillomaVirusandHPVVaccinesFAQ/hpv-faq.

after about four hours, and a few days later the warts begin to dry up and fall off. Sometimes more than one application is necessary. This procedure is relatively painless.

2. Warts may be removed by cryosurgery, a procedure in which an instrument treated with liquid nitrogen is held to the affected area, "freezing" the tissue. Within a few days, the warts fall off. This procedure can be painful.

3. Depending on size and location, some warts are removed by simple excision.

4. For larger warts, laser surgery is often used. This is a major procedure that normally requires general anesthesia. The frequency of laser use for wart removal is currently questioned by many health experts. (Precautions must also be taken during this procedure to shield medical staff from infection by viral spray.)

5. Creams containing 5-Fluoracil (an anticancer drug) are used to prevent further precancerous cell development.

6. For warts located externally, injections of interferon are sometimes given to keep the virus from spreading to healthy tissue. This treatment shows promise, but it is expensive and, when administered in large doses, can cause flu-like symptoms.

Prevention is clearly a better approach. What is true about protecting yourself from HIV infection is also true about protecting yourself from genital warts and other STIs (see the section on AIDS prevention later in this chapter).

Candidiasis (Moniliasis)

Unlike many of the other STIs caused by pathogens that come from outside the body, the yeast-like fungus caused by the *Candida albicans* organism normally inhabits the vaginal tract in most women. Only under certain conditions will these organisms multiply to abnormal quantities and begin to cause problems.

The likelihood of **candidiasis** (also known as moniliasis) is greatest if a woman has diabetes, if her immune system is overtaxed or malfunctioning, if she is taking birth control pills or other hormones, if she is pregnant, or if she is taking broad-spectrum antibiotics. All of the above factors decrease the acidity of the vagina, making conditions more favourable for the development of a yeast-like infection.

Symptoms of candidiasis include severe vaginal itching, a white, cheesy discharge, swelling of the vaginal tissue due to irritation, and a burning sensation. These symptoms are often collectively called **vaginitis**. When this microbe infects the mouth, whitish patches form and the condition is referred to as thrush.

This monilial infection also occurs in males and is easily transmitted between sexual partners.

Antifungal drugs applied on the surface or by suppository usually cure the infection in a few days. For approximately 10 percent of women, however, nothing seems to work, and the organism returns again and again. In women with this chronically recurring infection, symptoms are often aggravated by contact of the vagina with soaps, douches, perfumed toilet paper, chlorinated water, and spermicides. Further, tight-fitting jeans and pantyhose can provide the combination of moisture and irritant the organism thrives on. Some women report that a "natural" treatment with probiotics (yogurt or acidophilus capsules, either taken orally or used as a vaginal suppository) is effective for this problem.

Trichomoniasis

Unlike many of the other STIs, **trichomoniasis** is caused by a protozoan. Often infected individuals remain symptom free until their bodily defences are weakened. Men and women may transmit the disease, but women are the more likely candidates for infection. The "trich" infection can cause a foamy, yellowish discharge with an unpleasant odour that may be accompanied by a burning sensation, itching, and painful urination. These symptoms are most likely to occur during or shortly after menstruation, but they can appear at any time or be absent altogether. Treatment includes oral metronidazole, usually given to both sexual partners to avoid the possible "ping-pong" effect of repeated cross-infection typical of STIs.

General Urinary Tract Infections

Although general urinary tract infections (UTIs) can be caused by various factors, some forms are sexually transmitted. Any time invading organisms enter the genital area, there is a risk that they may travel up the urethra and enter the bladder. Similarly, organisms normally living in the rectum, urethra, or bladder can travel to the sexual organs and eventually be transmitted to another person.

You can also get a UTI through autoinoculation (transmission to yourself by yourself). This frequently occurs during the simple task of wiping yourself after defecating. Wiping from the anus forward may transmit organisms found in feces to the vaginal opening or to the urethra. Contact between the

Candidiasis Yeast-like fungal disease often transmitted sexually.

Vaginitis Set of symptoms characterized by vaginal itching, swelling, and burning.

Trichomoniasis Protozoan infection characterized by foamy, yellowish discharge and unpleasant odour.

hands and the urethra and between the urethra and other objects are also common means of autoinoculation of bacterial and viral pathogens. Women, with their shorter urethras, are more likely to contract UTIs. Treatment depends on the nature and type of pathogen.

Herpes

Herpes is a general term for a family of diseases characterized by sores or eruptions on the skin. Herpes infections range from mildly uncomfortable to extremely serious. One subcategory, herpes simplex, is caused by a virus. Herpes simplex virus type 1 (HSV-1) causes the cold sores and fever blisters that most of us have experienced at one time or another. The herpes simplex virus (HSV) is one of the most common infectious agents in Canada though its annual rates of infection are not actually known (Public Health Agency of Canada, 2013b). Still, it is believed that HSV infection has overtaken bacterial STI infection as the most common cause of genital ulceration worldwide. HSV-2 (genital herpes) is not a reportable STI in Canada; therefore, we have little baseline data available (Public Health Agency of Canada, 2013b; Rotermann et al., 2013). The data we do have suggest that genital herpes is as great a concern in Canada as in the rest of the world.

Genital herpes, caused by herpes simplex virus type 2 (HSV-2), is one of the most widespread STIs in the world. Typically, genital herpes is characterized by distinct phases. First, the herpes virus must gain entrance to the body, which it usually does through the mucous membranes of the genital area. Once these organisms invade, the infected individual will experience the prodromal (precursor) phase of the disease, characterized by a burning sensation and redness at the site of the infection. This phase is typically followed by the formation of a small blister filled with a clear fluid containing the virus. If you pick at this blister or otherwise spread this clear fluid with your hands, you can autoinoculate other body parts. Particularly dangerous is the possibility of spreading the infection to your eyes this way, because a herpes lesion on the eye can cause blindness.

Over a period of days, this unsightly blister will crust, dry, disappear, and the virus will travel to the base of an affected nerve supplying the area and become dormant. Only when the individual infected becomes overly stressed, when dietary intake is inadequate, when the immune system is overworked, or when there is excessive exposure to sunlight or other stressors will the virus reactivate (at the same site every time) and begin the blistering cycle all

Genital herpes STI caused by herpes simplex virus type 2.

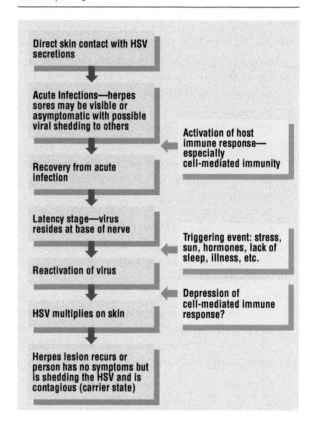

FIGURE 13.3

The Herpes Cycle

Direct skin contact with HSV secretions

Acute Infections—herpes sores may be visible or asymptomatic with possible viral shedding to others

Activation of host immune response— especially cell-mediated immunity

Recovery from acute infection

Latency stage—virus resides at base of nerve

Triggering event: stress, sun, hormones, lack of sleep, illness, etc.

Reactivation of virus

Depression of cell-mediated immune response?

HSV multiplies on skin

Herpes lesion recurs or person has no symptoms but is shedding the HSV and is contagious (carrier state)

over again. This cyclical recurrence can be painful, unsightly, and, most important, highly contagious. Fluids from these blisters can readily be transmitted to sexual partners. Through oral sex, herpes simplex type 2 can be transmitted to the mouth. Symptoms are similar to those of herpes simplex type 1. Figure 13.3 summarizes the herpes cycle.

Genital herpes is especially serious in pregnant women because of the danger of infecting the baby as it passes through the vagina during birth. For that reason, women who have herpes should be prescribed antiviral drugs before delivery; if they have active lesions at the time of labour, a Caesarean section will be recommended (Society of Obstetricians and Gynecologists of Canada, 2008). Additionally, women with a history of genital herpes also have a greater risk of developing cervical cancer.

Although there is no cure for herpes at present, certain drugs have shown some success in reducing symptoms. Unfortunately, they seem to work only if the infection is confirmed during the first few hours after contact. As you may guess, this is rather rare. In recent years, some treatments have been shown to be effective in managing herpes outbreaks. Although lip balms and cold-sore medications can provide

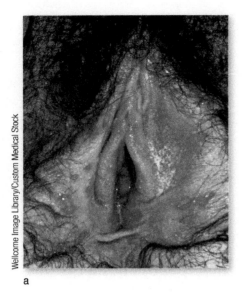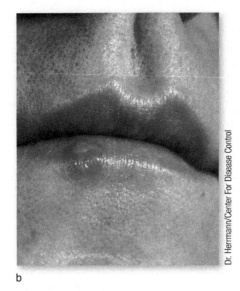

a. Genital herpes is a highly contagious and incurable STI. It is characterized by recurring cycles of painful blisters on the genitalia. b. Oral herpes, caused by the same virus as genital herpes, is extremely contagious and can cause painful sores and blisters around the mouth.

temporary anesthetic relief, it is useful to remember that rubbing anything on a herpes blister may spread herpes-laden fluids to other tissues or, via the hands, to other body parts.

Preventing Herpes

To prevent contracting or spreading the herpes virus, these precautions should be followed:

- Avoid any form of kissing if you notice a sore or blister on your or your partner's mouth. Kiss no one, not even a peck on the cheek, if you know that you have a herpes lesion. Allow a bit of time after the sores go away before you start kissing again.

- Be extremely cautious if you hook up frequently (i.e., have casual sex with different partners). Not every partner will feel obligated to tell you that he or she may have an STI. Protecting yourself against an infection is up to you.

- Wash your hands immediately with soap and water after any form of sexual contact.

- If you have herpes, reduce the risk of a herpes episode by avoiding excessive stress, sunlight, or whatever else appears to trigger a herpes outbreak in you.

- If you have questionable sores or lesions, seek medical help at once. Do not be afraid to name those you had sex with.

- Since the herpes organism dies quickly upon exposure to air, toilet seats, soap, and similar sources are not likely means of transmission.

- If you have herpes, be responsible in your sexual contact with others. If you have herpes lesions that put your partner at risk, let that person know. Although it is not necessary to announce openly a herpes problem, use common sense in determining the appropriate time and place for a candid herpes discussion with your partner.

ACQUIRED IMMUNE DEFICIENCY SYNDROME (AIDS)

Acquired immune deficiency syndrome (AIDS) is aptly named because it is a disease that is acquired. Since the virus suppresses the immune system, it is termed *immuno* and renders the body's immune system deficient; therefore, *deficiency* is the third word. Finally, because the symptoms of AIDS all occur together, it is called a *syndrome* (AIDS.GOV, 2012).

Since 1981, when the first case of AIDS was diagnosed, the number of AIDS-diagnosed individuals and people infected with **human immunodeficiency virus (HIV)** has skyrocketed in North America and worldwide. Few regions of the world have been spared.

Acquired immune deficiency syndrome (AIDS) Extremely virulent STI that renders the immune system inoperative.

Human immunodeficiency virus (HIV) The slow-acting virus that causes AIDS.

It has been estimated that more than 21 million people have died as a result of AIDS and that 57 million individuals had been infected with HIV. The World Health Organization (2015b) reported that in 2014 approximately 36.9 million people were living with HIV and/or AIDS. Individuals living in countries in southern and central Africa and South Asia account for three-quarters of these infections.

According to the Public Health Agency of Canada (2015c), 71 300 Canadians were living with HIV and/or AIDS in 2014. This is equivalent to 7.2 per 100 000 population. Of these cases nearly half (49.3 percent) acquired their infection through men having sex with men. Heterosexual contact was the next highest group at 18.7 percent, followed by injection drug users at 10.5 percent. One population group of particular concern in Canada is Aboriginal people as the rates are particularly high at 448 per 100 000 population (Public Health Agency of Canada, 2015c). Note that the actual number of individuals in Canada living with HIV is expected to be higher than these reported numbers because not all individuals infected with HIV have actually been tested for it (Public Health Agency of Canada, 2015c).

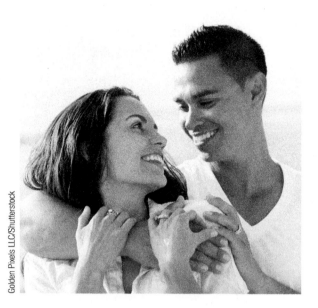

Golden Pixels LLC/Shutterstock

You cannot tell if someone has an STI, including HIV, just by looking at him or her. Being open and honest with your partners (and expecting the same from them) about sexual history and STI testing is an important part of prevention.

How HIV Is Transmitted

HIV typically enters the body when another person's infected body fluids (semen, vaginal secretions, blood, and so on) gain entry through a breach in body defences. Mucous membranes of the genital organs and the anus provide the easiest route of entry. If there is a break in the mucous membranes (as can occur during sexual intercourse, particularly anal intercourse), the virus enters and begins to multiply. After initial infection, the HIV typically begins to multiply rapidly in the body, invading the bloodstream and cerebrospinal fluid. It progressively destroys helper T-lymphocytes, weakening the body's resistance to disease. The virus also changes the genetic structure of the cells it attacks. In response to this invasion, the body quickly begins to produce antibodies.

HIV is not a highly contagious virus. Many studies of people living in households with a person with HIV/AIDS have turned up no documented cases of HIV infection due to casual contact (National Institute of Allergy and Infectious Diseases, 2005). Other investigations provide overwhelming evidence that insect bites do not transmit the virus. In fact, the virus is actually quite selective in the way it transmits itself from person to person.

Engaging in High-Risk Behaviours

HIV is not a disease of certain groups. People are not predestined to get the disease because they belong to a group or associate with a group. Thus, HIV is not a gay disease, or a disease of minority groups, or Haitians, or any other class of people. It is a disease that can result when you engage in high-risk behaviours. In other words, if you engage in these behaviours, you increase your risk for the disease. If you do not engage in these behaviours, your risk is minimal. Promiscuous sex—in males and females of all ages, ethnicities, sexual orientations, and socioeconomic conditions—is the greatest threat. Anyone who engages in unprotected sex at any time with a person who has engaged in high-risk behaviours is at risk. A celibate or monogamous gay man or a drug-injecting woman who never shares her needles is at very low risk for HIV. But a person who has had sex with someone who has, even once, had sex with an injecting drug user could be infected. You cannot tell by looking at someone; you cannot tell by questioning, unless the person has been tested recently and is HIV-negative.

Of course, the best method of protection is abstinence. If you do not exchange body fluids, you will not get the disease. As a second line of defence, your best option is to use a condom when you choose to be intimate. The following sections describe high-risk behaviours or situations.

Exchange of Body Fluids

The exchange of HIV-infected body fluids during sexual intercourse is the greatest risk factor. Substantial research indicates that blood, semen, and vaginal, cervical, and anal secretions are the major fluids involved. Although the virus was found in one person's saliva, saliva is not considered a high-risk body fluid.

Initially, breast milk was also considered a high-risk fluid because a small number of infants apparently contracted HIV while breastfeeding. However, the HIV transmission could have been caused by bleeding nipples rather than actual consumption of breast milk. Infection through contact with feces and urine is believed to be highly unlikely, though technically possible.

Receiving a Blood Transfusion Prior to 1986

A small group of people became infected with HIV as a result of a blood transfusion before 1986. Since then, the Canadian Red Cross has implemented a stringent testing program for all donated blood. Canada's blood supply is now controlled by Canadian Blood Services, which screens donors for a number of potential risks. Because of these massive screening efforts, the risk of receiving HIV-infected blood or any other blood-borne pathogen is almost nonexistent.

Injecting Drugs

Another source of infection is sharing or using HIV-contaminated needles. Injection drug use (IDU) has increasingly been a route of HIV transmission in Canada. As previously mentioned, in 2011, the percentage of new HIV infections in Canada estimated as a result of IDU was 17 percent (Public Health Agency of Canada, 2011b). This number has decreased significantly over the years due to increased attention focused on preventing HIV transmission in IDU, including various programs that distribute new and unused needles for free.

While illegal drug users are the people we usually think of in this category, it is important to remember that others may also share needles—for example, individuals with type 1 diabetes who inject insulin. People who share needles and engage in sexual activities with members of high-risk groups, such as those who exchange sex for drugs, increase their risks dramatically. Any needle prick with an HIV-contaminated needle provides a risk of infection. Thus, tattooing, body piercing, and any practice using unsterilized needles presents a potential risk. Similarly, dentists or physicians who work with HIV-positive individuals have increased risk of infection should there be any fluid transfer such as what might occur if their surgical gloves became torn and there were a cut or abrasion in the skin beneath.

Mother-to-Infant Transmission (Perinatal)

Infants can contract HIV from their infected mothers while in the womb or while passing through the vaginal tract during delivery.

Reducing Your Risks for HIV

Contracting HIV is not uncontrollable. HIV cannot, like cold or flu viruses, be caught casually. The transmission of HIV depends upon specific, generally high-risk, behaviours. Therefore, HIV infection can be prevented. The following suggestions will help you to reduce your risk:

- Avoid casual sexual partners. Ideally, have sex only in a long-term, mutually monogamous relationship and with a partner whose HIV status is known to be negative.

- Avoid unprotected sexual activity with people whose present or past behaviours put them (and ultimately you) at risk for infection. Do not be afraid to ask intimate questions about your partner's sexual history and past injection drug use. You have a right to know. You should also be willing to share similar information with your partner. You expose yourself to your partner's history whenever you choose to have sexual relations. Postpone sexual involvement until you are assured that he or she is not infected.

- Sexually active adults not in a lifelong monogamous relationship should practise safer sex by using latex condoms. Although, condoms do not provide 100-percent protection, they are the only protection available other than abstinence.

- Do not share injecting needles with anyone for any reason.

- Do not share any devices through which the exchange of blood could occur, including needles, razors, tattoo instruments, any body-piercing instruments, and any other sharp objects.

- Avoid injury to body tissue during sexual activity. HIV can enter the bloodstream through microscopic tears in anal or vaginal tissues.

- Avoid unprotected oral sex or any sexual activity in which semen, blood, or vaginal secretions could penetrate mucous membranes through breaks in the membrane. Always use a condom or a dental dam during all kinds of sex.

- Avoid using drugs that might dull your senses and affect your ability to make decisions about responsible precautions with potential sex partners.

- Wash your hands before and after sexual encounters. Urinate after sexual relations and, if possible, wash your genitals.

- Although total abstinence is the only absolute means of preventing the sexual transmission of HIV, abstinence can be a difficult choice to make. If you are in doubt about the potential risks of having sex, consider other means of intimacy, at least until you can ensure your safety. Enjoyable and safer alternatives include massage, dry kissing, hugging, holding and touching, and masturbation (alone or with a partner).

- When receiving care from medical professionals such as dentists or doctors, make sure they take appropriate precautions to prevent potential transmission, including washing their hands and wearing gloves and masks. Be sure that all equipment used for treatment is sterilized.

- If you are worried about your own HIV status, get tested!

- If you are a woman and HIV-positive, you should take the steps necessary to ensure that you do not become pregnant. However, in the event that a female infected with HIV does become pregnant, there a number of measures that can be taken to reduce the risk of HIV transmission from the mother to her infant.

- If you suspect that you may be infected or if you test positive for HIV antibodies, do not donate blood, semen, or body organs.

Symptoms of the Disease

A person may go for months or years after acquiring HIV before any significant symptoms appear. The incubation time varies greatly from person to person. Children have shorter incubation periods than adults. Newborns and infants are particularly vulnerable to HIV infection because they are not fully immunocompetent (that is, their immune system is not fully developed) until they are 6 to 15 months old. New information suggests that some very young children show the "adult" progression of the disease. In adults, the average length of time it takes the virus to cause the slow, degenerative changes in the immune system that result in AIDS is 10 years (Public Health Agency of Canada, 2012c). During this time, the person may experience a large number of opportunistic infections (infections that gain a foothold when the immune system is not functioning effectively). Colds, sore throats, fever, tiredness, nausea, night sweats, and other generally non-life-threatening conditions commonly appear.

Testing for HIV Antibodies

ELISA Blood test that detects the presence of antibodies to HIV.

Western blot More precise test than the ELISA to confirm presence of HIV antibodies.

Once antibodies have begun to form in reaction to the presence of HIV, a blood test known as the **ELISA** test might detect their presence. If sufficient antibodies are present, this test will be positive. When a person who previously tested negative (no HIV antibodies present) has a subsequent test that is positive, "seroconversion" is said to have occurred. In such a situation, the person would typically take another ELISA test, followed by a more expensive, more precise test known as the **Western blot**, to confirm the presence of HIV antibodies.

Although the ELISA is viewed as quite accurate, it is a conservative test in that it errs on the side of caution, meaning that it produces a large number of false positive results. It was deliberately designed to do this because it was intended as a test for screening the blood supply. There have also been instances of false negative results. Some health professionals believe there are chronic carriers of HIV who, for unknown reasons, continually show false negative results on the ELISA and the Western blot test. False negative HIV tests raise serious concerns about risks for these people's sexual partners. It should be noted that these tests are not AIDS tests per se. Rather, they detect antibodies for the disease, indicating the presence of HIV in the person's system. Whether or not the person will develop AIDS depends to some extent on the strength of the immune system. However, the vast majority of infected people do develop some form of the disease.

As testing for HIV antibodies improves, scientists have explored ways of making it easier for individuals to be tested. Health officials distinguish between reported and actual cases of HIV infection because it is believed that many people who are HIV-positive avoid being tested. One reason is fear of knowing the truth. Another is the fear of negative consequences or judgmental attitudes from employers, insurance companies, and health professionals. However, early detection and reporting are important, because immediate treatment for someone in the early stages of HIV infection is critical and necessary to prevent further spread of the virus.

Preventing HIV Infection

Although scientists have been searching for more than a decade for a vaccine to protect people from HIV infection, one has not been found. The only known effective prevention strategies relate to the means by which people contract HIV. HIV infection and AIDS are not uncontrollable conditions. As previously mentioned, you can reduce your risks by making responsible choices in your sexual and drug use behaviours.

Because the status of your immune system is an important factor in whether you are susceptible to any of the STIs, it is important that you do everything possible to protect yourself. Engaging in physical activity regularly, eating a healthy diet, getting enough sleep, managing your stress, taking time for yourself, ensuring that your vaccinations are up-to-date, and taking other preventive measures can do a great deal to ensure your long-term health.

NONINFECTIOUS DISEASES

Like others, you may think that the major ailments and diseases that affect people today are diseases such as cancer and heart disease. Although these diseases capture much of the media attention, you should be aware of other forms of chronic disease that also have the potential to cause substantial pain, suffering, and disability. Similar to heart disease and cancer, the majority of these diseases can be prevented or at the very least delayed.

To prevent or postpone the development of certain noninfectious and chronic diseases, you must identify their common characteristics. These diseases are not transmitted by any pathogen or by any form of personal contact. They usually develop over a long period of time, and result in progressive damage to human tissues. Although these conditions normally do not necessarily cause death, they can result in illness and considerable suffering. Lifestyle and personal health habits appear to be major contributing factors to the general increase observed in the incidence of chronic diseases in Canada in recent years. Education, reasonable changes in lifestyle behaviours, and public health efforts aimed at prevention and control could minimize the effects of many of these diseases.

RESPIRATORY DISORDERS

Allergy-Induced Problems

An **allergy** occurs as a part of the body's attempt to defend itself against a specific antigen or allergen by producing antibodies in response to its presence. When foreign pathogens such as bacteria or viruses invade the body, the body responds by producing antibodies to destroy them. Under normal conditions, the production of antibodies is a positive element in the body's defence system. However, for unknown reasons, in some people the body overreacts by developing an overly elaborate protective mechanism against relatively harmless allergens or antigens. The resultant hypersensitivity reaction to specific allergens or antigens in the environment is fairly common, as you can testify to if you have ever awakened with a runny nose or itchy eyes. Most commonly, these hypersensitive, or allergic, responses occur as a reaction to environmental antigens such as moulds, animal dander (hair and dead skin), pollen, ragweed, or dust. Once excessive antibodies to these antigens are produced, they trigger the release of **histamines**, chemical substances that dilate blood vessels, increase mucous secretions, cause tissues to swell, and produce other allergy-like symptoms (see Figure 13.4).

Although many people think of allergies as childhood diseases, in reality allergies

Allergy Hypersensitive reaction to a specific antigen or allergen in the environment in which the body produces excessive antibodies.

Histamines Chemical substances that dilate blood vessels, increase mucous secretions, and produce other allergy-like symptoms.

FIGURE 13.4

Steps of an Allergy Response

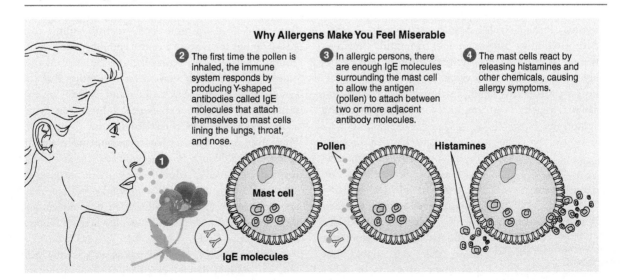

Why Allergens Make You Feel Miserable

2 The first time the pollen is inhaled, the immune system responds by producing Y-shaped antibodies called IgE molecules that attach themselves to mast cells lining the lungs, throat, and nose.

3 In allergic persons, there are enough IgE molecules surrounding the mast cell to allow the antigen (pollen) to attach between two or more adjacent antibody molecules.

4 The mast cells react by releasing histamines and other chemicals, causing allergy symptoms.

Pollen

Histamines

Mast cell

IgE molecules

tend to become progressively worse with time and with increased exposure to allergens. In these circumstances, allergic responses become chronic in nature, and treatment becomes difficult. Many people take allergy shots to reduce the severity of their symptoms. In most cases, once the offending antigen has disappeared, allergy-prone people suffer few symptoms. Although allergies cause numerous problems, the most significant are related to the immune system.

Hay Fever

Perhaps the best example of a chronic respiratory disease is **hay fever**. Usually considered a seasonally related disease (most prevalent when ragweed and flowers are blooming), hay fever is common throughout the world. Hay fever attacks, characterized by sneezing and itchy, watery eyes and nose, cause a great deal of misery for many people.

Hay fever appears to have a genetic component; thus, alterations to your lifestyle likely have little, if any, impact on its development. Instead, an overzealous immune system and an exposure to environmental allergens including pet dander, dust, pollen from various plants, and other substances appear to be the critical factors that determine vulnerability. For some people, a change in setting may help; for others, medical assistance in the form of injections or antihistamines may provide the only possibility of relief.

Asthma

If you suffer from hay fever, your condition may be complicated by the development of another chronic respiratory disease, **asthma**. Asthma is characterized by attacks of wheezing, difficulty breathing, shortness of breath, chest tightness, and coughing spasms (Public Health Agency of Canada, 2013a). Although most asthma attacks are mild, they can trigger bronchospasms (contractions of the bronchial tubes in the lungs) of such a severe nature that, unless treatment is rapid, death may occur. Between asthma attacks, you are likely to experience few symptoms.

Asthma attacks can be brought on by something as commonplace as engaging in moderate to vigorous physical activity. This type of asthma is called exercise-induced asthma (EIA). If you have EIA, it does not mean that you should not participate in sports or other

Hay fever A chronic respiratory disorder most prevalent when ragweed and flowers bloom.

Asthma A chronic respiratory disease characterized by attacks of wheezing, shortness of breath, and coughing spasms.

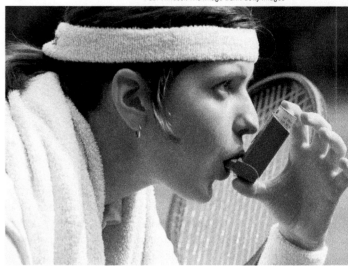

If you have exercise-induced asthma, you should be prepared for a reaction when engaged in physical activity.

physical activities, but rather that you should create a plan that allows you to take part while managing your asthma and its symptoms effectively.

Longitudinal research indicates that susceptibility to asthma is determined in utero and in the first three to five years of life (Public Health Agency of Canada, 2013a). This research has also identified the following risk factors:

- family history
- significant exposure to airborne allergens
- exposure to secondhand smoke, including in utero
- frequent respiratory infections early in life
- low birth weight and respiratory distress syndrome (Public Health Agency of Canada, 2013a).

Although women are more likely to have asthma than men, boys are more likely to have asthma than girls (Centers for Disease Control and Prevention, n.d.). Young adults are also more likely to be affected than older adults, providing support for the notion that you can outgrow asthma. Black adults and children are two times more likely to experience asthma than white adults and children (Centers for Disease Control and Prevention, n.d.). Further, socioeconomic status appears to have an influence in that individuals with a lower income and level of education are more likely to be affected. Finally, individuals who smoke and are obese are more likely to have asthma than nonsmokers and those at a healthy weight (Centers for Disease Control and Prevention, n.d.).

Although exposure to allergens such as dust, pollen, and animal dander can trigger many asthmatic episodes, emotional factors and excessive anxiety or stress can also trigger an attack. Relaxation techniques appear to help some individuals who have asthma. Drugs may be necessary for serious cases. Doctors warn against using over-the-counter inhalers without medical advice, as some over-the-counter products have serious side effects, depending on the type of asthma and other drugs used. Determining the specific allergen that provokes asthma attacks and taking steps to reduce your exposure, adjusting for triggers such as physical activity or stress, and finding the most effective medications are big steps in asthma control.

Emphysema

Emphysema involves the gradual destruction of the alveoli (tiny air sacs) of the lungs. As the **alveoli** are destroyed, the affected person finds it more and more difficult to exhale. The individual typically struggles to take in a fresh supply of air before the air held in the lungs has been expended. The chest cavity gradually begins to expand, producing the barrel-shaped chest characteristic of individuals with chronic emphysema.

The exact cause of emphysema is uncertain. Further, once established, little can be done to reverse its effects. There is, however, a strong relationship between the development of emphysema and long-term cigarette smoking and exposure to air pollution. Individuals with emphysema often suffer over a period of many years. What you likely take for granted—the easy, rhythmic flow of air in and out of your lungs—becomes a continuous struggle for people with emphysema. Inadequate oxygen supply, combined with the stress of overexertion on the heart, eventually takes its toll on the cardiovascular system and leads to premature death.

Chronic Bronchitis

Although often dismissed as "smoker's cough" or a bad case of the common cold, **chronic bronchitis** can be a serious, if not life-threatening, respiratory disorder. In this ailment, the bronchial tubes become so inflamed and swollen that normal respiratory function is impaired. Symptoms of chronic bronchitis include a productive cough and shortness of breath that persist for several weeks over the course of the year. Cigarette smoking is the major risk factor for this disease, although fumes, dust, and particulate matter in the air are also contributing factors. Individuals with chronic bronchitis must often use respiratory devices similar to those used by individuals with emphysema. They must also avoid factors—such as cigarette smoking—that contributed to the development of bronchitis. Bronchitis coupled with a severe cold can be serious enough to warrant immediate medical attention.

NEUROLOGICAL DISORDERS

Headaches

You most likely have experienced at least one major headache in your life, whether it is the mild, throbbing variety or the severe, pounding ache that makes you nauseated or dizzy. Not all headaches are equal, and more important, it is possible that not all headaches have the same cause, though all serious headaches may share the same basic causes and fall along a spectrum, with ordinary tension headaches at one end and full-blown migraines at the other (Allen, 1994). Headaches can result from dilated blood vessels within the brain, underlying organic problems, or excessive stress and anxiety. The following are the most common forms of headaches and the most effective methods of treatment.

Emphysema A respiratory disease in which the alveoli become distended or ruptured and no longer functional.

Alveoli Tiny air sacs of the lungs.

Chronic bronchitis A serious respiratory disorder in which the bronchial tubes become inflamed and swollen such that respiratory function is compromised.

Tension Headaches

Tension headaches are generally caused by muscle contractions or tension in the neck or head. This tension might

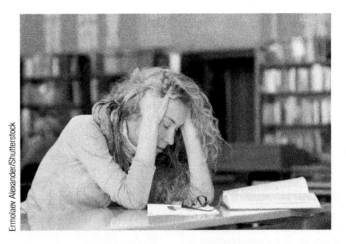

Tension headaches are triggered by many factors, including lack of sleep, stress, and strain on head and neck muscles.

be caused by actual strain placed on the neck or head muscles due to overuse, static positions held for long periods of time, or tension triggered by stress. The World Health Organization (2013b) noted that tension headaches are most likely a product of a more "generic mechanism" in which chemicals deep inside the brain cause the muscular tension, pain, and suffering often associated with them. Triggers for this chemical release might be red wine, lack of sleep, fasting, menstruation, or other factors, and the same symptoms (sensitivity to light and sound, nausea, and/or throbbing pain) may be characteristic of different types of headaches (World Health Organization, 2013b). Symptoms vary in intensity and duration. Relaxation, massage, quiet music, or a warm bubble bath may provide relief. Pain relievers such as Aspirin, Tylenol, and Advil may also provide relief.

Migraine Headaches

If you have ever experienced pulsating pain on one side of the head in combination with dizzy spells, nausea, and intolerance for light and noise, you probably suffer from **migraines**, a type of headache that has severe debilitating symptoms. Many migraine sufferers feel excruciatingly painful, recurring headaches that last for minutes, hours, or even days and may also experience some temporary visual impairment. Symptoms vary greatly by individual and typically last anywhere from 4 to 72 hours, with distinct phases. In about 20 percent of cases, migraines are preceded by a sensory warning sign known as an aura, such as flashes of light, flickering vision, blind spots, or tingling in the arms or legs, or sensations of odour or taste (National Headache Foundation, 2004). Symptoms of migraine include excruciating pain behind or around one eye and usually on the same side of the head. In some people, there is sinus pain, neck pain, or an aura without headache. Usually migraine incidence peaks in young adulthood (ages 20 to 45) although they commonly occur in those between 15 and 55 years of age and two to three times more frequently in women than men (Montgomery, n.d.; National Headache Foundation, 2004).

Migraines may occur when blood vessels dilate in the membrane that surrounds the brain. Historically, treatments centred on reversing or preventing this dilation. Critics of this theory question why only blood vessels of the head dilate in these circumstances. Others believe that migraines are started by disturbances that keep the pain-regulating chemical serotonin from doing its job.

Migraine A condition characterized by localized headaches that result from alternating dilation and constriction of blood vessels.

Epilepsy A neurological disorder caused by abnormal electrical brain activity; often accompanied by altered consciousness or convulsions.

When migraines occur, relaxation is minimally effective; rather, strong pain-relieving drugs prescribed by a physician are necessary.

Secondary Headaches

Secondary headaches arise as a result of some other underlying condition. An example is a person with a severe sinus blockage that causes pressure in the sinus cavity. This pressure can induce a headache. Hypertension, allergies, low blood sugar, diseases of the spine, the common cold, poorly fitted dentures, problems with eyesight, and other types of pain or injury can trigger this condition. Relaxation and pain relievers are of little help in treating secondary headaches. Rather, medications or other therapies designed to relieve the underlying organic cause of the headache must be included in the treatment regimen.

Psychological Headaches

With this type of headache, the "it's all in your head" diagnosis may, in fact, be correct. Rather than having a physical cause, psychological headaches stem from anxiety, depression, and other emotional factors. Psychological headaches result from the stress of emotional disturbances, particularly depression. Unlike tension headaches, no muscles or blood vessels appear to be involved, thereby making relaxation and painkillers ineffective as treatment. Only therapy designed to treat the underlying depression or emotional problem appears to be effective in reducing this kind of headache.

Seizure Disorders

The word **epilepsy** is derived from the Greek *epilepsia*, meaning "seizure." Reports of epilepsy appeared in Greek medical records as early as 300 BCE. Ancient peoples interpreted seizures as invasions of the body by evil spirits or as punishments by the gods. Although much of the mystery surrounding epileptic seizures has been solved in recent years, the stigma and lack of understanding remain. These disorders are generally caused by abnormal electrical activity in the brain and are characterized by loss of control of muscular activity and unconsciousness (World Health Organization, 2013a). Symptoms vary widely from person to person. There are several forms of seizure disorders. The most common are the following:

1. Grand mal, or major motor seizure: These seizures are often preceded by a shrill cry or a seizure aura (body sensations such as ringing in the ears or a

specific smell or taste). Convulsions and loss of consciousness generally occur and can last from 30 seconds to several minutes or more. Keeping track of the length of time elapsed is one aspect of first aid.

2. Petit mal, or minor seizure: These seizures involve no convulsions. Rather, a minor loss of consciousness that may go unnoticed occurs. Minor twitching of muscles may take place, usually for a shorter time than grand mal convulsions.

3. Psychomotor seizure: These seizures involve mental processes and muscular activity. Symptoms include mental confusion and a listless state characterized by activities such as lip smacking, chewing, and repetitive movements.

4. Jacksonian seizure: This is a progressive seizure that often begins in one part of the body, such as the fingers, and moves to other parts, such as the hand or arm. Usually only one side of the body is affected.

In the majority of cases, people with seizure disorders lead normal, seizure-free lives under medical supervision. Epilepsy is seldom fatal. The greatest risk for individuals with epilepsy whose seizures are uncontrolled is motor vehicle or other accidents. Public ignorance about these disorders is one of the most serious obstacles confronting individuals with seizure disorders. Improvements in medication and surgical interventions to reduce some causes of seizures are among the most promising treatments today.

SEX-RELATED DISORDERS

Fibrocystic Breast Disease

Fibrocystic breast disease, a common, noncancerous problem among women in Canada, is now referred to as generalized breast lumpiness (HealthLinkBC, 2013). Normal lumps in the breasts range in size from a small palpable lump to large masses of irregular tissue found in both breasts. Lumps can be found in either or both breasts around the nipple and in the upper, outer part of the breasts; these lumps can come and go and change size in just a few days (HealthLinkBC, 2013). The underlying causes of these lumps are unknown. Although some believe these breast lumps are related to hormonal changes during the normal menstrual cycle, many women report that their condition neither worsens nor improves during their cycles. In fact, in most cases, the condition appears to be genetic and becomes progressively worse with age, regardless of pregnancy or other hormonal disruptions, until menopause when

they often disappear (HealthLinkBC, 2013). Although the majority of these cyst formations consist of fibrous tissue, some are filled with fluid. Treatment often involves removal of fluid from the affected area or surgical removal of the cyst itself.

Premenstrual Syndrome (PMS)

Premenstrual syndrome (PMS) refers to as many as 150 physical and emotional symptoms that occur prior to menstruation in some women and vary from woman to woman and from month to month. It is estimated that as many as 80 percent of women experience a mild form of PMS and as many as 25 percent experience moderately severe symptoms (Kadian & O'Brien, 2012). It is further estimated that 3 to 8 percent of menstruating women experience a severe form of PMS called premenstrual dysphoric disorder (Kadian & O'Brien, 2012). These symptoms usually begin a week to 10 days before the menstrual period and include depression, tension, irritability, headaches, tender breasts, bloated abdomen, backache, abdominal cramps, acne, fluid retention, diarrhea, and fatigue. It is believed that women with PMS develop a predictable pattern of symptoms during the menstrual cycle and that the severity of their symptoms is influenced by external factors, such as stress.

Women usually experience PMS for the first time after the age of 20, though younger women can experience it too, and it may remain a regular part of their reproductive life unless they seek treatment. For many women, the first day of their period brings immediate relief. For others, the depressive symptoms persist all month and are simply heightened before the menstrual period.

Although the causes of PMS are not known, most believe that the most plausible cause is a hormonal imbalance related to the rise in estrogen levels preceding the menstrual period (Mayo Clinic, 2012). This theory is substantiated by the fact that women with PMS given prescriptions for progesterone often experience relief of symptoms (Baker & O'Brien, 2012). Other related factors include chemical changes in the brain such as fluctuations in serotonin, depression, stress, and poor eating habits that lead to low levels of vitamin and mineral intake, higher intakes of salty foods, and drinking alcohol and caffeinated beverages (Mayo Clinic, 2012).

Common treatments for PMS include hormonal therapy in addition to drugs and behaviours designed to relieve the symptoms. These include Aspirin for pain, diuretics for fluid retention, decreases in

Fibrocystic breast condition A common, noncancerous condition in women whose breasts contain fibrous or fluid-filled cysts.

Premenstrual syndrome (PMS) A series of physical and emotional symptoms that may occur in women prior to their menstrual periods.

caffeine and salt intake, increases in complex carbohydrate intake, stress-reduction techniques, and physical activity. Some women claim they find relief through alternative treatments such as traditional Chinese medicine (acupuncture and herbs).

Endometriosis

Whether the incidence of **endometriosis** is on the rise or whether the disorder is simply attracting more attention is difficult to determine. Women who develop endometriosis tend to be between the ages of 20 and 40 years. Symptoms include severe cramping during and between menstrual cycles, irregular periods, unusually heavy or light menstrual flow, abdominal bloating, fatigue, painful bowel movements with periods, painful intercourse, constipation, diarrhea, menstrual pain, infertility, and low back pain.

Although much remains unknown about the causes of endometriosis, it is known that the disease is characterized by the abnormal growth and development of endometrial tissue (the tissue lining the uterus) in regions of the body other than the uterus. Among the most widely accepted theories concerning the causes of endometriosis are the transmission of endometrial tissue to other regions of the body during surgery or through the birthing process; the movement of menstrual fluid backward through the fallopian tubes during menstruation; and abnormal cell migration through body-fluid movement. Women with cycles shorter than 27 days and those with flows lasting over a week are at increased risk. The more aerobic physical activity a woman engages in and the earlier she starts, the less likely she is to develop endometriosis.

Treatment of endometriosis ranges from bed rest and reduction in stressful activities to **hysterectomy** (the removal of the uterus) or the removal of one or both ovaries and the fallopian tubes. In some areas, where the rate of hysterectomy is high, physicians have been criticized for overreliance on this procedure. More conservative treatments that involve dilation and curettage—surgically scraping endometrial tissue off the fallopian tubes and other reproductive organs—and combinations of hormone therapy are considered more acceptable. Hormonal treatments include gonadotropin-releasing hormone (GnRH) analogues, various synthetic progesterone-like drugs (Provera), and oral contraceptives.

Endometriosis Abnormal development of endometrial tissue outside the uterus.

Hysterectomy Surgical removal of the uterus.

Diabetes A disease in which the pancreas fails to produce enough insulin (type 1) or the body fails to use insulin effectively (type 2).

Insulin A hormone produced by the pancreas; required by the body for the metabolism of carbohydrates.

Hyperglycemia Elevated blood sugar levels.

DIGESTION-RELATED DISORDERS

Diabetes

According to the Canadian Diabetes Association (2012), more than 9 million Canadians are living with **diabetes** or prediabetes; approximately 10 percent of all cases are type 1 diabetes and 90 percent are type 2. Aboriginal people are three to five times more likely to develop type 2 diabetes than the general population. The Canadian Diabetes Association (2012) also states that every hour, 20 more people in Canada will be diagnosed with diabetes. This increase in prevalence is expected because (1) the population is aging, (2) obesity rates are rising, (3) Canadian lifestyles are increasingly sedentary, and (4) 80 percent of new Canadians come from high-risk groups for developing type 2 diabetes (that is, those of Hispanic, Asian, South Asian, or African descent). Further, it should be pointed out that approximately one-third of persons with diabetes are undiagnosed (Health Canada, n.d.b).

Contrary to popular belief, diabetes does not result from eating too much sugar, although it does relate to insulin and the body's ability or inability to use sugar. In healthy people, the pancreas, a powerful enzyme-producing organ, produces the hormone **insulin** in sufficient quantities to allow the body to use or store glucose (blood sugar). When this organ fails to produce enough insulin to regulate sugar metabolism, or when the body fails to use insulin effectively, diabetes occurs. Individuals with diabetes exhibit **hyperglycemia**, or elevated blood sugar levels, and high glucose levels in their urine. Other symptoms include excessive thirst, frequent urination, hunger, tendency to tire easily, wounds that heal slowly, numbness or tingling in the extremities, changes in vision, skin eruptions, and, in women, a tendency toward vaginal yeast infections.

Many individuals with diabetes remain unaware of their condition until they begin to show overt symptoms. Type 1 (insulin-dependent) diabetes or diabetes mellitus usually begins early in life. Individuals with type 1 diabetes typically depend on insulin injections or oral medications for the rest of their lives, because insulin is not available in their bodies. Non–insulin dependent diabetes (formally termed "adult-onset"), or type 2 diabetes, in which insulin production is deficient, tends to develop in later life. Individuals with type 2 diabetes can often control the symptoms of their disease with minimal medical intervention through a healthy dietary intake, weight control, and regular physical activity (see Focus on Diabetes for more details). If they follow this regimen, they may be able to avoid oral medications or insulin indefinitely.

In addition to a genetic link, your risk of diabetes increases when you are obese and physically inactive (Public Health Agency of Canada, 2011e). Older people and mothers of babies weighing over 4 kilograms also run an increased risk. Approximately 80 percent of all individuals are overweight and sedentary at the time of their diagnosis with type 2 diabetes. Regular physical activity, irrespective of weight loss, is an important factor in lowering blood sugar and improving the efficiency of cellular use of insulin. Regular physical activity combined with weight (fat) loss can reduce the work of the pancreas and reduce the development of diabetes. Given the improvement in health care, people who develop diabetes today have a much better prognosis than those who developed it 20 or 25 years ago.

Many physicians attempt to control diabetes with a variety of insulin-related drugs. Most of these drugs are taken orally, although self-administered hypodermic injections are prescribed when oral treatments are inadequate. Recent breakthroughs in individual monitoring and the implanting of insulin monitors and insulin infusion pumps that regulate insulin intake "on demand" have provided many individuals with diabetes the opportunity to lead normal lives. Other individuals with diabetes find they can control their diabetes by eating foods rich in complex carbohydrates, low in sodium, and high in fibre, by losing weight, and by engaging in daily physical activity.

Colitis and Irritable Bowel Syndrome (IBS)

Ulcerative colitis is a disease of the large intestine in which the mucous membranes of the intestinal walls become inflamed. It is more localized than Crohn's disease in that this disease affects the large bowel, including the rectum and anus (Crohn's and Colitis Foundation of Canada, n.d.). Although Crohn's disease can occur anywhere in the gastrointestinal tract, from mouth to anus, the inflammation is most often found in the lower part of the small bowel and the upper end of the colon. In Crohn's disease, patches of inflammation are interspersed between healthy portions of the gut, and can penetrate the intestinal layers from inner to outer lining (Crohn's and Colitis Foundation of Canada, n.d.). Individuals with severe cases may have as many as 20 bouts of bloody diarrhea a day. Colitis can also produce severe stomach cramps, weight loss, nausea, sweating, and fever (Crohn's and Colitis Foundation of Canada, n.d.). Hypersensitivity reactions, particularly to milk and certain foods, are considered possible causes for colitis, though its exact cause is unknown. It is difficult to determine the cause of colitis because the disease goes into unexplained

remission and then recurs without apparent reason. This pattern often continues for years and may be related to the later development of colorectal cancer. Because the cause of colitis remains unknown, treatment focuses exclusively on relieving the symptoms. Effective measures include increasing fibre intake and taking anti-inflammatory drugs, steroids, and other medications designed to reduce inflammation and soothe irritated intestinal walls.

Many people develop a condition related to colitis known as **irritable bowel syndrome (IBS)**, in which nausea, pain, gas, diarrhea, or cramps occur after eating certain foods or when a person is under unusual stress. IBS symptoms commonly begin in early adulthood. Symptoms vary from week to week and fade for long periods of time only to return. The cause of IBS is unknown, but researchers suspect that people with IBS have digestive systems overly sensitive to certain foods and beverages, stress, and certain hormonal changes. They may also be more sensitive to pain signals from the stomach. Stress management, relaxation techniques, regular physical activity, and a healthy dietary intake can bring IBS under control in the vast majority of cases.

Diverticulosis

Diverticulosis occurs when the walls of the intestine become weakened for undetermined reasons and small pea-sized bulges develop. These bulges often fill with feces and, over time, become irritated and infected, causing pain and discomfort. Food particles, such as seeds that are small and not easily broken down, often trigger a diverticulosis attack. If this irritation persists, bleeding and chronic obstruction may occur, either of which can be life-threatening. If you have a persistent pain in the lower abdominal region, seek medical attention at once.

Peptic Ulcers

An ulcer is a lesion or wound that forms in body tissue as a result of some irritant. A **peptic ulcer** is a chronic ulcer that occurs in the lining of the stomach or the section of the small intestine known as the duodenum. Most peptic ulcers result from an infection from a common bacteria, *Helicobacter pylori*, and require powerful antibiotics to treat them. This is considerably different from the

Ulcerative colitis An inflammatory disorder that affects the mucous membranes of the large intestine, producing bloody diarrhea.

Irritable bowel syndrome (IBS) Nausea, pain, gas, or diarrhea caused by certain foods or stress.

Diverticulosis A condition in which bulges form in the walls of the intestine; results in irritation and infection of the intestine.

Peptic ulcer Damage to the stomach or intestinal lining, usually caused by digestive juices.

treatment in the past, which used acid-reducing drugs known as H2 blockers, such as cimetidine (Tagamet) or ranitidine (Zantac) because it was believed that digestive juices caused the damage to the stomach lining or the small intestine. The new treatment recommends a two-week course of antibiotics. H2 blockers are still used in ulcer cases in which excess stomach acid or overuse of drugs such as Aspirin and ibuprofen have caused the irritation.

In addition to a genetic contribution, ulcers tend to be more prevalent in people who are highly stressed over long periods of time and who consume high-fat foods or excessive alcohol. People with ulcers should reduce their consumption of high-fat foods, alcohol, and substances such as Aspirin that irritate organ linings or cause increased secretion of stomach acids and thereby exacerbate this condition. In some cases, surgery may be necessary to relieve persistent symptoms.

Gallbladder Disease

Gallbladder disease, also known as cholecystitis, occurs when the gallbladder has been repeatedly irritated by chemicals, infection, or overuse, thus reducing its ability to release bile for the digestion of fats. Usually, gallstones, consisting of calcium, cholesterol, and other minerals, form in the gallbladder itself. When the individual eats foods high in fats, the gallbladder contracts to release bile; these contractions cause pressure on the stone formations. One of the characteristic symptoms of gallbladder disease is acute pain in the upper right portion of the abdomen after eating fatty foods. This pain, which can last several hours, may feel like a heart attack or an ulcer attack and is often accompanied by nausea.

Not all gallstones cause acute pain. In fact, small stones that pass through one of the bile ducts and become lodged may be more painful than gallstones that are the size of golf balls. Many people find out that they have gallstones only after undergoing ultrasound and diagnostic X-rays to rule out other conditions. The absence of symptoms is significant because gallstones are considered a predisposing factor for gallbladder cancer.

Current treatment of gallbladder disease usually involves medication to reduce irritation, restriction of fat consumption, and surgery to remove the gallstones. There are medications available that are designed to dissolve small gallstones that can be used with some patients. Lithotripsy, in which a series of noninvasive shock waves break up small stones, can also be used. Lasers

Arthritis Painful inflammatory disease of the joints.

Osteoarthritis A progressive deterioration of bones and joints associated with the "wear and tear" of aging.

Rheumatoid arthritis A serious inflammatory joint disease.

and laparoscopic surgery is another effective technique that can be used with less risk than surgeries that involve large incisions.

MUSCULOSKELETAL DISEASES

Most of us will encounter some form of chronic musculoskeletal disease during our lifetime. Some form of arthritis will afflict half of us over the age of 65; low back pain hits most of us at some point in our life.

Arthritis

Arthritis is much more than occasional aches or pains; it is a serious and urgent problem in Canada. Currently, more than four million Canadians over the age of 15 years have from some form of arthritis (Health Canada, 2011). Although often thought of as a disease of age, 60 percent of those with arthritis are under the age of 64. **Osteoarthritis** is a progressive deterioration of bones and joints associated with the "wear and tear" of aging (Health Canada, 2008). As joints are used, they release enzymes that digest cartilage while other cells in the cartilage try to repair the damage. When the enzymatic breakdown overpowers cellular repair, the pain and swelling characteristic of arthritis may occur. Weather extremes, excessive strain, and injury often lead to osteoarthritis flare-ups. But a specific precipitating event does not seem to be necessary. It is estimated that most Canadians will be affected by osteoarthritis by age 70 (Health Canada, 2008). Although age and injury are undoubtedly factors in the development of osteoarthritis, heredity, abnormal use of the joint, dietary intake, abnormalities in joint structure, and impaired blood supply to the joint may also contribute. Osteoarthritis of the hands seems to have a particularly strong genetic component. Extreme disability as a result of osteoarthritis is rare. However, when joints become so distorted that they impair activity, surgical intervention is often necessary. Joint replacement and bone fusion are common surgical repair techniques. For most people, anti-inflammatory drugs, pain relievers, and cortisone-related agents ease discomfort. In some, applications of heat, mild physical activity, and massage can also relieve the pain.

Rheumatoid arthritis is similar to but far more serious than osteoarthritis. Rheumatoid arthritis is an inflammatory joint disease that can occur at any age, but most commonly appears between the ages of 20 and 45 years. It is three times more common among women than men during early adulthood but equally common among men and women in the over-70-years-of-age group. Symptoms may be gradually progressive or sporadic, with occasional unexplained remissions.

Rheumatoid arthritis typically attacks the synovial membrane, which produces the lubricating fluids for the joints. Advanced rheumatoid arthritis often involves destruction of the bony ends of joints. The remedy for this condition is typically bone fusion, which leaves the joint immobile. In some instances, joint replacement may be a viable alternative.

Although the exact cause of rheumatoid arthritis is unknown, it may be an autoimmune disorder, in which the body responds as if its own cells were the enemy, eventually destroying the affected body parts. Other theorists believe that rheumatoid arthritis is caused by some form of invading microorganism that takes over the joint. Certain toxic chemicals and stress have also been mentioned as possible causes. Regardless of the cause, treatment of rheumatoid arthritis is similar to that for osteoarthritis. Emphasis is placed on pain relief and attempts to improve the functional mobility of the patient. In some instances, immunosuppressant drugs are also given to reduce the inflammatory response.

Fibromyalgia

Fibromyalgia is a chronic, painful rheumatological-like disorder. Symptoms include widespread pain; stiffness and numerous tender points; weakness; swelling; and neurovascular complaints including coldness, numbness, tingling, mottled skin, headaches, auditory sensitivity, irritable bowel syndrome, sleep disorders, depression, and dysmenorrhea. The cause of fibromyalgia remains a mystery; acute sleep disturbances, muscular irregularities, and forms of psychopathological disturbance have been considered as possible culprits. Fibromyalgia primarily affects women (particularly in their 30s and 40s), and it causes more chronic pain and debilitation than other musculoskeletal disorders.

Systemic Lupus Erythematosus (SLE)

Lupus is a disease in which the immune system attacks the body, producing antibodies that destroy or injure organs such as the kidneys, brain, and heart. The symptoms vary from mild to severe and disappear for periods of time. A butterfly-shaped rash covering the bridge of the nose and both cheeks is common. Nearly all individuals with SLE have aching joints and muscles, and 60 percent develop redness and swelling that moves from joint to joint. Extensive research has not yet found a cure for this sometimes fatal disease.

Low Back Pain (LBP)

Most people (about 80 percent) will experience low back pain at some point during their life. Although some of these low back pain episodes result from muscular damage and can be short-lived and acute, others can involve dislocations, fractures, or other problems with spinal vertebrae or discs and be chronic or require surgery. LBP is epidemic throughout the world.

Risk Factors for Low Back Pain

The following factors contribute to LBP:

- advancing age
- certain body types
- poor posture
- poor muscular strength and endurance
- psychological factors
- occupational risks

Preventing Back Pain and Injury

Almost 90 percent of all back problems occur in the lumbar spine region (lower back). Consciously protecting this region of the body from blows, excessive strain, or sharp twists when muscles are not warmed up is essential. You can reduce your risk of LBP by consciously attempting to maintain good posture when sitting, standing, and sleeping. Recognize that you cannot sit or stand for long periods of time in the same position, so adjust your position frequently. You naturally move in your sleep. In addition, physical activity, particularly activities that strengthen the abdominal muscles and the muscles that support the spine and stretch the back muscles, is important. It is also important to sleep on a supportive mattress, to work in an ergonomically friendly environment (supportive chair with feet flat on the floor, computer at eye level, keyboard appropriately placed, and so on), to lift heavy objects with your knees rather than your back, to avoid high-heeled and otherwise poorly fitting shoes, and to engage in regular physical activity. If you injure your back, be sure to consult with several experts in rehabilitation and therapy to determine your best options. Consult an exercise physiologist, biomechanist, ergonomist, physical therapist, chiropractor, or physician specializing in bone and joint injuries for recommended physical activities.

Lupus A disease in which the immune system attacks the body.

OTHER MALADIES

During the last decade or so, numerous afflictions have surfaced that seem to be products of our times. Some of these health problems relate to specific groups of people, some are due to technological advances, and some are unexplainable. Still other diseases have been present for many years and continue to cause severe disability (see Table 13.6).

Among conditions that have received attention in recent years are chronic fatigue syndrome and disorders related to the use of video display terminals.

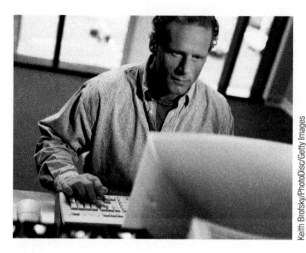

Working on your computer for several hours a day can put you at risk for eyestrain and back, neck, shoulder, and wrist pain.

Keith Brofsky/PhotoDisc/Getty Images

Chronic Fatigue Syndrome (CFS)

In the late 1980s, a characteristic set of symptoms was noted that included chronic fatigue, headaches, fever, sore throat, enlarged lymph nodes, depression, poor memory, general weakness, nausea, and symptoms remarkably similar to mononucleosis. Researchers initially believed that individuals were really talking about a series of symptoms caused by the Epstein-Barr virus, the same virus as mononucleosis. In some instances, the symptoms were so severe that individuals required hospitalization. Since those initial studies, researchers have all but ruled out the possibility of a mysterious form of the Epstein-Barr virus. Despite extensive testing, no viral cause has been found.

TABLE 13.6

Other Modern Afflictions

Disease	Description	Treatment
Parkinson's disease	Disease mostly affecting people over the age of 55. Symptoms include tremors, rigidity, slowed movement, loss of autonomic movements, and difficulty walking.	Unknown cause makes prevention difficult. Tranquillizers are useful in controlling nerve responses.
Multiple sclerosis	Disease that affects women more than men. Precise cause uncertain. Symptoms include vision problems, tingling and numbness in extremities, chronic fatigue, and neurological impairments.	Medication to control symptoms and slow progression of the disease. Stress management may be helpful.
Cystic fibrosis	Inherited disease occurring in 1 out of every 1600 births. Characterized by pooling of large amounts of mucus in lungs, digestive disturbances, and excessive sodium excretion. Results in premature death.	Most treatments are geared toward relief of symptoms. Antibiotics are administered for infection. Recent strides in genetic research suggest better treatments and potential cure in the near future.
Sickle cell disease	Inherited disease affecting mostly blacks. Disease affects hemoglobin, forming sickle shaped red blood cells that interfere with oxygenation. Results in severe pain, anemia, and premature death.	Reduce stress and attend to minor infections immediately. Seek genetic counselling.
Cerebral palsy	Disorder characterized by the loss of voluntary control over motor functioning. Believed to be caused by a lack of oxygen to the brain at birth, brain disorders or an accident before or after birth, poisoning, or brain infections.	Follow preventive actions to reduce accident risks; improved neonatal and birthing techniques.
Graves' disease	Thyroid disorder characterized by swelling of the eyes, staring gaze, and retraction of the eyelid. Can result in loss of sight. The cause is unknown and it can occur at any age.	Medication may help control symptoms. Radioactive iodine supplements also may be administered.

Today, in the absence of a known pathogen, many researchers believe that the illness, now commonly referred to as chronic fatigue syndrome (CFS), may have strong psychosocial roots.

The diagnosis of chronic fatigue syndrome depends on two major criteria and eight or more minor criteria. The major criteria are debilitating fatigue that persists for at least six months and the absence of diagnoses of other illnesses that could cause the symptoms. Minor criteria include headaches, fever, sore throat, painful lymph nodes, weakness, fatigue after physical activity, sleep problems, and rapid onset of these symptoms. Because an exact cause is not apparent, treatment of CFS focuses on improved dietary intake, rest, counselling for depression, judicious physical activity, and development of a strong support network.

Job-Related Disorders

During the last decade, a new potential health risk for computer users has been the topic of growing debate. Adverse health effects have been noted in people who work at computer video display terminals (VDTs) for several hours or more each day. Many post-secondary students are regular high-volume users of VDTs and are therefore at risk. Further adding to students' risk is their usage of cellphones.

Most of these problems relate to eyestrain and discomfort in the low back, neck, shoulders, and wrists. Questions about the danger posed by radiation from the electrical fields produced within the circuits of the VDT and about the potential effects on pregnant women and their fetuses remain unanswered.

Carpal tunnel syndrome is a common occupational injury in which the median nerve in the wrist becomes irritated, causing numbness, tingling, and pain in the fingers and hands. This condition is worsened by the repetitive typing motions made by computer users and is often classified as a common repetitive motion injury. For those who work on a computer for hours at a time, day after day, ergonomists recommend regular breaks. Remove your hands from the keyboard to move them about every 20 minutes; stretch other body parts such as the neck and shoulders periodically. Physically remove yourself from your computer at least once every hour for several minutes, perhaps walking around the room or doing some simple stretches. Paying attention to the design, height, and support of your chair, and placing your keyboard at a comfortable angle and height, can save hours of suffering—though these precautions do not remove the need to get up and move every so often.

Carpal tunnel syndrome A common occupational injury in which the median nerve in the wrist becomes irritated, causing numbness, tingling, and pain in the fingers and hands.

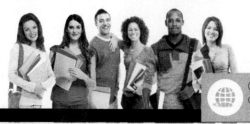

TAKING CHARGE: STI Attitude and Belief Scale

Read each statement. Circle T if you think the statement is true or F if you think the statement is false. Then consult the answer key that follows.

1. You can usually tell whether someone is infected with an STI, especially HIV.

        T   F

2. Chances are that if you do not have an STI by now, you probably have a natural immunity and will not get infected in the future.

        T   F

3. A person successfully treated for an STI does not need to worry about getting it again.

        T   F

4. So long as you keep yourself fit and healthy, you do not need to worry about STIs.

        T   F

5. The best way for sexually active people to protect themselves from STIs is to practise safer sex.

        T   F

6. The only way to catch an STI is to have sex with someone who has one.

        T   F

7. Talking about STIs with a partner is so embarrassing that you should not even bring it up.

        T   F

8. STIs are a problem only for people who are promiscuous.

        T   F

9. You do not need to worry about contracting an STI so long as you wash yourself thoroughly with soap and hot water immediately after sex.

        T   F

10. You do not need to worry about AIDS if no one you know has ever had it.

        T   F

Scoring Key

1. False. Several STIs, such as chlamydia, gonorrhea (especially in women), internal genital warts, and even HIV infection in its early stages, cause few if any obvious signs or symptoms.

2. False. There is no natural immunity to STIs, if you have not been practising safer sex methods, you have been lucky so far.

3. False. Successful treatment does not prevent reinfection.

4. False. Even people in prime physical condition can be affected by the tiniest of microbes that cause STIs.

5. True. If you are sexually active, practising safer sex is the best protection against contracting an STI. Abstinence is the only sure way to not contract an STI through sexual activity.

6. False. STIs can also be transmitted through non-sexual means, such as by sharing contaminated needles or, in some cases, through contact with disease-causing organisms on personal effects.

7. False. Do not let embarrassment prevent you from taking steps to protect your and your partner's welfare.

8. False. STIs can happen to anyone who is sexually active or an intravenous drug user.

9. False. While washing your genitals immediately after sex may have some protective value, it is no substitute for practising safer sex.

10. False. Symptoms of HIV infection may not appear for years after initial infection with the virus.

Interpreting Your Score

First, add up the number of items you got right, the number of 'trues' you have. A score of eight or better indicates that your attitudes, beliefs, and behaviours toward STIs should decrease your risk of contracting them. Yet even one wrong response on this test increases your risk of contracting an STI. Knowledge alone is not sufficient to protect yourself from STIs. You need to ask yourself how you are going to put knowledge into action by changing your behaviours to reduce your chances of contracting an STI.

(continued)

Source: Adapted from Jeffrey S. Nevid with Fern Gotfried, *Choices: Sex in the Age of STDs*, 10–13. © 1995 by Allyn & Bacon. Reprinted by permission.

Managing Your Disease Risks

Infectious diseases pose serious challenges throughout the world. Infectious diseases can be prevented by practising safe and responsible behaviours. In addition, many noninfectious diseases can be prevented or their onset delayed by making positive personal health choices.

Making Decisions for You

Protecting yourself from infectious diseases is not always easy. Because most pathogens are microscopic, exposure to one can occur without your knowledge. Therefore, you need to be aware of your risks. What can you do to improve your awareness of your potential exposure to disease-causing pathogens?

What are some actions you can take to reduce your risk of contracting an STI? What steps could you take right now to ensure the sexual health of your partners? Finally, if you thought you had been exposed to HIV, where would you seek testing? The following may help you to make better choices regarding your health:

- Be aware of factors that threaten your health. Know your disease and immunization history.
- Take the precautions needed to protect yourself from exposure to infectious pathogens.
- Know the health status of your intimate partners.
- Communicate openly and honestly with your partners about your feelings regarding sexual intimacy.
- Wash your hands frequently and thoroughly with soap and water.
- Avoid travel to places where outbreaks of infectious diseases have not been controlled. When travel to these places cannot be avoided, immunize yourself when possible for diseases that can be prevented.
- Maintain a healthy routine of adequate sleep, a healthy dietary intake following Eating Well with Canada's Food Guide, and regular physical activity.

- Cook foods at their appropriate temperatures. Keep hot foods hot and cold foods cold.
- Recognize the symptoms that indicate a possible infection and seek treatment immediately.
- Recognize your responsibility for the health of others.
- Behave in sexually responsible ways.
- Limit your sexual partners.
- Limit alcohol or other drug use during intimate sexual encounters.
- Assess your level of risk for acquiring an STI, including HIV.
- Respect the rights and needs of individuals affected by an infectious disease.
- Adopt personal health habits that will reduce your risk of a chronic disease.
- Identify actions you can take today to reduce your risks for the diseases and disorders discussed in this chapter.

Critical Thinking

You have been in a relationship for several months that has grown from a friendship to passionate sexual intimacy. During this time, a close and trusting bond has also developed. You have remained monogamous and believe that your partner has as well, although you have never discussed it. Nor has any discussion arisen about each other's sexual history or HIV status. You have been involved in sexual relationships in the past and have never been tested for HIV or any other STIs, and you are quite certain your partner is experienced as well. You trust your partner but recognize that, without complete information, you are both at risk for STIs. You want to take some precautionary steps but worry about insulting your partner's feelings.

Use the DECIDE model described in Chapter 1 to decide what you would do in this situation. Develop several different strategies and approaches for reaching the desired result.

Source: Adapted from Jeffrey S. Nevid with Fern Gotfried, *Choices: Sex in the Age of STDs*, 10–13. © 1995 by Allyn & Bacon. Reprinted by permission.

DISCUSSION QUESTIONS

1. What is a pathogen? What are the similarities and differences between pathogens and antigens?
2. What is the difference between natural and acquired immunity?
3. Identify five STIs and their symptoms in men and women. How do they develop? How are they treated? What are their potential long-term risks?
4. Why might it be inappropriate to identify groups as at high risk for HIV infection? Why might HIV infection be better referred to as a sexually transmissible infection than as a sexually transmitted infection?
5. What are some of the major noninfectious chronic diseases affecting Canadians today? What are the common risk factors? How are they treated?
6. List the common respiratory diseases affecting Canadians. Which of these has a genetic basis? An environmental basis? An individual basis?
7. Compare and contrast the different types of headaches, including their symptoms and treatments. What can be done to prevent them? Treat them?
8. Do you believe that PMS is a disorder or disease or simply a catchall name for many naturally occurring events in the menstrual cycle? Why?
9. What are the medical risks of fibrocystic breast condition and endometriosis? How can they be treated? Prevented?
10. Describe the symptoms and treatment of diabetes. What is the difference between type 1 and type 2 diabetes?
11. How can you tell whether your stomach is reacting to final exams or telling you that you have a serious medical condition?

APPLICATION EXERCISE

Reread the "Consider This . . ." scenario at the beginning of this chapter and answer the following questions.

1. What was your initial reaction to this scenario? Why?
2. How might you view the situation differently had it been Michael diagnose with an STI?
3. What are some legal issues that could arise or that already exist regarding all infectious diseases, including STIs? Why do the rights of all the individuals involved in relationships need to be considered?
4. What services exist on your campus for people living with HIV infection or AIDS? What services focus on informing people about STIs?

MASTERINGHEALTH

Go to MasteringHealth for Assignments, the eText, and the Study Area with case studies, self quizzing, and videos.

focus On
Diabetes

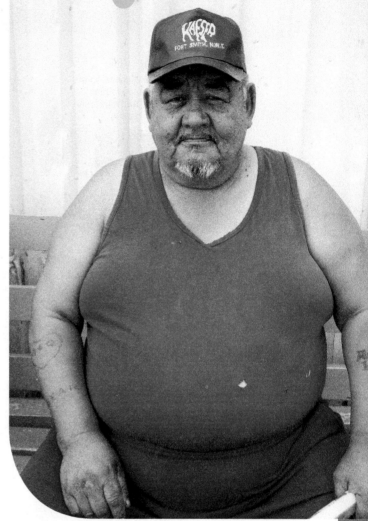

Ashley Cooper pics/Alamy

Like many college and university students, as well as most Canadian adults, Nora is overweight. She used to think it was no big deal—after all, there are lots of students like her and some are fatter! Nora planned to eat better and be more physically active as soon as she graduated and started to live "a normal life." But last week, her mom called and told Nora that she just found out that she has type 2 diabetes. Her mother's voice sounded shaky as she told Nora about her own mother's death from kidney failure—a complication of diabetes—at age 52, a few months before Nora was born. When Nora got off the phone, she searched online for information about diabetes. What she discovered made her feel scared, too; her Aboriginal ethnicity, family history, high stress level and lack of sleep, excessive weight, and sedentary lifestyle all increased her own risk for diabetes.

The next morning, Nora stopped off at the campus health centre and made an appointment for diabetes screening. She was instructed to fast the night before and was scheduled for an appointment first thing in the morning. At her visit, the nurse practitioner took a blood sample. A few days later, she called with the news: Nora has prediabetes, and needs to make changes to reduce her risk for developing type 2 diabetes like her mom.

DIABETES: INCIDENCE AND MORTALITY

Diabetes mellitus is a disease characterized by a persistently high level of sugar—technically glucose—in the blood. Another characteristic sign is the production of an unusually high volume of glucose-laden urine, a fact reflected in its name—*diabetes* is derived from a Greek word meaning "to flow through," and *mellitus* is the Latin word for "sweet." The high blood glucose levels—or **hyperglycemia**—seen in diabetes can lead to a variety of serious health problems and even premature death. Diabetes is actually a group of diseases, each with its own mechanisms. Diabetes is a serious, widespread, and costly chronic disease and if left untreated results in numerous health problems, including blindness, amputation, and kidney dysfunction, and ultimately, death.

Over the past 20 years, the number of Canadians 12 years and older diagnosed with diabetes has more than doubled. Current estimates (2012, the latest data available) indicate that 6.5 percent of the Canadian population has diabetes (Statistics Canada, 2013). At all ages except for 20 to 34 years, males are more likely to be diagnosed with diabetes than females. Further, diagnoses increase with age, with 8.6 percent of people between the ages of 45 and 64 years and 18.1 percent of all individuals over the age of 65 years having a positive diagnosis.

Diabetes mellitus A group of diseases characterized by elevated blood glucose levels.

Hyperglycemia Elevated blood glucose level.

FIGURE 1

Diabetes and How it Develops

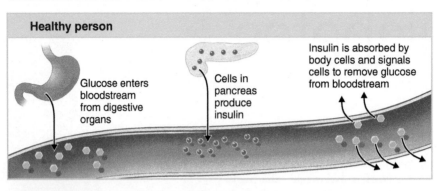

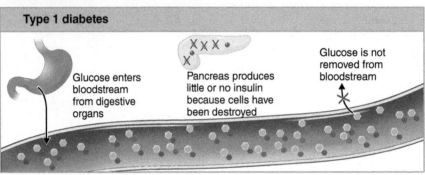

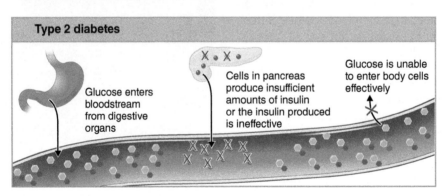

What causes diabetes? In healthy people, the pancreas, a powerful enzyme-producing organ, produces the hormone insulin in sufficient quantities to allow the body to use or store glucose. Further, in healthy people, glucose is taken up efficiently by body cells (Figure 1). When you eat, carbohydrates from foods are broken down into a monosaccharide called *glucose*. Once the digestive system releases it into the bloodstream, glucose becomes available to all body cells. Glucose is one of the main sources of energy for living organisms. When glucose levels drop below normal, certain mental functions may be impaired. You may feel "spacey" and unable to concentrate. Many cells within the body use glucose to fuel metabolism, movement, and other activities. When there is more glucose available than required to meet your body's immediate needs, the excess glucose is stored as glycogen in the liver and muscles for later use. Glucose cannot simply cross cell membranes on its own. Instead, cells have structures that transport it across in response to a signal. That signal is generated by the pancreas, an organ located just beneath the stomach. Whenever a surge of glucose enters the bloodstream, the pancreas secretes a hormone called insulin. Insulin stimulates cells to take up glucose from the bloodstream and carry it into the cell, where it is used for immediate energy. Conversion of glucose to glycogen for storage in the liver and muscles is also assisted by insulin. These actions lower the blood level of glucose, and in response, the pancreas stops secreting insulin—until the next influx of glucose arrives. When the pancreas fails to produce enough insulin to regulate sugar metabolism or when the body fails to use insulin effectively, diabetes develops. Individuals with diabetes exhibit hyperglycemia, or elevated blood sugar levels, and high glucose levels in their urine. Other symptoms include excessive thirst, frequent urination, hunger, a tendency to tire easily, wounds that heal slowly, numbness or tingling in the extremities, changes in vision, skin eruptions, and, in women, a tendency toward vaginal yeast infections.

Type 1 diabetes, also called insulin-dependent diabetes and formerly referred to as juvenile-onset diabetes, is an autoimmune disease in which the immune system destroys the insulin-making beta cells. It most often appears in childhood or adolescence, with rare cases diagnosed in early to mid-adult years. People with type 1 diabetes typically depend on insulin injections or oral medications because their body does not produce the insulin it needs.

In type 2 diabetes, also called non-insulin dependent diabetes and formerly called adult-onset diabetes, insulin production is deficient or the body is unable to utilize all available insulin. Type 2 diabetes accounts for 90 to 95 percent of all diabetes cases and in the past did not appear until after the age of 40 years—hence the term "adult-onset." Currently, type 2 diabetes is diagnosed across the age spectrum, including children and adolescents, and because of the frequency of diagnoses in younger individuals (reflective of current Canadian lifestyle), it can no longer be considered an adult-onset disease. Specifically, type 2 diabetes is linked to physical inactivity and obesity, both of which can be modified to control and prevent diabetes and improve health. Further, if people with type 2 diabetes change their lifestyle (that is, become more physically active, eat well, lose weight), they may be able to avoid the need for oral medications or insulin indefinitely.

A third type of diabetes, gestational diabetes, can develop in women during pregnancy. Although once believed to be only a transient event that disappeared after pregnancy, today experts realize that women with gestational diabetes have an increased risk of developing type 2 diabetes within 5 to 10 years of giving birth (Centers for Disease Control and Prevention, 2005). This is particularly true for women who do not lose the weight they gained during pregnancy and for those with subsequent pregnancies and weight gain with each one.

Understanding the Development of Type 2 Diabetes

In the early stages of type 2 diabetes, cells throughout the body begin to resist the effects of insulin. One culprit known to contribute to insulin resistance is an overabundance of free fatty acids concentrated in a person's fat cells (as may be the case in an obese individual). These free fatty acids directly inhibit glucose uptake by body cells. They also suppress the liver's sensitivity to insulin, so its ability to self-regulate its conversion of glucose into glycogen begins to fail. As a consequence of both problems, blood levels of glucose gradually rise. Detecting this elevated blood glucose, the pancreas attempts to compensate by producing more insulin.

The pancreas cannot maintain its hyperproduction of insulin indefinitely. As the progression to type 2 diabetes continues, more and more pancreatic insulin-producing cells become nonfunctional. As insulin output declines, blood glucose levels rise and warrant a diagnosis of type 2 diabetes.

Prediabetes—a measurable change in blood glucose levels—is one of the cluster of six conditions linked to overweight and obesity that together constitute a dangerous health risk known as *metabolic syndrome (MetS)*. Of the six conditions, prediabetes and central adiposity appear to be the dominant factors for MetS (American Heart Association, 2009). A person with MetS is five times more likely to develop type 2 diabetes than a person without the syndrome (National Heart Lung and Blood Institute, 2010).

Similar to heart disease and cancer (see Chapter 12), there are nonmodifiable and modifiable risk factors for type 2 diabetes. Nonmodifiable risks—those that you have no control over—include increased age, certain ethnicities, and genetic and biological factors. As previously mentioned, considerably more older Canadians have been diagnosed with diabetes; 8.6 percent of 45- to 64-year-olds and 18.1 percent of individuals over the age of 65 years (Statistics Canada, 2013). Individuals of African descent and Indigenous Canadians have much higher rates of type 2 diabetes than other Canadians, indicating an ethnic bias towards the disease. Similarly in the United States, Native Americans and non-Latino blacks have diabetes at a rate almost twice that of the white population (Centers for Disease Control and Prevention, 2011). Diabetes also tends to run in families (Brekke, Jansson, & Lenner, 2005). Having a close relative with type 2 diabetes is another significant risk factor. Type 2 has a strong genetic component. A small group of "type 2 diabetes genes" has been identified in a variety of studies so far (Das & Rao, 2007; Dedoussis, Kaliora, & Panagiotakos, 2007). Even though genetic susceptibility appears to play a role, the current increase in diagnoses of type 2 diabetes suggests that lifestyle factors, such as increased caloric intake and decreased physical activity, are more to blame. Modifiable risk factors include your body weight, dietary choices, and level of physical activity, as well as sleep patterns and level of stress. In children and adults, type 2 diabetes is linked to overweight and obesity. In adults, a body mass index (BMI) of 25 or greater increases the risk (see Chapter 6). In particular, excess weight carried around the waistline—102 or more cm in males or 89 or more cm in females—is highly correlated to the development of type 2 diabetes (New Mexico Health Care Takes on Diabetes, 2008).

A sedentary lifestyle and low levels of physical activity also increase the risk, not only because of the reduced calories used, but also because physical activity itself, and buildup of muscle tissue, improves insulin uptake by cells (American Diabetes Association, 2010). In fact, research indicates that regular, moderate intensity physical activity and a healthy diet can reduce a person's risk of type 2 diabetes significantly (Kriska, Hawkins, & Richardson, 2008).

Several recent studies suggest that sleep contributes to healthy metabolism, including healthy glucose control. In contrast, inadequate sleep may contribute to the development of type 2 diabetes, as well as obesity, as noted in the Focus on Sleep feature (Aronsohn et al., 2010; Cappuccio et al., 2010; Knutson et al., 2007). For example, people who routinely fail to get enough sleep have been shown to be at higher risk for metabolic syndrome (Hall et al., 2008).

Large epidemiologic studies provide evidence of a link between diabetes and psychological or physical stress (Fan et al., 2009; Pouwer, Kupper, & Adriaanse, 2010). The stress response can trigger a combination of increased blood glucose and inadequate production and release of insulin (Puustinen et al., 2011). Chronic, not acute, stress (see Chapter 3) contributes to the onset or progression of diabetes—another reason to manage your stress response (Chita & Steptoe, 2010).

Symptoms of Diabetes

The symptoms of diabetes are similar for both type 1 and type 2. The following are most common:

- **Thirst.** The kidneys filter excessive glucose from the blood. When they do, they dilute it with water so that it can be excreted in urine. This pulls too much water from the body and leaves the person dehydrated and thirsty.
- **Excessive urination.** Because a person is thirsty and drinking more, he or she experiences the need to urinate much more frequently than usual.
- **Weight loss.** Because so many calories are lost in the glucose that passes into urine, the person with diabetes often feels unusually hungry. Despite eating more, he or she typically loses weight.
- **Fatigue.** When glucose cannot enter cells, including brain cells and muscle cells, fatigue and weakness become inevitable.

- **Nerve damage.** A high glucose concentration damages the smallest blood vessels of the body, including those supplying nerves in the hands and feet. This can cause numbness and tingling.
- **Blurred vision.** Too much glucose causes body tissues to dry out. When this happens to the lens of the eye, vision deteriorates.
- **Poor wound healing and increased infections.** High levels of glucose can affect the body's ability to ward off infection and may affect overall immune system functioning.

Blood Tests Diagnose and Monitor Diabetes

Diabetes and prediabetes are diagnosed when a blood test reveals elevated blood glucose levels. Generally, your physician orders either of two blood tests to diagnose prediabetes or diabetes:

- The *fasting plasma glucose (FPG) test* requires the patient to fast overnight. Then, a small sample of blood is tested for glucose concentration. As you can see in Table 1, an FPG level greater than or equal to 5.55 mmol/L indicates prediabetes, and a level greater than or equal to 7.00 mmol/L indicates diabetes.
- The *oral glucose tolerance test (OGTT)* requires the patient to drink a fluid containing a significant level of concentrated glucose. A sample of blood is drawn for testing two hours after the patient drinks the solution. A reading greater than or equal to 7.77 mmol/L indicates prediabetes, whereas a reading greater than or equal to 11.1 mmol/L indicates diabetes.

TABLE 1

Blood Glucose Levels in Prediabetes and Untreated Diabetes (in mmol/L)*

	FPG Levels	OGTT Levels
Normal	< 5.55	< 7.77
Prediabetes	5.55–6.99	7.77–11.09
Diabetes	≥ 7.00	≥ 11.1

*The fasting plasma glucose (FPG) test measures levels of blood glucose after a person fasts overnight; the oral glucose tolerance test (OGTT) measures levels of blood glucose after a person consumes a concentrated amount of glucose.

Source: Based on data from American Diabetes Association, "How to Tell If You Have Pre-Diabetes." Copyright © 2010, American Diabetes Association.

Complications Associated with Diabetes

Depending on the type and severity of the disease, diabetes results in many complications (see Figure 2) as well as increasing the difficulty of existing conditions, including:

- **CVD.** Heart disease and stroke cause about 65 percent of deaths among people with diabetes. More than 70 percent of people with diabetes have hypertension.
- **Eye disease and blindness.** Diabetes is the leading cause of blindness.
- **Kidney disease.** The kidneys in many people with diabetes often fail. Dialysis is a common treatment for these individuals.
- **Amputations.** More than 60 percent of non-traumatic amputations of lower limbs are a result of diabetes. Foot care programs that include regular exams and patient education could prevent as many as 85 percent of these amputations.
- **Pregnancy complications.** Poorly controlled diabetes can cause major birth defects in 5 to 10 percent of all pregnancies and accounts for 15 to 20 percent of spontaneous abortions.
- **Flu- and pneumonia-related deaths.** People with diabetes have a threefold increase of dying as a result of complications from the flu or pneumonia compared to people without diabetes.

How Is Diabetes Treated?

Treatment options for people with prediabetes and diabetes vary according to the type that they have and how far the disease has progressed.

Lifestyle Changes Can Improve Glucose Levels

Studies have shown that people with prediabetes can prevent or delay the development of type 2 diabetes by up to 58 percent through changes to their lifestyle that include modest weight loss and regular exercise (American Diabetes Association, 2010). Further, if you have already been diagnosed with type 2 diabetes, lifestyle changes can sometimes prevent or delay your need for medication or insulin injections.

Weight Loss

The key to preventing type 2 diabetes in people with prediabetes is weight loss. A Diabetes Prevention Program (DPP) study showed that a loss of as little as 5 to 7 percent of current body weight significantly lowered the risk of progressing to diabetes (National Institute of Diabetes and Digestive and Kidney Diseases, 2008). Weight loss is also important for people currently diagnosed with type 2 diabetes.

FIGURE 2

Complications of Uncontrolled Diabetes: Amputation and Eye Disease

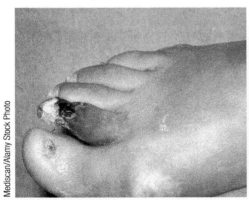

Infections in the feet and legs are common in people with diabetes, and healing is impaired, often resulting in amputations.

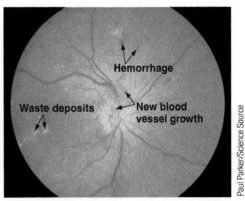

Possible damage to the eyes that may lead to blindness include swelling, leaking, and rupture of blood vessels, growth of new blood vessels, deposits of wastes, and scarring.

Eat Well

A variety of foods have an influence on blood glucose levels as noted below:

- **Whole grains.** A diet high in whole grains may reduce a person's risk of developing type 2 diabetes (de Munter et al., 2007).

- **High-fibre foods.** Eating foods high in fibre may reduce the risk of diabetes by improving blood sugar levels (Anderson et al., 2009). High-fibre foods include fruits, vegetables, beans, nuts, and seeds. See also Chapter 5.

- **Fatty fish.** An impressive body of evidence links the consumption of fatty fish such as salmon, which is high in omega-3 fatty acids, with decreased progression of insulin resistance (Dedoussis, Kaliora, & Panagiotakos, 2007; Lankinen et al., 2009).

It is also important for people with diabetes to pay attention to the glycemic index and glycemic load of the foods they eat to prevent surges in blood sugar. As noted in Chapter 5, the glycemic index compares the potential of foods containing the same amount of carbohydrate to raise blood glucose. A food's glycemic load is defined as its glycemic index multiplied by the number of grams of carbohydrate it provides, then divided by 100. The concept of glycemic load was developed by scientists to simultaneously describe the quality (glycemic index) and quantity of carbohydrate in a meal (Linus Pauling Institute, 2010). By learning to combine high and low glycemic index foods in order to avoid surges in blood glucose, a person with diabetes can help control his or her average blood glucose levels throughout the day. Paying attention to the amount of food consumed is also critical.

Increasing Physical Activity

As previously noted (Chapter 4), the Canadian Society for Exercise Physiology recommends that adults obtain a minimum of 150 minutes of moderate or more intense physical activity each week (Tremblay et al., 2011). Physical activity increases sensitivity to insulin. The more muscle you have and the more you use your muscles, the more efficiently cells utilize glucose for fuel, meaning there will be less glucose circulating in the bloodstream.

Oral Medications for Diabetes

When lifestyle changes fail to provide adequate control of type 2 diabetes, oral medications may be prescribed. These include several types, each of which influences blood glucose in a different way. Some medications reduce glucose production by the liver, whereas others

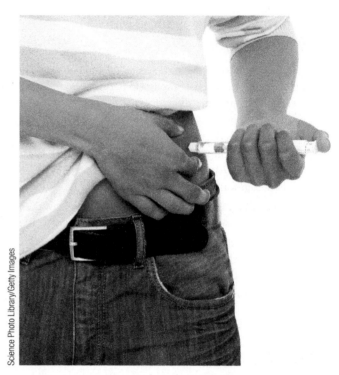

Science Photo Library/Getty Images

Individuals with type 1 diabetes may need to inject themselves with insulin daily or use an insulin pump. Your goal with type 2 diabetes should be to delay (or prevent) the need for injections through healthy lifestyle choices.

slow the absorption of carbohydrates from the small intestine. Other medications increase insulin production by the pancreas, whereas still others work to increase the insulin sensitivity of cells.

Insulin Injections May Be Necessary

Recall that in type 1 diabetes the pancreas can no longer produce adequate amounts of insulin. Thus, insulin injections are absolutely essential for those with type 1 diabetes. In addition, people with type 2 diabetes whose blood glucose levels cannot be adequately controlled with other treatment options might require insulin injections. Insulin cannot be taken in pill form because it is a protein and would be digested in the gastrointestinal tract. It must therefore be injected into the fat layer under the skin, from which it is absorbed into the bloodstream.

People with diabetes used to have to give themselves two or more insulin injections each day. Now, however, many individuals with diabetes use an insulin infusion pump. The external portion is only about the size of an MP3 player and can easily be hidden by clothes. It delivers insulin in minute amounts throughout the day through a thin tube and catheter inserted under the patient's skin. This infusion is more effective than delivering a few larger doses of insulin.

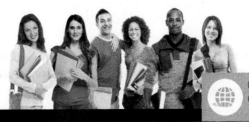

assess YOURSELF

Go to MasteringHealth to complete this questionnaire with automatic scoring

TAKING CHARGE: Managing Your Blood Glucose

As noted in this Focus On feature, certain characteristics—some modifiable, others not—place you at greater risk for diabetes. Still, you may not be aware of the symptoms of diabetes until after it has begun. The following Assess Yourself will help you to determine your risk for diabetes.

Are You at Risk for Diabetes?

Respond honestly to each of the questions below. If there is a question you do not know the answer to, you need to learn more about yourself or your family.

If you answer yes to three or more of these questions, consider seeking medical advice.

		Yes	No
1.	Do any of your primary relatives (parents, siblings, grandparents) have diabetes?	☐	☐
2.	Are you overweight or obese?	☐	☐
3.	Do you smoke?	☐	☐
4.	Have you been diagnosed with high blood pressure?	☐	☐
5.	Are you typically sedentary (seldom, if ever, engage in moderate or more intense physical activity)?	☐	☐
6.	Have you noticed an increase in your need for water or other beverages?	☐	☐
7.	Have you noticed that you have to urinate more frequently during a typical day than in the past?	☐	☐
8.	Have you noticed any tingling or numbness in your hands and feet, which might indicate circulatory problems?	☐	☐
9.	Do you often feel a gnawing hunger during the day, even though you eat regular meals and snacks?	☐	☐
10.	Are you often so tired that you find it difficult to stay awake?	☐	☐
11.	Have you noticed that you are losing weight although you are not doing anything in particular to make this happen?	☐	☐
12.	Have you noticed that you have skin irritations more frequently and that minor infections do not heal as quickly as they have in the past?	☐	☐
13.	Have you noticed any unusual changes in your vision (blurring, difficulty in focusing, and so on)?	☐	☐
14.	Have you noticed unusual pain or swelling in your joints?	☐	☐
15.	Do you often feel weak or nauseated when you wake in the morning, or if you wait too long to eat a meal?	☐	☐
16.	If you are a woman, have you had several vaginal yeast infections during the past year?	☐	☐

(continued)

The Assess Yourself activity asked you questions regarding your risk for diabetes. Each 'yes' response indicates a higher level of risk. Now that you have considered your results, you may need to take the following actions to better understand and address your risks:

- Call your parents and ask them if there is a history of diabetes mellitus in your family. If there is, ask which type (type 1, 2, or gestational) the family member(s) had.

- Consider all the risk factors you may have for diabetes—are you regularly physically active? Are you able to maintain your weight? Do you eat healthfully? Make a list of small steps you can take in the next day or two to address these potential risk factors.

- If you are at high risk for diabetes, make an appointment with your health-care provider to have your blood glucose levels tested. It is not only important to find out if you have diabetes, but also if you have prediabetes.

- If you smoke, devise a plan to quit. You may want to consult your doctor about medications or nicotine replacement therapies that could help you quit. Then quit.

- Gradually, over time (see Chapter 1), make the lifestyle changes that will reduce your risk. Make healthier choices regarding what you eat; increase your intake of whole grains, vegetables, and fruits; and decrease your consumption of saturated fats, trans fats, and sugar.

- Make physical activity and exercise part of your daily routine.

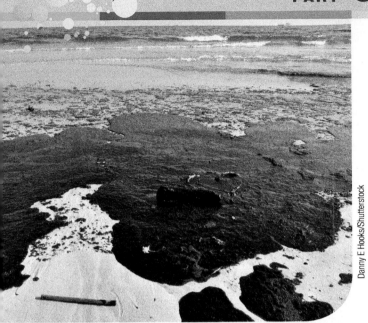

Danny E Hooks/Shutterstock

CHAPTER 14
CHOOSING HEALTHY LIVING FOR THE ENVIRONMENT

◄◉ CONSIDER THIS . . .

Leo decided to live off campus this year, so for the first time he is in charge of all aspects of his day-to-day living, including purchasing groceries and the cleaning of his apartment. Though environmentally conscious in his previous lifestyle habits (that is, he recycled as much as possible), he is not sure if there is a way to be more environmentally friendly when purchasing his groceries or what to look for when buying cleaning products, nor does he know where to look for help.

What suggestions would you give to Leo to be more environmentally friendly when purchasing groceries and to find more information and specific products he could purchase to clean effectively without causing too much damage to the environment?

LEARNING OUTCOMES

- Explain the impact of the growth of the global population on the environment.

- Identify the major causes of air pollution, including photochemical smog and acid rain, and make suggestions for reducing it.

- Identify major sources of water pollution and make suggestions for reducing it.

- Describe the consequences of noise pollution and what you can do to protect yourself.

- Identify the major causes of land pollution and what you can do to reduce it.

Human health, well-being, and survival are ultimately dependent on the integrity of the planet. Today, the natural world is under attack from the pressure of the number of people who live in it and the wide range of their activities. Effective management of the environment is critical to avoiding at least 25 percent of all preventable diseases worldwide (World Health Organization, n.d.a). In fact, as many as 13 million deaths could be prevented each year if we made our environment healthier. Worldwide, one-third of all diseases and about four million deaths of children under the age of five years are due to unsafe water and air pollution (World Health Organization, n.d.b). However, improved management of the environment could prevent as many as 40 percent of deaths from malaria, 41 percent from lower respiratory infections, and 94 percent from diarrhoeal disease—three of the world's biggest childhood killers. In the least developed countries, one-third of death and disease can be attributed to environmental causes. Though some environmental issues are managed better in developed countries, targeted interventions such as promoting safe household water storage, better hygiene measures, and the use of cleaner and safer fuels would reduce the incidence of cancers, cardiovascular diseases, asthma, lower respiratory infections, musculoskeletal diseases, road traffic injuries, poisoning, and drowning (World Health Organization, n.d.b).

Other interventions such as increasing the safety of buildings; promoting safe, careful use and management of toxic substances at home, at school, and in the workplace; and better water resource management would also result in improvements in population health and wellness (World Health Organization, n.d.b).

Canadians' concern about the environment has intensified since the initial outpouring on the first Earth Day in April 1970. Federal, provincial/territorial, and municipal governments share responsibility for the environment. Public health agencies are becoming more responsive to public concerns regarding the environment. While Canadians get most of their environmental information from the media, the majority look to public health professionals for answers to their concerns.

Health agencies are involved in defining the problems and seeking solutions in many of the approaches taken to address environmental health issues (Health Canada, 2009). This is supported by thousands of individual Canadians changing their habits and working to improve the environment. People are exposed to contaminants in water, air, food, and soil in various ways:

- Ingesting food, water, soil, objects, or liquids containing contaminants. The mouth, throat, stomach, and intestines can absorb ingested materials rapidly and at different rates, depending on the contaminant.

- Inhalation of a contaminated gas, vapour, or airborne particles. This includes small amounts of soil and dust inhaled into the lungs. The lungs often absorb gases and vapours quickly and efficiently.

- Dermal (skin) contact with contaminants in water, soil, or air. Some contaminants are absorbed through the skin, while in other cases the skin acts as an efficient barrier.

- Exposure to radioactivity can occur through penetration of the skin by radioactivity in the atmosphere or released from radionuclides in the air or on the ground. The radionuclide does not actually need to be in contact with the skin (Canadian Lung Association, 2012; Health Canada, 2009).

See Figure 14.1 for a diagram of major exposure pathways.

FIGURE 14.1

Major Pathways of Human Exposure to Environmental Contaminants

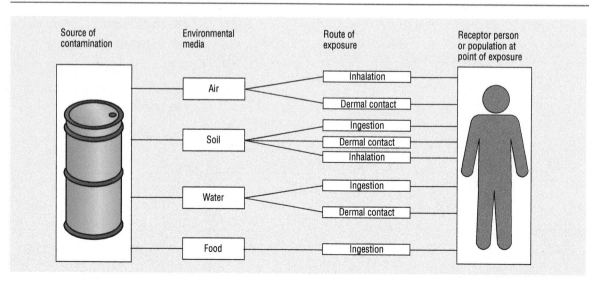

OVERPOPULATION

Our most challenging environmental problem is population growth. The anthropologist Margaret Mead wrote, "Every human society is faced with two population issues: how to beget and rear enough children and how not to beget and rear too many" (Caplan, 1990, p. 247).

The United Nations projects that the world population will grow from its current level of 7 billion to 9.3 billion by 2050 and exceed all previous projections, swelling to between 11 and 12.3 billion by 2100. Tomorrow's population will be more industrialized and consume more than those living in the world today.

Estimates for population growth are highly dependent upon predicted fertility rates (World Health Organization, 2009a). Overall global fertility has declined to an average of 2.5 births per woman in 2013, even though rates remain much higher in certain regions (Haub and Kaneda, 2014). While Europe, the United States, Mexico, China, and others have shown consistent declines in fertility rates in the last few decades, other countries, such as Niger (6.9 births per woman) and Somalia (6.1 births per woman) continue to have high fertility rates (Haub and Kaneda, 2014). While some argue that lower fertility rates mean slowing population growth, sheer population size can cause major increases, even if fertility rates remain constant or decline (Figure 14.2). Historically, in countries where women have little education and little control over reproductive choices, and where birth control is either not available or frowned upon, pregnancy rates continue to rise. However, as women become more educated, obtain higher socioeconomic status, and have more control over reproduction—as birth control becomes more accessible—fertility rates decline. Recognizing that population control will be essential in the decades ahead, many countries have enacted strict population control measures or have encouraged their citizens to limit the size of their families.

Mortality rates from chronic and infectious diseases have declined as a result of improved public health infrastructure, increased availability of drugs and vaccines, better disaster preparedness, and other factors. As people live longer, they add more years of resource consumption and add to the overall human footprint on the environment.

As the global population expands, so does the competition for the Earth's resources. Environmental degradation caused by loss of topsoil, pesticides, toxic residues, deforestation, global warming, air pollution, and acid rain seriously threatens the food supply

FIGURE 14.2

Global Fertility Rates, by Region

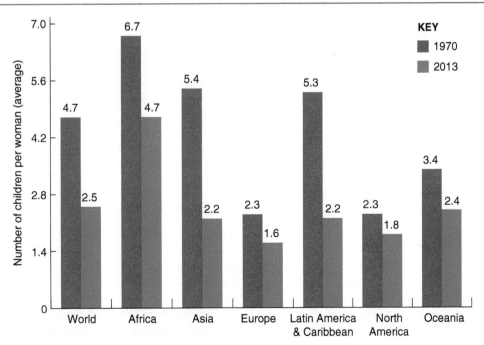

Average fertility rates (births per woman) have declined in all regions since 1970.

and undermines world health. However, population growth does not tell the whole story. North Americans consume more energy and raw materials per person than people from other regions of the world. Many of these resources come from other countries, and this consumption is depleting the resource balances of those countries. Therefore, we must start by living environmentally conscious lives.

AIR POLLUTION

As our population has grown, so have the number and volume of the environmental pollutants produced. It is estimated that urban air pollution causes approximately 1.3 million deaths worldwide per year (World Health Organization, 2013b). Concern about air quality prompted the Canadian Parliament to pass the Clean Air Act in 1970. This was consolidated in 1985 into the Canadian Environmental Protection Act (CEPA). CEPA was further updated and revised in 1999 and came into effect March 31, 2000 (Environment Canada, n.d.a). The Canadian Environmental Assessment Act (CEAA) provides a legal basis for federal environmental assessment and came into force on January 19, 2005 (Canadian Environmental Assessment Agency, n.d.). Various agreements (that is, high-level commitments entered into by two or more parties that identify the actions, roles, and commitments of the parties involved in dealing with environmental pollution) have also been established. The Canada-Wide Accord on Environmental Harmonization, Pollution Prevention Policy Agreement, Comprehensive Air Quality Management Framework for Canada, and the Canada–United States Air Quality Agreement are examples of agreements in place within the Canadian government and between the Canadian and U.S. governments (Environment Canada, n.d.b). These acts and agreements cover pollution prevention, management of toxic substances, clean air and water, control of pollution and waste, information gathering, and the setting of guidelines and enforcement of environmental laws and regulations.

Sources of Air Pollution

Sulphur Dioxide

Sulphur dioxide (SO2), a colourless gas and main ingredient of acid rain, smells like burnt matches (Canadian Lung Association, 2012). Sources of sulphur dioxide include:

- the burning of fossil fuels in petroleum refineries
- pulp and paper mill effluent

- steel mills
- coal-fired powered and electricity generating plants
- vehicles that use diesel
- volcanoes and hot springs (think of the sulphur hot springs at Banff, Alberta)

In humans, sulphur dioxide aggravates symptoms of heart and lung disease; leads to irritation in the nose and throat; obstructs breathing; and increases the incidence of respiratory diseases such as colds, asthma, bronchitis, and emphysema (Canadian Lung Association, 2012). It is toxic to plants, destroys some paint pigments, corrodes metals, impairs visibility, and is a precursor to acid rain.

Particulates

Particulates are tiny solid particles or liquid droplets suspended in the air. Cigarette smoke releases particulates. They are also by-products of some industrial processes and the internal combustion engine. Particulates irritate and carry heavy metals and cancer-causing agents deep into the lungs. When combined with sulphur dioxide, particulates exacerbate respiratory diseases. Particulates also corrode metals and obscure visibility.

Carbon Monoxide

Carbon monoxide is an odourless, colourless, tasteless gas that is poisonous at high concentrations (Canadian Lung Association, 2012). The major sources of carbon monoxide come from the burning of fossil fuels in vehicles, metal production, and emissions from heating devices. Carbon monoxide interferes with the blood's ability to absorb and carry oxygen and impairs thinking, leads to headaches and dizziness, slows reflexes, reduces perceptions, and causes drowsiness, unconsciousness, and death (Canadian Lung Association, 2012). When inhaled by a pregnant woman, it threatens the physical and mental growth and development of the fetus. Long-term exposure increases the severity of circulatory and respiratory diseases.

Nitrogen Oxides

Nitrogen oxides (NOx) are a group of reddish-brown gases with a foul smell (Canadian Lung Association, 2012). Sources of nitrogen oxides include the burning of fossil fuels in vehicles, homes, and industries; oil, gas, and coal-fired power plants; metal production; incineration; forest fires; lightning; and decaying vegetation (Canadian Lung Association, 2012). High concentrations of nitrogen dioxide can be fatal. Lower concentrations increase susceptibility to colds and flu, bronchitis, pneumonia, and other lung infections. Nitrogen dioxide is also toxic to plant life and causes a brown discolouration of the atmosphere. It is a precursor of ozone and, along with sulphur dioxide, of acid rain.

Ozone

Ozone is a form of oxygen produced when nitrogen dioxide reacts with hydrogen chloride. These gases release oxygen, which is altered by sunlight to produce ozone. In the lower atmosphere, ozone irritates the mucous membranes of the respiratory system, causing coughing and choking. It impairs lung functioning, reduces resistance to colds and pneumonia, and aggravates heart disease, asthma, bronchitis, and pneumonia. This ozone corrodes rubber and paint and injures or kills vegetation. It is also one of the irritants found in smog. A Canadian study concluded that there is no safe level of human exposure to ground-level ozone (Environment Canada, n.d.c).

The natural ozone found in the upper atmosphere serves as a protective layer against heat and radiation from the sun. This atmospheric layer, called the ozone layer, is discussed later in this chapter.

Lead

Lead is a metal pollutant found in the exhaust of motor vehicles powered by fuel containing lead and in the emissions from lead smelters and processing plants. Lead often contaminates drinking water systems in homes with plumbing installed before 1930. Lead negatively affects the circulatory, reproductive, and nervous systems and the blood and kidneys, and accumulates in bone and other tissues. Although lead is harmful to people of all ages, it is particularly detrimental to children and fetuses because of their increased rate of absorption, resulting in birth defects, behavioural abnormalities, and reduced intellectual development (Health Canada, 2013).

Hydrocarbons

Hydrocarbons encompass a wide variety of chemical pollutants in the air. **Hydrocarbons** are chemical compounds containing various combinations of carbon and hydrogen. The principal source of polluting hydrocarbons is the internal combustion engine. Most automobile engines emit hundreds of different types of hydrocarbon compounds. By themselves, hydrocarbons cause few problems, but when combined with sunlight and other pollutants they form such poisons as formaldehyde, various ketones, and peroxyacetylnitrate (PAN), all of which are respiratory irritants. Hydrocarbon combinations such as benzene and benzopyrene are carcinogenic (that is, cancer-causing). In addition, hydrocarbons play a major part in the formation of smog.

Smog

In the past, smog was the term used to describe a mixture of fog and smoke (Canadian Lung Association, 2012). Today, **smog**, also referred to as photochemical smog, is made up of several types of air pollution and is described as a brown, hazy mix of particulates and gases that forms when oxygen-containing compounds of nitrogen and hydrocarbons react in the presence of sunlight. Sometimes smog is easy to see when it forms as haze; other times it is invisible because the pollutants are too small to see (Canadian Lung Association, 2012). Another type of smog is called ozone pollution because ozone is created when vehicle exhaust reacts with sunlight. Such smog is most likely to develop on days with little wind and high traffic congestion. In most cases, it forms in areas that experience a **temperature inversion**, a weather condition in which a cool layer of air is trapped under a layer of warmer air, preventing air circulation. When gases such as hydrocarbons and nitrogen oxides are released into the cool air layer they cannot escape, and thus remain suspended until wind conditions move the warmer air layer. Sunlight filtering through the air causes chemical changes in the hydrocarbons and nitrogen oxides, which results in smog. Smog is more likely to be produced in valley regions blocked by hills or mountains.

The most noticeable adverse effects of exposure to smog relates to irritation in the eyes, nose, and throat, resulting in symptoms such as difficulty in breathing, burning eyes, headaches, coughing and wheezing, nausea, and reduced resistance to infections. Long-term exposure to smog poses serious health risks, particularly for children, the elderly, pregnant women, and people with chronic respiratory disorders such as asthma and emphysema. According to the Canadian Lung Association (2012), repeated exposure to smog accelerates the aging of the lungs and increases susceptibility to infections by hindering immune system functioning.

Acid Rain

Acid rain is precipitation that falls through acidic air pollutants, particularly those containing sulphur dioxides and nitrogen oxides. This precipitation, in the form of rain, snow, or fog, has a more acidic composition than unpolluted precipitation. In lakes and ponds, acid rain gradually acidifies the water. At a certain level, acid

Ozone A gas formed when nitrogen dioxide interacts with hydrogen chloride.

Hydrocarbons Chemical compounds that contain carbon and hydrogen.

Smog The brownish-yellow haze resulting from the combination of hydrocarbons and nitrogen oxides.

Temperature inversion A weather condition occurring when a layer of cool air is trapped under a layer of warmer air.

Acid rain Precipitation contaminated with acidic pollutants.

rain creates conditions in lakes and ponds where plants and animals cannot survive. Ironically, acidified lakes and ponds become a crystal-clear deep blue, creating an illusion of beauty and health.

Sources of Acid Rain

More than 95 percent of acid rain originates from human actions, chiefly the burning of fossil fuels. When industries burn fuels, the sulphur and nitrogen in the emissions combine with the oxygen and sunlight in the air to become sulphur dioxide and nitrogen oxides (precursors of sulphuric acid and nitric acids, respectively). Small acid particles are then carried by the wind and combine with moisture to produce acidic rain, snow, or fog. Because of higher concentrations of sunlight in the summer months, rain is more strongly acidic in the summertime. Additionally, the rain or snow that first falls is more acidic than that which falls later. Acid rain is a greater problem in Eastern Canada (Ontario, Quebec, New Brunswick, and Nova Scotia) because much of the water and soil lacks alkalinity—a lime base—and cannot neutralize acid naturally (Environment Canada, 2012).

Effects of Acid Rain

Damage to lake and pond habitats due to acid rain results in reduced capacity to support the variety of life that healthy lakes support (Environment Canada, 2012). As the waters become less habitable, the fish population decreases, partly because of mass mortalities during the spring snow melt and partly because of reduced female spawning (Environment Canada, 2012). Acid rain is also responsible for the destruction of millions of trees in forests in Europe and North America. Acid rain, acid fog, and acid vapour damage the trees and their growth in several ways, including inhibiting plant germination and reproduction as well as damage to the surface of leaves and needles and reducing the ability of the tree to withstand the cold (Environment Canada, 2012). Scientists concluded that 75 percent of Europe's forests are now experiencing damaging levels of sulphur deposition by acid rain. Forests in every country on the continent are affected including about 50 percent of Canada's eastern boreal forest (Environment Canada, 2012).

It is believed that acid rain aggravates and may even cause bronchitis, asthma, and other respiratory problems. The health effects may not be direct, as walking in acid rain or swimming in an acid lake will cause no more damage to your health than walking in clean rain or swimming in a clean lake or ocean (U.S. Environmental Protection Agency, 2012). It is the pollutants that comprise

Leach A process by which chemicals dissolve and filter through soil.

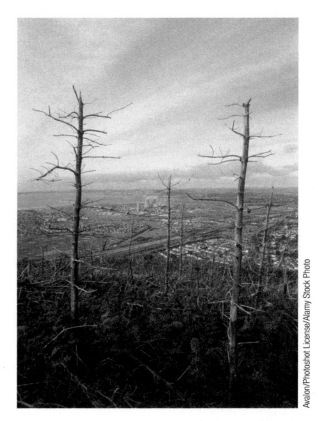

Avalon/Photoshot License/Alamy Stock Photo

Acid rain has many harmful effects on the environment and poses numerous health hazards, including the risk of cancer from heavy metals that can make their way into the food chain.

acid rain that relate to the health risks—sulfur dioxide and nitrogen oxides—described earlier.

Acidic precipitation can cause metals such as aluminum, cadmium, lead, and mercury to **leach** (dissolve and filter) out of the soil. If these metals make their way into water or food supplies (particularly fish), they can cause cancer in humans who consume them.

Acid rain is also responsible for crop damage, which, in turn, contributes to world hunger. Laboratory experiments showed that acid rain reduced seed yield by up to 23 percent. Actual crop losses are reported with increasing frequency. In May 1989, China's Hunan Province lost an estimated $260 million worth of crops and seedlings to acid rain. Similar losses have been reported in Chile, Brazil, and Mexico (French, 1990). Another consequence of acid rain is the destruction of public monuments and structures, with billions of dollars in damage each year (U.S. Environmental Protection Agency, 2012).

Indoor Air Pollution

A growing body of research indicates that the air within our homes and other buildings can be 10 to 40 times more hazardous than outdoor air even in the most industrialized cities (U.S. Environmental Protection Agency, 2002). This is a concern for the most vulnerable people in our population, particularly the young, the elderly, and the chronically ill, who spend most of their time indoors.

There are 20 to 100 potentially dangerous compounds in the average home. Most indoor pollution comes from sources that release gases or particles into the air (Canadian Centre for Occupational Health and Safety, 2011). Sources from building occupants include carbon dioxide, secondhand smoke, perfume, and body odours. Sources from building materials include dust, fibreglass, asbestos, and gases including formaldehyde. Toxic sources from cleaning agents come from cleansers, solvents, pesticides, disinfectants, and glue. Further contributors to indoor air pollution include gas emissions from furniture, carpets, and paints; dust mites from carpets, fabric, and foam chair cushions; microbial contaminants such as moulds, fungi, and bacteria from damp areas, stagnant water, and condensate pans; and ozone from photocopiers, electric motors, and electrostatic air cleaners (Canadian Centre for Occupational Health and Safety, 2011). Inadequate ventilation, particularly in heavily insulated buildings with airtight windows, can increase pollution by not allowing outside air in. Potential symptoms of indoor air pollution are listed below—if these appear in the first few hours in the building (at work or home) and then subside when you leave the building, there is strong support for the inside environment being at the core of your health issues:

- dryness and irritation of the eyes, nose, throat, and skin
- headache
- fatigue
- shortness of breath
- hypersensitivity and allergies
- sinus congestion
- coughing and sneezing
- dizziness
- nausea (Canadian Centre for Occupational Health and Safety, 2011)

Several factors affect risk for negative health outcomes due to air pollution including age; pre-existing medical conditions; individual sensitivity; room temperature and humidity; and liver, immune, and respiratory system functions (U.S. Environmental Protection Agency, 2002).

The U.S. Environmental Protection Agency (2002) suggests that the focus of reducing indoor air pollution should be on three main areas: source control (eliminating or reducing individual contaminants), ventilation improvements (increasing the amount of outdoor air coming indoors), and air cleaners (removing particulates from the air). Indoor air pollution comes primarily from woodstoves, furnaces, asbestos, passive smoke, formaldehyde, radon, and household chemicals and cleaners. In certain parts of Canada, mould can also be a significant source of air pollution.

Wood Stove Smoke

Wood stoves emit significant levels of particulates and carbon monoxide in addition to other pollutants, such as sulphur dioxide. If you rely on wood for heat, make sure your stove is properly installed, vented, and maintained. Proper adjustments and emission controls taken to recombust potential pollutants can help to reduce pollution levels from wood stoves. Burning seasoned wood also reduces the amount of particulates released into the air.

Furnaces

People who rely on oil- or gas-fired furnaces also need to make sure that these appliances are properly installed, ventilated, and maintained. Inadequate cleaning and maintenance can lead to a buildup of carbon monoxide in the home, which can be deadly.

Asbestos

Asbestos, previously mentioned as a contributor to indoor air pollution, poses serious threats to human health. **Asbestos** is a mineral commonly used in insulating materials in buildings constructed before 1970. When bonded to other materials, asbestos is relatively harmless, but if its tiny fibres become loosened and airborne, such as when asbestos is cut, ground up, or disturbed (i.e., removed from a building), they can embed themselves in the lungs and cannot be expelled (Canadian Lung Association, 2012). Their presence leads to cancer of the lungs, stomach, and chest lining, and is the cause of a fatal lung disease called mesothelioma (Canadian Lung Association, 2012).

Passive Smoke

Typically, **passive smoke** (or environmental tobacco smoke) is encountered as secondhand or sidestream smoke from cigarettes. Similar to active smoking, long-term exposure to passive smoke can cause serious negative health effects.

Asbestos A substance that separates into stringy fibres and lodges in lungs, where it cannot be expelled.

Passive smoke Secondhand or sidestream cigarette smoke.

Nonsmokers who live with smokers are at a higher risk for heart disease and some cancers. Passive smoke is a major cause of respiratory problems, especially in infants and children. Though widespread bans are now in place—limiting smokers from lighting up in restaurants, the workplace, shopping malls, schools, and in some cases while in a vehicle—many people, including children and youth, remain susceptible to passive smoke at home. Avoiding regular exposure to secondhand tobacco smoke will reduce your risks of heart and lung disease.

Formaldehyde

Formaldehyde, also previously mentioned as a contributor to indoor air pollution, is a colourless, strong-smelling gas present in some carpets, draperies, furniture, particle board, plywood, wood panelling, countertops, and many adhesives. It is released into the air in a process called outgassing. Outgassing is greatest in new products, but the process can continue for many years. Exposure to formaldehyde can cause respiratory problems, dizziness, fatigue, nausea, and rashes. Exposure at high concentrations may lead to burning sensations in the eyes, nose, and throat (Health Canada, 2012). Long-term exposure can lead to central nervous system disorders and cancer of the nasal cavity. These health risks are not likely to be experienced from exposure in your home, but rather in industry workers (Health Canada, 2012).

Radon

Radon, an odourless, colourless gas, is the natural by-product of uranium or radium decay in the soil. Radon can penetrate homes through cracks, pipes, sump pits, and other openings in the foundation. Although at toxic levels it can cause lung cancer, Health Canada (2012) does not consider radon pollution a widespread problem in Canadian homes. In fact, studies indicate that less than one-tenth of 1 percent of all homes in Canada could have levels of radon sufficiently high to warrant efforts aimed at lowering the level. Still, it is prudent to lower your home's radon level as much as possible. Guidelines for radon levels and if repairs are needed can be found on the Canadian Lung Association (2012) website at www.lung.ca/protect-protegez/pollution-pollution/indoor-interieur/radon-radon_e.php.

Household Chemicals

Cleansers and other cleaning products should be used only in well-ventilated rooms.

Formaldehyde A colourless, strong-smelling gas released from products through outgassing.

Radon A naturally occurring radioactive gas resulting from the decay of certain radioactive elements.

Chlorofluorocarbons (CFCs) Chemicals that contribute to the depletion of the ozone layer.

Further, regular cleaning will reduce the need to use potentially harmful cleaning products. Reduce your dry cleaning as much as possible as the chemicals used by many cleaners can cause cancer. If your newly cleaned clothes smell of dry cleaning chemicals, either return them to the cleaner or hang them in the open air until the smell is gone. Avoid the use of household air freshener products containing the cancer-causing agent dichlorobenzene. It is recommended that you clean with nontoxic, phosphate-free, and environmentally friendly products.

Ozone Layer Depletion

We earlier defined ozone as a chemical produced when oxygen interacts with sunlight. In people, ozone can lead to respiratory distress. Farther away from the earth, it forms a protective membrane-like layer in the earth's stratosphere—the highest level of the earth's atmosphere, located from 20 to 50 kilometres above the earth's surface. The ozone layer in the stratosphere protects the planet and its inhabitants from ultraviolet B (UV-B) radiation, a primary cause of skin cancer. Ultraviolet B radiation can also damage DNA and has been linked to weakened immune system functioning in humans and animals.

In the early 1970s, scientists began to warn of a depletion of the earth's stratospheric ozone layer. Special instruments developed to test atmospheric contents indicated that specific chemicals used on the earth contributed to the rapid depletion of this vital protective layer. These chemicals are called **chlorofluorocarbons (CFCs)** (see Figure 14.3). In 1979, a satellite measurement showing a large hole in the ozone layer over Antarctica shocked scientists. Since then, satellite measurements of the ozone layer have regularly shown increases in the size of the hole. As a result, Canada banned the production of CFCs in 1993 and their importation in 1996. Methyl chloroform was also banned in 1996.

In 2001, the Government of Canada published its Interim Plan 2001 on Particulate Matter and Ozone to share its plans to achieve Canada-wide standards for particulate matter and ozone. Five years later, a progress report indicated that major advances had been made in reducing smog-producing pollutants in the transportation sector, transboundary sources of air pollution, and establishing strong air quality monitoring networks across the country (Environment Canada, 2012). This plan continues to guide actions regarding achieving previous Canada-wide standards regarding particulate matter and ozone. The report can be obtained from Environment Canada (2012) at www.ec.gc.ca/air/default.asp?lang=En&n=0768F92F-1&offset=9&toc=show.

FIGURE 14.3

An Illustration of the Depletion of the Stratospheric Ozone Layer

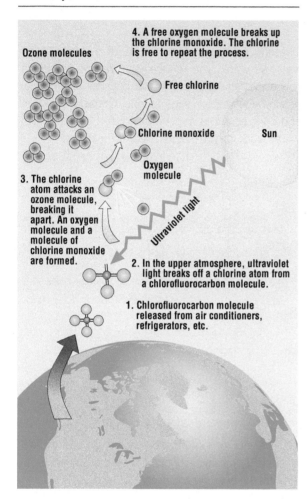

Ozone molecules

4. A free oxygen molecule breaks up the chlorine monoxide. The chlorine is free to repeat the process.

Free chlorine

Chlorine monoxide

Sun

Oxygen molecule

3. The chlorine atom attacks an ozone molecule, breaking it apart. An oxygen molecule and a molecule of chlorine monoxide are formed.

Ultraviolet light

2. In the upper atmosphere, ultraviolet light breaks off a chlorine atom from a chlorofluorocarbon molecule.

1. Chlorofluorocarbon molecule released from air conditioners, refrigerators, etc.

FIGURE 14.4

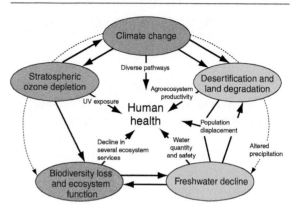

Large-scale and global environmental hazards to human health include climate change, stratospheric ozone depletion, loss of biodiversity, changes in hydrological systems and the supplies of fresh water, land degradation, and stresses on food-producing systems.

Source: Reprinted from Publication Millennium Ecosystem Assessment, Global environmental change, © 2005.

Global Warming

More than 100 years ago, scientists theorized that carbon dioxide emissions from fossil-fuel burning would create a buildup of "greenhouse" gases in the earth's atmosphere and that this accumulation would have a warming effect on the earth's surface. The century-old predictions are now coming true, with alarming effects. Average global temperatures are higher today than at any time since global temperatures were first recorded, and the change in atmospheric temperature may be taking a heavy toll on humans and crops. Climate researchers predicted in 1975 that the buildup of greenhouse gases would produce life-threatening natural phenomena, including drought, severe forest fires, flooding, extended heat waves over large areas of the earth, and killer hurricanes. Figure 14.4 illustrates the complex interactions and the influence of climate change on human health.

Greenhouse gases include carbon dioxide, CFCs, ground-level ozone, nitrous oxide, and methane. These chemicals become part of a gaseous layer that encircles the earth, allowing solar heat to pass through and then trapping it close to the earth's surface (as if in a greenhouse). The most predominant of these chemicals is carbon dioxide, which accounts for 49 percent of all greenhouse gases. Eastern Europe and North America are responsible for approximately half of all carbon dioxide emissions. Since the late nineteenth century, carbon dioxide concentrations in the atmosphere have increased 25 percent, with half of this increase occurring since the 1950s. Not surprisingly, these greater concentrations coincide with world industrial growth.

Rapid deforestation of the tropical rainforests of Central and South America, Africa, and Southeast Asia is also contributing to the rapid rise of greenhouse gases. Trees take in carbon dioxide, transform it, store the carbon for food, and then release oxygen into the air. Thus, as we lose forests, we lose the capacity to dissipate carbon dioxide.

The potential consequences of global warming are dire. The rising atmospheric concentration of greenhouse gases may be the most economically disruptive and costly change of our modern industrial society. Ground-level ozone causes damage to leaf tissue, inhibiting photosynthesis, the process by which plants use light energy for growth (Environment Canada, 2012). Some forest species at risk include

Greenhouse gases Gases that contribute to global warming by trapping heat near the earth's surface.

point of view

REDUCING AIR POLLUTION: Active Transportation?

One way that you can contribute positively to the environment, and reduce air pollution, is by reducing your personal use of a vehicle. There are several ways that you can do this. The obvious one is to engage in active forms of transportation, where you use your own energy to power your transportation. Have you considered the possibility of walking, cycling, or wheeling as your primary mode of transportation? Not only would you reduce your vehicle emissions you would also obtain positive physical and mental health benefits from your actions. Consider the pros and cons of active transportation and decide which would work for you—at least part of the time.

PROS

- reduced vehicle emissions
- costs savings (gas and parking fees)
- physical and mental health benefits
- the possibility of getting to know the area and community within which you live, work, and go to school better
- the opportunity to enjoy time outside
- for short distances may save time (distances of less than one kilometre, particularly when parking is an issue)
- provides a form of stress relief (particularly after work or school)

CONS

- takes more time (for distances greater than one kilometre)
- the need to shower afterwards
- if showering, the need to plan ahead for work/school clothes
- costs associated with having appropriate walking shoes, bicycle and helmet, skateboard, scooter, etc.
- poor weather—rain, snow, sleet, ice, etc.

Other more environmentally friendly ideas for those of you that really do live too far from work or school are to take the bus or carpool. These options also take careful planning and involve a commitment to the environment.

It is your responsibility to consider the environment before you jump into your car to drive short distances. In terms of the environment, every little bit helps.

northern red oak, eastern white pine, black oak, and sugar maple. Ground-level ozone has been linked to the forest decline observed in Germany and other European countries (Canadian Lung Association, 2012).

Reducing Air Pollution

Canada's air pollution problems are rooted in our energy, transportation, and industrial practices. Comprehensive national strategies are required to reduce air pollution and clean the air for future generations. You should support policies that encourage the use of renewable resources such as solar, wind, and water power as the providers of more, if not most, of the world's energy. The atmosphere has no borders.

Most experts agree that shifting away from gasoline-powered automobiles as the primary source of transportation is the only way to reduce air pollution significantly, which would reduce the greenhouse effect and, consequently, global warming. Some cities have taken steps in this direction by setting high parking fees, imposing bans on city driving, and establishing high road-usage tolls. Other positive efforts include tax benefits for the use of public transportation.

Automakers must be encouraged to manufacture automobiles that provide excellent fuel economy and low rates of toxic emissions. Incentives given to manufacturers to produce such vehicles, tax breaks for purchasers who buy them, and "gas-guzzler" taxes on inefficient vehicles are three promising suggestions that may effectively help to reduce air pollution.

Similarly, primary suppliers of gasoline have been encouraged and regulated to reduce the proportion of benzene in their products. In Canada, the Benzene in Gasoline Regulations came into effect on July 1, 1999. These regulations state that concentration of benzene in gasoline may only be 1 percent by volume and that the aromatics (or equivalent tailpipe emissions) must be frozen at 1994 levels (Thompson, El-Solh, & McGuire, 2006).

WATER POLLUTION

Although 75 percent of the earth is covered with water in the form of oceans, seas, lakes, rivers, streams, and wetlands, only 3 percent of this water is suitable for drinking water and most of that is found in glaciers, polar icecaps, and in deep underground aquifers resulting in only 1 percent of the water actually being available for drinking. It is not a surprising then that lack of water affects 40 percent of the world's population (World Health Organization, 2009b). Beneath the landmass are reservoirs of groundwater. We draw our drinking water either from this underground source or from surface freshwater sources. The status of our water supply reflects the pollution level of our communities and, ultimately, the whole earth.

The federal government passed the Canada Water Act in 1970 and created the Department of the Environment in 1971, entrusting the Inland Waters Directorate with providing national leadership for freshwater management. Under the Constitution Act (1867), the provinces are "owners" of the water resources within their boundaries and have wide responsibilities in their day-to-day management.

Water Contamination

Any substance that gets into the soil has the potential to get into the water supply. Contaminants from industrial air pollution and acid rain eventually work their way into the soil and then into the groundwater. Pesticides sprayed on crops wash through the soil into the groundwater. Oil spills and other hazardous wastes flow into local rivers and streams. Underground storage tanks for gasoline may develop leaks. The list continues.

Pollutants can enter waterways through a number of routes. These routes may be divided into two general categories: point-source and non-point-source. Pollutants that enter a waterway at a specific single point, through a pipe, ditch, culvert, or other such conduit, are referred to as **point-source pollutants** (Environment Canada, 2010). The two major sources of this type of pollution are sewage treatment plants and

industrial facilities. Other sources include on-site septic systems, leaky tanks or pipelines containing petroleum, leaks or spills from industrial manufacturing facilities, underground injection wells, landfills, livestock waste, leaky sewer lines, chemical use at wood preservation facilities, mill tailings in mining areas, fly ash from coal-fired power plants, sludge disposal from petroleum refineries, graveyards, road salt storage areas, wells for disposal of liquid wastes, runoff of salt and other chemicals from roads, spills related to highway accidents, coal tar at old coal gasification sites, and asphalt production and cleaning sites (Environment Canada, 2010).

Non-point-source pollutants—commonly called runoff and sedimentation—refer to pollutants entering groundwater from more than one point; thus, they may seep into waterways from broad areas of land rather than through a discrete pipe or conduit. Non-point sources include fertilizers on agricultural lands, pesticides on agricultural and forest lands, and contaminants in rain, snow, and dry atmospheric fallout (Environment Canada, 2010). It is estimated that 99 percent of the sediment in our waterways, 98 percent of the bacterial contaminants, 84 percent of the phosphorus, and 82 percent of the nitrogen come from non-point sources (Nadakavukaren, 1990). Non-point-source pollution results from a variety of human land-use practices including soil erosion and sedimentation, construction wastes, pesticide and fertilizer runoff, urban street runoff, wastes from engineering projects, acid mine drainage, leakage from septic tanks, and sewage sludge (Griffin, 1991). (See Figure 14.5.)

Septic Systems

Bacteria from human waste can leach into the water supply from improperly installed septic systems. Toxic chemicals disposed of directly into septic systems also get into the groundwater supply.

Landfills

Landfills and dumps generate a liquid called leachate, a mixture of soluble chemicals that come from household garbage and office, biologic, and industrial waste. If a landfill has not been properly lined, leachate trickles through the layers of garbage and eventually into the water supply.

Gasoline and Petroleum Products

Underground storage tanks for gasoline and petroleum products are common; most are located at gasoline filling stations. Tanks that have been leaking have been replaced over time; many were installed 45 to 50 years ago and were made of

Point-source pollutants Pollutants that enter waterways at a specific point.

Non-point-source pollutants Pollutants that seep into waterways from broad areas of land.

FIGURE 14.5
Sources of Groundwater Contamination

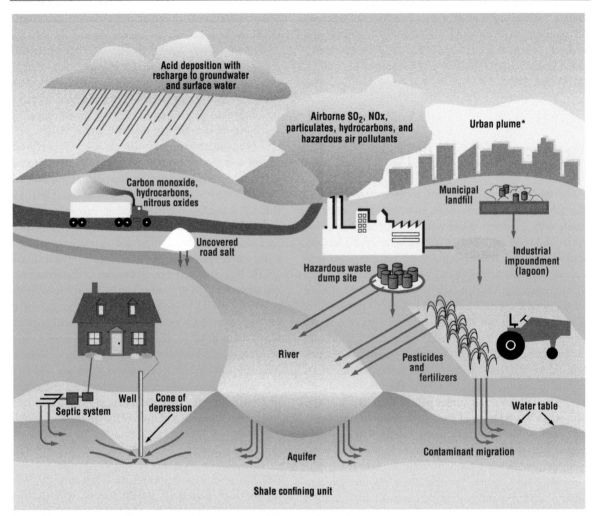

*Rising air at lower altitudes caused by urban areas being warmer than surrounding areas.

fabricated steel that was unprotected from corrosion. As a result, over time pinpoint holes developed in the steel and the petroleum products stored in the tanks leaked into the groundwater. The most common way to detect the presence of petroleum products in the water supply is to test for benzene, a component of oil and gasoline. Benzene is highly toxic and associated with cancer development.

Dioxins

Dioxins are chlorinated hydrocarbons contained in herbicides (chemicals used to kill vegetation) and produced during certain industrial processes. Dioxins have the ability to bioaccumulate, which means the body does not excrete them but instead

Dioxins Highly toxic chlorinated hydrocarbons contained in herbicides and produced during certain industrial processes.

stores them in fatty tissues and the liver, and are much more toxic than PCBs (see below).

Chemical Contaminants

Most chemicals designed to dissolve grease and oil are called organic solvents. These extremely toxic substances, such as carbon tetrachloride, tetrachloroethylene, and trichloroethylene (TCE), are used to clean clothing, painting equipment, plastics, and metal parts. Many household products, such as stain and spot removers, degreasers, drain cleaners, septic system cleaners, and paint removers, also contain these toxic chemicals.

Organic solvents work their way into the water supply in different ways. Consumers often dump leftover products into the toilet. One example of this is pharmaceuticals; many consumers dispose of unused medications by flushing them—whereas they should be returned to pharmacies. Another example is paint thinner; some consumers will flush this as well. Industries pour leftovers into large barrels, which are then buried. After a while, the chemicals eat their way out of the barrels and leach into the groundwater. All of these products can and should be properly discarded. When faced with the decision to get rid of these sorts of things, find a more appropriate way to do so.

A related group of toxic substances contains chlorinated hydrocarbons. The most notorious of these substances are the polychlorinated biphenyls (PCBs), their cousins the polybromated biphenyls (PBBs), and the dioxins.

PCBs

Polychlorinated biphenyls, commonly known as chlorobiphenyls or PCBs, are industrial chemicals that were synthesized and commercialized since the late 1920s and used in the manufacturing of electrical equipment, including high voltage transformers, heat exchangers, hydraulic systems, and other specialized applications for about 50 years (Environment Canada, 2010). The import, manufacture, and sale (for reuse) of PCBs were made illegal in Canada in 1977 and the release of PCBs to the environment illegal in 1985. However, PCB equipment owners were allowed to use their equipment until the end of their equipment's serviceable life.

PCBs also bioaccumulate. PCBs are associated with birth defects and known to cause cancer. PCBs have not been manufactured in North America since the late 1970s, but millions of kilograms of PCBs have been dumped into landfills and waterways, where they continue to pose an environmental threat (Nadakavukaren, 1990). However, in recent years the Canadian government has committed millions of dollars to cleaning up Canadian waterways and placed large fines on dumping toxic substances in waterways.

The long-term effects of bioaccumulation of these toxic substances include possible damage to the immune system, increased risk of infection, and elevated risk of cancer. Exposure to high concentrations of PCBs or dioxins for a short period of time can also have severe consequences, including nausea, vomiting, diarrhea, painful rashes and sores, and chloracne, an ailment in which the skin develops hard, black, painful pimples that may never go away.

Pesticides

Pesticides are chemicals designed to kill insects, rodents, plants, and fungi. Canadians use millions of kilograms of pesticides each year, with only 10 percent actually reaching the targeted organisms. The remaining pesticides settle on the land and in the water. Pesticide residues also cling to many fresh fruits and vegetables and are ingested when people eat them. Most pesticides accumulate in the body. Health effects from pesticide exposure can occur immediately, within several hours, or longer term with symptoms described in categories of mild, moderate, and severe poisoning (Canadian Centre for Occupational Health and Safety, 2010). Potential hazards associated with long-term exposure to pesticides include birth defects, cancer, liver and kidney damage, and nervous system disorders. Thus, many municipalities across Canada are banning the use of pesticides.

Trihalomethanes

Most Canadians drink water treated with chlorine to kill harmful bacteria. Trihalomethanes (THMs) are synthetic organic chemicals formed at water treatment plants when the added chlorine reacts with natural organic compounds in the water. Any chlorinated drinking water supply is likely to contain THMs, which include such substances as chloroform, bromoform, and dichlorobromomethane. Short-term exposure to chloroform relates to central nervous system depression, while long-term exposure relates to hepatitis, jaundice and other negative effects on the liver, and central nervous system effects including depression and irritability (U.S. Environmental Protection Agency, 2007). Further, chloroform in high doses is known to cause liver and kidney disorders, central nervous system problems, birth defects, and cancer. THM concentrations can be substantially reduced by adjusting the chlorine dose, improving filtration practices to remove organic material, or adding chlorine after filtration rather than before.

Lead

Lead can be ingested in household water that comes through lead pipes. Water, particularly acidic water, will leach some of the lead from the pipes. One way to reduce the possibility of ingesting lead if it does exist in your home's water system is to run tap water for several minutes to flush out water that has been standing overnight. Health Canada is mandated, under the Government of Canada's Hazardous Products Act and Regulations, to protect Canadians from potential health hazards in consumer products. Although leaded paints and ceramic glazes also pose health risks, particularly for small children who put toys in their mouths, the use of leads in such products has been effectively reduced in recent years.

Chronic low-level exposure to lead may result in serious health consequences such as anemia, malaise, and damage to the nervous system (World Health Association, 2013c). As

Polychlorinated biphenyls (PCBs) Toxic chemicals once used as insulating materials in high-voltage electrical equipment.

Pesticides Chemicals designed to kill insects and other pests that interfere with growth of a particular product (for instance, grass).

mentioned, children are particularly vulnerable as even low-level exposure can reduce their IQ and result in learning disabilities, poor school performance, and violent behaviour (World Health Association, 2013c).

NOISE POLLUTION

Loud noise has become commonplace. We are often painfully aware of construction crews working on our streets, jet airplanes roaring overhead, stereos blaring next door, and trucks rumbling down nearby freeways. We also use various devices to listen to music privately with earphones directly in our ears. Your body has a physiologic response to loud sounds, and when they are perceived as noise, they can become a source of physical and mental distress (Canadian Centre for Occupational Health and Safety, 2007).

Prolonged exposure to some noises results in hearing loss. Short-term exposure reduces productivity, concentration levels, and attention spans, and can affect mental and emotional health. Symptoms of noise-related distress include disturbed sleep patterns, headaches, and tension. Physically, our bodies respond to noises in a variety of ways and the effects can be temporary or permanent (Canadian Centre for Occupational Health and Safety, 2007). Blood pressure increases, blood vessels in the brain dilate, and vessels in other parts of the body constrict. The pupils of the eyes dilate. Cholesterol levels in the blood rise and some endocrine glands secrete additional stimulating hormones, such as adrenaline, into the bloodstream.

At this point, it is necessary to distinguish between sound and noise. Sound is anything that can be heard. Noise is sound that can damage the hearing or cause mental or emotional distress. When sound becomes distracting or annoying, it becomes noise.

Despite increased awareness that noise pollution is more than a nuisance, government representatives continue to give noise-control programs low priority. In order to prevent hearing loss, it is important that you avoid exposure to excessive noise. Playing stereos in your vehicle, home, and in your ear at reasonable levels, wearing earplugs when you use power equipment, and establishing barriers (closed windows, and so on) between you and noise will help prevent hearing loss.

Municipal solid waste Includes durable goods; nondurable goods; containers and packaging; food waste; yard waste; and miscellaneous waste from residential, commercial, institutional, and industrial sources.

Hazardous waste Solid waste that poses a hazard to humans or the environment.

LAND POLLUTION

Many communities in Canada face serious problems in safely and effectively managing their garbage.

Solid Waste

Municipal solid waste is outstripping available landfill sites, and the opening of new landfill sites is usually controversial as people become more aware of the hazards they pose to nearby land and water. Toronto, for instance, has had to scramble to find communities in other parts of Ontario that would take its overflow garbage.

Part of the answer to this worsening problem is increased personal commitment to reducing, reusing, and recycling. Experts believe that as much as 90 percent of our garbage is ultimately reusable or recyclable.

Hazardous Waste

Hazardous wastes are defined as wastes with properties that make them capable of harming human health or the environment.

The Canadian Environmental Protection Agency (CEPA) established an overall program to deal with hazardous wastes. The CEPA divides hazardous materials into two groups for elimination or reduction. Persistent, bioaccumulative, toxic hazardous wastes that are primarily the result of human activity will be targeted for virtual elimination from the environment; substances that do not meet these criteria are candidates for full life-cycle management to prevent or minimize their release into the environment (Environment Canada, 1995).

Industry education and cooperation are important for achieving a safer environment with less hazardous waste. In cooperation with provincial/territorial and municipal authorities, the following procedures are in place:

- Many wastes are banned from land disposal or treated in such a way that their toxicity is reduced before they are dumped.

- Hazardous-waste handlers must clean up contamination resulting from past waste management practices in addition to current activities.

- CEPA is exploring ways to create economic incentives to encourage ingenuity in hazardous waste minimization practices and recycling.

Organizations such as the Recycling Council of Ontario are dedicated to improving waste reduction and recycling in communities across Canada.

RADIATION

A substance is considered radioactive when it emits high-energy particles from the nuclei of its atoms. There are three types of radiation: alpha particles, beta

Are Cell Phones Hazardous to Your Health?

You, like most students, are likely to have a cellphone. You may even be lost without it. Have you considered the risk associated with your cell-phone use? Potential health risks exist—particularly if you use your phone a lot. Further, the type of use (testing, game-playing, talking, and so on) you give your phone also influences your risk. Depending on how close your cell phone is to your head, as much as 60 percent of the radiation emitted by the phone can penetrate the area around your head, some of it reaching an inch to an inch-and-a-half into your brain.

At high power levels, radio-frequency energy (the energy used in cell phones) can rapidly heat biological tissue and cause damage. That said, it should be pointed out that cell phones operate at power levels well below the level at which such heating occurs. Many countries, including the United States, Canada, and most European nations, use standards set by the Federal Communications Commission (FCC) for radio-frequency energy based on research by several scientific groups. These groups identified a whole-body *specific absorption rate (SAR)* value for exposure to radio-frequency energy. Four watts per kilogram was identified as a threshold level of exposure at which harmful biological effects may occur. The FCC requires wireless phones to comply with a safety limit of 1.6 watts per kg.

The World Health Organization and other major health agencies agree that the research to date has not shown radio-frequency energy emitted from cell phones to be harmful. However, they also point to the need for more research, because cell phones have only been in widespread use for less than two decades, and no long-term studies have been done to determine if cell phones are risk free. Three large studies have compared cell phone use among brain cancer patients and individuals free of brain cancer, finding no correlation between cell phone use and brain tumours. However, preliminary results from smaller, well-designed studies continue to raise questions suggesting the need for more longitudinal and prospective research.

To lower any potential risk of health problems related to your cell phone use, limit your usage, and purchase a hands-free device that keeps the phone farther from your head. Send text messages or e-mail rather than talking on the phone. Better yet, talk in person. In addition, check the SAR level of your phone (for instructions, see www.fcc.gov/cgb/sar). Purchase one with a lower level if yours is near the FCC limit.

Sources: Based on American Cancer Society (2008). "Cellular Phones," www.cancer.org/docroot/PED/content/PED_1_3X_Cellular_Phones.asp; Committee on Identification of Research Needs Relating to Potential Biological or Adverse Health Effects of Wireless Communications Devices, National Research Council (Washington, DC: National Academies Press, 2008); National Cancer Institute (2011). Cell Phones and Cancer Risk. www.cancer.gov/cancertopics/factsheet/Risk/cellphones.

particles, and gamma rays (Canadian Nuclear Association, 2009). Alpha particles are relatively massive particles produced by the radioactive decay of heavy elements such as uranium and are not capable of penetrating human skin. They pose health hazards only when inhaled or ingested. Beta particles are derived from the transformation of a neutron to a proton in the nucleus of an atom and are capable of slight penetration of the skin and are harmful when ingested or inhaled. Gamma rays are electromagnetic radiation similar to X-rays and are the most dangerous radioactive particles because they pass right through the skin, causing serious damage to organs and other vital structures (Canadian Nuclear Association, 2009).

Ionizing Radiation

Exposure to ionizing radiation is an inescapable part of life. **Ionizing radiation** is caused by the release of particles and electromagnetic rays from atomic nuclei during the normal process of disintegration. Some naturally occurring elements, such as uranium, emit radiation. Other radiation-producing elements, such as deuterium, develop as part of the decay process of uranium or are created by scientists in laboratories. Radiation, whether naturally occurring or human-made, can damage genetic material in the reproductive cells of living organisms. It can also cause mutations, miscarriages, physical and mental deformities, cancer, eye cataracts, gastrointestinal illnesses, and shortened life expectancies.

Scientists cannot agree on a safe level of radiation. Reactions to radiation differ from person to person. Exposure is measured in radiation absorbed doses, or "rads" (also called roentgens). Recommended maximum "safe" dosages range from 0.5 to 5 rads per year. Approximately 50 percent of the radiation we are exposed to comes from natural sources, such as building materials. Another 45 percent comes from medical and dental X-rays. The remaining 5 percent comes from computer screens, microwave

Ionizing radiation Radiation produced by photons with enough energy to ionize atoms.

ovens, television sets, luminous watch dials, and radar screens and waves. Most of us are exposed to far less radiation than the "safe" maximum dosage per year.

Radiation can cause damage at dosages as low as 100 to 200 rads. At this level, signs of radiation sickness include nausea, diarrhea, fatigue, anemia, sore throat, and hair loss. Death is unlikely at this dosage. At 350 to 500 rads, the previously mentioned symptoms increase in severity, and death may result because bone marrow production of the white blood cells that we need to protect us from disease is hindered. Dosages above 600 to 700 rads are invariably fatal. The effects of long-term exposure to relatively low levels of radiation are unknown. Some scientists believe that such exposure can cause lung cancer, leukemia, skin cancer, bone cancer, and skeletal deformities.

Nonionizing Radiation

The lower-energy portions of the electromagnetic spectrum, ranging from lower-energy ultraviolet radiation down through infrared, radar, radio, and the electric and magnetic fields associated with many household appliances and electric power lines, are **nonionizing radiation**. Although the biological effects of ionizing radiation have been recognized for some time, we still do not know very much about the effects of certain types of nonionizing radiation—in particular, the photons associated with electric and magnetic fields. Techniques for assessing radiation from many such sources continue to evolve (Moeller, 1992). Currently there are four interrelated units for measuring radiation: radioactivity, exposure, absorbed dose, and dose equivalent.

Nuclear Power Plants

Nuclear power plants account for less than 1 percent of the total radiation we are exposed to. Other producers of radioactive wastes include medical facilities that use radioactive materials for treatment and diagnostic procedures (for instance, MRI, CT scans, and so on) and nuclear weapons production facilities.

Proponents of nuclear energy believe it is a safe and efficient way to generate electricity. Initial costs of building nuclear power plants are high, but actual power generation is relatively inexpensive. A 1000-megawatt reactor produces enough energy for 600 000 homes and saves 1590 million litres of fossil fuels each year. In some areas where nuclear power plants were decommissioned, electricity bills tripled when power companies turned to hydroelectric or fossil fuel sources.

Nonionizing radiation Radiation produced by photons associated with lower-energy portions.

Meltdown An accident that results when the temperature in the core of a nuclear reactor increases sufficiently to melt the nuclear fuel and its containment vessel.

Nuclear reactors also discharge fewer carbon oxides into the air than fossil fuel-powered generators. Advocates believe that conversion to nuclear power could slow the global warming trend (Flavin, 1990). Some have gone as far to say that nuclear fission energy has the potential eliminate greenhouse gases altogether (Brook, 2012).

All of these advantages of nuclear energy must be weighed against the disadvantages. First, disposal of nuclear wastes is extremely problematic for the entire world, partly because the radioactive half-life is 10 000 years. Additionally, the chances of a reactor core meltdown pose serious threats to the immediate environment of nuclear plants—and to the world in general.

A nuclear **meltdown** occurs when the temperature of the core of the reactor increases to a point that it melts the nuclear fuel and its containment vessel. Most modern facilities seal their reactors and containment vessels in concrete buildings with pools of cold water on the bottom. Then, if a meltdown occurs, the building and the pool should prevent the radioactive release.

Human error and mechanical failure were the reported causes of the 1986 reactor core fire and explosion at the Chernobyl nuclear power plant in Russia as well as the nuclear disaster in Fukushima in 2011. In just four and a half seconds, the temperature in the reactor rose to 120 times normal, causing an explosion. Eighteen people were killed immediately, thirty died later from radiation sickness, and two hundred others were hospitalized for severe radiation sickness. Officials evacuated people living near the plant. Some medical workers estimate that the eventual death toll from radiation-induced cancers exceeded 100 000. Direct costs of the disaster were more than $13 billion, including lost agricultural output and the cost of replacing the power plant.

Opponents of nuclear energy believe that there is no safe place to dispose of, contain, or store the escalating supply of nuclear waste.

FOOD QUALITY

For most Canadians, food accounts for 80 to 95 percent of their daily intake of the most persistent toxic contaminants, while air contributes 10 to 15 percent, and drinking water contributes very little. Compared with other countries, the food available in Canada is some of the safest. Still, contamination remains a concern. Aside from microbial contamination, as discussed in Chapter 5, environmental contamination can occur in several fashions. Chemical contaminants enter the food supply through uptake from water or soil, and by air deposition on leaves and fruit. Worldwide there have been a number of instances where people have been exposed to high levels of chemical contaminants

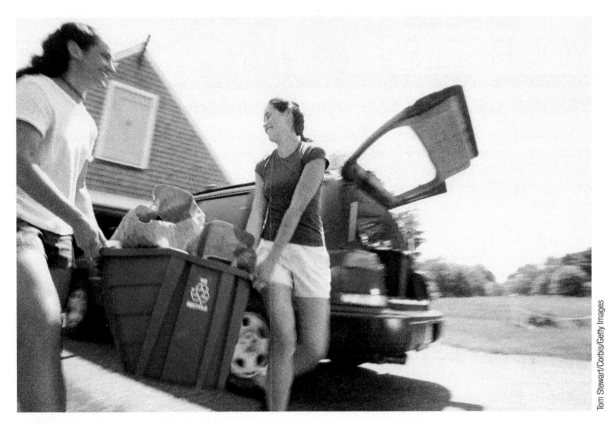

While we may feel that many of the environmental problems facing the world today are beyond individual control, we can play a significant role in keeping our own little part of it clean, green, and beautiful.

Tom Stewart/Corbis/Getty Images

(World Health Organization, 2014). Dioxins, already discussed, can accumulate in the food chain, mainly in the fatty tissue of animals. One such example occurred in 1999, where high levels of dioxins were found in poultry and eggs from Belgium. These contaminated products were then detected in several other countries. The cause was traced to animal feed contaminated with illegally disposed PCB-based waste industrial oil. Another well known incident occurred in 1976 in Seveso, Italy, when large amounts of dioxins were accidentally released at a chemical factory. The chemicals released contaminated an area of 15 square kilometres where 37 000 people lived. The short-term exposure of humans to high levels of dioxins may result in skin lesions, patchy darkening of the skin, and altered liver function (World Health Organization, 2002). Less well known are the long-term impacts of dioxin exposure. Studies have shown links to impairment of the immune system, the developing nervous system, the endocrine system, and reproductive functions (World Health Organization, 2003). Moreover, research among animals indicates that chronic exposure to dioxins results in several types of cancer (Baan et al., 2009). Extensive studies in the affected population are continuing to determine the long-term human health effects from this incident. Some contaminants can bioaccumulate to become more toxic when at the top of the food chain, as with mercury concentration in game fish in a number of Canadian water systems. Also, chemicals used in food production and handling can leave residues on food products—for example, the hormones and antibiotics used to increase meat and dairy production, or the substances used to preserve freshness or enhance flavour (Health Canada, n.d.). Refer back to "Food Borne Illness" in Chapter 5 for steps you can take to reduce your risk.

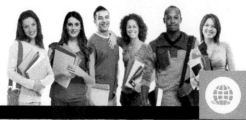

assess
YOURSELF

Go to MasteringHealth to complete this questionnaire with automatic scoring

TAKING CHARGE: Managing Environmental Pollution

Environmental health begins at home. You and your classmates must overcome the inertia exhibited in society and make efforts and/or sacrifices that contribute to the good of the planet. By understanding how political and economic issues affect the environment, you can pressure corporations and elected representatives to change policies harmful to the environment. For example, environmentalists pressured the World Bank to stop issuing development loans leading to the destruction of rainforests. Discussing issues with lawmakers and making decisions at the polls are two ways you can influence environmental policy.

You also can—and should—be making more personal efforts to reduce your environmental impact. Before you can do that, you need to be aware of your attitudes and behaviours towards the environment. Complete the following, being honest with yourself.

It Is Not Easy Being Green

Circle the number of each item that describes what you have done or are doing for the environment.

1. When spending time at parks and beaches, I never leave anything behind.
2. I ride my bike, walk, or use other forms of active transportation or I carpool or use public transportation whenever possible.
3. I write my municipal, provincial/territorial, and federal representatives about environmental issues.
4. I avoid or limit turning on the air conditioner or increasing the heat whenever possible.
5. I take short showers instead of baths.
6. My shower has a low-flow shower head.
7. I do not run the water while brushing my teeth, shaving, or hand-washing clothes.
8. My sink taps have aerators installed in them.
9. I have a water displacement device in my toilet(s) or I have low-flow toilet(s).
10. I snip or rip plastic six-pack rings before I throw them out.
11. I choose recycled and recyclable products as often as possible.
12. I avoid noise pollutants. (I sit away from speakers at concerts, select an apartment away from busy streets or airports, and so on.)
13. I make sure my car is tuned with functional emission control equipment.

14. I try to avoid known carcinogens such as vinyl chloride, asbestos, benzene, mercury, X-rays, and so on.
15. When shopping, I choose products with the least amount of packaging.
16. I dispose of hazardous materials (used batteries, paint, oil, and antifreeze) at appropriate sites.
17. If or when I have children, I will use cloth rather than disposable diapers.
18. I store food in reusable containers rather than using plastic wrap. I pack my lunch in a reusable bag.
19. I use as few paper products as possible.
20. I take my own reusable bag(s) along when I go shopping for groceries and other things. If I do not need a bag, I tell the salesclerk I will go without.
21. I avoid products packaged in plastic and unrecycled aluminum.
22. I recycle newspapers, glass, cans, plastics, other paper, and all other recyclables.
23. I run the clothes dryer only as long as it takes my clothes to dry. I dry as many clothes as possible outdoors or indoors on a laundry line or drying rack.
24. I turn off lights and appliances, including my computer, when not in use.
25. I compost organic wastes.

Scoring and Interpretation

Count how many items you have circled; ideally, you should be doing all these things. Interpret your score as follows:

20–25: Good contributions to maintaining the environment.

14–19: Moderate contributions to maintaining the environment.

Below 13: Need to reconsider your approach to the environment and make changes for the sustainability of the environment.

Considering Your Personal Choices Regarding the Environment

One of the most significant decisions you will make as a consumer is whether to pay more for environmentally safe products. As a student on a tight budget, are you willing to pay more for products such as environmentally friendly soap and laundry detergent? If so, how much more? If not, are you willing to buy a *less* environmentally unfriendly product? If not, will you purchase more environmentally friendly products when your finances allow it? While it is not likely that you can increase your budget enough to buy all environmentally safe products, you can start now. Think about the products you buy: Which could you substitute with more environmentally friendly brands? Could you use less of the environmentally damaging products?

Other questions you might ask yourself regarding the environment include the following:

- Do you vote in municipal, provincial, and federal elections? Do you know the difference between rhetoric and reality when it comes to environmental issues? Do you ask questions of the candidates regarding the environment?

- Do you conserve water? Do you fix leaky taps quickly? Do you wash only full loads? Do you overwater lawns or gardens?

- Do you think before you throw household chemicals away? Finish them, give them away, or save them for a household hazardous waste collection. Consider nonhazardous substitutes.

- Do you recycle used oil? Oil dumped down storm drains or on the ground can pollute streams, killing insects, fish, birds, and wildlife.

- Do you recycle tin cans, glass, newspaper, paper, plastic, and cardboard?

- Have you considered reporting people who litter?

- Have you considered walking, riding the bus, using your bike, wheeling, or carpooling whenever possible?

- Have you thought about the amount of fertilizers and pesticides you or your family use? Rain can wash them off lawns and carry them into lakes and streams. Use low-phosphorus fertilizers.

- Do you ask yourself, your family, and your friends if you (or they) really need a product before purchasing it?

- Do you consider whether a product is practical and durable, well made, and of timeless design?

- Do you buy used and rebuilt products whenever possible? Do you sell unused/lightly used items at yard or garage sales or donate them to charities?

- Do you compost leaves, grass clippings, and kitchen scraps?

- What do you do, or will you do, when you return home for the summer? What will you do with the various items you purchased to be at college or university? Will you find a new home for them? What efforts will you make to NOT throw reusable items away?

Critical Thinking

Your health teacher is leading a protest next week to the corporate headquarters of "one of the country's worst polluters." You are told that this company has a terrible record of point- and non-point-source pollutants and that the "corporate bigwigs refuse to do anything about it." After hearing the brief appeal to join the protest, you decide it is your duty as a citizen to go. As your teacher hands out maps to the protest site, you realize that the company in question is your employer! Now you are really confused: your company claims to have spent billions of dollars to reduce pollution and considers itself an innovator in cleaning up sites it polluted in the past. You are upset because only one side of the story is being told. Should you speak up in class? What else could you do?

Using the DECIDE model in Chapter 1, decide what you would do. First, decide why you are upset. Then decide what you would like to accomplish by speaking up. In addition, consider the best setting to communicate your message to your teacher (in class, during office hours, by email, and so on).

DISCUSSION QUESTIONS

1. Describe the issues surrounding global population and how they differ among the developed, developing, and least developed regions. How can the developing world be encouraged and assisted to be 'environmental' in their development?

2. How does an increasing global population affect the environment locally, provincially, nationally, and globally?

3. List the primary sources of air pollution, acid rain, and indoor air pollution in Canada. What can be done individually and collectively to reduce each type of pollution?

4. What are the environmental consequences of global warming? What can Canadian citizens do to slow the deforestation of tropical rainforests?

5. Explain point- and non-point sources of water pollution. Discuss how water pollution can be reduced or prevented altogether in Canada. What actions can you as a student take?

6. Given all the open land in Canada, do you think solid waste disposal is a problem? Why or why not?

7. Are the advantages of nuclear power worth the risks involved with storage? Put another way, if you lived near a nuclear power plant, would you be willing to pay two or three times as much for electricity in order to have the nuclear power plant closed? Why or why not?

APPLICATION EXERCISE

Reread the "Consider This . . . " scenario at the beginning of the chapter and answer the following questions.

1. What resources are available on your campus to help students such as Leo become environmentally friendly in their day-to-day living? In your community?

2. How much time and effort are students willing to put into conserving the environment? Is it seen as a real issue? Why or why not?

MASTERINGHEALTH

Go to MasteringHealth for Assignments, the eText, and the Study Area with case studies, self quizzing, and videos.

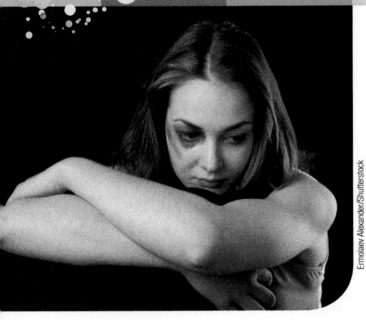

Ermolaev Alexander/Shutterstock

CHAPTER 15
PREVENTING VIOLENCE, ABUSE, AND INJURY

CONSIDER THIS . . .

Will is awakened by the sound of loud voices. His parents are fighting again. His father is calling his mother nasty names. She is shouting back. Will creeps to the top of the stairs. They are just below him. He hears a sickening "whack" as his father hits his mother. Then his father kicks her. There is a knock at the door. The police were called by the neighbours. They take his father away and talk to his mother. Will goes back to his room, where he lies awake wondering what has happened, why it happened, and what he could—or should—have done differently. He wonders, was this his fault? Should he have done something to stop his father? Should he have tried to intervene to get his parents to stop fighting? What would happen now? Would his father go to jail? What will his mother do?

What factors in Canadian society contribute to our increased awareness of violence, particularly violence in the family? What attitudes and beliefs do you have regarding family violence? Do you think violence in the home is increasing? Decreasing? What is the effect of family violence—on the perpetrator? The victim? The other family members? Society as a whole?

LEARNING OUTCOMES

- Describe the various forms of violence in Canada and who is involved. Include homicide, suicide, youth violence, and hate and bias crimes.

- Identify domestic violence (abuse against women, children, men, and the elderly committed by their family members) and its causes.

- Describe sexual victimization, including sexual assault, and the culture surrounding it at your university or college and in your home community.

- Identify attitudes and actions to prevent date rape from both the victim and perpetrator perspective.

- Describe the steps you can take to prevent personal assaults in your home, on your street, or in your car.

Chances are that if you turn on the TV, open a newspaper, watch a movie or music video, or play a video game, you will see graphic images of violent acts and their outcomes. Some of these will be real and others created for our entertainment. We live in a world caught in an epidemic of violence. The Violence Protection Alliance of the World Health Organization (2013a) defines **violence** as "the intentional use of physical force or power, threatened or actual, against oneself, another person or against a community, that either results in or has a high likelihood of resulting in injury, death, psychological harm, maldevelopment or deprivation." Violence can take many forms including terrorist activities (such as bombings and beheadings), government coups and extreme control of citizens, rape, abuse (human and animal), and hate crimes. The focus of this chapter is the kinds of violence that might have particular relevance to you.

VIOLENCE IN CANADA

Violence is a worldwide problem. Each year, more than 1.6 million people lose their lives to violence (World Health Organization, 2013b). Worldwide, violence is among the leading causes of death for individuals between the ages of 15 and 44, accounting for 14 percent of male and 7 percent of female deaths. Further, for every person who dies as a result of violence, many more are injured, resulting in a myriad of physical, sexual, social, spiritual, and mental health problems. Children and adults with disabilities and adults with mental health issues are at much greater risk of violence than those without disabilities (World Health Organization, 2013b).

Although violent incidents may not be as common in Canada as other countries, we have experienced riots and various levels of bedlam after sporting events and political and academic confrontations: the 2016 school shootings in La Loche, Saskatchewan, the 2012 student protests regarding proposed tuition changes in Quebec, the 2011 riots following the Stanley Cup final in Vancouver, the 2000 melee at the Ontario provincial legislature, and the 1995 standoff at Gustafson Lake in British Columbia are notable examples. We have also had police strikes with no change in the crime rate, and most cities are relatively safe to work, play, and live in. Canadians are less likely to take precautions against crime when going out than people in other industrialized countries (van Dijk, Mayhew, & Killias, 1990). Yet violence exists here, in overt forms

Violence Refers to intentional behaviours that produce injuries, as well as the outcomes of these behaviours (the injuries themselves).

such as assault or homicide and in more subtle but nonetheless intimidating forms such as stalking. Violence can flare up between groups—as it did at Oka in 1990, between First Nations peoples and the town of Oka over disputed land—or in families, as in child, spousal, and elder abuse. In fact, the most violent setting in Canadian society today is the family. In 2014, police reported that there were 87 820 victims of family violence in Canada, with almost half of the violent acts occurring between current or former spouses (Statistics Canada, 2015a).

Statistics Canada collects data regularly on crime using two different yet complementary surveys: the General Social Survey on Victimization and the Uniform Crime Reporting survey (Perreault & Brennan, 2015). The latest General Social Survey (from 2014) found that just over one-fifth of Canadians reported being a victim of a crime in the past 12 months (Perreault & Brennan, 2015). Victimization rates have decreased over the last 10 years, with the exception of sexual assault which remained stable. Violent victimization rates fell by 28 percent, while the household victimization rate decreased by 42 percent, and the rate of theft of personal property declined by 21 percent. The majority (65 percent) of those incidents were non-violent. Theft of personal property was the crime most frequently reported, representing one-third (34 percent) of all victimization incidents. Among violent crimes, physical assault was the most common violent crime, at 22 percent. Next was theft of household property (12 percent), sexual assault (10 percent), vandalism (9 percent), break and enter (7 percent), theft of motor vehicle or parts (4 percent) and robbery (3 percent). Although most Canadians who had been victimized reported only a single incident, more than one-third (37 percent) of victims reported having been the target of at least two victimization incidents in the preceding 12 months.

Vulnerable groups, such as women, children, the elderly, and individuals with disabilities, witnessing or experiencing violence in families is of concern. The issue of violence by men toward women and children and by adult children toward their parents is recognized as a major social problem in Canadian society. The opening of sexual assault centres and battered women's shelters in the 1970s made this type of violence more visible to the public and indicates some of the efforts made to treat the effects of it. Still, not enough is done for prevention, and there remains a need to raise awareness of the various types of violence that continue to be pervasive in our society today.

Violence does not just happen in the home. Elderly Canadians in long-term care facilities have been subjected to violence as have children and youth in foster or other types of care. Further, in a 1995 report, the

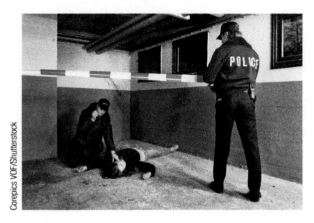

Violence in the form of fatal stabbings; beatings; and spousal, child, and elder abuse is a major cause of death and physical and emotional disability in Canada.

Department of Justice noted that Canada has a long history of violence toward ethnic and visible minorities. Some might think that we have a long way to go to become a truly just and caring society.

Acts of violence result in injuries and deaths as well as the subtler forms of damage caused by actual or threatened violence, such as stress, poor mental health, conduct disorders, and lack of social and emotional responsiveness. In addition to these social and emotional costs, the economic costs of violence are very high (Suderman & Jaffe, 1996).

Although the underlying causes of violence and abuse are as varied as the individual crimes and people involved, several social, cultural, and individual factors increase the likelihood of violence occurring. Poverty, unemployment, hopelessness, lack of education, inadequate housing, poor parental role models, cultural beliefs that objectify women and allow men to act as aggressors, lack of social support systems, discrimination, ignorance about people who are different, religious self-righteousness, breakdowns in the criminal justice system, stress, economic uncertainty, and a host of other factors can precipitate violent acts.

By learning more about the root causes of homicide, suicide, and other violent acts, you will reduce your risk of becoming a victim or perpetrator and protect your health. Further, by taking steps to prevent violence against others, you will safeguard the health of society.

Homicide

There were 516 **homicides** in Canada in 2014, four more than in the previous year. The homicide rate, however, was stable in 2014 (1.45 per 100 000 population) (Statistics Canada, 2015b). Figure 15.1 shows that Nunavut (10.93 per 100 000 people) has the highest rate of homicides, The lowest homicide rates were in Newfoundland and Labrador (0.38 per 100 000) and Nova Scotia (0.64 per 100 000). In Canada, stabbing (38 percent), shooting (31 percent), or beating (19 percent) continue to be the most common (combined 88 percent) forms of homicide (Statistics Canada, 2015b). Males continue to make up the majority of both homicide victims (72 percent) and accused (87 percent) and these rates are highest among males 18 to 24 years of age. Moreover, of the

Homicide Death as a result of another's intent to injure or kill.

FIGURE 15.1

Rate of Homicide Offences, by Province and Territory (Rate of Homicides per 100 000 Persons in 2014)

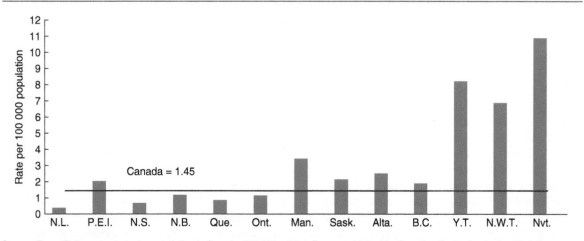

Source: From "Police-reported crime statistics in Canada, 2014" by Jillian Boyce, published by Canadian Centre for Justice Statistics, © 2015.

FIGURE 15.2

Rate of Female Homicides, by Aboriginal Identity, Provinces, and Territories, 2001 to 2014

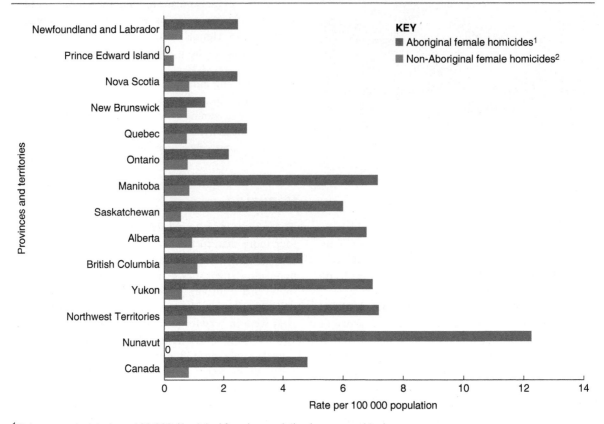

KEY
■ Aboriginal female homicides[1]
■ Non-Aboriginal female homicides[2]

[1]Rates are calculated per 100 000 Aboriginal female population by geographical area.

[2]Rates are calculated per 100 000 non-Aboriginal female population by geographical area.

Note: Population projections were not available prior to 2001 for this report; therefore rates could not be calculated for this time period. Population counts were provided by Statistics Canada's Demography Division. The counts for Aboriginal and non-Aboriginal populations are based on Aboriginal identity; for the years 2001 to 2011, they are derived from an interpolation between the censuses of population and the National Household Survey adjusted for net under coverage, partially enumerated reserves, and population living in collective dwellings; the population counts from 2012 to 2014 are based on custom population projections.

Source: From Homicide survey, published by Canadian Centre for Justice Statistics, © 2012.

516 homicide victims, almost one quarter (23 percent) were Indigenous. Homicides involving Indigenous female victims in the three territories were higher than the overall rate in Canada (Figure 15.2) Despite popular fears of the violent stranger, a homicide is most likely to be committed by someone known to the victim (37 percent killed by an acquaintance or 34 percent killed by a family member) (Statistics Canada, 2015b)

Canadians who own a firearm must register it. Currently, there are about 1.94 million valid firearm licences issued to individuals under the Firearms Act; 627 621 are possession only licences (allows the holder to possess, but not acquire firearms, and to possess and acquire ammunition), 1 301 792 are possession and acquisition licences (holder is allowed to possess

and acquire firearms and ammunition), and 8464 are minors' licences (for individuals under the age of 18) (Royal Canadian Mounted Police, 2013).

Suicide

When anger, rage, and hopelessness turn inward rather than outward, violence against the self results. Suicide is the most extreme form of this violence. As discussed in Chapter 2, suicide attempts occur for a number of reasons. They can be "a cry for help" and/or a signal of extreme distress and emotional pain. The physical pain of self-injury distracts the person from what is perceived as never-ending emotional pain. A suicide attempt may be an explosive outburst of rage at the self; such attempts are usually fatal. Or, the suicide may be motivated by sadness, resignation, and a desire for dignity, in the case of a terminally ill person. Why some people choose suicide is unclear.

According to the World Health Organization (2013b), about one million people kill themselves each year—a rate equivalent to 16.0 per 100 000 people, or roughly one suicide every 40 seconds. The most recent Statistics Canada (2012) data (from 2009) indicate that there were 3890 suicides in Canada that year, equivalent to 11.5 per 100 000 people. As shown in Figure 15.3, those aged 45 to 54 years have the highest rates of suicide (Statistics Canada, 2012). The rate for suicide ranges from a low of 1.3 per 100 000 in men between 10 to 14 years and a high of 30.6 per 100 000 in men between the ages of 85 and 89 years. The rate for suicide ranges from a low of 1.2 per 100 000 in women between the ages of 10 to 14 years and a high of 8.7 per 100 000 in women between the ages of 50 and 54 years.

Suicides accounted for 70 to 80 percent of all firearm deaths in Canada, with the proportion of suicides involving firearms declining over the last three decades (Dauvergne & De Socio, 2009). According to the Royal Canadian Mounted Police (2010), the proportion of completed suicides is highest with a firearm (92 percent) and suicides are five times more likely in homes where there is a firearm.

Those who attempt suicide are a mixed group and may differ markedly from those who complete suicide. The rate of suicide in men is four times greater than in women; however, there are two times as many women than men who attempt suicide (Health Canada, 2009).

This difference may relate to the reality that men have a greater access to more lethal means, including firearms. Women are more likely to choose an overdose of pills which allows for intervention to save their lives. Almost all people who commit suicide have a mental illness such as major depression, bipolar disorder, schizophrenia, or borderline personality disorder. Predisposing factors for suicide include:

- mental illness
- abuse
- loss of a loved one early in life
- family history of suicide
- long-term difficulty with peer relationships (Health Canada, 2009)

There is a need to understand suicide more completely so we can respond more appropriately.

The suicide rate among Canadian Indigenous people is at least two times that of the general population (Clifford, Doran, & Tsey, 2013). Canadian Indigenous youth are at an even greater risk, committing suicide at a rate five to six times greater than non-Indigenous youth (Health Canada, 2013). The main risk factors for suicide among Indigenous peoples are mental health disorders, stressful life events, and substance abuse (Clifford, Doran, & Tsey, 2013). These findings are a warning that Indigenous people and, in particular, Indigenous youth need more support, recognition, respect, and hope for the future, and that society as a whole must rethink the way we work with and serve Indigenous peoples.

FIGURE 15.3

Suicide Rates by Age in Canada for 2012

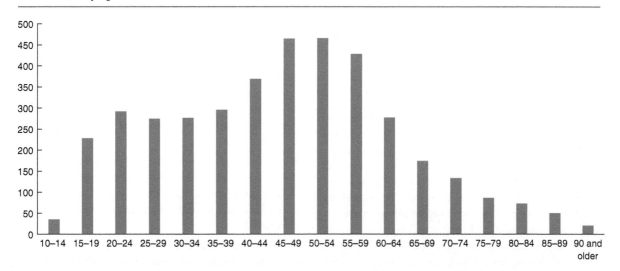

Source: From "Suicides and suicide rate, by sex and by age group, 2012," published by Canadian Centre for Justice Statistics, © 2012.

Youth Violence

Violence continues to be among the leading causes of death for people aged 15 to 44 worldwide, accounting for 14 percent of all male deaths and 7 percent of all female deaths (World Health Organization, 2013b). Also, as noted previously, the greatest number of male homicides and the greatest number of males accused of homicide in Canada in 2014 occurred in those between the ages of 18 and 24 (Statistics Canada, 2015b).

In 2013–2014, Canada's youth courts reported close to 40 000 cases. The number of completed youth court cases declined by 12 percent from the previous year (2011–2012). Over time, the rate of youth court cases has increased for females and decreased for males (Brennan, 2012a).

Historically, youth were more likely to be formally charged with their criminal offences in Canada than to be dealt with by other means. This changed in 2003, prior to which youth were more likely to be diverted (57 versus 43 percent) from the formal justice system if charged with a criminal offence, when the Youth Criminal Justice Act came into effect (Statistics Canada, 2013).

Youth crime rates tend to peak during late adolescence and early adulthood (Brennan, 2012a). In fact in 2013–2014, 16- and 17-year-olds continued to make up the largest proportion of accused persons, representing 62 percent of cases completed in youth court, while 12- to 15-year-olds accounted for 38 percent of cases.

The Violence of Hate

Canada has always welcomed people from other cultures—while marginalizing Indigenous people. The degree of acceptance, however, decreases with the immigrants' physical and cultural differences from Northern European peoples. Much as you may think otherwise or that people have come a long way in their acceptance of those different from them, prejudice and racism have always been and continue to be a part of Canadian society.

Historically, established leaders in Canadian society (individual and institutional) have made key contributions to interracial violence—for example, the anti-Chinese riot of 1887 and the anti-Chinese and Japanese riot of 1907 in Vancouver. In both cases, the local newspapers, respectable individuals (businessmen, clergymen, politicians), and organizations played a very prominent role in at least preparing the groundwork and instigating the violence, which claimed scores of Chinese lives. The timing of the riots seems to have been related to white workers' alleged fears of economic competition, especially at a time of recession (Patel, 1980). How much are things the same today? Different? Why do you think bias and prejudice remain? Why in some and not in others?

Preventing Hate and Bias Crimes

Violence can and does happen anywhere—at home, at school, at work, and at play—and it takes many forms. When we think of violence, we often think of physical violence and underestimate the effect of psychological violence, such as verbal putdowns and degrading gestures. Many people endure emotional, psychological, economic, social, physical, and sexual violence in silence. Women, Indigenous peoples, visible minorities, and members of the LGBTQ community confront systemic forms of violence almost every day of their lives. This is the harsh reality of the violence that permeates our society.

Canadian data relating to hate-motivated conduct are not collected and reported systematically by police forces on a national scale. Other countries, such as England, France, and the United States, have reporting mechanisms that provide a more comprehensive national picture of the scale of hate-motivated behaviours in their respective countries. Thus, it is difficult to say how much of an issue remains in Canada or where the hate and bias crimes are more prevalent.

Although the causes of intolerance range among individuals, it is believed that much of it stems from a fear of change and a desire to blame others when forces such as the economy and crime seem to be out of control. Think about yourself, your family, your friends, and your community, and your interactions with them. How do you—and they—talk about and treat others? Does this differ based upon colour of skin? Age? Sex? Accent? What can you do to reduce the violence of hate in your home, on campus, and in your community? The following suggestions may help to direct your personal and collective efforts to reduce intolerance.

- Support educational programs designed to foster understanding and appreciation for differences in people. Many colleges and universities require diversity classes as part of their academic curriculum.

- Examine your attitudes and behaviours. Are you intolerant of others? Do you have beliefs about a particular group? Do you engage in behaviours or hold any attitudes that demean any group or individuals?

- Discourage racist, sexist, ageist, and homophobic jokes and other forms of social or ethnic bigotry. Do not participate in such attitudes and behaviours and express your dissatisfaction with others who do. Silence condones others' attitudes and behaviours. It takes courage to speak out—even though it is the right thing to do.

- Vote for community leaders who respect the rights of others, value diversity, and do not have racially or ethnically motivated hidden agendas.

- Educate yourself. Read, interact with, and try to understand people who appear to be different from you. Respecting people's right to be different is part of being a healthy, integrated individual.

- Examine your values in determining the relative worth of your friends and the others in your life. Are you judgmental? Are you somewhat intolerant of others' differences? Do you expect others to think and act as you do? How do you resolve your tendencies to be judgmental and bigoted? Do you judge people on appearances? Do you take time to get to know who they are as individuals? Do you respect them as individuals?

Violence against Women

Canadians were shocked out of denying the existence of violence toward women by the Montreal Massacre at École Polytechnique in Montreal in 1989, when a young man shot and killed 14 women at the school because, as his writings amply explained, he hated women.

The first major empirical study on violence toward women noted that one in ten women living with a man are abused each year (McLeod, 1980). This figure, which was initially ridiculed, is now accepted as an underestimate; 12 percent of all violent crime in Canada, or about 40 000 arrests, result from domestic violence and, given that only 22 percent of all incidents are reported, the real number is much higher (Canadian Women's Foundation, n.d.). It is further estimated that every six days in Canada, a woman is murdered by her current or former partner. Domestic violence is eight times more likely in a relationship of less than 2 years than in partnerships lasting more than 20 years. Almost half (45 percent) of assault cases result in physical injury to the woman. Research shows us that women are particularly vulnerable during times of crisis, when women's shelters may have to close, and social services are stretched by increased demand (Parkinson & Zara, 2013). Given that Canada has its share of natural disasters, such as the 2016 wildfires in Fort McMurray, Alberta, the 2013 flood in Calgary, or the Manitoba floods of 2009 and 2011, this research points to the need for increased awareness and services related to domestic violence during these crises (Canadian Women's Foundation, 2016).

The shelter movement (begun in England in 1972 and in Canada in 1974) lobbied for zero tolerance of abuse and mandatory charging of abusers. This policy was adopted in virtually all jurisdictions in Canada in 1982, when Canada's attorney general urged police to lay charges in all cases of suspected wife abuse. The Royal Canadian Mounted Police introduced a formal policy in 1984 specifically instructing its members to lay charges in all cases where there were "reasonable and probable grounds" to believe that assault occurred. The abusive partner may be charged under the assault sections of the Criminal Code of Canada. A police charge not only highlights the criminal nature of the act but also relieves the victim of the burden of laying charges (Solicitor General, n.d.).

Discrimination and violence toward women is a global issue. At the urging of Canada and other nations, the United Nations Convention on the Elimination of All Forms of Discrimination Against Women adopted a resolution in 1992 accepting that states are responsible for acts of domestic violence between individuals. In December 1993, the United Nations passed a Declaration Against Violence Against Women.

How many times have you heard of a woman being repeatedly beaten by her partner or spouse and wondered, "Why doesn't she just leave him?" There are many reasons women find it difficult, if not impossible, to leave their abusers (Joerger, 1992). Many women, particularly those with small children, are financially dependent on the abuser. Others fear retaliation against themselves or their children. Some women hope that the situation will change with time (it rarely does). Other women feel that the good times are so very good that they think they can put up with the bad times. Some women stay because of their cultural or religious beliefs that forbid divorce. Finally, there are women who still love their partner despite the abuse and are concerned about what will happen to him if they leave. Regardless of the reasons women do not—or cannot—leave, it is not their fault that they suffer abuse at the hands of their partner.

Cycle of Violence Theory

Psychologist Lenore Walker developed a theory known as the "cycle of violence" to explain how women (and men) can get caught in a downward spiral without knowing what is happening to them (West, 1992). The cycle has three phases:

- Phase One: Tension Building. In this phase, minor battering occurs, and the victim may become more nurturant, more pleasing, and more intent on anticipating the abuser's needs in order to forestall another violent scene. The victim assumes guilt for doing something to provoke the abuser and tries hard to avoid doing it again.

- Phase Two: Acute Battering. At this stage, pleasing the abuser does not help and the victim can no longer control or predict the abuse. Usually, the abuser claims to be trying to "teach a lesson," and will not stop until enough pain has been inflicted. When the acute attack is over, the abuser may respond with shock and denial about his or her behaviours. Usually, both the abuser and the victim soft-pedal or deny the seriousness of the attacks and the resulting physical and mental damage.

- Phase Three: Remorse/Reconciliation. During this "honeymoon" period, the abuser may be kind, loving, and apologetic, swearing to never act violently again. The abuser may "behave" for several weeks or months, and the victim may question whether she (or in some cases he) overrated the seriousness of past abuse. Then the kind of tension that precipitated abusive incidents in the past resurfaces, the abuser loses control again, and once more beats his or her partner. Unless some form of intervention breaks this downward cycle of abuse, contrition, further abuse, denial, and contrition, it will repeat again and again, ending perhaps only when the abuser kills the victim or, less often, when the victim kills the abuser.

It is very hard for most people who get caught in this cycle of violence (which may include forced sexual relations and psychological and economic abuse as well as physical beatings) to find the courage and resolution to extricate themselves. Most need effective outside intervention. Some die at the hands of their abuser.

Domestic Violence

The extent of spousal violence has only been well documented since 1993, when Statistics Canada conducted its first Violence Against Women survey; since 1998, an annual report is released as part of the larger federal Family Violence Initiative to document the extent of family violence in Canada (Sinha, 2012). The first Violence Against Women survey noted that 29 percent of Canadian women experienced violence at the hands of a current or past marital partner. Between 1974 and 1992, 1435 women were killed by their husbands and 451 men were killed by their wives (Statistics Canada, 1995). In 2013, there were more than 90 300 victims of police-reported violence by an intimate partner (including spousal and dating partners) accounting for over one quarter of all police-reported victims of violent offences (Statistics Canada, 2015a). Dating violence was higher than spousal violence with a rate greater than any other relationship categories.

Domestic violence The use of force to control and maintain power over another person in the home environment; it includes actual physical harm or psychological harm and the threat of harm.

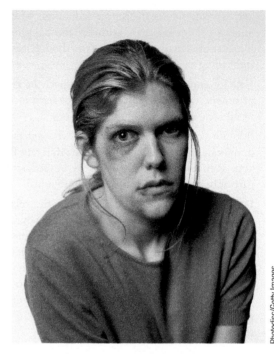

Despite obvious physiological and psychological injury, it can be difficult for a woman to leave her abusive partner.

Moreover, individuals who experience spousal violence were likely to have been victimized first as a child.

Women tend to be victims of intimate partner violence more often than males, particularly those between the ages of 15 and 24 years. Rates of intimate partner homicides against women were highest for victims aged 20 to 44, ranging from 6 to 8 victims per million population (Statistics Canada, 2015a). In general, 75 percent of intimate partner violence victims are physically assaulted.

Causes of Domestic Violence

There is no single explanation for why people tend to be abusive in relationships. Although alcohol abuse is often associated with **domestic violence**, marital dissatisfaction seems to predict physical abuse more effectively than any other variable (Pan, Malone, & Tyree, 1994). Numerous studies also point to differences in the communication patterns between abusive relationships and non-abusive relationships (Wilson, 1996). While some argue that the hormone testosterone is the cause of male aggression, studies have failed to show a strong association between physical abuse in relationships and this hormone (Wilson, 1996). Thus, it is more likely that men who engage in severe violence are more likely than other men to suffer from personality disorders (Wilson, 1996).

The dynamics that people bring to a relationship may increase risk of violence. Obtaining help from community support and counselling services may help to determine the underlying basis of the problem and help the victim and the abuser come to a better understanding of the actions necessary to stop the cycle of abuse. The Assess Yourself at the end of the chapter may help you to determine if you are a victim (or perpetrator) of abuse.

Violence against Children

Child abuse is found in all societies and is almost always a highly guarded secret wherever it takes place. The World Health Organization (2010) uses the term *child maltreatment* and defines it as ". . . the abuse and neglect that occurs to children under 18 years of age. It includes all types of physical and/or emotional ill-treatment, sexual abuse, neglect, negligence and commercial or other exploitation, which results in actual or potential harm to the child's health, survival, development or dignity in the context of a relationship of responsibility, trust or power."

In countries with reliable mortality reporting, the WHO estimates that as many as 1 in 5000 to 1 in 10 000 children under the age of five die each year from physical violence. In the same countries, every year from 1 in 1000 to 1 in 180 children are either taken to a health-care facility or are reported to child welfare services as a consequence of abuse.

A second nation-wide study of reported child maltreatment in Canada estimated that, of the estimated 217 319 investigations, 47 percent were substantiated—equivalent to an incidence rate of 21.71 per 1000 cases of maltreatment in children (Trocomé et al., 2005). It was pointed out in this report that only cases investigated by child welfare services were included, and those that were screened out or only investigated by the police were not reported. Further, it was noted that there was a change in reporting that may relate to the increase in rates of investigated and substantiated cases of maltreatment between 1998 and 2003. Of the confirmed cases of maltreatment, 15 percent involved emotional maltreatment, 28 percent of the children were exposed to domestic violence (that is, witnessing violence against another family member), 3 percent were sexually abused, 24 percent were physically abused, and 30 percent were neglected.

Physical violence often originates when there is a lack of parenting skills. Typically, parents who are abusive are unable to respond to a young child's needs and have unrealistic expectations for the stage of a child's development. Another factor is the cultural acceptance of corporal punishment and violence within a society.

Other stresses contributing to child maltreatment may include an unwanted child, an unsupported single-parent household, the absence of social support, financial pressures, and unemployment. Child maltreatment can be aggravated by substance abuse on the part

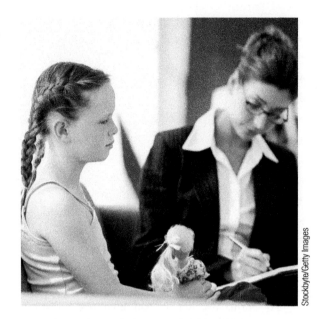

Stockbyte/Getty Images

Sympathetic and sensitive therapy can help abused children cope with the mental and physical pain inflicted on them.

of the parent or guardian. Families in which there is substance abuse are also likely to experience physical violence, sexual abuse, and domestic violence. Further, these violent acts are most often directed at family members, particularly women and young children.

The perpetrators of violence against or sexual abuse of children are often trusted individuals in a position of authority, usually males, and often family members (World Health Organization, 2010). In fact, one-quarter of violent incidents that children and youth experience are family violence (Sinha, 2012). As in previous years, girls (relative to boys) continued to be victimized at a higher rate by family members in 2013. More specifically, the rate of police-reported victimization by family members was about 1.5 times higher for girls than for boys (298.2 per 100 000 versus 191.5 per 100 000) (Statistics Canada, 2015a). Although females experience higher rates of victimization for all types of violence, this is particularly true of sexual assault. In 2013 female children were four times more likely than males to be the victim of a sexual assault. Physical violence and sexual abuse in the home is a factor contributing to the phenomenon of street children in developed and developing countries. Further abuse on the street is an everyday reality (World Health Organization, 2010).

Child victims of violence or sexual abuse have a high risk of becoming perpetrators of similar forms of abuse toward younger children. In later years, they may be abusive toward children in their care or toward their own children (Royal Canadian Mounted Police, 2012).

Child abuse The systematic harming of a child by a caregiver, generally a parent.

Maltreatment as a child disrupts early brain development and puts these children, when they become adults, at risk of:

- perpetrating or being a victim of violence
- depression
- smoking
- obesity
- high-risk sexual behaviours
- sexually transmitted infections
- unintended pregnancy
- alcohol and drug misuse
- suicide
- heart disease
- cancer (World Health Organization, 2010)

The normal reactions to child abuse are the expression of anger and pain. The child who is abused is usually forbidden or unable to express anger and cannot bear to endure the pain alone. To survive, the child must repress his or her feelings as well as the memories of what happened. The repressed emotions will gain expression in destructive acts—against others, as in criminal behaviours and even mass murder, or self-directed, as with drug and alcohol abuse (Miller, 1992). Suppressed memories of child abuse can also surface later in adult years, with post-traumatic stress experienced as a result (see Chapter 2).

The use of threat and power by an adult against a child breaks the trust the child has in the adult. That the adult would turn against the child is unthinkable, and so the child divorces awareness of the abuse from everyday thoughts and manages to forget the trauma. But the fear influences the child's attitudes, behaviours, and interactions with others, often in destructive ways. Later in life, when it is safer, the memory may resurface and the person can begin to heal.

Not all child violence is physical. A child's health can be severely affected by psychological violence—assaults on personality, character, competence, independence, or general dignity as a human being. The negative consequences of this kind of victimization in close relationships can be harder to discern and therefore harder to combat. They include depression, lowered self-esteem, sub-optimal growth and development (Malina, Bouchard, & Bar-Or, 2004), and a pervasive fear of doing something that will offend the abuser.

Factors that Contribute to Family Violence

There is no single cause of family violence, and all people—regardless of status—are vulnerable to it (Department of Justice Canada, 2009). Most believe that violence is linked to inequalities and power imbalances in our society. Family violence is linked to inequalities in the family since most abusers are in a position of power over their victims and are exerting that power in their abuse.

Your vulnerability to abuse may be increased by factors such as dislocation, racism, sexism, ageism, homophobia, disability, poverty, isolation, and by lack of access to community services and support and the child welfare and criminal justice systems (Department of Justice Canada, 2009). Historically, churches, residential schools, and orphanages have been places where many children from marginalized groups in our society experienced various forms of abuse.

What Are the Consequences of Family Violence?

Individuals who experience—or are exposed to—family violence often experience psychological, physiological, behavioural, academic, sexual, interpersonal, self-perceptual, or spiritual consequences, which are fatal in some cases (Department of Justice Canada, 2009). Also as previously noted, children who have been abused have a greater likelihood than children who have not been abused of becoming abusive themselves as adults.

Consequences for Abusers

In many cases, abusers have been abused as children—or were exposed to abuse—themselves. Either experience leads to learned attitudes and behaviours about abuse as a way of exerting power and control over others (Department of Justice Canada, 2009). They may continue to harm others even when it destroys their relationships or has other negative consequences for their lives.

Societal Consequences

Family violence has enormous economic costs for Canadian society (Department of Justice Canada, 2009). The first research study to estimate the costs of various forms of violence against women, including abuse in intimate relationships, found it costs Canadian society an estimated $4.2 billion per year in social services, education, criminal justice, labour, employment, health, and medical costs. Personal costs cannot be estimated.

Preventing and Responding to Family Violence

Victims and abusers are involved in intimate or dependent relationships, and often have strong emotional ties (Department of Justice Canada, 2009). Community

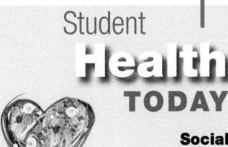

Health
TODAY

Social Networking Safety

At any given time, millions of people are chatting away on social networking sites with friends, family, and strangers, and posting photos and personal information that may be available to people they barely know or do not know at all, sometimes placing themselves at considerable risk. These sites raise some concerns about potential risks—from stalking and identity theft to embarrassment and defamation. For example:

- The highly publicized story of the Canadian teen from British Columbia, Amanda Todd, who took her own life after she was cyber bullied, harassed, and stalked online.

- A Carleton University student, 18-year-old Nadia Kajouji, jumped into a frozen Rideau River in 2008. Following an investigation into her death, it was revealed that she was encouraged to take her own life by 52-year-old William Melchert-Dinkel, whom she met and communicated with online.

- Hiring and firing decisions have been influenced by information employees and job applicants made publicly available on Facebook and Twitter.

- Underage users may pose as adults, leading to claims of inappropriate sexual contact with minors and other criminal offences on the part of people interacting with them online.

Although very real threats to health, reputation, financial security, and future employment lie in wait for those who post indiscriminately and unwisely, social networking sites are far from wholly dangerous. To safely enjoy the benefits and to avoid the risks of social networking sites, you should practise a little caution and use some common sense. The following tips will help you to remain safe, protect your identity, and feel free to express yourself without fear of repercussions:

- Do not post anything on the Web that you would not want someone to pick out of your trash can and read. Your address, phone numbers, banking information, calendar, family secrets, and other information should be kept off the sites.

- Do not post compromising pictures, videos, or other things that you would not want your mother or co-workers to see.

- Never meet a stranger in person whom you met only online without bringing a trusted friend along, or at the very least notifying a close friend of where you will be and when you will return. Arrange a ride home with a friend in advance and choose a well-established, public place to meet during daylight hours. Do not give your address or traceable phone numbers to the person you are meeting.

---

services and supports for victims, such as shelters, are essential. All levels of government need to continue to work together to ensure that the criminal justice system responds effectively to protect victims and hold abusers accountable and responsible for their actions via legal reform, public and professional education, research, and support for programs and services.

Violence against Men

While women are most often the targets of violence by men, men can also be the target. In 1999, males committed 85.5 percent of violent crimes. Thirty-nine percent of violent crimes in 1999 involved males attacking other males. Men under the age of 34 are more likely to be perpetrators in major assaults (65 percent). In only 6 percent of reported cases did a woman commit a violent act toward a man (Statistics Canada, 1995). Thus, the task of overcoming violence in our society is largely a male issue. The principal reason seems to be that boys are taught—overtly or subtly—that competitiveness, power, and control are valued male attributes. Violence can be seen as an expression of frustration and stress.

Violence against Older Adults

Violence toward older adults (elder abuse) has been getting attention recently. The first national survey of abuse toward the elderly was done in 1989 at Ryerson University; the researchers found that 4 percent of Canadians over 65 living in private dwellings (or 98 000 seniors) reported experiencing at least one type of abuse in the last 12 months. The most prevalent types of abuse reported (listed in order of prevalence) were

FIGURE 15.4

Senior Victims of Police-Reported Family Violence, by Sex of Victim and and Accused–Victim Relationship, Canada, 2013

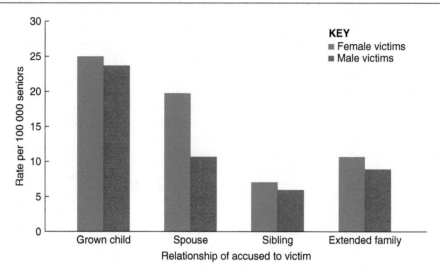

Note: Grown child includes biological, step, adoptive and foster children. Includes a small number of victims aged 65 years and older where the relationship of the accused to the victim was miscoded as 'parent' (including 'step-parent') and was therefore recoded as 'child' (including 'step-child'). Spouses include legally married, separated, divorced, common-law, and same-sex partners. Sibling includes biological, step, adoptive, and foster brothers and sisters. Extended family includes all other family member related by blood, marriage, or adoption. Excludes incidents where the victim's sex and/or age was unknown. Rates are calculated on the basis of 100 000 population of seniors aged 65 to 89. Victims aged 90 years and older are excluded from Statistics Canada, Demography Division.

Source: From "Incident based crime reporting survey," published by Canadian Centre for Justice Statistics, © 2012.

material abuse (such as forcing older adults to hand over money or valuable goods), chronic verbal aggression, physical abuse, and neglect (Health Canada, n.d.). The victim was more often female (67 percent), and the abuser was most frequently a spouse or a child of the victim. The General Social Survey is now consistently used to provide a national perspective on violence against older adults. In this survey, adults over the age of 55 are included as 'older adults' partially to include populations, such as Indigenous peoples, who have a shorter life span (Brennan, 2012b). Most recent statistics indicate that nearly 8900 Canadian seniors (aged 65 years and older) were victims of a violent crime in 2013. One third of violent crimes committed against seniors were carried out by family members; as indicated in Figure 15.4, among family members, grown children were the most common perpetrators (Statistics Canada, 2015a).

SEXUAL VICTIMIZATION

Sexual Assault

Sexual assault Any act in which one person is sexually intimate with another person without consent.

Sexual assault can be understood in terms of a power imbalance in society "in which violence is implicit" as the base upon which sexual exploitation is built (Sinha, 2012). In Canada, sexual assault is defined as incidents of unwanted sexual activity, including sexual attacks and sexual touching (Brennan & Taylor-Butts, n.d.). According to Statistics Canada (2013), the number of self-reported sexual assaults was the same for 1999, 2004, and 2009, with 21 to 24 per 1000 people reported. Further, according to the General Social Survey, more than 80 percent of the sexual assaults reported are considered minor offences such as sexual touching, unwanted grabbing, kissing, or fondling. In 2014, the police reported about 20 700 sexual assault or 58 sexual assaults per 100 000 population (Statistics Canada, 2015b). The difference between these two sets of data provides clear evidence of the lack of reporting of sexual assault. Various reasons are given for not reporting sexual assaults including the belief that the incident was not significant enough, it was a private matter, and it was dealt with in another way (Brennan, 2013). A survey of more than 6000 post-secondary students found that 84 percent of women who had been sexually assaulted knew their attacker and that 57 percent of the rapes happened on a date (Health Canada, 1993). Of male offenders, 19 percent were between the ages of 18 and 24, 32 percent were between 25 and 34, and 23 percent were between 35 and 44. Many universities coordinate "safe walk" programs, during which a person can be accompanied at night on campus from building to building or to and from the parking lots. Self-defence courses can provide some protection against attackers as well as improve self-confidence.

Why Some Males Sexually Assault Women

Over the years, psychologists and others have proposed many theories to explain why so many males sexually victimize women. One study found that almost two-thirds of the male respondents had engaged in sexual activity that was unwanted by the woman, primarily because of male peer pressure (Berkowitz, 1992). This attitude was also noted in research aimed at preventing sexual assault on college and university campuses given that men at this stage of their life are more likely to be perpetrators of sexual assault (Thompson et al., 2011). This research noted positive change when rape-supportive beliefs were diminished in men's social groups. In other words, perceptions that a person's peer group disapproved of sexual assault were related to a reduced likelihood of committing sexual assault (Thompson et al., 2011).

Peer pressure is certainly a strong factor in such behaviours, but a growing body of research suggests that sexual assault is encouraged by the normal socialization processes that males experience daily (Berkowitz, 1992). One Canadian study investigated the characteristics of stalkers (Morrison, 2008). A physically violent stalker is more likely to have had a strong previous attachment with the victim, be highly fixated on the victim, have a higher degree of perceived negative affect toward the victim, engage in significant verbal threats to the victim, and have a history of battering or abusing the victim. Overall, the author describes the physically violent stalker as someone with significant anger, vengeance, emotional arousal, humiliation, projection of blame, and insecure attachment. Another Canadian study examined male erotomania, a particularly dangerous form of sexual harassment. These men have a severely paranoid thought disorder that combines jealously, projection, and interpretation. The typical behaviour of these men is characterized by escalating violence in their contact with women who they believe love them (Gagné & Desparois, 1995).

Social Assumptions

According to many experts, certain common assumptions in our society prevent the recognition by the perpetrator and the wider public of the true nature of

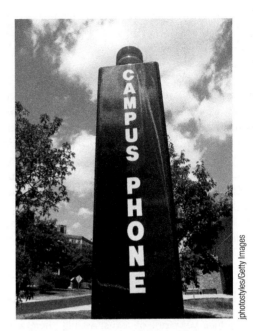

Emergency call boxes should be available on college and university campuses for students.

sexual assault (Benson, Charlton, & Goodhart, 1992). The most important of these assumptions are:

- Minimization: It is assumed that sexual assault of women is rare because official crime statistics show relatively few offences; however, sexual assault is the most underreported of all serious crimes—with 91 percent not reported in Canada!

- Trivialization: Incredibly, sexual assault of women is often not viewed as a major issue; in fact, it is often treated in a jocular matter by many men.

- Blaming the victim: Many discussions of sexual violence against women display a sometimes unconscious assumption that the woman did something to provoke the attack—that she dressed too revealingly or flirted too much or she put herself in a compromising position (Whittaker, 1992).

- "Boys will be boys": This is the assumption that men cannot control themselves once they become aroused. The myth that men cannot stop once they start is millennia old and typically suggests that males are slaves to their sexual organs or that physical harm can happen to the unfortunate male denied ejaculation. These notions can be countered by pointing out the following: (a) If a woman's parents walked into the room where sex was occurring, it's a sure bet that the man could stop; and (b) there has never been a documented case where a male died due to coitus interruptus.

PREVENTING PERSONAL ASSAULTS

After a violent act is committed against someone we know, we acknowledge the horror of the event, express sympathy for the victim, and then go on with our lives. But the brutalized person often takes a longer time to recover—and sometimes complete recovery from the assault is not possible (see Table 15.1 for a summary of the most common consequences of victimization). In this section, we discuss prevention of violence and abuse rather extensively because it is far better to stop a violent act than to have to recover from it.

Self-Defence against Sexual Assault

To reduce your risk of sexual assault, there are some common-sense self-defence tactics that you can learn. Self-defence is a process that includes increased awareness, learning self-defence techniques, taking reasonable precautions, and developing the self-confidence and judgment needed to determine appropriate responses to different situations.

Taking Control

Most sexual assaults by assailants unknown to the victim are planned in advance. They are frequently preceded by a casual, friendly conversation. Although many victimized women said that they started to feel uneasy during such a conversation, they denied the possibility of an attack on themselves until it was too late. Listen to your feelings and trust your intuition. Be assertive and direct to someone who is getting out of line or threatening—this may convince the would-be assailant to back off. Stifle your tendency to be "nice," and don't be afraid of making a scene. Let him or her know that you mean what you say and are prepared to defend yourself:

- Speak in a strong voice and use statements like "Leave me alone" rather than questions like "Will you please leave me alone?" Avoid apologies and excuses.
- Maintain eye contact with the would-be attacker.
- Mean what you say. Speak assertively.
- Stand up straight, be confident, and remain alert. Walk as if you own the sidewalk.

Many assailants use certain ploys to initiate their attacks. Among the most common are:

- Request for help. This allows the assailant to get close—to enter your house to use the phone, for instance.
- Offer of help. This can also help the assailant to gain entrance to your home: "Let me help you carry that package."
- Guilt trip. "Gee, no one is friendly nowadays . . . I cannot believe you will not talk with me for just a little while."
- Authority. Some victims have been fooled by the "police officer at the door" ruse. If anyone comes to your door dressed in the uniform of a police officer, firefighter, repair person, or any other individual, ask

TABLE 15.1

Common Consequences of Victimization

Psychological	Medical
Recurrent and intrusive recollections, dreams, or flashbacks involving traumatic incidents	Death
Generalized anxiety, mistrust, and/or social isolation	Sexual/reproductive symptoms/consequences: chronic pelvic pain, HIV infection, urinary tract infections, premenstrual pain, fertility problems, trauma-specific pain, orgasmic difficulty
Difficulty in forming or maintaining non-exploitive intimate relationships	Battering-related symptoms: bruises, black eyes, fractured ribs, broken teeth, subdural hematomas, detached retinas, other head injuries
Chronic depression	Stress-mediated symptoms: headaches, backaches, TMJ symptoms, high blood pressure, hyperalertness, sleep disorders, gastrointestinal disorders
Dissociative reactions: phobic avoidance, often generalized to apparently unrelated situations; feelings of "badness," stigma, and guilt; impulsive or self-defeating behaviour	Eating disorders
	Self-mutilation

Source: From Continuum of Violence Against Women: Psychological and Physical Consequences, *Journal of American College Health* Volume:40 Issue:4 by Marjorie Whitaker Leidig, published by Department of Justice.

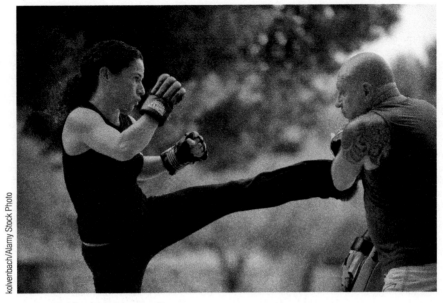

Take self-defence classes so that you can learn the techniques that may help you should you be assaulted.

him or her to show you his or her ID before you unlock the door. You can also call the employer to get a confirmation on his or her ID.

If you are attacked, act immediately:

- Do not worry about causing a scene. Draw attention to yourself and your assailant. Scream for help.
- Report the attack to the appropriate authorities immediately.

To prevent an attack from occurring:

- Always be vigilant. Even the safest cities and towns have sexual and physical assaults. Do not be fooled by a sleepy, little-town atmosphere.
- Use campus escort services whenever possible.
- Be assertive in demanding a well-lit campus and safe-walk programs.
- Do not use the same routes all the time. Think about your movement patterns and vary them accordingly.
- Do not leave a bar alone with a friendly stranger. Stay with your friends, and let the friendly stranger come along. Do not give your address or phone number to anyone you do not know.
- Never accept a drink from another person unless you watched it being made. Do not leave your drink unattended, not even with the safety personnel watching the bathroom doors. Rohypnol (often called the date rape drug) is odourless and colourless and you cannot tell when it has been put in your drink.

- When you and your friends go out, you may have a 'safe' word that must be used if one of you is leaving early unexpectedly with someone who is not a partner or close friend. If the word is not used, do not let your friend go—he or she may be drugged or incapable of taking care of him- or herself.
- Let friends or family know where you are going, what route you plan to take, and when to expect your return.
- Stay close to others. Avoid shortcuts through dark or unlit paths. Do not be the last one to leave the lab or library late at night.
- Keep your windows and doors locked. Do not answer the door to strangers (Schneider, 1992).

Preventing Date Rape

Men and women need to proactively protect themselves from date rape in their potential roles as perpetrators and victims. The following suggestions—created specifically and separately for women and men—help to reduce the risk of date rape.

What to Do When a Sexual Assault Occurs

If you are a victim of sexual assault, it should be you who reports the attack. This gives you a sense of control. Call 9-1-1 immediately. Do not bathe, shower, douche, clean up, or touch anything the attacker may have touched. Do not throw away or launder the clothes you were

Women	Men
• Decide ahead of time how far you are willing to go. Remember that it is your game, your rules, and no one should pressure or force you to go beyond your limits.	• Take stock of your past behaviours in sexual situations and in potentially sexual situations. How have you behaved, what have been the outcomes of the encounters, etc.? Have you felt uncomfortable about pushing too hard to have sex with your dates in the past? Have you felt pushed yourself?
• Think ahead and try to avoid "compromising" situations. If you have not implicitly decided to have sex, stay out of your date's bedroom, the back seat of the car, or other quiet spots away from the rest of the crowd where intimacy can result.	• Know and express your sexual limits. If you feel that you are beginning to lose control in an intimate situation, communicate your feelings and indicate why it is time to stop.
• Communicate directly. Do not be wishy-washy. If things start to go farther than you want them to, say "no" loudly and with conviction. Do not worry about hurting feelings, disappointing your partner, or seeming aggressive. Be firm and stick to your words.	• Understand that NO means NO—and that it is not a sign of rejection. Respect your partner's right to say no, regardless of how far you have gone or what you thought she might have wanted. Stop NOW and do not try "another line." Think about how you would want your sister, brother, or close friend to be treated by another guy in a similar situation.
• Be aware that some people, in some situations, will interpret a low-cut, sexy dress or other clothing as a come-on. Although this is obviously wrong on their part, it is important that you do not naïvely assume that everyone is enlightened. Be direct and firm with anyone who seems to be assuming too much from your attire or interactions.	• Just because you may have been intimate with this person before does not mean it is okay now. When you hear the word NO, or if your partner struggles in any way, STOP.
• Limit your consumption of alcohol and other drugs that reduce your ability to think clearly. Do not accept a drink from anyone. Do not leave your drink unattended.	• Limit alcohol and other drugs that cause you to think less clearly. Do not accept a drink from anyone or leave your drink unattended. Do not purchase a drink for someone unless he or she asks for it.
• Pay attention to the nonverbal and verbal cues that your date is giving you. If he or she is indicating that he or she is interested in more, let him or her know that you are not.	• Avoid situations likely to get you into trouble. Until you are sure of your intentions and your date's intentions, stay out of bedrooms, the back seats of cars, or any other places away from people where there is the potential to be intimate.
• Be concerned about any of the following behaviours or expressions exhibited by your date:	• If you encounter a particularly aggressive date, it is not unmanly to tell her or him you do not want to have sex and are not interested in being intimate in any way. Say NO and avoid situations that may cause you to be caught in a compromising position. Forget about what she or he may say or what your friends will say. Remember, it is up to you whether or not you have sex.
• Continued suggestive or dirty language indicating disrespect for you and others.	
• Failure to listen to or to value your opinions about where to go, whom to spend time with, etc.	
• Unusual displays of jealousy or rage concerning your interactions with others.	
• Unusual roughness and forceful pushing or shoving to get you to comply with his or her wishes.	
• Wild anger and violent acts toward others.	
• Inability to control drinking and to display appropriate behaviours.	
• Lack of concern for your feelings; laughter or derisive comments when you say no.	

wearing. They will be needed as evidence. Bring a clean change of clothes to the clinic or hospital. Contact the Rape Crisis Centre in your area and ask for advice on therapists or counselling for additional support.

If you want to help a victim of sexual assault, the best thing you can do is to believe her or him. Do not ask questions that appear to implicate the victim in the assault. Your hindsight may find some questionable judgment on her or his behalf, but that does not mean he or she's to blame. Sexual assault is a violent act against someone; the victim was certainly not looking or asking for it. Encourage the victim to talk, and when she or he does, listen. Hold back on advice.

Encourage the victim to see a doctor immediately, as she or he may have medical needs but be too embarrassed to seek help. Be supportive of reporting the crime. Continue to be a friend. It may take six months to a year for emotional recovery, and you should be empathetic during this time. Encourage the victim to seek counselling if problems persist.

Preventing Assaults in Your Home

In your home, there are several precautions you can take to reduce your risk of being assaulted:

- Get deadbolts and peepholes installed, if possible, and make sure the entryway to your house is well lit and free of shrubs.
- Put a lock on your door, if possible, install a solid-core door, and bring your cellphone to your bedroom.
- Get to know your neighbours and organize a neighbourhood watch.
- Do not hide your keys under a fake rock, under your door mat, over your door, or in any other obvious place. These are dead giveaways to experienced criminals.
- Do not open your door to anyone you do not know.
- Ask for identification from repair people, police officers, firefighters, and any others who come to your door offering services. If you are not expecting one of these individuals, call to verify that he or she was sent to your place on official business.
- Keep lights on in at least one room other than the one you are in to make it look as if you are not home alone. If you live alone or are alone frequently, alternate which lights you put on.
- Do not put your full name on your mailbox or in the phone book; use your initials instead. Shred mail that has your name and address on it.
- Use a "Beware of Dog" sign to deter assailants. If you have a dog or cat, be careful of "doggy doors." Many assailants have entered a house through a pet door (Schneider, 1992).

Preventing Assaults When You Are Away from Home

There are several suggestions to prevent an assault when you walk or jog:

- Walk or jog at a steady pace. Be confident and alert to your surroundings. If you are listening to music through ear buds, consider using only one, so that you can be aware of the sounds around you.
- Walk or jog with others. There is safety in numbers.
- Vary your running or walking routes.
- At night, avoid dark parking lots, wooded areas, and all other places where an assailant could hide.
- Listen for footsteps and voices. Change the pace of your walk if you think you are being followed to see if the person behind you does likewise. If you are being followed, walk down the middle of the street, staying near the streetlights. Run and yell if you feel threatened.
- Be aware of cars that keep driving around in your area. Report these vehicles if they persist (Schneider, 1992).

Preventing Assaults When You Are in Your Car

Carjackings and murders of individuals driving expensive cars, rental cars, and other vehicles point out the necessity for personal actions to prevent assaults when you are in your car:

- Keep your doors locked and your windows shut.
- Do not stop for vehicles in distress. Drive on and call for help.
- If your car breaks down, lock the doors and wait for help from the police. Do not accept assistance from strangers, particularly from individuals on isolated roads.
- If you think someone is following you, do something to attract attention. Stay in your car with locked windows and doors and drive to a fire station, police station, all-night grocery, restaurant, or other place where there are people. If you are forced to stop on a deserted road, leave your engine running and in gear. Wait until your pursuer gets out of his or her car, then drive away as fast as you safely can.
- Stick to well-travelled routes. Avoid dark, isolated shortcuts.
- Fill your car with gas and keep it in good running order.
- Do not put your name and address on your key ring.
- Before getting into your car, walk around it and check the back seat, floor, and undercarriage.
- On long trips, do not make it obvious that you are travelling alone. Never take a map into a restaurant.
- Do not sleep in your car along the highway. This may not be safe.
- When you stop at a traffic light, leave a car's length ahead of you so that if you are approached you will have room to pull out. If someone does approach, blow your horn and attract attention.
- If someone bumps into you, never get out of the car until a police officer arrives. Murders and carjackings have involved assailants ramming victims' cars from behind and then shooting or attacking those who investigate (Schneider, 1992).

VIOLENCE AND HEALTH

If the health sector is to adequately understand and respond to violence, greater emphasis is needed on the Population Health Model adopted by the various levels of government, which views health as embracing not only medical services and personal health practices; but also the physical, social, and economic environment (see Chapter 1). Prevention of violence must be based on the creation of life conditions that reduce the occurrence of violence and lessen its effects.

Clearly, a violence-free environment is a prerequisite for health. Violence is a barrier to health and a consequence of an unhealthy environment. The Ottawa Charter for Health Promotion (Public Health Agency of Canada, 1986) (an international statement on health promotion) states:

> The fundamental conditions and resources for health are peace, shelter, education, food, income, a stable ecosystem, sustainable resources, social justice and equity. Improvement in health requires a secure foundation in these basic prerequisites.

Injury Prevention

Intentional acts of violence and abuse receive more media coverage and public awareness than unintentional injuries, which disable and kill Canadians every day. Unintentional injuries—the result of falls, motor vehicle crashes, railway and pedestrian injuries, drowning and suffocation, poisoning, and fires—are the leading cause of death among Canadians up to the age of 44, and they kill more young people between the ages of 1 and 20 than all other causes of death combined. Why, then, do we not view injury as a serious population health problem? It is likely because we tend to call unintentional injuries "accidents." This suggests that the injury was due to some unavoidable circumstance over which the individual had no control. However, most injuries are predictable and preventable. Not wearing seatbelts or bicycle helmets drastically increases the risk of injury. Falls account for about 40 percent of the total injuries to Canadians, while motor vehicle crashes account for about 20 percent.

Who Are the Victims of Unintentional Injury?

The injury rate resulting in death or hospitalization is higher for seniors than for any other age group in Canada, and is expected to grow as the population ages. The most common cause of injury among seniors is falls. More than $980 million is spent each year to cover the cost of direct medical care to treat these falls. Canadians of all ages face hazards in their everyday environment that might cause falls—ice-coated sidewalks and stairs, loose banisters, and unsafe play or work equipment.

Falls are by far the most common reason that Canadians are admitted to hospital for injury. The Canadian Institute for Health Information (2012) reports that falls account for more than 50 percent of all people admitted to hospital, 67 percent of all days spent in hospital due to trauma, and 75 percent of all people who die in hospital due to trauma.

Preventable injuries account for almost 70 percent of injury-related deaths among children and youth. Of the 3000 people per year who die in motor vehicle crashes in Canada, 40 percent (1200 deaths) are attributed to alcohol. Up to $25 billion is spent annually for emergency care, rehabilitation, and other costs resulting from traffic collisions.

point of view

BANNING PHONE USE WHILE DRIVING:
Good Idea or Going Too Far?

Okay, fess up: How often in recent history have you chatted on the phone while driving, tried to read a text message, or switched the music on your iPod? Even though it is illegal to do so in all Canadian provinces? For many the answer is more than once—even though we know better and may even know of someone seriously injured or killed when texting and driving. According to research in the United States, texting drivers make up 31 percent of all drivers between the ages of 16 and 24 years, 41 percent of drivers between the ages of 25 and 39 years, and 5 percent of drivers 55 years of age and older. In addition, 70 percent of all drivers report talking on their cellphones regularly while driving. So, what is the problem? The fact is that driving while distracted is deadly. Talking on your phone is distracting. Texting is distracting. (There are other behaviours that are distracting too, but we are only focused on cellphone use here.)

Recognizing that increased reliance on cellphones could be contributing to motor vehicle accidents, laws have been enacted to restrict their use when driving. Are these laws worth the effort, or have they gone too far?

ARGUMENTS FAVOURING BANNING CELLPHONE USE WHILE DRIVING:

Other laws to improve public safety while driving, such as laws against drunk driving or mandating seatbelt use, have saved millions of lives. Cellphone bans could do the same.

Statistics have shown that texting while driving is about six times more likely to result in an accident than driving while intoxicated, and drivers who use hand-held devices are four times as likely to get into crashes resulting in injury than those who do not use them.

ARGUMENTS OPPOSING BANNING CELLPHONE USE WHILE DRIVING:

Although distracted driving from phone calls and texting is a problem, there are many other distractions that are just as serious: talking with passengers, eating, working a GPS device, putting on makeup, changing the radio station, and more. Why ban cellphones without banning the others?

These laws will be difficult to enforce and will spend tax dollars that might be better spent improving traffic safety in other ways.

Where Do You Stand?

○ Do you currently use a cellphone while driving? If so, would a law make you stop? Even if it was not made illegal, would you or could you stop?

○ Do you think cellphone use while driving should be banned? If so, all forms or only certain things like texting? Why or why not?

○ What about other distractions? Do you think they are as dangerous as cellphone use? Why or why not? How could you avoid getting distracted while driving?

Sources: Based on Governors Highway Safety Association, Cell Phone and Texting Laws: May 2011, Accessed May 10, 2011, www.ghsa.org/html/stateinfo/laws/cellphone_laws.html; Distraction.gov. U.S. Department of Transportation, Statistics and Facts about Distracted Driving, Accessed May 10, 2011, www.distraction.gov/stats-and-facts/index.html; M. Reardon, "Study: Distractions, Not Phones, Cause Car Crashes" in CNET.com Signal Strength, January 29, 2010, http://news.cnet.com/8301-30686_3-10444717-266.html.

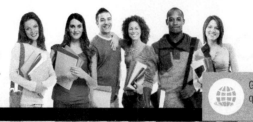

assess
YOURSELF

Go to MasteringHealth to complete this questionnaire with automatic scoring

TAKING CHARGE: Managing Yourself to Reduce Your Experiences with Violence

This chapter covered a variety of topics related to violence—murder, suicide, physical and sexual assault, hate and bias crimes, and so on. Unless immersed or living with these topics, they may be issues that you do not consider as part of your overall health. Even if not directly involved, each of these issues has a potential to influence your health because of the role these issues play in your home, school, and local community. We finish this chapter challenging you to think about yourself, first to assess yourself and identify if you are a victim of abuse. We make some suggestions at the end of this questionnaire should you be in a position where you are abused.

Following the Assess Yourself questionnaire is a section regarding safety on your campus. Although you may not feel it is your direct responsibility to create a safe environment where you live on campus, if you do not raise awareness about it, who will? Read this section carefully and consider what actions you will take.

Are You a Victim of Abuse?

Ask yourself if you are being abused. Start with the following questions, responding yes or no. Be honest.

1. Does your partner continually criticize what you wear, what you say, how you act, and how you look? _____
2. Does your partner often call you insulting or degrading names? _____
3. Do you feel like you need to ask permission to go out and see your friends and family? _____
4. Do you feel that no matter what you do, everything is your fault? _____
5. Do you feel like you're walking on eggshells trying to avoid an argument? _____
6. When you are late getting home, does your partner harass you about where you were and whom you were with? _____
7. Is your partner so jealous that you are always being accused of having affairs? _____
8. Has your partner threatened to hurt you or the children if you leave? _____
9. Does your partner force you to have sex? _____
10. Has your partner threatened to hit you? _____
11. Has your partner ever pushed, shoved, or slapped you? _____

12. Has your partner ever purposely broken anything of value to you? _____

If you answered yes to one or more of these questions, you may be suffering abuse.

Where to Go for Support Services

- Transition house or shelter
- Police department/RCMP unit
- Distress centre
- Sexual assault centre/women's resource centre
- Social service agency
- Health centre/doctor's office
- Hospital emergency department

Telephone numbers can be found at the front of your phone book or online.

Do You Want to Learn More?

If you are looking for further information and resources focusing on family violence, the Family Violence Initiative, led by the Public Health Agency of Canada, has been the federal government's main collaborative forum for addressing family violence since 1988. The Family Violence Initiative brings together 15 partner departments and agencies to prevent and respond to family violence. Visit their website at www.phac-aspc.gc.ca/sfv-avf/index-eng.php.

Source: Deborah Prieur and Mary Rowles, *Taking Action: A Union Guide to Ending Violence Against Women* (BC Federation of Labour and the Women's Research Centre, 1992) 14. Reprinted by permission of the BC Federation of Labour. http://chodarr.org/sites/default/files/chodarr0693.pdf.

Consider the Safety of Your Campus

University and college campuses today may be healthy places for student interactions, or they may be settings for violent and aggressive interactions between students. Most campuses have initiated programs, services, and policies designed to protect students from possible violations of their personal health and safety. Respond to the following to determine yours and your college administrators' degree of interest in and commitment to proactive violence protection and to a violence-free setting.

CHOICES for Change: Making Personal Choices

Setting limits on where you go, at what time, and with whom seems to be a running theme of this chapter. What types of limits do you set for yourself? What precautions do you take when you head out of your room or house? Think for a moment about your next night out with friends or with your lover.

- What limits will you set for yourself?
- Will you decide ahead of time how much you will drink?
- What time do you want to be home? How will you get home?
- How far will you go sexually? Will you use condoms?
- Do you travel in groups whenever possible?
- Do you avoid being out alone at night?
- Do you avoid high-crime areas?
- Have you and your friends created a 'safe' word?
- Do you and your friends look out for one another? For example, do you take turns where one of you stays sober and thinking clearly on a night of partying?

CHOICES for Change: Making Community Choices

The safety—or lack thereof—of your campus is important too. You may want to personally become involved in making changes to make your campus safer—or at the very least make your student government aware of the changes that need to be made. Consider the following questions as you evaluate the safety of your campus.

- Does your campus have a student health centre with a trained staff?
- Does your health centre offer workshops on prevention of sexual assault?
- Does your campus offer courses focusing on understanding human diversity?
- Does your campus offer workshops or seminars for men to help them understand their sexuality

and refrain from all forms of sexual assault against women?
- Does your campus offer workshops and information for students to help them avoid situations that put them at risk for violent sexual or other interactions?
- Does your campus offer confidential counselling or assistance to victims of sexual assault?
- Does your campus offer workshops or educational sessions dealing with suicide?
- Does your campus offer information, workshops, or services dealing with domestic violence?
- Does your campus offer information, workshops, or services dealing with child abuse and/or sexual abuse?
- Does your campus offer workshops or seminars that help males learn how to confront peers who express attitudes supportive of "overcoming" women sexually?
- Does your campus have strict substance-use policies designed to reduce the likelihood of sexual assaults?
- Are sessions designed to negate myths and to increase understanding between the sexes offered in "safe" environments where discussions are open and positive role models encourage positive actions?
- Are services such as rides and escort services available to students after hours to prevent assaults? Do security guards patrol the campus?
- Is your campus well-lit and open in the evenings?
- Are campus health educators, counsellors, and other professionals trained to spot victimization in clients and recommend appropriate services?
- Does your campus have a code of conduct that mandates swift and prudent punishment for alcohol and other drug abuse and acts of campus violence?

Critical Thinking

Your best friend and roommate was accused of date rape; if the charge is substantiated, he could be dismissed. The way your friend tells it, they had a few drinks, started making out, and eventually had sex. He claims that she did not try to stop him. Your friend asks you to talk to the girl; after all, she is a friend of yours from high school and you introduced them. He wants you to "find holes in her story" and see if you can get her to "forget about the whole thing." It is hard to believe your best friend is a rapist. But then you have not talked to the accuser yet.

Using the DECIDE model described in Chapter 1, decide what you will do. Reconsider the information about date rape in the chapter. Would it make a difference if she came to you to talk?

DISCUSSION QUESTIONS

1. Identify the types of violence in Canada and the prevalence of each.

2. What are the health issues of violence on your campus? And in society?

3. What leads to domestic violence? Compare spousal abuse against men and women: What are the differences? What are the similarities?

4. What puts a child at risk for abuse? What can be done to prevent or to decrease the amount of child abuse?

5. How, when, and where can we stop the cycle of abuse where an abused child becomes a child abuser in his or her adult years?

6. Detail the actions you can take to protect yourself from personal assault in your home, on the streets, or in your car.

7. If your friend called to tell you she or he was just sexually assaulted, what would you do? What would you suggest that she or he do?

8. Think about a time when you did something risky. Was it a smart or foolish risk? What steps did you take to manage or limit the risk? If you had the same opportunity, what, if anything, would you do differently?

APPLICATION EXERCISE

Reread the "Consider This . . . " scenario at the beginning of the chapter and answer the following questions.

1. From what you have read in this chapter, do you think what Will has witnessed is common in Canadian society?

2. How do you think Will might react to the police taking his father away?

3. How might Will react to his mother?

4. How can Will break the cycle of violence and not become an abuser himself?

5. Where can Will go for help for himself?

MASTERINGHEALTH

Go to MasteringHealth for Assignments, the eText, and the Study Area with case studies, self quizzing, and videos.

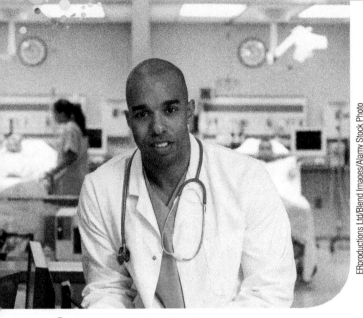

ERproductions Ltd/Blend Images/Alamy Stock Photo

CHAPTER 16

BECOMING A WISE CONSUMER OF HEALTH SERVICES

CONSIDER THIS . . .

Petra is 25 years old with a history of chronically painful menstrual periods and excessive bleeding. She seeks care from a gynecologist, who immediately tells her that she must have a hysterectomy. Because she has not yet had children and does not want to risk early menopause, Petra seeks a second opinion from the gynecologist's colleague. Without giving her much of an exam, the second doctor agrees with the first, so Petra seeks yet another opinion—but this time from a gynecologist outside the original group's practice. This third doctor adamantly disagrees and suggests a more conservative treatment not involving surgery.

Which doctor's advice should Petra follow? Is it appropriate to seek more than one opinion? Is it appropriate to seek more than two opinions? How much say should the individual have about his or her course of treatment?

LEARNING OUTCOMES

- Describe the funding and expenses of Canada's health system.

- Outline a method for making informed health-care choices, including evaluating online medical sources of information.

- Explain when self-diagnosis and self-care are appropriate, when to seek medical care, and how to assess the quality and care of health professionals.

- Create guidelines for choosing a family physician or other health-care personnel.

- Compare and contrast allopathic and non-allopathic medicine, including the types of treatments that fall into each category.

There are many reasons for you to be an informed health-care consumer. Most important, you have only one mind and body, and it is up to you to maintain them. Doing everything you can to be healthy and to recover rapidly when not healthy enhances every other part of your life. Canada's history reflects a commitment to sharing the liability of illness and injury among the entire population because our health-care system is based on shared values of equity, fairness, compassion, and respect for the dignity of all (Health Canada, 2012). This is not the case in many other countries.

In the 1990s, the federal government cut its health-care transfer payments to the provinces, in stages, from a 50–50 share to a 15–85 share as part of its deficit reduction strategy. This shift had—and continues to have—a profound impact on the provinces and territories, which are responsible for providing health care. In 2002, the Commission on the Future of Healthcare in Canada made recommendations aimed at sustaining our publicly funded health system by balancing investments in prevention and health maintenance with those directed to care and treatment (Commission on the Future of Health Care in Canada, n.d.). As head of the Commission, Roy Romanow recommended comprehensive changes to ensure that our health-care system would be sustainable.

As we scrutinize the evolution and progression of our health-care system, trends continue to emerge—including a shift from centralized governing bodies to regional health authorities, a shift in emphasis from institutionally focused care to community-based care, decision making based on need and the best available evidence, and funding of health services at sustainable levels (Health Canada, 1999). Despite these changes, health care remains very important to Canadians, with 63 percent of those polled in a 2005 study indicating that health care should receive the greatest attention from the country's leaders (Canadian Institute for Health Information, n.d.). At the same time, approximately 20 percent and fewer than 10 percent thought education and the economy, respectively, should be the main issue for Canada's leaders.

Even though health and health care are often treated as a social good to which everyone is entitled, you should be knowledgeable about what resources are available and when to be assertive to obtain services in your best interests. Almost all Canadians use some type of health services each year.

Not surprisingly, medical and health-care services are much harder to evaluate than clothing or fruit and vegetables. That said, 85 percent of Canadians were very or somewhat satisfied with the care they received in the past 12 months (Canadian Institute for Health Information, n.d.). Further, most Canadians rated the quality of care as excellent or very good. Although men and women throughout the country report similar levels of satisfaction overall regarding their health care when responses for 'somewhat satisfied' and 'very satisfied' are combined, more women reported being very satisfied with their health care. In response to questions about access to health care, most Canadians (84 percent) did not have difficulty in accessing care (Canadian Institute for Health Information, n.d.). The most common challenges to accessing health care were waiting too long to get an appointment, waiting too long in doctors' offices, and problems in contacting a physician. Another issue highlighted in the 2006 Statistics Canada survey included access time for elective or non-emergency surgeries, with almost 20 percent waiting more than three months (Canadian Institute for Health Information, n.d.).

The federal and provincial governments have responded to the need to adapt the system to meet Canadians' needs, notably by

- adopting a "determinant of health" framework that recognizes that, while health care is obviously an important contributor to health, its role must be placed in context as only one component of a much broader set of determinants of health

- shifting the emphasis of the health-care system away from institutionally based delivery models (that is, physicians and hospital-based care) to integrated community-based models that place increased emphasis on prevention and health promotion

- developing strategies for the coordinated management of the health-care workforce, including the remuneration, geographical distribution, and appropriate use of various health-care providers

- reducing wait times for cancer care, cardiac care, hip and knee replacements, cataract surgery, and diagnostic imaging (Canadian Institute for Health Information, n.d.)

This chapter will help you to become proactive in making decisions that affect your health and health care. Canada's health-care system is a shared responsibility of the federal, provincial, and territorial governments. It includes hospitals, home-care agencies, long-term care facilities, and people (physicians, nurses, social workers, midwives, and other health-care providers) (Public Health Agency of Canada, n.d.). Total health expenditure in Canada is projected to be $219.1 billion in 2015, for a broad range of services including physician visits, immunizations, prescriptions, lab tests, and hospital stays.

This was a 1.6 percent increase in spending from 2014 (Canadian Institute for Health Information, 2016). The federal government funding provides about 3.5 percent in the form of direct health spending, while provincial/territorial support is 65.2 percent of all health expenditures. Thus, a significant portion remains to be covered from federal Canada Health Transfer support (Health Canada, 2011).

MAKING INFORMED HEALTH-CARE CHOICES

Perhaps the single greatest difficulty that we face as consumers is the magnitude of options available. Many companies aggressively market health products and services to the public. Even medical professionals sometimes feel overwhelmed, confused, and frustrated by the many options. Informed consumers are aware that there is always more to learn about their health-care related options. Wise consumers use every means at their disposal to ensure that they are acting responsibly in their own health-care choices.

Evaluating Online Medical Resources

The internet has increasingly become a source of health information for many Canadians. How can we be sure that the information we read on websites is credible? The National Centre for Complementary and Alternative Medicine (n.d.) suggests that we ask ourselves the following questions:

- Who maintains the site? Any reputable site will make it easy for you to find out who is responsible for the information presented on it.

- Who financially supports the site? The source for the website's funding should be clearly stated. You should know how a website pays for its existence. Does it sell advertising? Is it sponsored by a pharmaceutical company? The source of funding might influence how information is presented.

- What is the purpose of the site? This is related to who runs and pays for the site. The site's purpose should be clearly stated and help you in evaluating the trustworthiness of the information included.

- Where does the information come from? If the information does not come from the website creator, the original source(s) should be identified.

- What is the basis of the information? In addition to providing a complete citation list, the site should describe what the materials presented are based upon. Facts and figures presented should have credible references. Opinions should be set apart from evidence-based information.

- How is the information selected? Was the presented material peer-reviewed? That is, did other appropriate health professionals review the material prior to posting?

- How current is the information? Good health websites are reviewed and updated on a regular basis to ensure that the information presented is current. The date when the website was most recently updated should be clearly stated.

- How does the site choose links to other sites? Credible websites have policies regarding what links they will establish.

- How does the site manage interaction with visitors? A credible site will provide a way for you to contact the site owner if you have any problems, questions, or feedback.

Financing Health Care

Canada has a predominantly publicly funded, privately delivered health-care system that rests on an interlocking set of 10 provincial and three territorial health insurance plans. The Canada Health Act, informally known to Canadians as Medicare, is the system that provides access to universal, comprehensive coverage for medically necessary hospital, inpatient, and outpatient physician services. This structure results from the constitutional assignment of jurisdiction over most aspects of health care to provincial governments. The system is referred to as a "national" health insurance system because all provincial or territorial hospital and medical insurance plans are linked through adherence to national principles set at the federal level. The provinces and territories plan, finance, and evaluate the provision of hospital, physician, and allied health care, some aspects of prescription care, and public health (Health Canada, 1999).

Accepting Responsibility for Your Health Care

While income should not be a barrier to universally insured medical services, disparities in access to insured and uninsured health services remain. Dental care, vision care, counselling services, and most allopathic medicines are not covered in our current national health care—though they were in the past. Access to these services is essential to basic health, yet many have restricted or no access to these services because of lack of private or publicly assisted insurance (Health Canada, 1999), particularly for those who cannot afford the services personally. Further, obtaining insured health-care services can be a struggle for those with limited accessibility for many reasons whether it is transportation, need for childcare, lack of understanding how to use services, and so on.

Even though most health care you need is publicly funded, you still need to learn how, when, and where to enter the system and how to obtain the care you need without incurring unnecessary risk or wasting resources. Acting responsibly in times of illness can be difficult, and the person best able to act on your behalf is you. Being knowledgeable about self-care and its limits is critical for responsible and effective consumerism.

Why Some False Claims May Seem True

Many marketing strategies revolve around trendy news items. A good example of this is the concern about trans fat. While food advertisements and product labels previously focused on "low calories," "low cholesterol," "low fat," or "low in saturated fat," they now emphasize "0 trans fat." The risk here is that many of the products, despite having 0 grams of trans fat, have high levels of saturated fats—which puts an individual at risk for heart disease. When it comes to gathering health information, it is your responsibility to approach advertisers' claims with a "buyer beware" mindset firmly in place. Further, you need to 'read' beyond the glamourized information presented.

The same skepticism should be used when evaluating advertising for medical cures. Because of Canadian restrictions and limitations on pharmaceutical advertising, we have not experienced as much of this as people in the United States have, whose laws in this regard are not as stringent. People often fall victim to false health-care claims because they mistakenly believe that a product or provider has helped them. This belief often arises from two conditions: spontaneous remission and the placebo effect.

Spontaneous remission The disappearance of symptoms without any apparent cause or treatment.

Placebo effect An apparent cure or improved state of health brought about by a substance or product with no medicinal value.

Spontaneous Remission

It is commonly said that if you treat a cold, it will disappear in a week, but if you leave it alone, it will last seven days. A **spontaneous remission** from an ailment refers to the disappearance of symptoms without any apparent cause or treatment. Many illnesses, like the common cold and even back strain, are self-limiting and will improve in time, with or without treatment. Other illnesses, such as multiple sclerosis and some cancers, are characterized by alternating periods of severe symptoms and sudden remissions. Because of this phenomenon, people seeking profit exploit consumers by claiming that their particular treatment, procedure, or drug cured the condition. People experiencing spontaneous remissions can easily attribute their "cure" to a treatment, drug, or provider that had no real effect on the disease or condition.

Placebo Effect

The **placebo effect** is an apparent cure or improved state of health brought about by a substance, product, or procedure that has no therapeutic value. It is not uncommon for people to report improvements or reduced symptoms based on what they expected, desired, or were told would happen after taking simple sugar pills believed to be powerful drugs. About 10 percent of the population is believed to be exceptionally susceptible to the power of suggestion; the remainder might be influenced to varying degrees. Those most susceptible to the placebo effect can be victimized by aggressive marketing of products and services. Although the placebo effect is often harmless, it does account for the expenditure of millions of dollars on worthless health products and services every year.

SELF-CARE

Individuals can practise behaviours that promote health and reduce the risk of disease as well as treat minor afflictions without seeking professional help. Self-care consists of knowing your body, paying attention to its signals, and taking appropriate action to stop the progression of illness or injury. Common forms of self-care include the following:

- Diagnosing symptoms or conditions that occur frequently but might not require physician visits (for example, the common cold, minor abrasions)
- Using over-the-counter remedies to treat mild, infrequent, and unambiguous pain and other symptoms
- Performing first aid for common, uncomplicated injuries and conditions

- Checking blood pressure, pulse, and temperature
- Performing monthly breast or testicular self-examinations
- Doing periodic checks for blood glucose, cholesterol, or other levels as prescribed by a physician
- Learning from reliable self-help books, websites, and videos
- Performing meditation and other relaxation techniques
- Maintaining a healthful diet, getting adequate rest, and exercising.

In addition, a vast array of at-home diagnostic kits are now available to test for pregnancy, allergies, HIV, possible prediabetes and type 2 diabetes based on A1C levels, genetic disorders, and many other conditions.

Taking prescription drugs used for a previous illness to treat your current illness, using unproven self-treatment or using other people's medications are examples of inappropriate self-care.

Using self-care methods appropriately takes effort, education, and the ability to make informed decisions based on scientific evidence.

When to Seek Help

Effective self-care requires the knowledge of when to seek professional medical attention rather than treat a condition on your own. Generally, consult a physician if you experience any of the following:

- a serious accident or injury
- sudden or severe chest pains resulting in difficulty breathing
- trauma to the head or spine accompanied by a headache, blurred vision, loss of consciousness, vomiting, convulsions, or paralysis
- sudden high fever or recurring high temperature (over 38.5°C for adults and 39.5°C for children) or sweats
- tingling sensation in the arm accompanied by slurred speech or impaired thought processes
- adverse reactions to a drug or insect bite (shortness of breath, throat constriction, severe swelling, itchiness, or dizziness)
- unexplained bleeding or loss of bodily fluid from any body opening
- unexplained and sudden weight loss
- persistent or recurrent diarrhea or vomiting
- blue-coloured lips, eyelids, or nail beds
- any lump, swelling, thickness, or sore that does not subside or that grows for over a month
- any marked change in or pain accompanying bowel or bladder habits
- yellowing of the skin or the whites of the eyes
- any unusual symptom that recurs over time
- signs that suggest possible pregnancy including morning nausea, tender breasts, and a missed period

With the vast array of home diagnostic devices currently available, it appears to be relatively easy for most people to take care of themselves. A strong word of caution is in order: although many of these devices are valuable for making an initial diagnosis, home health tests should not be a substitute for regular, complete examinations by a trained practitioner whether that is done in person or through one of the provincial telehealth centres. The next section offers valuable information about taking an active part in your health care.

Being Proactive in Your Health Care

Personal involvement in your wellness is critical. Taking a proactive approach to practising preventive behaviours goes a long way toward ensuring a long and healthy life. Sometimes, regardless of the steps taken to care for yourself, you still get sick. At such a time, it is important that you continue to be involved in your care. The more you know about your body and the factors that affect your health, the better you are able to communicate with your doctor or other health professional. It also helps you to make informed decisions and to recognize when a certain treatment may not be right for you. The following points may be helpful.

- Know your and your family's medical history.
- Be knowledgeable about your condition—causes, physiological effects, possible treatments, prognosis. Do not rely only on the doctor or other health professional for this information. Do some research of your own.
- Bring a friend or relative along for medical appointments to help you review what is said and possibly write down the answers to your questions.
- Ask the practitioner to explain the problem and appropriate treatments, tests, and drugs in a way that you understand.
- If the doctor prescribes medications, ask about the prescription, how long the drug has been on the market, if you are being prescribed the generic

Student
Health
TODAY

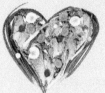

Finding a Personal Physician

Asking the right questions at the right time can save you personal suffering. Many individuals find that writing their questions down ahead of time helps them to get all their inquiries answered. You should not accept a defensive or hostile response; asking questions is your right as a patient. The following section will help you to find your own physician or other health professional if you do not already have one or more in place.

Consider the following situation. Corry wakes one morning with a chest cold. In a few days, the cold worsens and she thinks she has developed bronchitis. Corry knows she should see a doctor, but she does not have a primary care physician, so she decides to let the cold take its course, without medical attention. Unfortunately for Corry, this approach does not work, as her cold worsens, resulting in pneumonia and a much longer recovery time.

Unfortunately, many people hesitate to seek early care because they do not have a physician. In these cases, emergency room care or drop-in clinics are used. As a result, no long-term relationship is established between the health-care practitioner and patient. If Corry (and others) had a primary care physician, she could have called him or her as soon as her symptoms worsened.

One of the most important decisions a person or family makes is choosing a primary care physician. Your physician plays a critical role in the prevention and treatment of illnesses. When you are ill or develop symptoms that need attention, having someone to contact in whom you have confidence can relieve a great deal of anxiety. Yet, despite the importance of identifying and regularly visiting a primary care physician, a great many people wait until they are ill to seek a doctor. Depending on the severity of the illness, waiting too long might limit your options. Selecting a doctor before an illness develops allows you to identify and interview several doctors to find the one who best fits your needs and with whom you feel the most comfortable. In Canada, you may have easier access to a primary care physician (general or family practitioner) if another family member visits that practitioner or if you are new to the area. It can be difficult to change doctors when remaining in the same location. This difficulty makes it all the more important to properly assess a doctor at the outset. Another issue to keep in mind is that there is a physician shortage in many areas in Canada, with some physicians not taking new patients.

The following guidelines may help you to find the health professionals that are right for you.

1. First, consider the following questions:

   - Would you feel more comfortable with a male or female health professional? Why?

   - Is the age of your health-care professional an important factor to you? If so, why?

   - Do you have a pre-existing condition for which a health-care specialist may be needed?

   - Do you prefer to see primarily one physician or are you comfortable visiting a service with a team of doctors (as you would find in a health clinic or team practice)?

2. Once you have considered your responses to the previous questions, assemble a list of names of doctors in your area. Names of potential physicians or other health professionals can be identified by

   - Asking friends and colleagues for recommendations. These are often your best sources of information about a doctor's availability and promptness as well as for providing their perception of the doctor's overall general concern for his or her patients' well-being.

   - Calling the local medical association, local health advocacy groups (many communities provide references as a service), or the local hospital for names of doctors accepting new patients.

   - Researching medical directories at your local library or online. The *Canadian Medical Directory*, for example, includes information about every physician who belongs to the CMA (Canadian Medical Association).

3. Call the offices of the physicians on your list and explain that you are seeking a primary care physician. Ask the receptionist about the doctor's hospital affiliation, office hours, and the kind of coverage the physician has for emergency situations outside normal office hours. Take into consideration the receptionist's tone and how your questions are answered. Find out how much time is allotted for appointments (30 to 45 minutes for a routine physical is average).

4. Narrow the list to two or three physicians and make appointments for brief consultations.

5. While visiting with each doctor, you should find answers to the following questions:

   - Is the doctor's educational and experiential background appropriate?

   - While visiting, do you feel that he or she cares about you as a person?

   - Do you feel relaxed in his or her presence?

   - Are you encouraged to ask questions? Are answers explained clearly?

   - Does the physician use a lot of medical jargon? If so, how does that make you feel?

   - Does the doctor use a condescending tone?

   - Does the physician attend to you personally or does he or she serve primarily as a "gatekeeper" to specialists?

6. Develop some direct questions about treatment that identify the physician's philosophy on care. For example, you could ask how the physician would treat a terminally ill patient or about his or her willingness to accommodate your religious beliefs.

7. Once you choose a physician, get the most from your visits by creating and maintaining an open line of communication. You can do this by:

   - Being prepared for appointments. Know your medical and family history and be specific and detailed about the symptoms you experience.

   - Not bringing up irrelevant questions regarding your partner's, children's, or parent's health when the appointment is about you.

   - Being an educated patient. Expect and insist on a diagnosis explained in a way that you fully understand. Never leave your doctor's office with questions unanswered.

   - Taking a proactive and reactive role in your health care. Treatment will work only if you follow it. Listen to and follow instructions, find out when you can call with follow-up questions, and be sure that the doctor reports any test results to you promptly. "No news is good news" is not an appropriate adage to follow.

   - Communicating your needs to the doctor. If you have concerns about communication or treatment, speak up.

brand and, if so, how it might be different than the name brand, when you should expect a change in your symptoms, and so on.

- Ask for a written summary of the results of your visit and any lab tests.

- If you have any doubt about the doctor's recommended treatment, seek a second opinion.

Afterward:

- Write down an account of what happened and what was said. Be sure to include the names of the doctor or health professional and all other people involved in your care, the date, and the place.

- Shop around at various drugstores for the best prices in the same way that you would when shopping for clothes.

- When filling prescriptions, ask to see the pharmacist's package inserts that list medical considerations concerning the prescribed drug and any possible interactions. Ask the pharmacist questions about main and side effects (see Chapter 9). Talk to the pharmacist about other drugs you take. What are the risks for interactions?

- Have clear instructions written on the label to avoid risk to others who may take the drug in error.

Doctors and other health professionals are human; their decisions are based on the best information available to them and may be influenced by a number of factors including—but not limited to—workload, limited information, and personal views. Therefore, in addition to the fore-mentioned practical steps, being proactively involved in your health care also means that you should be aware of your rights as a patient. The following are the basic rights of all individuals seeking care from a health-care professional. You have the right to

1. Informed consent. Before receiving any care, you have the right to be fully informed of what is planned, the risks and potential benefits, and possible alternative forms of treatment, including the option of no treatment. Your consent must be voluntary and without any form of coercion. It is critical that you read consent forms carefully and amend them as necessary before signing.

2. Know whether the treatment you receive is standard or experimental. In experimental conditions, you have the legal and ethical right to know if the study is one in which some people receive treatment while others do not and if a drug is used in the research project for a purpose not approved by the Health Protection Branch of Health Canada.

3. Privacy, which includes protecting your right to make personal decisions concerning all reproductive matters.

4. Refuse or stop treatment at any time.

5. Receive care.

6. Access your medical records.

7. Maintain confidentiality of your records.

8. Seek the opinions of other health-care professionals regarding your condition.

Assessing Health Professionals

Suppose you decide that you do need medical attention. You must then identify what type you need, where to obtain it, and who to obtain it from. Initially, selecting a doctor or other health professional may seem a simple matter, yet many people have no idea how to assess the qualifications of a medical practitioner. Knowledge of traditional medical specialties and alternative medicine is critical to making intelligent selections. You also need to be aware of criteria for evaluating a health professional. Studies indicate that many people's greatest concerns when choosing a doctor have less to do with medical qualifications than with availability and personality. While a warm and caring personality is certainly a valuable attribute, doctors who lack in bedside manner may, in fact, be better trained and qualified than more cordial practitioners (Sims & Tsai, 2015). That being said, it is critical to find a physician who is willing and able to listen to your concerns. Carefully consider the following factors about prospective health-care providers:

- What professional education/training do they have? What licence or board certification do they hold?

- Are they affiliated with an accredited medical facility or institution? Accreditation Canada requires these institutions to verify all education, licensing, and training claims of their affiliated practitioners.

- Do they indicate clearly how long a given treatment may last, or do they have you returning week after week with no apparent end in sight?

- Do their diagnoses, treatments, and general statements appear to be consistent with established scientific theory and practice?

- Do they listen to you, appear to respect you as an individual, and give you time to ask questions?

Allopathic medicine Traditional, Western medical practice; based on scientifically validated methods and procedures.

Primary care practitioner A medical practitioner who treats routine ailments, advises on preventive care, gives general medical advice, and makes appropriate referrals when necessary.

CHOICES OF MEDICAL CARE

Familiarizing yourself with the various health professions and health subspecialties will help you choose the right provider for your needs. There are more than 77 000 physicians and 406 817 registered nurses in Canada. The number of physicians per population (220 per 100 000) is the highest ever recorded (Canadian Institute for Health Information, 2014a, 2014b). Those you are most familiar with probably subscribe to allopathic medical procedures. Most people believe that **allopathic medicine**, or traditional, Western medical practice is based on scientifically validated methods, but you should consider that only about 20 percent of all allopathic treatments have been found to be clinically effective in research trials. Medical practitioners who adhere to allopathic principles are bound by a professional code of ethics.

Traditional (Allopathic) Medicine

Selecting a **primary care practitioner**—a medical practitioner whom you can go to for routine ailments, preventive care, general medical advice, and appropriate referrals—is not an easy task, particularly given the shortage of general practitioners in various parts of Canada. The primary care practitioner for most people is a family practitioner. Others use nontraditional providers as their primary source of care. The common denominator is continuity in services over a period of time. Having a "usual source of care" is important to the quality of care you receive.

Some of what is done in medicine either does not improve health outcomes or creates iatrogenic disease (illness caused by the medical treatment itself). An essential part of medical care is informed consent. This refers to your right to have explained to you—in language you can understand—possible side effects, benefits, and consequences of a specific procedure and treatment regimen, as well as available alternatives (Evans, n.d.). It also means that you have the right to refuse a specific treatment or to seek a second or even third opinion from unbiased, noninvolved health-care providers (Evans, n.d.).

Informed consent implies that you have the right to ask questions such as:

- What will happen if you choose not to have this particular test or treatment?

- Can other tests be performed instead? What are their risks? Why should you choose this test instead of something else?

- How often has the health professional you are consulting with performed this test, surgery, or procedure, and with what success?

- Are the risks from the proposed treatment greater than the risks from the condition?

- What are the side effects of the diagnostic tests? Can these side effects be prevented, treated, or reduced?

- Does this procedure require an overnight stay at a hospital or can it be performed on an outpatient basis or in a health professional's office?

- Why has this test been ordered? What will this test find or exclude?

- Are these medications necessary? What are their possible side effects? What will happen if you decide not to take them? What alternatives are available? Is there a generic version that costs less? Will they interact with the other drugs you currently consume (other prescription or OTC drug, caffeine, alcohol, or any other drug that I may be taking)?

- Why do I have this problem? What can you do to prevent it from happening again?

Allied Professionals

Canada lags behind other countries in its creative and integrative use of allied health professionals, including nurses. **Nurses** are highly trained and strictly regulated health practitioners who provide a wide range of services for patients and their families, including patient education, counselling, community health and disease prevention information, and administration of medications. They have the designation RN (registered nurse). Although the number of RNs eligible to practise in Canada increased 6.1 percent between 2007 and 2009, the number of RNs per 100 000 people has remained about the same, increasing from 783 to 785 (Canadian Institute for Health Information, 2013). In addition to working in health service organizations (HSOs), clinics, doctors' offices, student health centres, nursing homes, public health departments, schools, businesses, and other health-care settings, many nurses are employed in the hospital setting. There has, however, been an increasing trend away from hospital-based employment as the demand for nurses in other settings has increased.

Nurse practitioners are professional nurses with advanced training obtained through a master's degree program. Nurse practitioners have the training and authority to conduct diagnostic tests and prescribe medications. They work in a variety of settings, particularly in hospitals, clinics, and client homes. They have become an increasingly popular source of health care in recent years. Nurses may also earn a bachelor of science and nursing degree (BScN), a master of science and nursing (MScN), or a research-based PhD in nursing. Clinical nurse specialist is another advanced practice role.

Complementary and Alternative Medicine

While people in other parts of the world consider **complementary and alternative Medicine (CAM)** (also known as non-allopathic) medicine the "traditional" form of treatment, in Canada we tend to think of non-allopathic medicine as "alternative medicine." These are practises and products commonly used together with traditional medicine; however they can also be used in place of traditional medicine. As the government, private payers, and consumers evaluate the costs, effectiveness, and quality of traditional (allopathic) health care, many have found it wanting. The two core services under the Canada Health Act, hospital and physician services, count for 10.9 percent of the total health spending of $219 billion in 2015 (Canadian Institute for Health Information, 2016).

Although these two core services account for a smaller part of the total health-care spending than in the past, they have increased more than 51 percent since 1994. However, it should be pointed out that the increase in spending on public health and administration (6 percent of the total) outpaced increases for hospital and physician services. Further, the cost of prescription and OTC drugs has been the fastest-growing component of the total bill.

Partly as a result of dissatisfaction with traditional methods of care and the financing of the health-care system, each year more people seek CAM services from providers other than licensed medical doctors. More than 70 percent of Canadians regularly use CAM therapies such as vitamins and minerals, herbal products, and homeopathic medicines and other natural health products to stay healthy and improve their quality of life (Public Health Agency of Canada, 2008).

More women than men are likely to seek non-allopathic forms of treatment (Statistics Canada, 2005). Further, individuals who are midlife versus the very young or very old are more likely to choose nontraditional forms of treatment. Individuals of a higher income or higher level of education are also more likely to seek non-allopathic forms of medicine (Statistics Canada, 2005). The most sought CAM treatments are chiropractory, massage therapy, acupuncture, and homeopathic or naturopathic care.

Nurse Health practitioner who provides many services and may work in a variety of settings.

Complementary and alternative medicine (non-allopathic medicine) A group of health care practices and products that are not considered part of traditional (allopathic) medicine.

Numerous non-allopathic alternatives are available. Many people turn to CAM only after more traditional methods have failed to improve their conditions. Because they are often "providers of last resort," these unconventional treatments may appear to produce more negative outcomes overall than traditional medicine. This has given these types of care a bad reputation even though it was the failure of successful treatment through traditional medicine that sent many to non-allopathic practitioners in the first place. Although some alternative therapies—similar to traditional therapies—are controversial and may be dangerous, many offer significant benefits at reasonable costs. It is your role to ascertain the credentials of CAM practitioners whom you choose to engage with, because not all are licensed or regulated; this job of verifying credentials may, therefore, be even more difficult than in traditional medicine. Similar to self-care and accessing traditional practitioners, you must be assertive in asking CAM providers their training, licensing (if relevant), and affiliations (see "Finding a Personal Physician earlier"). You should also ask how many patients with your specific condition they have treated and what their success rate is. A potential danger in seeking the assistance of an alternative medical practitioner is that it may keep you from obtaining effective conventional treatment (if any is available).

As such, consider the possibility of combining traditional and CAM forms of treatment.

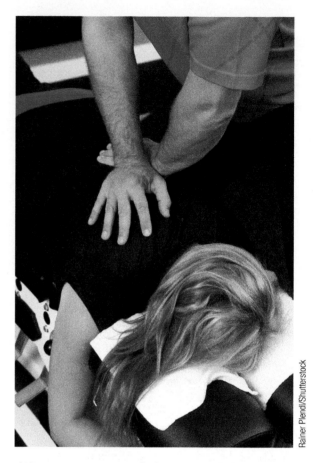

A chiropractor uses a variety of techniques to manipulate the spine into alignment.

Chiropractic Treatment

Chiropractic medicine has been practised for many years. Although there have always been medical doctors who collaborate with chiropractic doctors, their numbers have recently increased. Some chiropractic treatments are covered by provincial health insurance, and many private insurance companies pay for treatment if a medical doctor recommends it.

Chiropractic medicine is based on the premise that a life-giving energy flows through the spine via the nervous system. Ill health occurs then if the spine is subluxated (partly misaligned or dislocated) because that force is disrupted. Chiropractors, in their treatment, use a variety of techniques to manipulate the spine back into alignment, so the life-giving energy can flow unimpeded through the nervous system. It has been established that their treatment is effective for chronic low back pain, neck pain, and headaches.

The average chiropractic training program requires four years of intensive courses in biochemistry, anatomy, physiology, diagnostics, pathology, nutrition, and related topics, combined with hands-on clinical training. Currently, the only school in Canada where you can learn to become a chiropractor is the Canadian Memorial Chiropractic College, located in Toronto. Many chiropractors continue their training to obtain specialized certification—for example, in women's health, gerontology, or pediatrics.

You should investigate and question a chiropractor as carefully as you would a medical doctor. As with many health-care professionals, you may note vast differences in technique among specialists. It is recommended that you choose a chiropractor who follows standard chiropractic regimens for treating musculoskeletal conditions. Further, it is recommended that you choose a chiropractor who is willing to listen to you and provide treatment complete with explanations that you can understand.

Massage Therapy

Massage therapy refers to the assessment and treatment of the body's soft tissues (Newfoundland and Labrador Massage Therapy Association, n.d.). More specifically,

Chiropractic medicine A form of medical treatment that emphasizes the manipulation of the spinal column.

Rainer Plendl/Shutterstock

massage therapy is used to treat soft-tissue injuries and dysfunctions (whiplash, sprains, strains, muscle spasms), diseases and disorders (osteoarthritis, rheumatoid arthritis, bronchitis); painful conditions such as low back or neck pain; and conditions with psychological implications such as stress, anxiety, or depression. The Mayo Clinic (n.d.) describes the work of a massage therapist as follows: "during a massage, a certified massage therapist or medical professional manipulates your body's soft tissues (muscle, connective tissue, tendons, ligaments and skin), using varying degrees of pressure and movement." The Canadian Massage Therapy Alliance recommends a two-year intensive program, equivalent to approximately 2200 hours of training. All provinces and territories have different requirements to become a registered massage therapist. Check out the Canadian Massage Therapist Alliance website at www.cmta.ca for the specific requirements related to where you live.

Acupuncture and Acupressure

Acupuncture is the ancient (more than 2000 years old) Chinese art of inserting fine needles at points on the skin that fall along 14 major meridians, or pathways of energy (called *qi*), that flow through the body. These points and meridians are thought to be associated with particular internal organs and bodily functions. Proponents of acupuncture believe that the vital forces of life—the yin and the yang—are restored to equilibrium when these points are stimulated. Western practitioners believe that acupuncture may be effective in relieving pain because the acupuncture points stimulate nerves, muscles, and connective tissues that increase blood flow and boost the release of the body's natural painkillers (Mayo Clinic, 2012). Acupuncturists treat complaints as diverse as back and neck pain, menstrual cramps, morning sickness, addiction, asthma, headaches and migraines, infections, fibromyalgia, and osteoarthritis. They also help women in labour and people who want to quit smoking.

The Acupuncture Foundation of Canada Institute (www.afcinstitute.com) teaches licensed health practitioners about acupuncture. Some licensed MDs, physiotherapists, and chiropractors have also trained in acupuncture. If you decide to have acupuncture, it is very important to ensure that the needles the acupuncturist uses are disposable or properly sterilized using an autoclave, because needles reused without sterilization can transmit hepatitis and HIV.

Acupressure is similar to acupuncture, but does not use needles. Instead, the practitioner applies pressure to points critical to balancing yin and yang. Practitioners must have the same basic understanding of energy pathways as acupuncturists. Acupressure should not be applied by an untrained person to pregnant women or anyone with a chronic condition.

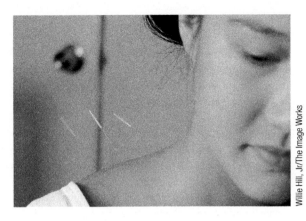

Acupuncture can be an effective treatment for a variety of conditions.

Herbalists and Homeopaths

Herbalists practise herbal medicine, which is based on the medicinal qualities of plants or herbs. Homeopaths use herbal medicine (as well as minerals and chemicals), and at the root of their practice is the theory that administering extremely diluted doses of potent natural agents that produce disease symptoms in healthy persons will cure the disease in the sick. Herbal and homeopathic medicines are common in Europe, Asia, and Canada, with 73 percent of Canadians reporting their use (Health Canada, 2015).

Herbal Remedies and Other Supplements

People have been using herbal remedies for thousands of years. Herbs are the sources for compounds found in approximately 25 percent of the pharmaceutical drugs we use today, including aspirin (white willow bark), the heart medication digitalis (foxglove), and the cancer treatment Taxol (Pacific yew tree). Scientists continue to make pharmacological advances by studying the herbal remedies used in cultures throughout the world. With conventional science now recognizing the benefits of herbs, it is no wonder that more and more consumers are turning to herbal products.

However, herbal remedies are not to be taken lightly. Just because a product has a natural source does not necessarily mean that it is safe. For example, the FDA has warned that certain herbal products containing kava may be associated with severe liver damage (National Center for Complementary and Alternative Medicine, 2010). Even rigorously tested products can be risky. Many plants are poisonous, and some can be toxic if ingested in high doses. Others may be dangerous when combined with prescription or over-the-counter drugs, can disrupt the normal action of the drugs, or can cause unusual side effects (Mayo

Clinic Staff, 2009). Properly trained herbalists and homeopaths have received graduate-level training in special programs such as herbal nutrition or traditional Chinese medicine. These practitioners are trained in diagnosis, properties of herbs, correct concentrations and dosages, and follow-up care.

Do Herbal Remedies Have Risks or Side Effects?
Herbs do have the potential to cause negative side effects. St. John's wort, for example, has potentially dangerous interactions with some prescription antidepressants and should never be taken with them. Other herbs, such as kava, can have negative effects even when taken alone.

Herbal remedies come in several different forms. *Tinctures* (extracts of fresh or dried plants) usually contain a high percentage of grain alcohol to prevent spoilage and can be a high-quality option. *Freeze-dried extracts* are stable and can offer good value for the cost. *Standardized extracts*, often available as pills or capsules, are also among the more reliable forms of herbal preparations. Herbal teas are also widely available. Increasingly, herbal preparations are being offered by companies that produce them in an environmentally responsible manner.

Herbal medicines tend to be milder than synthetic drugs and produce their effects more slowly; they also are much less likely to cause toxicity because they are usually less concentrated forms. Regardless of how natural they are, herbs still contain many of the same chemicals as synthetic drugs. Too much of any herb, particularly one from nonstandardized extracts, can cause health-related issues.

Not all supplements on the market are derived from plant sources. Various vitamins, minerals, amino acids, and other biological compounds have been promoted as providing certain health benefits. Some of these claims have been validated by research, and some have not.

Table 16.1 provides an overview of some common herbal supplements. Table 16.2 lists supplements that should be avoided because of previously identified safety concerns.

Although plants have been used for medicinal purposes for centuries and form the basis of many modern "wonder drugs," herbal medicine should not be taken lightly. Because something is natural—or grows on its own—does not necessarily mean that it is safe. Many plants are poisonous, and others can be toxic if consumed in high doses. One of the greatest dangers with this kind of therapy is that practitioners who mix their own tonics do not use standardized measures. Further, the actual potency of each herb varies with each season and its growing conditions (similar to marijuana—see Chapter 11). It is therefore imperative that you carefully investigate the chemical properties of herbs, including potential main and side effects yourself before you ingest them.

Naturopathy

According to the Canadian Association of Naturopathic Doctors (2013), "naturopathic medicine is a distinct primary health care system that blends modern scientific knowledge with traditional and natural forms of medicine." Naturopaths believe that illness results from violations of natural principles of life in modern societies. They view diseases as the body's effort to ward off impurities and harmful substances from the environment. Naturopathic treatment uses substances and forces found in nature: water, magnets, gravity, heat, crystals and minerals, herbs, and even the sun. Practitioners argue that returning to a natural, purified state will restore health.

The Canadian Association of Naturopathic Doctors (www.cand.ca) shares information regarding finding a naturopathic doctor as well as where individuals are trained in naturopathic medicine in Canada. Those who receive a naturopathic doctor (ND) degree typically have been through at least a four-year graduate program that emphasizes humanistically oriented family medicine. Similar to other health professionals, if you decide to be treated by a naturopath, you should carefully check his or her credentials.

Other Alternative Therapies

Many other therapies exist, including reflexology (zone therapy), iridology (light therapy), aromatherapy, and auramassage. Although these forms of non-allopathic medicine may work, they have yet to be substantiated scientifically. Until you can sort through the proliferation of new therapies, it is a good idea to follow the maxim "buyer beware."

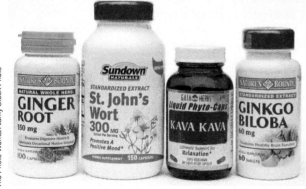

Herbal remedies, like all other drugs, should be used with caution.

TABLE 16.1

Common Supplements: Benefits, Research, and Risks

	Herb	Claims of Benefits	Research Findings	Potential Risks
Elena Elisseeva/Shutterstock	Echinacea (purple coneflower, *Echinacea purpurea*, *E. angustifolia*, *E. pallida*)	Stimulates the immune system and increases the effectiveness of white blood cells that attack bacteria and viruses. Useful in preventing and treating colds or the flu.	Many studies in Europe have provided preliminary evidence of its effectiveness, but two recent studies in the United States indicated that it is no more effective than a placebo in preventing or treating a cold.	Allergic reactions, including rashes, increased asthma, gastrointestinal problems, and anaphylaxis (a life-threatening allergic reaction). Pregnant women and those with diabetes, autoimmune disorders, or multiple sclerosis should avoid it.
Shapiso/Shutterstock	Flaxseed (*Linum usitatissimum*)	Useful as a laxative and for hot flashes and breast pain; the oil is used for arthritis; both flaxseed and flaxseed oil have been used for cholesterol level reduction and cancer prevention.	Study results are mixed on whether flaxseed decreases hot flashes or lowers cholesterol levels.	Delays absorption of medicines, but otherwise has few side effects. Should be taken with plenty of water.
Joanna Wnuk/Shutterstock	Ginkgo (*Ginkgo biloba*)	Useful for depression, impotence, premenstrual syndrome, dementia and Alzheimer's disease, diseases of the eye, and general vascular disease.	Some promising results have been seen for Alzheimer's disease and dementia, and research continues on its ability to enhance memory and reduce the incidence of cardiovascular disease.	Gastric irritation, headache, nausea, dizziness, difficulty thinking, memory loss, and allergic reactions.
Choo Poh Guan/123RF	Ginseng (*Panax ginseng*)	Affects the pituitary gland, increasing resistance to stress, affecting metabolism, aiding skin, muscle tone, and sex drive; improves concentration and muscle strength.	Studies have raised questions about appropriate dosages. Because the potency of plants varies considerably, dosage is difficult to control and side effects are fairly common.	Nervousness, insomnia, high blood pressure, headaches, chest pain, depression, and abnormal vaginal bleeding.
eAlisa/Shutterstock	Green tea (*Camellia sinensis*)	Useful for lowering cholesterol and risk of some cancers, protecting the skin from sun damage, bolstering mental alertness, and boosting heart health.	Although some studies have shown promising links between green and white tea consumption and cancer prevention, recent research questions the ability of tea to significantly reduce the risk of breast, lung, or prostate cancer.	Insomnia, liver problems, anxiety, irritability, upset stomach, nausea, diarrhea, or frequent urination.
Astrid & Hanns Frieder Michler/Science Source	Zinc (mineral)	Supports immune system, used to lessen duration and severity of cold symptoms, aids wound healing.	Research results are mixed, possibly due to the wide variety of cold viruses and differences of formulations and dosages in zinc lozenges.	Excessive intake associated with reduced immune function, reduced levels of high-density lipoproteins ("good" cholesterol).

Sources: Based on National Center for Complementary and Alternative Medicine, "Herbs at a Glance," April 2011, http://nccam.nih.gov/health/herbsataglance.htm; Office of Dietary Supplements, National Institutes of Health, "Dietary Supplement Fact Sheets," 2011, http://ods.od.nih.gov/factsheets/list-all/; American Cancer Society, "Green Tea," 2008, www.cancer.org/docroot/ETO/content/ETO_5_3x_Green_Tea.asp.

TABLE 16.2

Supplements That Should Be Avoided

Name (also known as)	Uses	Possible Dangers	Actions/Conclusions
Aconite (aconiti tuber, aconitum, *Radix aconiti*)	Inflammation, joint pain, wounds, gout	Toxicity, nausea, vomiting, low blood pressure, respiratory-system paralysis, heart-rhythm disorders, death	Unsafe. Aconite is the most common cause of severe herbal poisoning in Hong Kong.
Bitter Orange (aurantii fructus, *Citrus aurantium*, zhi shi)	Weight loss, nasal congestion, allergies	Fainting, heart-rhythm disorders, heart attack, stroke, death	Possibly unsafe. Contains synephrine, which is similar to ephedrine, banned by the FDA in 2004. Risks might be higher when taken with herbs that contain caffeine.
Chaparral (creosote bush, *Larrea divaricata*, larreastat)	Colds, weight loss, infections, inflammation, cancer, detoxification	Liver damage, kidney problems	Likely unsafe. The FDA advises people not to take chaparral.
Colloidal Silver (ionic silver, native silver, silver in suspending agent)	Fungal and other infections, Lyme disease, rosacea, psoriasis, food poisoning, chronic fatigue syndrome, HIV/AIDS	Bluish skin, mucous membrane discoloration, neurological problems, kidney damage	Likely unsafe. The FDA advised consumers about the risk of discoloration on Oct. 6, 2009.
Coltsfoot (coughwort, farfarae folium leaf, foalswort)	Cough, sore throat, laryngitis, bronchitis, asthma	Liver damage, cancer	Likely unsafe
Comfrey (blackwort, common comfrey, slippery root)	Cough, heavy menstrual periods, chest pain, cancer	Liver damage, cancer	Likely unsafe. The FDA advised manufacturers to remove comfrey products from the market in July 2001.
Country Mallow (heartleaf, *Sida cordifolia*, silky white mallow)	Nasal congestion, allergies, asthma, weight loss, bronchitis	Heart attack, heart arrhythmia, stroke, death	Likely unsafe. Possible dangers linked with its ephedrine alkaloids banned by the FDA in 2004.
Germanium (Ge, Ge-132, germanium-132)	Pain, infections, glaucoma, liver problems, arthritis, osteoporosis, heart disease, HIV/AIDS, cancer	Kidney damage, death	Likely unsafe. The FDA warned in 1993 that it was linked to serious adverse events.
Greater Celandine (celandine, chelidonii herba, *Chelidonium majus*)	Upset stomach, irritable bowel syndrome, liver disorders, detoxification, cancer	Liver damage	Possibly unsafe
Kava (awa, *Piper methysticum*, kava-kava)	Anxiety (possibly effective)	Liver damage	Possibly unsafe. The FDA issued a warning to consumers in March 2002. Banned in Germany, Canada, and Switzerland.
Lobelia (asthma weed, Lobelia inflata, pukeweed, vomit wort)	Coughing, bronchitis, asthma, smoking cessation (possibly ineffective)	Toxicity; overdose can cause fast heartbeat, very low blood pressure, coma, possibly death.	Likely unsafe. The FDA warned in 1993 that it was linked to serious adverse events.
Yohimbe (yohimbine, *Corynanthe yohimbi*, Corynanthe johimbi)	Aphrodisiac, chest pain, diabetic complications, depression; erectile dysfunction (possibly effective)	Usual doses can cause high blood pressure, rapid heart rate; high doses can cause severe low blood pressure, heart problems, death.	Possibly unsafe for use without medical supervision because it contains a prescription drug, yohimbine. The FDA warned in 1993 that reports of serious adverse events were under investigation.

TABLE 16.2

Supplements That Should Be Avoided (*continued*)

Name (also known as)	Uses	Possible Dangers	Actions/Conclusions
St. John's Wort (SJW, Klamath weed, *Hypericum perforatum*)	Depression, anxiety, and sleep disorders	Interacts with many medications and can interfere with their intended effects, including birth control pills, some heart medications, seizure control drugs, drugs used to treat cancer, and HIV drugs.	The FDA is working closely with manufacturers to ensure proper labeling of St. John's wort and the possibility for drug interactions.
Ephedra (ma huang, Chinese ephedra, Ephedra sinica)	Weight loss and athletic performance	Heart attack, stroke, heart palpitations, psychiatric problems, upper gastrointestinal effects, tremor, insomnia, and death	The FDA has banned the sale of supplements containing ephedra.
Aristolochia (aristolochic acid)	Weight loss, wound treatment	Can cause kidney damage leading to the need for kidney dialysis and kidney transplant. It also greatly increases the risk of bladder cancer and other urological tract cancers.	The FDA has issued a safety warning; banned in many countries.

Sources: Based on *Consumer Reports*, 2010, www.consumerreports.org/health/natural-health/dietary-supplements/supplement-side-effects/index .htm; National Center for Complementary and Alternative Medicine, "Ephedra," Updated July 2010, http://nccam.nih.gov/health/ephedra/; U.S. Food and Drug Administration, "Risk of Drug Interactions with St. John's Wort and Indinavir and Other Drugs," Updated 2009; National Center for Complementary and Alternative Medicine, "St. John's Wort," Updated July 2010, http://nccam.nih.gov/health/stjohnswort/ataglance.htm; U.S. Food and Drug Administration, "Letter to Health Professionals Regarding Safety Concerns Related to the Use of Botanical Products Containing Aristolochic Acid," 2009, www.fda.gov/Food/DietarySupplements/Alerts/ucm111200.htm; Emedicinehealth, "Aristolochia," 2011, www.emedicinehealth.com/ aristolochia-page2/vitamins-supplements.htm.

TYPES OF MEDICAL PRACTICES

Many health-care providers combine resources into a **group practice**, which can be single- or multi-specialty. Physicians share their offices, equipment, utility bills, and staff costs. Proponents of group practice maintain that it reduces unnecessary duplication of equipment and improves the quality of health care through peer review. **Solo practitioners** are medical providers who practise independently.

Hospitals and Clinics

Hospitals and clinics provide a range of health-care services. These include emergency treatment, diagnostic tests, and inpatient and outpatient (ambulatory) care.

There are several ways to classify hospitals: by profit status (nonprofit or for-profit), by ownership (private, public), by specialty (children's, chronic care, psychiatric, general, acute), by teaching status (teaching-affiliated or not), and by size. **Nonprofit (voluntary) hospitals**

have traditionally been administered by religious or other humanitarian groups. Before universal health care, such hospitals cared for patients whether they could pay or not. Today, some hospitals retain religious ties and orientations; others are administered by independent hospital boards. There are few **for-profit (proprietary) hospitals** in Canada, though they are increasing in number as our health-care system continues to struggle to balance needs and services in a timely manner. For-profit hospitals do not receive tax breaks and tend to focus on particular specialties.

More treatments or services, including surgery, are delivered on an **outpatient (ambulatory) care** basis (care which does not involve an overnight stay) by hospitals, traditional clinics, student health clinics, and nontraditional clinical centres. One type of ambulatory facility is the surgicentre—a

Group practice A group of physicians who combine resources, including offices, equipment, and staff, to render care to patients.

Solo practitioner Physician who renders care to patients independently of others.

Nonprofit (voluntary) hospitals Hospitals funded by the people through taxes.

For-profit (proprietary) hospitals Hospitals that provide a return on earnings to the investors; not funded by the government.

Outpatient (ambulatory) care Treatment that does not involve an overnight stay in a hospital.

place where minor, low-risk procedures such as vasec-tomies, tubal ligations, tissue biopsies, cosmetic surgery, abortions, and minor eye operations are performed.

Hospitals have made efforts to improve the quality of care and patient outcomes. Many hospitals are now designated as trauma centres. They have helicopters available to transport patients to the hospital quickly, specialty physicians in-house (not just on call) around the clock, and specialized diagnostic equipment. This combination of rapid transport and readily available specialty equipment and staff has dramatically reduced mortality rates for trauma patients. One drawback, however, is that trauma centres are exceptionally expensive to run.

PROMISES AND PROBLEMS OF CANADA'S HEALTH-CARE SYSTEM

From its initiation, Canada's health-care system has been a work in progress (Health Canada, n.d.). Over the past 50 plus years, reforms have been made and will continue to be made to our health-care system in response to changes within medicine and demands from society. Regardless, the underlying concepts of Canada's health-care system, known to Canadians as "Medicare," remain the same: universal coverage for medically necessary health-care services provided on the basis of need, rather than the ability to pay.

Even though we have one of the best health-care systems in the world, there are problems with the system. First, several levels of government are involved in delivering the services. The federal government funds health care, provided the provinces meet the established guidelines. The federal government also funds and administers health programs for special groups such as Indigenous peoples, war veterans, and federal prisoners. Using federal dollars, the provinces allot monies to health care. As governments struggle to reduce deficits and/or manage their various financial pressures, there is less money available even though health-care costs continue to rise. Reduced or limited health-care spending often results in downsizing and restructuring. These organizational divisions and increased fiscal pressures add tension between the federal and provincial governments over power, dollars, and responsibilities.

Physicians and provincial governments have also been in conflict. The provinces are responsible for medical programs and the allocation of dollars, while physicians control access to programs and institutions. Some provinces provide bonuses for physicians working in remote areas or reduce payments to physicians working in over-serviced areas. As well, other stakeholders, such as midwives, nurses, and dietitians, vie for financial resources and recognition for their contributions to the health status of Canadians.

Another source of pressure for funding is the many voluntary organizations that help Canadians, some long-established. For example, the Canadian National Institute for the Blind has been in operation since before Confederation. These organizations (for instance, Heart and Stroke Foundation, Canadian Cancer Society, and so on) also solicit funds from the general population.

Health research is also supported by federal monies. Direct-care health services (hospitals and physicians, for example) compete for dollars with research and prevention.

Access

Your access to health care is determined by numerous factors, including the supply of providers and facilities and your health status. Doctors are generally not well distributed by specialty and geographic area. Some rural areas face constant shortages of physicians and other practitioners.

Quality Assurance

The Canadian health-care system employs several mechanisms for ensuring quality services overall: education, licensure, certification or registration, accreditation, peer review, and, as a last resort, the legal system of malpractice litigation. Some of these mechanisms are mandatory before a professional organization may provide care, while others are purely voluntary. Consumers should note that licensure, although provincially mandated for some practitioners and facilities, is only a minimum guarantee of quality.

Detecting Fraud and Abuse in the System

Becoming knowledgeable and acting responsibly when selecting health-care providers and payers reduces the likelihood of financial or physical abuse. Nevertheless, with the number of options in health products and services available, even the most careful consumer can be victimized. Individual provinces maintain boards for quality assurance in the medical system. If you find yourself in a situation you cannot deal with, remember that the Health Protection Branch of Health Canada, the provincial ministries of health, and the colleges/ universities of various professions are responsible for protecting you and other health consumers. Do not hesitate to contact them if you have suspicions about a provider, service, or product.

point of view

SHOULD CANADA PRIVATIZE ITS HEALTH CARE?

You, like most students your age, do not remember a time when you had to pay for services from your family physician. Your parents also may not remember, as the Medicare system became nation-wide when the Yukon Territory was the last to join in 1972. Prior to Medicare, Canada had a health-care system similar to that in the United States—partly public, partly private, partly for-profit, and partly nonprofit. In both countries, a number of its citizens were uninsured. Costs were about the same, as were outcomes, though Canadian's life expectancy was one year longer. These things changed when Canada implemented its Medicare system for the delivery of health care. Costs escalated in the United States to double the cost in Canada, more Americans were uninsured, and the gap in life expectancy widened to 2.5 years.

As you know, not all health-care services are covered by Medicare and that is how the Canadian government manages the costs. According to the Medical Care Act, all Canadians are insured for physician and hospital services, but not for other health-care services including home care, care in long-term facilities, or prescription drugs. The costs for these and other benefits were left to the individual provinces to cover, if they were covered at all. By not covering all health-care costs, the government was able to keep the expenses in check. Examples of services not covered include imaging and surgical facilities and the specialist physicians necessary to carry out these procedures. The result was the waiting lists for some procedures. And for this reason, some Canadians think they would be better served by a user-pay system.

What Do You Think?

○ Would you be willing to pay for health-care services if in doing so your wait times were reduced?

○ Do you think in creating a user-pay system that it would be better to create a two-tiered system (that is, those who can afford to pay will pay and get their services on demand, while those who cannot afford to pay will wait and get their services later)?

○ Is our current model of health care sustainable?

○ What are your thoughts on the user-pay system in the United States?

Source: Based on Privatizing health care is not the answer: lessons from the United States, by Marcia Angell, published by Canadian Medical Association, 2008.

HEALTH SERVICE ORGANIZATIONS: A NEW MODEL OF HEALTH CARE

The dominant model of medicine in Canada is fee-for-service. A practitioner, most often a physician, performs a service and bills the provincial health plan. Planners have been searching for other models that would contain costs while providing improved services and encouraging prevention and shared responsibility. One model already in place is the health service organization (HSO). The patient registers with the organization, which is funded a set amount per patient per year (capitation) and is responsible for the patient's overall care. The originators of this model believed it would encourage practitioners and patients alike to emphasize prevention.

There are currently 87 HSOs in Ontario alone, serving more than half a million patients. Many are run by community-based boards. In Ontario, the community health branch of the provincial Ministry of Health is responsible for the HSOs, and defines the program's objectives as follows:

- to create an atmosphere that supports physicians and other health-care personnel, and that allows flexibility in responding to health-care needs

- to develop a coordinated system of health-care delivery that makes the most appropriate use of health-care resources and is accessible, efficient, and economical

- to provide special attention to health maintenance and illness prevention

- to decrease institutional health care by giving emphasis to outpatient care, self-care, and home care

HSOs may offer a more comprehensive range of services than the conventional system. For example, counselling is available through HSOs as part of the service. If you live in Ontario, your physician may be a member of an HSO, so additional services may be available at no cost to you.

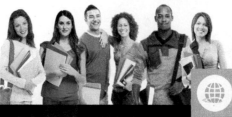

TAKING CHARGE: Managing Your Health-Care Needs

Throughout this text, we have emphasized behaviours important for keeping you healthy. Now we focus your attention on your attitudes and behaviours about when and how to seek medical attention. Most people wait until a problem arises to seek medical care and take the first available physician or medical facility. But by looking ahead to future needs, you can take charge of your choices and make positive moves toward getting more effective and efficient health care.

Are You a Good Health-Care Consumer?

Select the response that best describes your typical health behaviours. After completing this survey, total your points and assess your competence regarding health-care products and services.

1 I never act this way   **3** I act this way most of the time

2 I sometimes act this way   **4** I always act this way

1. When moving to a new location, I seek recommendations from friends and ask for referrals from physicians who treated me in the past, before I get ill.	1 2 3 4
2. I schedule an interview with health-care professionals prior to treatment to determine if I am comfortable with them.	1 2 3 4
3. I ask about costs of health-care procedures.	1 2 3 4
4. I carefully assess my symptoms and go to the doctor only when necessary.	1 2 3 4
5. I get second opinions when I am unsure of what my physician tells me.	1 2 3 4
6. I ask my physician why a test is given and what my options are before I allow that test to be performed.	1 2 3 4
7. I follow recommended guidelines for health exams, inoculations, and self-care.	1 2 3 4
8. Whenever I receive a prescription drug, I follow the directions exactly, including finishing the medication in the prescribed time period.	1 2 3 4
9. I am aware of differences in prices at various pharmacies and comparison-shop whenever possible.	1 2 3 4
10. When my peers make obviously incorrect statements about "health alternatives," I tactfully point out their errors.	1 2 3 4
11. I am aware of my body and seek medical care quickly when unusual changes occur.	1 2 3 4
12. I try to get my health information from reputable sources.	1 2 3 4
13. I carefully scrutinize health-related advertisements and news items.	1 2 3 4
14. I read the labels of health products and follow instructions carefully.	1 2 3 4

Interpreting your Score

14–19: Health consumer skills dangerously weak

20–29: Health consumer skills below average

30–44: Health consumer skills about average, not adequate for many situations

45–56: Very good health consumer skills

Beyond Interpretation

- Given your results above, where do you need the most improvement?
- What can you do to improve in these areas?

Making Decisions for You

As you have seen in this chapter, many health-care decisions are dictated by physicians and government agencies. Still, many decisions rest with you.

Checklist for Change: Making Personal Choices

Considering the following questions may help you in obtaining excellent health care from your medical practitioner.

- How long did you have to wait before getting an appointment?
- How long did you have to wait in the waiting room before being seen?
- Do the clerical staff convey their concern for you when delays occur?
- Are there educational materials available in the waiting areas?
- Are the medical practitioner's credentials clearly displayed?
- Does the medical practitioner treat you as if he or she is concerned about you?
- Do you feel comfortable discussing your problems with the medical practitioner?
- Are you confident that your medical practitioner knows what he or she is talking about?

- Is the medical practitioner willing to talk about issues such as credentials, hospital affiliations, and qualifications or referrals for special needs?
- Are you able to understand answers to your questions? Does the medical practitioner seem interested in whether you understand? Seem willing to answer questions? Encourage you to ask questions?
- Does the medical practitioner tell you why one test is being given rather than another? About risks of the test? About preparation for the tests? About what to expect concerning certain results?
- Does the medical practitioner support you in obtaining a second opinion, or does he or she seem irritated with such a request?
- If you became seriously ill and had to see a lot of this medical practitioner, would you feel comfortable with him or her, or would you rather have someone else?

Checklist for Change: Making Community Choices

The following questions may help you in determining the level of health-care service available in your community.

- What health-care services are located in your community?
- How long has your doctor been practising in your community?
- How many hospitals are within a 30-minute drive of your home? Are any of them teaching hospitals?

DISCUSSION QUESTIONS

1. Describe one dubious claim made by a health-care product (such as fat-reducing creams, hair-growth tonics, muscle-building milkshakes, and so on). Why do marketers use such claims when advertising their products? Why do consumers buy such products?

2. List some conditions (resulting from illness or accident) for which you do not need to seek medical help. If the symptoms increase in severity, at what point would you seek medical attention? How do you decide to whom and where to go for treatment?

3. What are the differences in education between allopathic and non-allopathic practitioners? Under what circumstances would you seek treatment from a non-allopathic practitioner? Which types of non-allopathic medicine appeal to you? Why? Which types of non-allopathic medicine do not appeal to you? Why not?

4. What are the benefits and risks of group practices?

5. Discuss the problems of the Canadian health-care system. If you were Minister of Health, what would you propose as a solution—provincially and/or nationally? Which groups might oppose your plan? Which groups might support it?

6. Should governments dictate costs for various medical tests and procedures in an attempt to manage the finances of the health-care system?

APPLICATION EXERCISE

Reread the "Consider This . . ." scenario at the beginning of the chapter and answer the following questions.

1. When you have a medical problem like Petra's, where do you go for medical attention? How do you know if you are getting good advice?

2. Make up a list of questions for Petra to ask each physician so that she has a better understanding of her diagnosis and the recommended treatment plan.

MASTERINGHEALTH

Go to MasteringHealth for Assignments, the eText, and the Study Area with case studies, self quizzing, and videos.

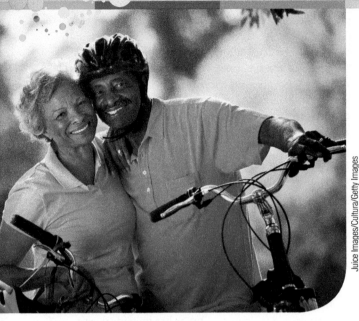

Juice Images/Cultura/Getty Images

CHAPTER 17

PREPARING FOR AGING, DYING, AND DEATH

→ CONSIDER THIS . . .

Choi, aged 82, is a springboard diver. She walks 10 blocks every morning to the city pool, where she practises her diving and swims for about an hour. Alyson, aged 79, is an internationally recognized expert in family dysfunction. She travels extensively, giving several lectures a week, volunteering her services to community groups and maintaining an active social life. Riccardo, aged 83, is a professional writer who recently purchased an iPad and loaded it with various new apps that provide him hours of entertainment. He also uses his iPad to keep in touch with his children and grandchildren.

What do all these people have in common? Are these people atypical? Why or why not? What factors do you think contributed to their healthy aging? Do you know any elderly people like them? How do these people compare to your parents or grandparents?

LEARNING OUTCOMES

- Define aging, and explain the related concepts of biological, psychological, social, legal, and functional age.

- Discuss the biological and psychosocial theories of aging along with the major physiological and psychological changes that occur as a result of the aging process.

- Define the various types of death.

- Describe the grief process, grief work, and strategies for coping more effectively.

- Identify the ethical concerns that arise from the concepts of the right to die and rational suicide.

Although growing old often involves declining physical and mental health, the rate of decline can be mitigated through healthier living choices. Health promotion, disease prevention, and wellness-oriented activities prolong vigour and productivity, even among those who may not have always led an ideal lifestyle or made healthy choices a priority. Thus, getting older can mean getting better socially, psychologically, spiritually, and intellectually.

The manner in which you view aging (either as a natural part of living or as an inevitable move toward disease and death) is an important factor in how successfully you will adapt to life's transitions. If you view these transitions as opportunities for growth—as changes that lead to improved mental, emotional, spiritual, and physical phases in your development as a human being—your journey will be smooth. You will have the chance to explore your knowledge of aging in the Assess Yourself box at the end of the chapter.

Aging has traditionally been described as the patterns of life changes that occur in members of all species as they grow older. Some believe that it begins at the moment of conception. Others contend that it starts at birth. Still others believe that true aging does not begin until we reach our 40s. Typically, your chronologic age (that is, your age based on your birthdate) is used to assign you to a particular life-cycle stage. However, people of different chronologic ages view age very differently. To the four-year-old, a university or college student seems quite old. To the 20-year-old (you perhaps?), parents in their 40s are over the hill. Have you ever heard your 65-year-old grandparents talking about "those old people down the street"—and those 'old people' may even be their age? Views of aging are also often coloured by occupation. For example, a professional linebacker may find himself too old to play football in his mid-30s. Airline pilots and police officers often retire in their 50s, while professors, senators, and prime ministers work well into their 70s.

REDEFINING AGING

Discrimination against people based on age is known as **ageism**. According to the Ontario Human Rights Commission (n.d.), ageism refers to "a socially constructed way of thinking about older persons based on negative attitudes and stereotypes about aging and a tendency to structure society based on an assumption that everyone is young, thereby failing to respond appropriately to the

real needs of older persons." When directed against the elderly, this type of discrimination carries with it social ostracism and negative portrayals of older people, in addition to services, programs, and facilities that do not adequately meet their needs. A developmental task approach to life-span changes tends to reduce the potential for ageist or negatively biased perceptions about what occurs as a person ages chronologically. The study of individual and collective aging processes, called **gerontology**, explores the reasons for aging and the ways in which people cope with and adapt to this process. Gerontologists have identified several types of age-related characteristics that should be used to determine where a person is in terms of biological, psychological, social, legal, and functional life-stage development:

- *Biological age* refers to the relative age or condition of the person's organs and body systems. Arthritis and other chronic conditions often accelerate biologic age.
- *Psychological age* refers to a person's adaptive capacities, such as coping abilities and intelligence, and to the person's awareness of his or her individual capabilities, self-efficacy, and general ability to adapt to a given situation.
- *Social age* refers to a person's habits and roles relative to society's expectations. People in a particular life stage often share similar tastes in music, television shows, and decor.
- *Legal or chronological age* is probably the most common definition of age in Canada. Legal age is based on chronological years (that is, the current date – your birthdate) and is used to determine such things as voting rights, driving privileges, drinking age, eligibility for Old Age Security and Canada Pension Plan benefits, and a host of other rights and obligations.
- *Functional age* refers to the ways in which people compare to others of a similar age. It is difficult to separate functional aging from other types of aging, particularly chronological and biological aging (Hayslip & Panek, 1992).

WHAT IS NORMAL AGING?

Contemporary gerontologists analyze the vast majority of people who continue to live full and productive lives throughout their later years. Many people in our society view the onset of the physiological changes of aging as something to be dreaded. In this regard, the aging process is seen primarily from a pathological (disease)

Aging The patterns of life changes that occur in a species as they grow older.

Ageism Discrimination based on age.

Gerontology The study of individual and collective aging processes.

perspective, and, therefore, as a time of decline. It is possible to see aging in another way, where the focus is on the gains and positive aspects of normal adult development throughout the life span. Many of these positive developments occur in the areas of emotional and social life as older adults learn to cope with and adapt to the many changes and crises that life has in store for them.

Gerontologists have devised several categories for specific age-related characteristics. For example, people who reach the age of 65 years are considered to fit the general category of "old age." They receive special consideration in the form of government assistance programs such as the Old Age Pension. Further definitions of 'old' are provided by Jeangsawang, et al. (2012):

- 60 to 69 years = **young-old**
- 70 to 79 years = **middle-old**
- 80 to 89 years = **old-old**
- 90+ years = **oldest-old**

Another perspective in objectively defining aging asks the question of how much life a person has packed into his or her chronological years. This quality-of-life index, combined with the inevitable chronological process, appears to be the best indicator of the "aging gracefully" phenomenon. The eternal question that results is, "How can I age gracefully?" Most experts agree that the best way to experience a productive, full, and satisfying old age is to take appropriate action to lead a productive, full, and satisfying life *prior* to old age. Essentially, older people are the product of their lifelong experiences, moulded over years of happiness, heartbreak, and day-to-day existence.

WHO ARE THE ELDERLY?

Contrary to popular belief, the elderly are not and never will be the "forgotten minority." The 65-and-over age group will unquestionably continue to be a major force in the social, political, and economic plans of the nation because of their sheer numbers and buying power. Canadian seniors are living longer lives in better health than in the past. In 2010, a whole generation of 1960s "flower children," who once proclaimed that no one over 30 could be trusted, became 65 years old. While people aged 65 and older made up less than 10 percent of the population in 1981, they are projected to make up more than 20 percent by 2031. In 2015 it was reported that nearly one in six Canadians (16.1 percent) were at least 65 years old (Statistics Canada, 2015).

For a more detailed profile of today's elderly, review "Canada's Aging Population," a report prepared by Health Canada in collaboration with the Interdepartmental Committee on Aging and Seniors Issues, at www.globalaging.org/elderrights/world/canada.pdf (Health Canada, 1999a).

THEORIES ON AGING

Biological Theories

Explanations about the biological causes of aging include:

- The wear-and-tear theory, which states that, like everything else in the universe, the human body wears out. Inherent in this theory is the idea that the more you do not treat your body as well as you can, the faster it will wear out.

- The cellular theory, which states that at birth we have only a certain number of usable cells, and these cells are genetically programmed to divide or reproduce only a limited number of times. Once these cells reach the end of their reproductive cycle, they begin to die and the organs they make up begin to show signs of deterioration. The rate of deterioration varies from person to person, and the impact of the deterioration depends on the system involved.

- The autoimmune theory, which attributes aging to the decline of the body's immunological system. Studies indicate that as we age, our immune systems become less effective in fighting disease. Lifestyle can contribute negatively to this process in bodies subjected to too much stress, lack of sleep, a poor dietary intake, inactivity, and so on. Although autoimmune diseases occur in all age groups, some gerontologists believe that they increase in frequency and severity with age.

- The genetic mutation theory, which proposes that the number of cells exhibiting unusual or different characteristics increases with age. In this theory, it is believed that aging relates to the amount of mutational damage within the genes. The greater the mutation, the greater the chance that cells will not function properly, leading to eventual dysfunction of body organs and systems.

Psychosocial Theories

Numerous psychological and sociological factors also have a strong influence on the manner in which people age. Psychologists have formulated theories of

Young-old People aged 60 to 69 years.

Middle-old People aged 70 to 79 years.

Old-old People aged 80 to 89 years.

Oldest-old People aged 90 years and over.

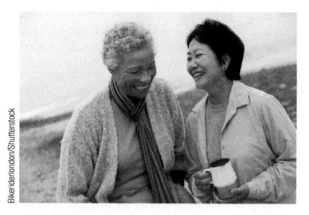
For many, the secret to aging well is to remain physically active, eat well, and enjoy the company of good friends.

that despite physical changes that occur, 76 percent of seniors 65 to 74 years old and 68 percent of seniors over 75 years of age reported their health to be "good," "very good," or "excellent" (National Advisory Council on Aging, n.d.).

Physical Changes

Although the physiological consequences of aging differ in their severity and timing from person to person, there are standard changes that occur to the skin, bones and joints, the head, the urinary tract, heart and lungs, eyesight, hearing, taste, smell and touch, mobility, sexual organs, and body comfort. Each of these is described in the following sections.

The Skin

As we age, the skin becomes thinner and loses elasticity, particularly in the outer surfaces. Fat deposits, which add to the soft lines and shape of the skin, begin to diminish with age, as does the water content of the body. Starting at about age 30, lines develop on the forehead as a result of smiling, squinting, and other facial expressions. These lines become more pronounced, with added "crow's-feet" around the eyes, during the 40s. During your 50s and 60s, you can expect your skin to sag and lose colour, leading to an overall pallor in your 70s. Body fat in underlying layers of skin continues to be redistributed away from the limbs and extremities into the trunk region of the body. Age spots become more numerous because of excessive pigment accumulation under the skin. The sun tends to increase pigment production, leading to more age spots.

personality development that encompass the human life span. These theories emphasize adaptation and adjustment. In the developmental model, it is noted that people must progress through eight critical stages during their lifetime. If a person does not receive adequate stimulation or develop effective methods of coping with life's stresses from infancy onward, problems are likely to develop later in life. According to this theory, attitudes, behaviours, and beliefs related to maladjustments in old age are often a result of problems encountered in earlier stages of a person's life. Specifically, the developmental theory focuses on the crucial issues of middle and old age because it is believed that during these periods people face a series of increasingly stressful tasks. Those who are poorly adjusted psychologically or who have not developed appropriate coping skills are likely to undergo a painful aging process.

A key element in these theories is the incorporation of age-related factors into lifelong behaviour patterns. Both models (biological and psychosocial) emphasize that successful aging involves maintaining emotional as well as physical well-being. Most probably, a combination of psychosocial and biological factors as well as environmental "trigger mechanisms" cause each of us to age in a unique manner.

CHANGES IN THE BODY AND MIND

Answers to the question of what is "typical" or "normal" when applied to aging are highly speculative. In order to assess the typical aging process, we should ask ourselves what we can reasonably expect to happen to our bodies as we grow older (Figure 17.1). Keep in mind

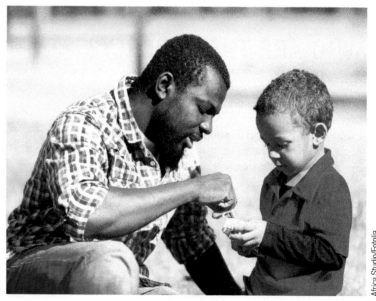
Learning to cope with challenges and make effective decisions early in life develops attitudes and skills that contribute to a full and satisfying old age.

FIGURE 17.1

Normal Effects of Aging on the Body

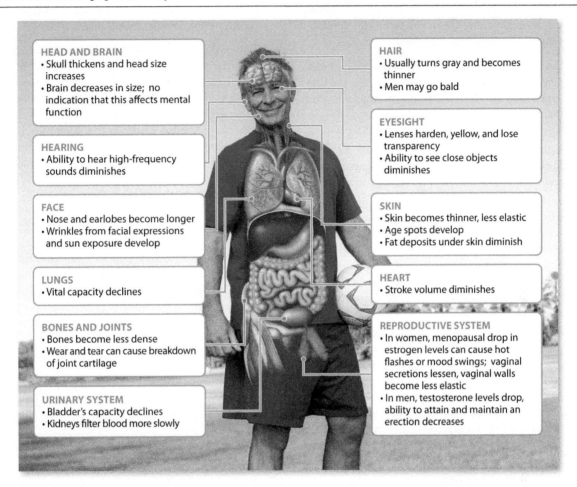

HEAD AND BRAIN
- Skull thickens and head size increases
- Brain decreases in size; no indication that this affects mental function

HEARING
- Ability to hear high-frequency sounds diminishes

FACE
- Nose and earlobes become longer
- Wrinkles from facial expressions and sun exposure develop

LUNGS
- Vital capacity declines

BONES AND JOINTS
- Bones become less dense
- Wear and tear can cause breakdown of joint cartilage

URINARY SYSTEM
- Bladder's capacity declines
- Kidneys filter blood more slowly

HAIR
- Usually turns gray and becomes thinner
- Men may go bald

EYESIGHT
- Lenses harden, yellow, and lose transparency
- Ability to see close objects diminishes

SKIN
- Skin becomes thinner, less elastic
- Age spots develop
- Fat deposits under skin diminish

HEART
- Stroke volume diminishes

REPRODUCTIVE SYSTEM
- In women, menopausal drop in estrogen levels can cause hot flashes or mood swings; vaginal secretions lessen, vaginal walls become less elastic
- In men, testosterone levels drop, ability to attain and maintain an erection decreases

Bones and Joints

Bones are the most metabolically active tissue in our bodies, in a continual state of modelling or remodelling (Malina, Bouchard, & Bar-Or, 2004). Bone mineral accrual exceeds bone mineral loss during our growing years. Then, once we are fully grown, our bone mineral accrual and loss are at about the same rate, with our bones maintaining their integrity and strength. Then, in mid-to-late adult life, generally during menopause in women, and a little later in men, bone mineral loss exceeds bone mineral accumulation, resulting in deterioration of bone tissue in which bones become fragile and brittle and at an increased risk of fracture. This loss of bone mineral content occurs in men and women, although it tends to occur at a faster rate in women, especially after menopause. Loss of bone mineral content contributes to **osteoporosis**, a condition characterized by low bone mass and deterioration of bone tissue (Osteoporosis Canada, 2012).

Although many people consider osteoporosis a disease of the elderly, it is actually a progressive disorder with roots firmly established in childhood and adolescence (Malina, Bouchard, & Bar-Or, 2004). In fact, osteoporosis prevention begins in childhood by developing the strongest bones possible with the greatest reservoir of bone mineral content to draw upon when needed. When you hear of osteoporosis, you likely envision a slumped-over individual with a characteristic "dowager's hump" in the upper back, but this is the rare extreme. Bone loss occurs over many years and without symptoms until fractures occur. The spine, hips, shoulders, and wrists are the most common sites of fractures, though other bones of the body can be involved (Osteoporosis Canada, 2012).

Osteoporotic fractures of the hip, vertebrae, proximal humerus, pelvis, and wrist increase in incidence with age and are more common among women. It is estimated that one in four women aged 60 years and over will have an osteoporotic fracture (National Advisory Council on

Osteoporosis A degenerative bone disease characterized by loss of bone mineral content and density, resulting in an increased fracture risk.

Aging, n.d.). Further, about one-third of all women aged 65 and over will experience vertebral osteoporosis. About 70 percent of all fractures among individuals over the age of 45 result from osteoporosis. Although there is no single cause, several risk factors for developing osteoporosis have been identified:

- Sex: Women's risk is four times greater than men's. Their peak bone mass is lower than men's, and they experience an accelerated rate of bone loss after menopause.

- Age: After the third and fourth decade of life, most individuals begin to lose bone mass and are more susceptible—particularly if sedentary. Generally, men and women over the age of 50 are at greater risk.

- Low bone mass: Low bone mass is one of the strongest predictors of osteoporosis. Measurement of bone density is an important aspect of risk assessment. Low bone mass is often a result of inadequate bone-growth stimulation (inactivity), poor dietary intake (lack of total calories and insufficient calcium intake), estrogen suppression (delayed onset of menarche, amenorrhea), and smoking.

- Early menopause: The early occurrence of menopause, whether natural or caused by surgery, means that the positive effects of estrogen occur for a shorter period of time. (Decreases in sex hormones—estrogen in females and testosterone in males—increase risk for osteoporosis.) Menstrual disturbances, such as those caused by anorexia nervosa, bulimia nervosa, or excessive exercise without an adequate dietary intake, can similarly result in an early loss of bone minerals.

- Thin, small-framed body: Petite, thin women usually have a relatively low bone mass and are therefore at greater risk for osteoporosis. Also, a risk factor is weight loss greater than 10 percent of total body weight since the age of 25 years.

- Ethnicity: Caucasians and Asians are at higher risk of developing osteoporosis than individuals of African descent. Individuals of African descent have greater bone density, on average, than individuals of Caucasian or Asian descent. And women of African descent have about half the incidence of hip fractures of women of Caucasian descent.

- Lack of calcium and vitamin D: A lifetime of low calcium and vitamin D intake can result in a lower than expected peak bone mineral content and above-average loss of bone mineral content throughout adulthood.

- Lack of physical activity: Immobilized, bedridden, and inactive people have less muscle and bone mass.

- Cigarette smoking: Since cigarette smoking suppresses estrogen, bone mineral accrual is negatively affected.

- Alcohol intake of three or more drinks per day.

- Heredity: Hereditary factors may play a role in the development of osteoporosis; these factors relate to body size as well as the body's efficiency at using calcium and other minerals to build bone (Health Canada, 2008; Osteoporosis Canada, 2012).

The goal of treatment and prevention of osteoporosis is to decrease the likelihood and severity of bone fractures. Treatment of established osteoporosis includes enhancing calcium and vitamin D intake, engaging in regular weight-bearing and strength enhancing physical activities, fall-prevention measures, and, potentially, hormonal supplementation (in individuals not at high risk for certain forms of cancer) (International Osteoporosis Foundation, 2013). Increasing calcium intake to 1380 mg per day—an amount that exceeds the current DRI for calcium—may be effective at reducing bone loss and increasing bone mineralization in women aged 58 to 77 (National Research Council, 1989). Other therapies for osteoporosis, such as sodium fluoride, various metabolites of vitamin D, and bisphosphonates, are also recommended (International Osteoporosis Foundation, 2013).

The most effective method of preventing osteoporosis is to develop strong, dense bones during growth. Critical to developing strong bones is sufficient calcium intake during childhood and young adulthood as well as weight-bearing or weight resistance (that is, bone-growth-stimulating) physical activity (Malina, Bouchard, & Bar-Or, 2004). For adolescent males and females (ages 15 to 18 years), an adequate intake of calcium is 1200 to 1500 mg per day (American Academy of Pediatrics: Committee on Nutrition, 1999). Children and adolescents should also do at least 60 minutes of moderate or more intense physical activities almost every day (Canadian Society for Exercise Physiology, 2013). Once strong bones are developed, the next critical step is to maintain them and delay the onset of bone mineral loss. Regular physical activity of weight-bearing joints, maintenance of muscular strength and flexibility, and an adequate intake of calcium are probably your best routes of osteoporosis prevention during early, middle, and late adulthood.

Another bone condition that affects a large number of people is osteoarthritis, a disease of the joints and surrounding tissue (Osteoporosis Canada, 2012). This common condition most often affects middle-aged to elderly people. Factors that cause osteoarthritis include genetics, gender, previous injuries, and so on. Osteoarthritis also becomes more common with age and is another leading cause of disability.

The Head

With age, features of the head enlarge and become more noticeable. Increased cartilage and fatty tissue cause the nose to grow 1.25 cm wider and another 1.25 cm longer. Earlobes get thicker and grow longer, while overall head circumference increases 0.6 cm per decade, even though the brain itself shrinks.

The Urinary Tract

One problem often associated with aging is **urinary incontinence**, which ranges from passing a few drops of urine while laughing or sneezing to having little or no control when and where urination takes place. As such, urinary incontinence is classified in three categories: stress, urge, and mixed, with 10 percent of Canadians experiencing one of these levels (Bettez et al., 2012). Stress incontinence, which represents 50 percent of all cases, is defined as leakage that occurs with exertion, sneezing, or coughing. Urgency incontinence is defined by leakage that is immediately preceded by a sudden desire to void and represents about 14 percent of the cases. The mixture of the two symptions is called mixed urinary incontinence and includes about one-third of all cases (Bettez et al., 2012). Incontinence has the potential to create social, physical, and emotional problems for the elderly. Embarrassment and fear of wetting oneself can cause an older person to become isolated and avoid social functions. Caregivers might become frustrated. Prolonged wetness and the inability to properly care for oneself can lead to irritation, infections, and other problems. However, incontinence is not an inevitable part of the aging process. Most cases are caused by highly treatable underlying neurological problems that affect the central nervous system, medications, infections of the pelvic muscles, weakness in the pelvic walls, or other problems. Many causes are easily treatable (Mayo Clinic, 2011). For the men and women who cannot be successfully treated, there are well-designed, discreet options available for urinary incontinence to allow for full participation in social functions and all other aspects of life.

The Heart and Lungs

Assuming physical fitness levels do not fluctuate dramatically, resting heart rate remains about the same during an adult's life. Stroke volume (the amount of blood the muscle pumps per beat), however, diminishes as the aging heart muscles deteriorate. Vital capacity, or the amount of air that moves when you inhale and exhale at maximum effort, also declines with age. As a result, overall cardiorespiratory capacity decreases with age, at a rate of about 10 percent per decade after the age of 30 (see also Chapter 4). Regular aerobic physical activity is effective at reducing and slowing the age-related deterioration expected in heart and lung function.

Eyesight

By the age of 30, the lens of the eye begins to harden, causing specific problems by the early 40s. The lens begins to yellow and loses transparency, while the pupil of the eye begins to shrink, allowing less light to penetrate. Activities such as reading become more difficult, particularly in dim light. By age 60, depth perception declines and farsightedness often develops. A need for glasses usually develops in the 40s that evolves into a need for bifocals in the 50s and trifocals in the 60s. **Cataracts** (clouding of the lens) and **glaucoma** (elevation of pressure within the eyeball) become more likely. Both conditions can be treated. There may eventually be a tendency toward colour-blindness, especially for shades of blue and green. **Macular degeneration** is the breakdown of the light-sensitive part of the retina responsible for the sharp, direct vision needed to read or drive. Its effects can be devastating to independent older adults.

Hearing

Our ability to hear high-frequency consonants (for example, *s*, *t*, and *z*) diminishes with age. Much of the actual hearing loss experienced as we age relates to our inability to distinguish extreme ranges of sound from normal conversational tones—which can make it harder for older individuals to hear what someone is saying if the surrounding environment is noisy, compared to younger people in the same situation.

Taste

Our sense of taste declines as we age. At age 30, each tiny elevation on the tongue (called papilla) has 245 taste buds. By the age of 70, there are only 88 left. The mouth gets drier as salivary glands secrete less fluid. The ability to distinguish sweet, sour, bitter, and salty diminishes. Thus, many older people compensate for their diminished sense of taste by adding salt, sugar, and other flavour enhancers to their food. Caution is warranted regarding the addition of salt and sugar, with preference given to spices and herbs that do not relate to increased health risk.

Smell and Touch

Our sense of smell also diminishes with age. As a result of this loss and a reduced capacity in taste, food is often less appealing when we get older. This lack of appeal may be one factor that contributes to the tendency for the older population to be malnourished. Pain receptors also become less effective with age and our tactile senses decline.

Urinary incontinence The inability to control urination.

Cataracts Clouding of the lens that interrupts the focusing of light on the retina, results in blurred vision or eventual blindness.

Glaucoma Elevation of pressure within the eyeball, leading to hardening of the eyeball, impaired vision, and possible blindness.

Macular degeneration Disease that breaks down the macula, the light-sensitive part of the retina responsible for sharp, direct vision.

Mobility

Nearly half of older Canadians report some disability, usually related to mobility and agility; one-third require help with housework and shopping. The incidence and severity of disability typically increases with age.

Sexual Changes

As people age, they experience noticeable changes in sexual function. The degree and rate of change varies from person to person. As men age, the following changes generally occur:

- The ability to get and maintain an erection diminishes.
- The length of the refractory period between orgasms increases.
- The orgasm itself becomes shorter.

Women experience the following changes with age:

- Menopause usually occurs between the ages of 45 and 55. At this time, women may experience hot flashes, mood swings, weight gain, development of facial hair, and other hormone-related problems.
- The walls of the vagina become less elastic, and the epithelium thins, making sexual activity less comfortable.
- Vaginal secretions diminish, particularly during sexual activity (though this problem can be reduced with the use of a lubricant).
- The breasts decrease in firmness. Loss of fat in various areas leads to fewer curves, and a decrease in the soft lines of the body.

While these physiological changes may sound discouraging, the fact is that many older people can and do enjoy satisfying sexual activity throughout their lives (Philadelphia Corporation for Aging, 2013). Indeed, one study refuted long-held beliefs that sexual desire decreases with age with results indicating that nearly half the population over 60 years of age engaged in sexual activity at least once a month, and 40 percent would like to have sex more frequently (National Council on Aging, n.d.).

Body Comfort

Because of the loss of body fat, thinning of the epithelium, and diminished glandular activity, elderly people generally have greater difficulty regulating body temperature. This change means that their ability to withstand extreme cold or heat may be limited, resulting in an increased risk of hypothermia, heat stroke, and heat exhaustion.

Many of these changes related to body comfort are exacerbated by poor nutrition. For a variety of reasons, obtaining adequate nutrition is a problem for many adults later in life (Ramage-Morin & Garriguet, 2013). Diminished appetite and impaired senses (as previously mentioned), reduced mobility, and various social and economic factors, as well as issues related to the digestion and absorption of nutrients contribute to the nutrient risk of the older Canadian population (Ramage-Morin & Garriguet, 2013). Women tend to be at greater risk than men (38 versus 29 percent), particularly older women (over 75 years = 41 percent) (Ramage-Morin & Garriguet, 2013). The limited data on frailer seniors suggest that their dietary intake is much worse. The Public Health Agency of Canada (2010) estimates that as many as 60 percent of older adults living in nursing homes or hospital environments may be malnourished. Poor nutrition elevates the impact of chronic disease, reduces resistance to infections, slows healing, and increases use of the health-care system. Identifying older adults at risk for malnutrition is important to enable them to maintain an optimal quality of life and age successfully.

Mental Changes

Intelligence

Stereotypes concerning inevitable intellectual decline among the elderly have been largely refuted. Research demonstrated that much of our previous knowledge about elderly intelligence was based on inappropriate testing procedures. Given an appropriate length of time, elderly people can learn and develop skills in a similar manner to younger people. Researchers have also determined that what many elderly people lack in speed of learning, they make up for in practical knowledge—that is, the "wisdom of experience."

Memory

Have you ever wondered why your grandfather seems unable to remember what he did last weekend even though he can graphically depict the details of a social event that occurred 40 years ago? This phenomenon is not unusual among the elderly. Research indicates that although short-term memory may fluctuate on a daily basis, the ability to remember events from past decades remains largely unchanged.

Adaptability

Although it is widely believed that people become more like one another as they age, nothing could be further from the truth. Having lived through a multitude of experiences and faced diverse joys, sorrows, and obstacles, the typical older person has developed unique methods of coping. These unique adaptive variations make for interesting differences in how the elderly confront the many changes brought on by the aging process. Thus, as a group, older Canadians are heterogeneous.

Depression

Most adults continue to lead healthy, fulfilling lives as they grow older. Some research indicates, however, that depression may be the most common psychological problem as we age. Although fewer older Canadians (65+) report very good or excellent mental health compared to younger Canadians, the rate of depression is higher in those aged 25 to 44 years (approximately 10 percent) than those older than 65 (5 percent) (Statistics Canada, 2013). The rate of suicide is also higher among middle-aged individuals (40–59 years of age) compared to seniors (65 years and older).

Dementia

Over the years, older people have often been the victims of ageist attitudes. People chronologically old were often labelled "senile" whenever they displayed memory failure, errors in judgment, disorientation, or erratic behaviours. (The term *senile* is seldom used today except to describe a very small group of organic disorders.) Today, it is recognized that these same symptoms can occur at any age and for various reasons, including disease or as a side effect from the use of OTC or prescription drugs. When the underlying problems are corrected, memory loss and disorientation also improve.

Alzheimer's Disease

Dementia refers to progressive brain impairments that interfere with memory and normal intellectual functioning. Although there are many types of **dementia**, one of the most common forms is **Alzheimer's disease**. Alzheimer's affects an estimated one in twenty people between the ages of 65 and 75 and one in five people over the age of 80. The total number of people with cognitive impairment, including Alzheimer's disease, is expected to increase from 747 000 where it stands currently to 1.4 million in 2031 (Alzheimer Society of Canada, 2012). This possibility presents a real economic burden for the future. While the disease is associated in most people's minds strictly with the elderly, it has been diagnosed in people as young as their late 40s. In fact, about 5 percent of all cases occur before age 65.

Alzheimer's refers to a degenerative disease of the brain in which nerve cells stop communicating with one another. Ordinarily, brain cells communicate by releasing chemicals that allow the cells to receive and transmit messages for various behaviours. In Alzheimer's patients, the brain does not produce enough of these chemicals, cells cannot communicate, and eventually the cells die.

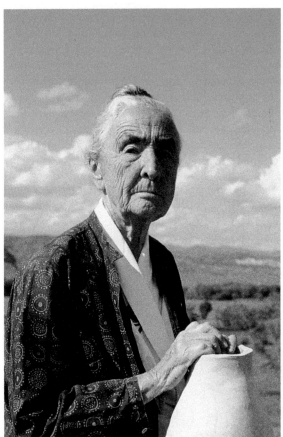

Georgia O'Keeffe retained her intellectual and artistic abilities into old age.

Joe Munroe/Science Source

This degeneration happens in the sections of the brain that affect memory, speech, and personality, leaving the parts that control other bodily functions, such as heartbeat and breathing, working fine. Thus, the mind's ability to function decreases while the body continues to work more or less as it should. Alzheimer's happens slowly and progressively, and it may be as long as 20 years before symptoms are noticed. It is generally detected first by family members, who note memory lapses and personality changes. Medical tests rule out other underlying causes and neurological tests confirm the diagnosis.

What are the symptoms of Alzheimer's? Alzheimer's disease is characteristically diagnosed in three stages. During the first stage, symptoms include:

* forgetfulness
* memory loss
* impaired judgment
* increasing inability to handle routine tasks
* disorientation
* lack of interest in one's surroundings
* depression.

Dementia Refers to mental deterioration, loss of memory, and judgment and orientation problems.

Alzheimer's disease A chronic condition involving changes in nerve fibres of the brain; results in mental deterioration.

These symptoms accelerate in the second stage, which also includes agitation and restlessness (especially at night), loss of sensory perceptions, muscle twitching, and repetitive actions. Many patients become depressed at this stage and there is a tendency to be combative and aggressive. In the final stage, disorientation is often complete. The person becomes completely dependent on others for eating, dressing, and other activities. Identity loss and speech problems are common symptoms. Eventually, control of bodily functions may be lost.

Once Alzheimer's disease strikes, the remaining life expectancy is cut in half. Treatment includes several prescription drugs. Some physicians prescribe vitamin E because it may help protect brain cells from free radical damage. Researchers are also examining anti-inflammatory drugs, theorizing that Alzheimer's may develop in response to an inflammatory ailment. Others are focusing on stimulating the brains of those prone to Alzheimer's, believing that as people learn, more connections between brain cells are formed that might offset those that are lost.

HEALTH CHALLENGES OF OLDER CANADIANS

The elderly are disproportionately victimized by a number of societally induced problems. Other problems come from a perceived loss of control in older people over the circumstances of their lives—when they watch loved ones die, are forced to retire, face problems with personal health, and confront an uncertain economy on a fixed income. Developing adequate coping and decision-making skills in your earlier years, as well as strong social supports, may significantly reduce your risk for problems in old age.

Alcohol Use and Abuse

A person prone to alcoholism during his or her younger and middle years is more likely to continue drinking during his or her later years. The older individual addicted to alcohol is no more common than the younger person, despite the stereotype of the old, lost soul hiding his or her sorrows in a bottle. Alcohol abuse is five times more likely in older men than in older women. Almost half of all older men and even more older women do not drink at all. Those who do drink may do so more frequently, but generally consume less than younger persons (see Chapter 10).

Sarcopenia Age-related declines in the quality and quantity of muscle tissue.

Prescription Drug Use: Unique Problems for Older Canadians

It is extremely rare for older people to use illicit drugs, but some do overuse, misuse, and grow dependent upon—even addicted to—prescription and OTC drugs. Beset with numerous aches, pains, and inexplicable as well as diagnosable maladies, some older Canadians take between four and six prescription drugs a day in addition to vitamin and/or mineral supplements and regular use of OTCs such as Aspirin. Anyone who combines drugs runs the risk of dangerous and/or uncomfortable drug interactions. The risks of adverse effects are greater for people with circulation impairments and declining kidney and liver functions. Older people displaying symptoms of these drug-induced effects, including bizarre behaviour patterns or an appearance of being out of touch, are often misdiagnosed as experiencing dementia.

Over-the-Counter Remedies

Although older Canadians today appear to be more receptive to medical treatment than previous generations, a substantial segment of the over-60 population avoids orthodox medical treatment, viewing it as only a last resort. Still, as might be expected, ASA and laxatives head the list of commonly used OTC medications for relief of arthritic pain and the irregular bowel activity sometimes experienced by older Canadians.

Physical Activity

An inevitable physical change the body undergoes as it ages is **sarcopenia**, age-related declines in muscle mass. The less muscle you have, the less energy you require, even when physically active. The lower your metabolic rate, the more likely you will gain weight—particularly when your caloric intake remains the same. Regular moderate-intensity physical activity that gets your heart beating faster will help to reduce the expected age-related declines in quality and quantity of muscle (see also Chapter 4). Further, regular resistance training will increase (or maintain) muscle mass, boost metabolism, strengthen your bones, prevent osteoporosis, and in general help older Canadians to feel better and function more effectively and efficiently.

The Canadian Society for Exercise Physiology (2013) recommends that older adults choose a variety of endurance, flexibility, and strength and balance activities such that they accumulate 150 minutes of moderate-intensity physical activity each week. It is further noted that these activities can be accumulated in 10-minute blocks of time.

Dietary Concerns

As with many bodily processes, the digestion of food slows with age. Nevertheless, the body still requires nutrients consumed in moderate quantities and in the right combination. Certain nutrients are especially important to healthy aging:

- Calcium: Many elderly people do not consume adequate calcium, or they may take it as an individual supplement without vitamin D, which is necessary for calcium absorption in the body. Adequate calcium intake should be part of a lifelong regimen of preventive health care to reduce loss of bone mineral content. For individuals over the age of 50, a calcium intake of 1200 mg per day is recommended (Thompson, Manore, & Sheeska, 2007).

- Vitamin D: As noted previously, vitamin D is essential to enable adequate calcium absorption. As people age, particularly in and beyond their 50s and 60s, they do not absorb vitamin D as readily from foods. More recently, vitamin D has been identified as protection from a number of chronic diseases.

Further, it is clear, particularly during the winter months in Canada, that most Canadians cannot obtain sufficient vitamin D from the sun. Supplementation may therefore be warranted.

- Protein: As their budgets shrink, some older adults often cut back on protein. Meat costs more, takes longer to cook, and has a "fat" stigma associated with it. Many older people cut back on protein to a point below the DRIs. Because protein is necessary to maintain muscle mass, deficiencies in this nutrient can lead to health issues.

Gender Issues: Caring for Older Canadians

Older women continue to fill a disproportionate place in Canadian society. In 2012 (the latest population data available), for example, 55.2 percent of Canadians over the age of 65 years were women (Statistics Canada, 2012). This difference in the number of older women increases with age; women made up 56.0 percent of people aged 75 to 84 years, 67 percent of those aged 85 to 100 years, and 80 percent of Canadian centenarians. This is also a relatively new phenomenon—as recently as 1950, there were more older men than women (Health Canada, 1999b). Because women live longer than men on average, older women are more likely than older men to be living alone, and thus to lack the support in the home that helps keep them independent.

Although a considerable percentage of men and women over the age of 65 years reported formal or informal home care in 2009 (the latest data available), women tend to be greater users (30 versus 18 percent) (Hoover & Retermann, 2012). Not unexpectedly, the use of home care services increases with the age of the population such that 44 percent of men and 59 percent of women over the age of 85 years use it (Hoover & Retermann, 2012).

The rate of institutionalization is twice as high among older people without a spouse as for married older people; one reason is that a married person has a built-in potential caretaker. Further, women are more likely than men to experience poverty and multiple chronic health problems, a situation referred to as **comorbidity**. Consequently, more older women than men are likely to need assistance from children, other relatives, friends, and neighbours.

UNDERSTANDING DEATH AND DYING

Death eventually comes to everyone. Although this can be a depressing thought, we must accept the inevitable. The acceptance of death shapes our attitudes about the importance of life. Throughout history, humans have attempted to determine the nature and meaning of death. This questioning continues today. Although we will briefly discuss moral, spiritual, and philosophical questions about death, we will not explore such issues in depth in this chapter or in this textbook. Rather, our primary focus is to present dying and death as a normal part of life and to discuss how we can cope effectively with it.

Confrontations with death elicit different feelings depending on many factors, including age, religious beliefs, family orientation, health, personal experience, and the circumstances of the death itself. To cope effectively with dying and death, we must address the individual needs of those involved. Further, we need to consider why it is that we wish to deny, or even postpone, death.

Comorbidity The presence of more than one disease at the same time.

Dying The process of decline in body functions resulting in the death of an organism.

Death The "final cessation of the vital functions" and the state in which these functions are "incapable of being restored."

Defining Death

Dying is the process of decline in body functions resulting in the death of an organism. **Death** can be defined as the "final cessation of the vital functions" and refers to a state in which these functions are "incapable of being restored" (Oxford English Dictionary, 1969, pp. 72, 334, 735). This definition has become more significant as medical and scientific advances have made it increasingly possible to postpone death. Although irreversible cessation of circulatory and respiratory functions acceptably defines death, irreversible cessation of brain function is also equivalent to death even though the heart continues to beat if the individual is on a respirator.

In 1968, following the publication of the Harvard criteria for the diagnosis of brain death, the Canadian Medical Association (CMA) provided guidelines, revised in 1974 and 1975. In 1976, guidelines were established in the United Kingdom, and in 1981, revised guidelines were published in the *Journal of the American Medical Association*. In all of these guidelines, brain death must be determined clinically by an experienced physician in accordance with accepted medical standards (Canadian Medical Association, 1987). The following definitions facilitate classification of various phases of biological death:

- Cell death: The gradual death of a cell after all metabolic activity has ceased. The rate of cellular death varies according to the tissue involved. For example, higher-functioning brain cells die five to eight minutes after respiration ceases; striated muscle cells die two to four hours later; kidney cells die after about seven hours; and epithelial cells (hair and nails) die several days later. Rigor mortis, the temporary stiffening of muscles, is associated with cell death.

- Local death: The death of a body part or portion of an organ without the death of the entire organism. For example, a kidney may fail, part of the heart muscle may die, or a limb or section of intestine may die as a result of loss of circulation—each of these occurs without the death of the overall body.

- Somatic death: The death of the entire organism, as opposed to death of a part of an organ or an extremity.

- Apparent death: The cessation of vital physiological functions, particularly spontaneous cardiac and respiratory activities, which produces a state simulating actual death but from which recovery is possible through resuscitative efforts.

- Functional death: Extensive and irreversible damage to the central nervous system, with respiration and circulatory function maintained by artificial means.

- Brain death: The cessation of brain function, as evidenced by loss of all reflexes and electrical activity of the brain or by irreversible coma. Brain death is confirmed by an **electroencephalogram** reading of electrical activity of brain cells.

The Canadian Medical Association (1987) established the following criteria for the clinical diagnosis of brain death:

1. An etiology has been established capable of causing brain death, and potentially reversible conditions have been excluded (drug intoxication, treatable metabolic disorders, core temperature less than 32.2°C, shock, and peripheral nerve or muscle dysfunction due to disease or neuromuscular-blocking drugs).

2. The patient is in deep coma and shows no response within the cranial nerve distribution to stimulation of any part of the body. In particular, there should be no motor response within the cranial nerve distribution to stimuli applied to any body regions. There should be no spontaneous or elicited movements arising from the brain. However, various spinal reflexes may persist in brain death.

3. Brain-stem reflexes are absent. Pupillary light and corneal, vestibulo-ocular, and pharyngeal reflexes must be absent. The pupils should be midsize or larger and must be unresponsive to light. Care should be taken that atropine or related drugs that could block the pupillary response to light have not been given to the patient.

4. The patient does not breathe when taken off the respirator for an appropriate time.

5. The conditions listed above persist when the patient is reassessed after a suitable interval to ensure that the nonfunctioning state of the brain is persistent and to reduce the possibility of observer error.*

The CMA also suggests that a physician consult with another experienced physician before determining death.

Denying Death

We can look at our attitudes toward death as falling on a continuum. At one end of the continuum, death is viewed as the enemy of humankind. Medical science promotes this idea of death. At the other end of the continuum, death is accepted and welcomed (Aiken, 1994). For people whose attitudes fall at this end, often those with a deep religious faith or spiritual belief, death is a passage to a better state of being. Most of us perceive ourselves somewhere in the middle of this

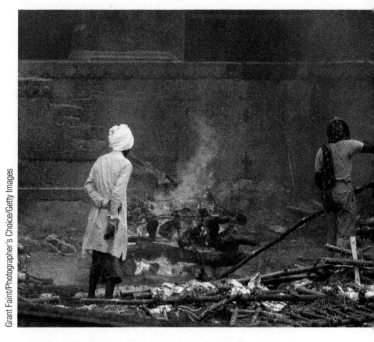

In some cultures, death is not feared but viewed as a passage to a better state of being that is to be celebrated.

continuum. From this perspective, death is a bewildering mystery that elicits fear and apprehension, as well as profoundly influencing our attitudes, beliefs, and actions throughout our lives.

In most Canadians, a high level of discomfort is associated with dying and death. As a result, we often avoid speaking about it. You may be denying death if you:

- avoid people who are grieving after the death of a loved one because you do not know what to say and therefore do not want to talk about it

- fail to validate a dying person's situation by talking to the person as if nothing is wrong

- substitute euphemisms for the word *death* (a few examples are "passed away," "kicked the bucket," "no longer with us," "gone to heaven," or "gone to a better place")

- give false reassurances to dying people by saying things like "everything is going to be okay" or "you are not going to die"

- shut off conversation about death by silencing people trying to talk about it

- avoid touching or talking to a dying person

Although some experts indicate that the denial of death has always been a predominant characteristic of our society, you must keep in mind that societal norms contribute

electroencephalogram (EEG) is a test that measures and records the electrical activity of the brain through electrodes or sensors attached to the head.

*Based on "Guidelines for the Diagnosis of Brain Death, Vol. 136." Published by Canadian Medical Association, 1987.

to this denial. The miraculous feats of science and medicine during the first half of the century created an attitude closer to death-defying than to death-denying. However, the pendulum appears to be swinging back. Today, a growing number of people are rejecting "high-tech" death—death postponed through the use of life-support technology—in favour of more personal, and perhaps more humane, alternatives. The concept of death as an enemy may be giving way to acceptance of dying as a natural part of life.

THE PROCESS OF DYING

Dying is a complex process that includes physical, intellectual, mental, social, spiritual, and emotional dimensions. Accordingly, we must consider the process of dying from several perspectives. The preceding section primarily examined the physical indicators of death. It is also essential to consider the emotional aspects of dying and "social death" in establishing an appreciation for the multifaceted nature of life and death.

Coping Emotionally with Death

Science and medicine enable us to understand changes associated with growth, development, aging, and social roles throughout the life span, but they have not revealed the nature of death. This may partially explain why the transition from life to death evokes mystery and emotion. Although emotional reactions to dying vary, there seem to be many similarities in this process.

Much of our knowledge about reactions to dying stems from the work of Elisabeth Kübler-Ross, a major figure in modern **thanatology**, the study of death and dying. In 1969, Kübler-Ross published *On Death and Dying,* a sensitive analysis of the reactions of terminally ill patients. This pioneering work encouraged the development of death education as a discipline and prompted efforts to improve the care of patients who were dying. In her book, Kübler-Ross (1969) identified five psychological stages that terminally ill patients often experience as they approach death: denial, anger, bargaining, depression, and acceptance. Health professions immediately embraced this "stage theory" and hastily applied it in clinical settings (Kübler-Ross, 1969). However, research evidence supporting or refuting the concept of stages of grief is neither extensive nor convincing. Although it is normal to grieve when a severe loss has been sustained, some people never go through this process and instead remain emotionally calm. Others pass back and forth between the stages.

Thanatology The study of death and dying.

A summation of Kübler-Ross's (1969) five stages follows:

- Denial: ("Not me, there must be a mistake.") This is usually the first stage, experienced as a sensation of shock and disbelief. A person intellectually accepts his or her impending death but rejects it emotionally. The individual is too confused and stunned to comprehend "not being" and thus rejects the idea. When this anxiety level diminishes, the individual is able to sort through the powerful web of emotions surrounding his or her impending death.

- Anger: ("Why me?") Anger is another common reaction to the realization of imminent death. The person becomes angry at the prospect of dying when others, including loved ones, are healthy and not threatened. The person dying perceives the situation as "unfair" or "senseless" and may be hostile to friends, family, physicians, and/or the world in general.

- Bargaining: ("If I am allowed to live, I promise . . .") This stage generally occurs at about the middle of the progression toward acceptance of death. During this stage, the dying person may resolve to be a better person in return for an extension of life or may secretly pray for a short reprieve from death in order to experience a special event, such as a family wedding or birth.

- Depression: ("It is really going to happen to me and I cannot do anything about it.") Depression eventually sets in as vitality diminishes and the person begins to experience distressing symptoms with increasing frequency. The individual's deteriorating condition becomes impossible for him or her to deny, and feelings of doom and tremendous loss may become unbearably pervasive. Feelings of worthlessness and guilt are also common in this depressed state because the person dying may feel responsible for the emotional suffering of loved ones and the arduous but seemingly futile efforts of caregivers.

- Acceptance: ("I am ready.") This is often the final stage. The individual stops battling with emotions and becomes tired and weak. The need to sleep increases, and wakeful periods become shorter and less frequent. With acceptance, the person does not "give up" and become sullen or resentfully resigned to death, but rather becomes passive. According to one dying person, the acceptance stage is "almost void of feelings . . . as if the pain had gone, the struggle is over, and there comes a time for the final rest before the long journey." As he or she lets go, the dying person may no longer welcome visitors and may not wish to engage in conversation. Death usually occurs quietly and painlessly while the individual is unconscious.

Subsequent research indicated that each individual has a distinct mix and process of grieving. A person may move from denial to depression, to anger, to denial again, and so on. Even if it is not accurate in all its particulars, Kübler-Ross's (1969) theory offers valuable insights for those seeking to understand or cope with the process of dying.

Social Death

The need for recognition and appreciation within a social group is nearly universal. Although the size and nature of the social group may vary widely, the need to belong exists in all of us. Loss of value or of appreciation by others can lead to **social death**, an often irreversible situation in which a person is not treated like an active member of society. Dramatic examples of social death include the exile of nonconformists from their native countries or the excommunication of dissident members of religious orders. More often, however, social death is inflicted by avoidance of social interaction. Numerous studies indicate that people are treated differently when they are dying. The isolation that accompanies social death in terminally ill patients may be exacerbated by the following (Kastenbaum, 1995):

- The dying person is referred to as if he or she were already dead.
- The dying person may be inadvertently excluded from conversations.
- Dying patients are often moved to terminal wards and given minimal care.
- Bereaved family members are avoided, often for extended periods, because friends and neighbours are afraid of feeling uncomfortable in the presence of grief.
- Medical personnel may make degrading comments about patients in their presence.

A decrease in meaningful social interaction often strips dying and bereaved people of recognition as valued members of society at a time when belonging is critical. Some dying people choose not to speak of their inevitable fate in an attempt to make others feel more comfortable and thus preserve vital relationships.

Near-Death Experiences

We cannot speak of the process of dying without mentioning near-death experiences. Thousands of similar reports have been given by people who almost died or were actually pronounced dead and subsequently recovered. The descriptions of feelings, perceptions, and visions associated with being near death have many common features. Three phases have been identified: resistance, life review, and transcendence. During the initial phase, resistance, the dying person is aware of extreme danger and struggles desperately to escape from the unseen threat. Many people report a sensation of expanding fear. The second phase, life review, has been described as a feeling of being outside one's body and beyond danger. During this period, the dying person feels a sensation of security while observing his or her physical body from an emotionally detached perspective. The dying person's life experiences may also seem to pass by in rapid review. The last phase, transcendence, is characterized by a reported feeling of euphoria, contentment, and even ecstasy. Some people recall a sensation of being unified with nature and of having an awareness of infinity. In February 2000, Pam Barrett, long-time leader of the Alberta New Democratic Party, abruptly resigned from politics after a near-death experience due to an allergic reaction. She termed the experience "a spiritual awakening," and said that it had forced her to re-evaluate all aspects of her life. Given the number of books available on this topic, you can choose to read more about near-death experiences if interested.

Coping with Loss

The death of a loved one can be extremely difficult to cope with. The dying person, as well as close family and friends, frequently suffers emotionally and physically from the impending loss of critical relationships and roles. Words used to describe feelings and behaviours related to losses resulting from death include bereavement, grief, grief work, and mourning. These terms are related but not identical. A discussion of them may help you to understand the emotional processes associated with loss and the cultural constraints that often inhibit normal coping behaviours (see Figure 17.2).

Bereavement is generally defined as the loss or deprivation experienced by a survivor when a loved one dies. Because relationships vary in type and intensity, reactions vary. The death of a parent, spouse, sibling, child, friend, or pet will result in different kinds of feelings. The death of loved ones will leave "holes" in the lives of the bereaved or of close survivors. We can think of bereavement as the awareness of these holes. Time and courage are necessary to fill these spaces.

When a person experiences a loss that cannot be openly acknowledged, publicly mourned, or socially supported, coping may be much more difficult. This type of

Social death An often irreversible situation in which a person is not treated as an active member of society.

Bereavement The loss or deprivation experienced when a loved one dies.

FIGURE 17.2

The Stages and Tasks of Grief

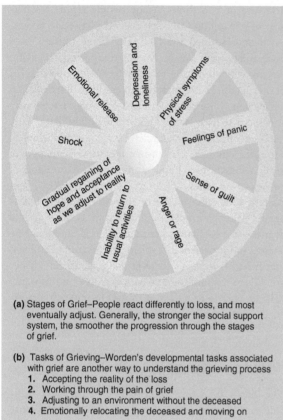

(a) Stages of Grief–People react differently to loss, and most eventually adjust. Generally, the stronger the social support system, the smoother the progression through the stages of grief.

(b) Tasks of Grieving–Worden's developmental tasks associated with grief are another way to understand the grieving process
1. Accepting the reality of the loss
2. Working through the pain of grief
3. Adjusting to an environment without the deceased
4. Emotionally relocating the deceased and moving on

grief is referred to as **disenfranchised grief** (Doka, 1989). Some examples of a death that may lead to disenfranchised grief include

- Death of a divorced spouse: Unresolved anger and hurt along with fond memories are conflicting feelings that may prevent the resolution of feelings surrounding the ex-spouse's death.

- Death of a secret lover: When a lover dies and no one but the partner knew of the relationship, grief is often hidden. Examples would include a partner in an extramarital relationship or a lover of a gay person who is not openly gay.

- Miscarriage: The loss of a pregnancy can be traumatic because often the parents are not given time to grieve, and their sadness is dismissed with words such as, "You are still young and have time to have another child."

Disenfranchised grief Grief concerning a loss that cannot be openly acknowledged, publicly mourned, or socially supported.

Grief The mental state of distress that occurs in reaction to significant loss.

Mourning The culturally prescribed behaviour patterns for the expression of grief.

A special case of bereavement occurs in old age. Death is an intrinsic part of growing old. The longer we live, the more deaths we are likely to experience. These deaths include physical, social, spiritual, and emotional losses as our bodies deteriorate and more and more of our loved ones die. The theory of bereavement overload has been proposed to explain the effects of multiple deaths and the accumulation of sorrow in the lives of some elderly people. This theory suggests that the gloomy outlook, disturbing behaviour patterns, and apparent apathy that characterize these people may be related more to bereavement overload than to intrinsic physiological degeneration in old age (Kastenbaum, 1995).

Grief is a mental state of distress that occurs in reaction to significant loss, including one's own impending death, the death of a loved one, or a quasi-death experience. Grief reactions include any adjustments needed for one to "make it through the day" and may include changes in patterns of eating, physical activity, sleeping, working, and even thinking.

The term **mourning** is often incorrectly equated with the term *grief*. As we have noted, grief refers to a wide variety of feelings and actions that occur in response to bereavement. *Mourning*, in contrast, refers to culturally prescribed and accepted time periods and behaviour patterns for the expression of grief. In Judaism, for example, "sitting shivah" is a designated mourning period of seven days that involves prescribed rituals and prayers. Depending on a person's relationship with the deceased, various other rituals may continue for up to a year.

By accepting dying as a part of the continuum of life, many people are able to make necessary readjustments after the death of a loved one. This holistic concept, which accepts dying as a part of the total life experience, is shared by believers and nonbelievers.

What Is "Normal" Grief?

Grief responses vary widely from person to person. Despite these differences, a classic acute grief syndrome often occurs when a person acknowledges a death. This common grief reaction can include the following:

- periodic waves of physical distress lasting from 20 minutes to an hour
- a feeling of tightness in the throat
- choking and shortness of breath
- a frequent need to sigh
- a feeling of emptiness
- a feeling of muscular weakness
- an intense feeling of anxiety described as actually painful

Other common symptoms of grief include insomnia, memory lapse, loss of appetite, difficulty in concentrating, a tendency to engage in repetitive or purposeless behaviours, an "observer" sensation or feeling of unreality, difficulty in making decisions, lack of organization, excessive speech, social withdrawal or hostility, guilt feelings, and preoccupation with the image of the deceased. Susceptibility to disease increases with grief and may even be life-threatening in severe and enduring cases.

Coping with Grief

A bereaved person can suffer emotional pain and exhibit a variety of grief responses for many months after the death of a loved one. The rate of healing depends on the amount and quality of "grief work" that a person does. **Grief work** is the process of integrating the reality of the death with everyday life and learning to feel better. Often, the bereaved person must deliberately and systematically work at reducing denial and coping with the pain that results from memories of the deceased. This process takes time and requires emotional effort.

Worden's Model of Grieving Tasks

William Worden, a researcher of the death process, developed an active grieving model suggesting four developmental tasks to complete in the grief work process (refer also to Figure 17.2) (Worden, 2001):

1. Accept the reality of the loss. This task requires acknowledging and realizing that the person is dead. Traditional rituals, such as the funeral, help many bereaved people move toward this acceptance.

2. Work through the pain of grief. It is necessary to acknowledge and work through the pain associated with loss or it will manifest itself in other symptoms or behaviours.

3. Adjust to an environment in which the deceased is missing. The bereaved may feel lonely and uncertain about their identity without the person who has died. This loss brings the challenge of adjusting to their own sense of self.

4. Emotionally relocate the deceased and move on with life. Individuals never lose memories of a significant relationship. They may need help in letting go of the emotional energy that used to be invested in the person who has died, finding an appropriate place for the deceased in their emotional lives.

Models of the grief process can be viewed as "generalized maps"—each theory is an attempt by an

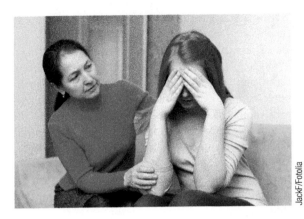

Teenage suicide affects many people, with siblings and friends—who generally have little experience with death—especially challenged in coping with their grief.

investigator to understand and guide grieving people through their pain. However, each individual will travel through grief at his or her own speed using an appropriate route.

When an Infant or a Child Dies

The death of a child is terribly painful for the whole family. For several reasons, siblings of the deceased child have a particularly hard time with grief work. Bereaved children usually have limited experience with death and therefore have not learned how to deal with it. Children may feel uncomfortable talking about death, may have difficulty understanding it, and may also receive less social support and sympathy than their parents. Because so much attention and energy are devoted to the deceased child, the surviving children may also feel emotionally abandoned.

QUASI-DEATH EXPERIENCES

Social and emotional support for the bereaved in the aftermath of death is supported by many cultures. Typically, however, there is little support for many other significant losses in life. Losses that in many ways resemble death and carry with them a heavy burden of grief include a child running away from home, an abduction or kidnapping, a divorce, a move to a distant place, a move to a long-term care facility, the loss of a romance or an intimate friendship, retirement, job termination, finishing a

Grief work The process of accepting the reality of a person's death and coping with memories of the deceased.

"terminal" academic degree, or ending an athletic career.

These **quasi-death experiences** (Kamerman, 1988) resemble death in that they involve separation, termination, loss, and a change in identity or self-perception. If grief results from these losses, the pattern of the grief response will probably follow the same course as responses to death. Factors that complicate the grieving process associated with quasi-death experiences include uncomfortable contact with the object of loss (for example, an ex-spouse or ex-partner) and a lack of adequate social and institutional support.

LIFE-AND-DEATH DECISION MAKING

Life-and-death decisions are serious, complex, and often expensive. We will not attempt to present the "answers" to death-related moral and philosophical questions. Instead, we offer topics for your consideration. We hope that discussion of the needs of the dying person and the bereaved will help you to make difficult decisions in the future. Problematic or controversial issues include questions concerning the right to die and euthanasia. On February 6, 2015, the Supreme Court of Canada made a unanimous decision to remove the federal prohibition of physician-assisted dying, stating that the old law violates the Canadian Charter of Rights and Freedoms. The federal government's new assisted dying law received royal assent on June 17, 2016. Currently the following types of medical assistance in dying are permitted in Canada:

- A physician or nurse practitioner can directly administer a substance that causes the death of the person who has requested it, and

- A physician or nurse practitioner can give or prescribe to a patient a substance that they can self-administer to cause their own death. For more information visit Dying with Dignity Canada at www.dyingwithdignity.ca/.

The right to self-determination is situated within the context of society, health and illness, and human rights and freedoms. Considerations of the economic, social, spiritual, and moral impact of the individual's choice are often involved in decision making. A living will, discussed in the Point of View box, is one way in which people can express their wishes about life-and-death choices.

Quasi-death experiences Losses or experiences that resemble death in that they involve separation, termination, significant loss, a change of personal identity, and grief.

Palliative Care

The needs of terminally ill patients are different from those of other patients. They require another approach and different services defined by different criteria. Palliative care is a compassionate form of health care for patients approaching the end of their life. Pain and symptom management and social, psychological, and spiritual support are components of palliative care. We need to understand more fully the meaning that death and dying have to seniors, and how to provide effective pain management for those experiencing the symptoms of several health conditions simultaneously.

Several models of care have been explored all over the world: St. Christopher's in London, the Maison Michel Sarrazin in Quebec, and the Elizabeth Bruyère Centre in Ottawa, for example, are highly specialized in pain control and offer supportive care and attention to dying patients. Friends and family are welcome at all times and special training is given to volunteers who can then assist the patients, their families, and the caregivers on staff.

In-home palliative care services are provided in collaboration with a care facility. If treatment is balanced, this type of service can ensure the full continuum of care and nurturing needed to allow terminally ill individuals to remain in their familiar surroundings for as long as possible. The family also needs to be supported and kept informed by being given clear explanations and directives. For individuals to derive maximum benefit from this situation, the home atmosphere needs to be calm and serene, and services must be of the same

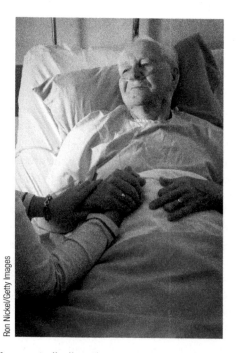

Ron Nickel/Getty Images

Many terminally ill people spend their last days in a hospice where maximum involvement of loved ones is emphasized.

point of view

MAKING HEALTH CARE DECISIONS NOW

When You Have The Capacity To Do So

This textbox, unlike other "Point of View" textboxes in this textbook, does not lightheartedly encourage you to consider two sides to a topic, but rather presents a deep topic that you ought to think and talk about. You may not feel ready to engage in thoughts about 'what if'—but who is? The reality is we do not know when tragedy will befall us. Creating a personal directive (or living will), although difficult, provides you with an opportunity to provide input for the 'what if' scenarios.

Personal Directive or Living Will

A personal directive is a written document in which you clearly identify your wishes for health care in the event that, sometime in the future, you are unable to make decisions regarding your treatment. Personal directives deal with health care. They do not deal with property or assets. Personal directives are needed if you are unable to consent when have a terminal illness or are seriously injured and unlikely to recover. In such cases, medical staff will ask your partner or family as to what measures you do or do not wish them to take in their care for you.

There are no guarantees that every term of your personal directive will be followed. In your personal directive, you will identify a delegate who in consultation with medical staff will make the decisions regarding your health care taking into account the existing circumstances, as well as your previously written expressed wishes. (A delegate is the person [or persons] you have appointed to make decisions about your health care should you become unable to consent or make those decisions.) A personal directive can ease the emotional burden for your partner or family members since someone has been directed to make decisions about your health. It is important to share your personal directive, not only with your delegate, but also your partner (if not your delegate) and other family members so that they are aware of your wishes regarding health care when you are not capable of making those decisions yourself. Most people consider a personal directive morally binding, especially if it has been discussed with them beforehand.

As mentioned, it is important for you to share with your partner (if you have one) and your family your wishes should you become incapacitated and medical attention is required. In fact, this is a conversation to have with your parents as well. Are you aware of their expressed wishes regarding end-of-life care? For that matter, do you know if your parents have a will, preferences for a funeral or end of life services? Cremation or burial? These are topics of conversation that should be talked about too. You may also ask who is identified as a delegate for your parents regarding a personal directive.

A personal directive is not a request to take steps to end your life. Euthanasia, or mercy killing, as it is sometimes called, is the term used when someone takes steps to end your life in order to relieve suffering. Assisted suicide is a term used when someone, at your request, takes steps to end your life, because your illness or condition prevents you from committing suicide. Euthanasia and assisted suicide have recently become legal in Canada.

A personal directive must include your name, address, and the date. It should clearly identify a delegate who will consent to treatment on your behalf should you become unable to do so as well as what kind of life-sustaining treatments you would want in certain circumstances if you are incapable of consenting at the time. For your delegate, choose someone whom you trust to carry out your wishes—and be sure to discuss your personal directive with him or her. This person must be at least 19 years of age and does not have to be your in your biological family. In your personal directive, you might also include whether or not you wish to donate any or all of your viable organs as well as whether or not you would donate your body to science. Finally, you may include in your personal directive, your wishes regarding cremation or burial and the type of funeral or services you prefer. You sign and date your personal directive in the presence of two adult witnesses. These witnesses should also provide their addresses.

Source: Data f.rom The Legal Information Society of Nova Scotia (LISNS), Living Wills, www.legalinfo.org.

quality as those offered in hospital. If you are terminally ill, you can make your wishes regarding your care known in several ways:

- If you are facing a life-threatening illness, you should talk over your wishes with your family and let them know what you want.

- You can also put your wishes in writing so that, in the event you are unable to say what you want, your family and health-care providers will know. Such documents are called advance personal directives or living wills (see the Point of View box). You should seek advice within your community about advance directives, as the laws concerning them vary from province to province.

- Your public library might have material on palliative care. You can also access information online, such as from the Canadian Hospice Palliative Care Association, www.chpca .net and Virtual Hospice, www.virtualhospice.ca/ en_US/Main+Site+Navigation/Home.aspx.

Dyathanasia is a form of "mercy killing" in which life-prolonging treatments are withheld or life-sustaining medical support is withdrawn, thereby allowing the person to die. It is believed that withholding food and water from terminally ill individuals may actually ease their suffering. **Euthanasia** is the active form of "mercy killing." An example of euthanasia is direct administration of a lethal drug overdose with the objective of hastening the death of a suffering person. Euthanasia is illegal and considered murder in Canada, if carried out by an individual who is not a physician or nurse practitioner. After years of legal run-ins, the well-known American euthanasia proponent Dr. Jack Kevorkian was convicted of murder for assisting in euthanasia ("assisted suicide") in the late 1990s. Similarly, Robert Latimer was found guilty for killing his daughter who was severely disabled. However, a bill was passed recently, making this legal in Canada. Euthanasia is also legal in some countries as well as in four states in the United States. In fact, it is believed that some doctors induce euthanasia upon the request of the patient. This type of euthanasia is accomplished by administering large doses of painkillers that depress the central nervous system to the extent that basic life-sustaining regulatory centres cease to function. The heart stops beating, breathing ceases, and total brain death follows shortly.

Dyathanasia The passive form of "mercy killing" in which life-prolonging treatments or interventions are withheld, thereby allowing a terminally ill person to die naturally.

Euthanasia The active form of "mercy killing" in which a person or organization knowingly acts to hasten the death of a terminally ill person.

assess
YOURSELF

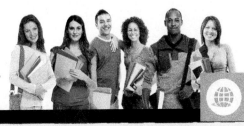

Go to MasteringHealth to complete this questionnaire with automatic scoring

TAKING CHARGE: Managing Your Health in Your Older Years

This chapter covers a number of things regarding your health that you may not have thought much about. You are young, though aging as you read this book. Time passes too quickly (much too quickly) and before you know it, you will be in your 40s and 50s and starting to feel the effect of age. Not only is it good to understand what to expect for yourself, you can also think about your parents and grandparents as you think about the material presented in this chapter. We finish this chapter with an Aging Quiz. Complete the questionnaire, responding to each question honestly so that you can gauge your understanding of the aging process.

Aging Quiz

Test your knowledge of healthy aging by taking the following test. Answer true or false to each statement. The answers are listed below.

1. Men usually outlive women.

             T   F

2. If your parents had Alzheimer's disease, you will also get it.

             T   F

3. Dietary intake and physical activity can reduce the risk of developing osteoporosis.

             T   F

4. Heart disease affects women as much as men.

             T   F

5. The older you get, the less sleep you need.

             T   F

6. People should reduce their caloric intake as they age.

             T   F

7. People take more medications as they age.

             T   F

8. As your body changes with age, so does your personality.

             T   F

9. Intelligence declines with age.

             T   F

10. Most older people live alone.

              T   F

11. Most people become "senile" if they live long enough.

              T   F

12. Physical strength tends to decline with age.

              T   F

13. Most older adults limit their travel to be closer to home.

              T   F

14. Older adults have the lowest income of all adult groups.

              T   F

15. Most older adults have no interest in, or capacity for, sexual activity.

              T   F

16. People tend to become more religious with age.

              T   F

17. People tend to change their driving habits as they age.

              T   F

18. Older people are more likely to commit suicide than younger people.

              T   F

19. Many older people are preoccupied with death.

              T   F

20. Most older people new to Canada speak neither English nor French.

              T   F

Answers

1. False. Women have an average life expectancy greater than men. A boy born in 2003 is expected to live to 77.4 years, while a girl born in the same year is expected to live to 82.4 years or 5 years longer.

2. False. Between 90 and 95 percent of people with Alzheimer's disease have a form of the disease not necessarily linked to family history. Only 5 percent of Alzheimer's cases are a result of a genetic link.

3. True. Bone loss can be reduced by eating foods rich in calcium (for example, milk and other dairy products; dark green, leafy vegetables; canned salmon; sardines; and tofu) and engaging in regular, weight-bearing physical activity, such as walking and resistance training.

4. True. Heart disease is one of the leading causes of death for men and women.

5. False. Although quality of sleep declines when we age, required sleep time does not. Further, sleep tends to get more fragmented as we get older.

6. True. Older people need fewer calories because of decreases in metabolic function and physical activity. If an involuntary weight gain or loss of 5 kilograms or more occurs in six months, a physician should be consulted.

7. True. Most Canadian older adults take some form of prescription or over-the-counter medication. Further, older adults (85+) are more likely than younger older adults (65–74) to take more than one medication (65 versus 52 percent).

8. False. Other than personality changes associated with Alzheimer's disease and other forms of dementia, personality does not change appreciably as you age.

9. False. Although studies show that the elderly have a slower reaction time and take longer to learn something new, their intellect is maintained and can be improved as they get older.

10. False. The majority of Canadian older adults (69 percent) live with their family or extended family.

11. False. Dementia (*senility* is not the correct term) is not a normal part of aging. One in fifty older adults between the ages of 65 and 74, one in nine older adults between the ages of 75 and 84, and one in three older adults over the age of 85 will develop dementia.

12. True. Physical strength does decrease with age—as does the quality of the muscles. Decreases in strength can be reduced by regular participation in physical activity, including resistance training.

13. False. In fact, some older adults are more likely to travel abroad than younger adults.

14. True. In 1997, 19 percent of all older adults (65+) had an income below the low-income cut-off. Women (24 percent) are more likely than men (11.7 percent) to have a low income.

15. False. Aging does not equal a loss of interest in or capacity for sex.

16. False. Despite a perception that people tend to become more religious with age, this is not true. This perception may reflect a difference between generations rather than a characteristic of aging.

17. True. To accommodate the changes associated with aging, many older adults modify their driving behaviour by planning their trips, driving less, limiting highway travel, and avoiding driving in poor weather or at night.

18. False. Overall, older adults in Canada are less likely to commit suicide than younger adults.

19. False. Older adults' attitudes toward death are variable, though some trends can be noted. Specifically, older adults are less anxious and more matter-of-fact about death. Most young adults avoid thinking about or discussing death.

20. True. The majority (61 percent) of older immigrants to Ontario from 1996 to 1999 spoke neither English nor French.

Source: Adapted from the Ontario Gerontology Association, "Aging Quiz." Retrieved on May 16, 2006, from http://ontgerontology.on.ca.

DISCUSSION QUESTIONS

1. Discuss the various definitions of aging. At what age would you place your parents or grandparents in each category? Yourself?

2. As the population of older people grows, what implications are there for you? Would you be willing to pay higher taxes to support social programs for older Canadians? Why or why not?

3. List the major physiological changes that occur with aging. Which of these, if any, can you change? Which can you slow down? Specifically address dietary intake, physical activity, and sedentary behaviours in your response.

4. Identify the major physical and mental health challenges that older Canadians face.

5. List the varied definitions of death. How do they relate to one another?

6. Discuss why we deny death. How could death become a more socially accepted topic to discuss?

7. What are the stages that terminally ill patients theoretically experience? Do you agree with the five-stage theory? Explain why or why not.

APPLICATION EXERCISE

Reread the "Consider This . . . " scenario at the beginning of the chapter and answer the following questions.

1. Do you think the individuals in the scenario are normal for their age? What is normal for a particular age? How is "normal" defined?

2. What changes have made it easier for older people to lead healthy lives? What changes have made it more difficult?

3. What can be done to reduce ageism in your community?

MASTERINGHEALTH

Go to MasteringHealth for Assignments, the eText, and the Study Area with case studies, self quizzing, and videos.

focus On
Financial Health

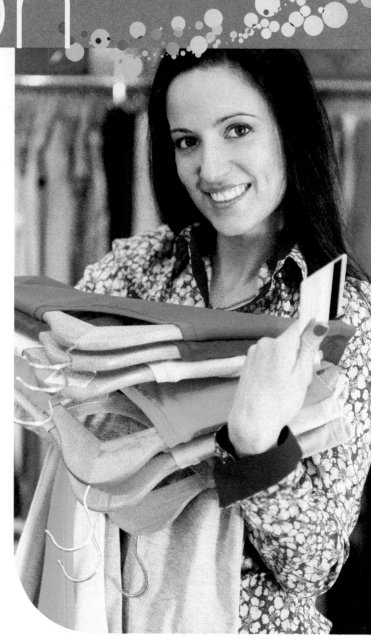

Spass/Shutterstock

It is the last month of classes in the second term and August's money from his student loan has run out. August is also not likely to get any more hours working in event management from the Athletics Department because the varsity athletic season is over for all of the teams. As a result, August is not sure where he will get the money to buy groceries, pay his cellphone and other bills, or to go out with his friends. He thinks back to his run away spending habits earlier in the school year when his loan came in—it seemed then that he had an endless supply of money to do all that he wanted to do. August ate out frequently, partied, went to the movies, and bought what he wanted, when he wanted it—after all, he deserves the good life, right? And with his student loan, he had the money to pay for it.

How familiar does this sound? How many students run out of money before the end of the school term, relying on others—including food banks—to get them through to the end of the school year? How many students do you know who seem to have an endless supply of money and seem to spend considerable amounts eating out, buying alcohol to consume at home and when out, for clothing and shoes, and for various forms of entertainment? Spending more than you have can lead to financial distress, particularly when you are supporting the costs of your own education through student loans, part-time work during the school year, and (hopefully) full-time work during the summers.

This sort of financial behaviour is also common in working adults (Movenblog, n.d.). Think of what most people do when given a raise—they go out for dinner or buy a bottle of wine and celebrate, deservedly. Many then continue to spend what they earn living paycheque to paycheque, seldom getting ahead with their finances. In these circumstances, financial risk may result, particularly if you start to think that you are entitled to spend more money, just because you make more of it—or because your student loan came in. You may then lose context, consistency, and control of your finances (Movenblog, n.d.).

FINANCIAL WELLNESS

In addition to the components of wellness discussed in Chapter 1 (physical, social, mental, environmental, spiritual, intellectual, and occupational), some suggest there should be another dimension—financial wellness. Financial wellness has been defined as "a 'state' of wealth that can be achieved by individuals or families—irrespective of income levels" (Capital Wellness, 2010).

The BusinessDictionary.com (n.d.) defined financial health as "A way in which to measure the overall financial aspect of an individual that includes the amount of assets they own and how much income they must pay out to cover regular and other expenses." Thus, to be financially well, you need to understand your financial situation and manage it in such a way to be prepared for fluctuations in income and spending. Further, when you are financially well, you understand that money can be created, saved, and lost (Capital Wellness, 2010). Similar to other aspects of wellness, your level of financial wellness varies depending upon your personal circumstances, and will likely fluctuate throughout your lifetime. Further, when you are aware of your debts and assets, or what you owe and the value of what you own, you can create a picture of your personal financial net worth and have two of the necessary ingredients for creating your financial wellness. When you understand what you owe and what you own, as well as what your income is, you can create a personal budget and plan, short- and long-term, to spend within your means (Capital Wellness, 2010). Financial wellness is not about having a certain amount of money in the bank but rather about spending, saving, and living better within your financial reality (Movenblog, n.d.). As such, financial wellness can be achieved by people with all levels of income. According to InvestorWords.com (n.d.), "[s]omeone with good financial health usually deals well with their finances, makes their payments on time, and knows how to manage their money. Someone in poor financial health usually owes a lot of money and is not making their payments on time."

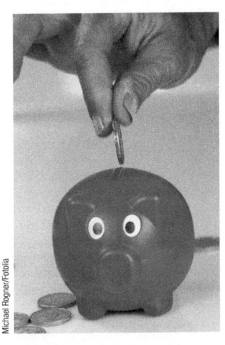

Saving for future expenses and enjoying short-term indulgences is part of financial wellness.

Students and Their Financial Wellness

It is not surprising that today's college and university students face considerable stresses on their financial wellness. Given the pressure of competing for grades, scholarships, bursaries, athletic positions, and jobs and internships, it can be difficult for many students to work part- or full-time to pay the bills. Further, summer employment (even if full-time) seldom covers the costs of an academic year. Recent economic setbacks and relatively high levels of unemployment also challenge students' ability to work. Fear over slim job opportunities, debt from student loans, and a host of other financial concerns test students' financial wellness as they approach each year of their education, their graduation, and an uncertain professional future.

The cost of higher education results in significant personal financial burden for many students. Nearly two-thirds of students indicated that they have "some" or "major" concerns regarding their ability to pay for their education (Pryor et al., 2010). The economic downturn of the past few years is likely pushing already financially stretched students further toward the breaking point. Personal financial debt can lead to extensive stress in students today with considerable potential to negatively influence their physical and mental health (Krisher, 2011). Similar to other sources of stress (as noted in Chapter 3), symptoms of financial stress include headaches, hair loss, hypervigilance, insomnia, social withdrawal, low self-esteem, depression, anxiety, drug or alcohol dependency, violence, and increased potential for suicide (Krishner, 2011). Further, people with unmanaged financial stress typically do not eat well nor do they engage in sufficient physical activity, which can lead to other health risks as noted in Chapters 4 and 5 (Working Toward Wellness, 2010). If you experience duress as a result of your financial situation, it is recommended that you:

- Do not hide from your personal financial stress.
- Be realistic and recognize that all stress, especially financial stress, cannot be completely eliminated. In addition to examining your personal attitudes and behaviours regarding your finances, you can also manage your response to the stress.
- Try to recognize stress from financial overload early, as this can help you to take steps early enough to minimize the harmful effects (Working Toward Wellness, 2010).

Several factors are converging to increase today's students' financial worries. First, a recession resulted in many of their parents losing their jobs. Faced with dwindling resources at home, many students are forced to look for part-time or even full-time work—not just in the summer months, but also during the school year. These students may encounter increasing competition for even the lowest-paying jobs as displaced workers are also competing for these jobs to remain financially afloat. As a result, many students rely on their provincial government to provide them with substantial student loans. For some, these loans may not cover their entire expenses, and students are forced to establish student lines of credit. Both loans require repayment, with payments to begin usually about six months after graduating (or six months after the most recently completed term). Already known to carry a disproportionate level of credit card debt, students are resorting to using plastic to pay for essentials, leading to more debt and higher financial stress. Given these pressures, you (similar to working adults) are recommended to take a serious look at your financial situation and come up with a plan to develop your financial health and reduce your financial stress. The suggestions below may help:

- **Develop a realistic budget.** Track your expenses for one month. Are you spending way too much in certain categories? Are you able to juggle some of your spending? Online budget tracking systems such as www.mint.com can help you learn about where you spend your money and then you can reflect upon what you really need and what you could do without.

- **Pay bills immediately and consider electronic banking.** Late fees and other penalties unnecessarily deplete your bank account and are easily avoided by paying bills as soon as you get them. Sign up for an online account to pay bills quickly and easily. If possible, set up your bills for automatic payment. Whenever possible, pay the entire bill; interest charges are exorbitant and should be avoided whenever possible. If you cannot pay your bills in their entirety, consider a line of credit, as the interest charges are considerably less.

- **Educate yourself about how to manage your money.** Take advantage of campus or community workshops on financial aid and money management. Take a course in personal financial planning.

- **Avoid tempting credit card offers.** You need only one or two credit cards. Shred extra offers you get in the mail. Do not be lured by discounts you get when opening up credit cards at department stores. Be careful of using credit cards simply for the 'reward' benefits.

- **Do not get into debt.** Pay the entire balance of your credit card each month—do not let interest accumulate. If you do not have the money for an item now, do not buy it on credit; put aside a certain amount every month until you have enough to afford it.

Personality and Financial Health—Is There a Connection?

There are three personality characteristics as well as a few personality disorders that may influence your spending patterns and ultimately your financial health: a loss of perspective, an addictive personality, and a loss of control (Movenblog, n.d.).

A Loss of Perspective

Can you recall the first time you were paid for the work you had done—maybe it was babysitting or doing yardwork or shovelling snow for a neighbour? Do you remember how great it felt to get paid? You likely thought that you had a lot of money, and it was yours to do what you wanted with it. You may have initially felt the same way when you received your first paycheque from a 'regular' job—that you could do what you wanted with your money, until you remembered the bills that needed to be paid—your rent, cellphone bill, groceries, car loan, gas, and so on. Suddenly, your money does not go so far. It is important to keep this reality in perspective, especially when your student loan first arrives, because it has to last you eight months— much longer than your monthly paycheque did!

People who are manic often lose perspective (Movenblog, n.d.). In these cases, the inflated view of self, including an elevated self-esteem, may lead to the misconception of greater financial means than what exist in reality, as well as an inability to recognize the consequences of overspending. As such, individuals who are manic often overspend, resulting in poor financial health.

One way to keep your perspective regarding your finances is to learn about your "daily spend" (Movenblog, n.d.). Your daily spend refers to your take home pay minus all of your required living expenses divided by 30 (assuming you are paid once per month). You can do this with your student loan too; take your student loan and subtract all your expenses (tuition, books, meal card, bus pass, cellphone bill, and so on) then divide it by the number of days in your school term. The value you determine is your "daily spend" or the amount you can spend each day without going into debt. When you want to purchase an item that costs more than your daily spend, you need to compensate by having several days (or weeks) without spending to cover the actual cost. In this way, the daily spend can be effective in helping you to keep perspective as to how much money you really have available—and you might think twice when you recognize how many days, or weeks, a particular item costs.

An Addictive Personality

There are times you may catch yourself or your friends saying "I am addicted to . . .". Chances are you are not really an addict, nor do you have an addictive personality. Still, you should consider the financial consequences of some of your daily habits—particularly those that cost money. Choosing to purchase a latte or smoothie each day can add up over the term. Think about it, a large latte may cost as much as $5—if you buy one each school day, that is $25 per week and there are typically 13 weeks of classes each term (not counting exams)—so $325 for lattes for one term!

Although buying a coffee, smoothie, lunch, or snack each day clearly does not classify you as an addict, when you total the costs, it should lead to some personal reflection regarding your spending and, therefore, your financial health (Movenblog, n.d.). You may even ask yourself if you really need your daily purchase. You may also ask yourself if there is an alternative that makes more financial sense. For example, you could make and take a coffee from home and pack yourself a healthy lunch, including extra items for snacks. Individuals who have an addictive personality or who are compulsive shoppers (see also Chapter 9) may not be able to rationalize their spending as they will be driven to shop simply for the need to feel normal.

To avoid—or limit—damage to your financial health from your daily purchases, keep track of your spending for a month, including what, when, and how much it costs (Movenblog, n.d.). Reflect upon this diary and critically evaluate if you are spending your money in 'healthy' ways. If you are not, make the changes necessary to protect your financial health.

A Loss of Control

Do you have control of your shopping? Would others describe you as a "shopaholic?" To determine if your

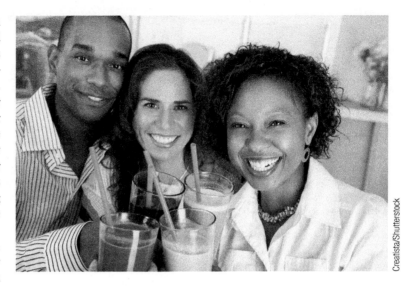

Purchasing a smoothie or latte each day can add up to a considerable amount of money over the week, month, or year.

shopping has a negative influence on your financial health and potentially your relationships, ask yourself the following using a Likert-type scale of rarely, sometimes, often, always:

1. How much of your time is spent buying things or thinking about buying things?

2. How often do you feel guilt, depression, or shame because of your discretionary purchases?

3. How often do your discretionary purchases impair your ability to pay for basic necessities?

If your answer is always to one of these, or often to two of the above, you should seek help for your shopping tendencies and behaviours. Most people respond rarely or sometimes to these questions, so there should be no concern if those were your responses (Movenblog, n.d.). Again, your responses to these questions can help you to better understand the pressures on your financial health as well as to whether or not your approach to shopping is healthy.

NOTES

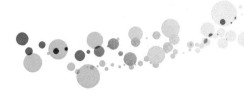

CHAPTER 1

Ajzen, I. (1991). The theory of planned behavior. *Organizational Behavior and Human Decision Processes, 50,* 179–211.

Barbiero, G., Berto R., & Pasini, M. (2011). Biophilia in practice: Children perceive the restorative value of nature and this improves performance in attention test. *University Research Catalogue*. Retrieved from www.univr.it/main?ent=catalogoaol&id=383411&page=dettaglioPubblicazione

Beckington, C. F. (1975). The World Health Organization. In *World Health*. New York: Longman, 149.

Bishop, G. D. (1994). *Health psychology*. Needham Heights, MA: Allyn & Bacon, 84–86.

Canadian Cancer Society. (2013). Breast cancer statistics at a glance. Retrieved from www.cancer.ca/canada-wide/about%20cancer/cancer%20statistics/stats%20at%20a%20glance/breast%20cancer.aspx

Daniels, S. R. (2006). The consequences of childhood overweight and obesity. *Future Child, 16*(1), 47–67.

DiGiuseppe, R. A. (2010). Rational-emotive behavior therapies. In N. Kazantzis, M. A. Reinecke, & A. Freeman (Eds.), *Cognitive and behavioral theories in clinical practices*. Retrieved from http://books.google.ca/books?hl=en&lr=&id=y4SOyU12iTYC&oi=fnd&pg=PA115&d-q=Rational-Emotive+Therapy&ots=chuc_iKeO_&sig=AEMqxRk-zLbZ2KK1B50f3mvezKc0#v=onepage&q=Rational-Emotive%20Therapy&f=false

DiMatteo, M. (1994). *The psychology of health, illness, and medical care: An individual perspective*. Pacific Grove, CA: Brooks/Cole, 101–103.

Dubos, R. (1968). *So human an animal*. New York: Scribners, 15.

Eichler, M., Reisman, A. L., & Borins, E. M. (1992). Gender bias in medical research, *Women and Therapy, 12,* 61–70.

Franks, P. W., Hanson, R. L., Knowler, W. C., Sievers, M. L., Bennett, P. H., & Looker, H. C. (2010). Childhood obesity, other cardiovascular risk factors, and premature death. *New England Journal of Medicine, 362,* 485–493. doi:10.1056/NEJMoa0904130

Gould, T., Fleming, M. L., & Parker, E. A. (2012). Advocacy for health: Revisiting the role of health promotion. *Health Promotion Journal of Australia, 23*(3), 165–170.

Harakeh, Z., Scholte, R. H. J., & Vermulst, A. A. (2010). The relations between parents' smoking, general parenting, parental smoking communication, and adolescents' smoking. *Journal of Research on Adolescence, 20*(1), 140–165. doi:10.1111/j.1532-7795.2009.00626.x

Hatzigeorgiadis, A., Zourbanos, N., Galanis, E., & Theodorakis, Y. (2011). Self-talk and sports performance: A meta-analysis. *Perspectives on Psychological Science, 6,* 348.

Hill, K. G., Hawkins, J. D., Catalano, R. F., Abbott, R. D., & Guo, J. (2005). Family influences on the risk of daily smoking initiation. *Journal of Adolescent Health, 37*(3), 202–210.

Medicinenet.com. (n.d.). Women's health (cont). Retrieved from www.medicinenet.com/womens_health/page4.htm

Miller, L. (1994). Medical schools put women in curricula. *Wall Street Journal,* May 24, pp. B1, B7.

PolzerCasarez, R. L., & Engebretson, J. C. (2012). Ethical issues of incorporating spiritual care into clinical practice. *Journal of Clinical Nursing,* (21), 2099–2107. doi:10.1111/j.1365-2702.2012.04168.x

Prochaska, J. O., & DiClemente, C. C. (1983). Stages and processes of self-change of smoking: Toward an integrative model of change. *Journal of Consulting and Clinical Psychology, 51,* 390–395.

Public Health Agency of Canada. (2010). Overview of the Pan Canadian Healthy Living Strategy. Retrieved from www.phac-aspc.gc.ca/hp-ps/hl-mvs/ipchls-spimmvs-eng.php

Public Health Agency of Canada. (2011a). Curbing childhood obesity: An overview of the federal, provincial, and territorial framework for action to promote healthy weights. Retrieved from www.phac-aspc.gc.ca/hp-ps/hl-mvs/framework-cadre/intro-eng.php

Public Health Agency of Canada. (2011b). United Nations NCD Summit 2011. Retrieved from www.phac-aspc.gc.ca/media/nr-rp/2011/2011_0919-bg-di-eng.php

Ruiz, M. T., & Verbrugge, L. M. (1997). A two way view of gender bias in medicine. *Journal of Epidemiology and Community Health*, 51(2), 106–109.

Sarafino, E. P. (1990). *Health psychology*. New York: John Wiley & Sons, 189–191.

Scherrer, J. F., Xian, H., Pan, H., Pergadia, M. L., Madden, P. A. F., Grant, J. D., … Bucholz, K. K. (2012). Parent, sibling and peer influences on smoking initiation, regular smoking and nicotine dependence. Results from a genetically informative design. *Addictive Behaviors, 37*(3), 240–247.

Statistics Canada. (1997). *Canada year book 1997*. Ottawa: Minister of Industry, Cat. No. 402 XPE, (1996), 116.

Statistics Canada. (2011). Centenarians in Canada. Retrieved from www12.statcan.gc.ca/census-recensement/2011/as-sa/98-311-x/98-311-x2011003_1-eng.pdf

Statistics Canada. (2012). Deaths. *The Daily*, Thursday, May 31, 2012. Retrieved from www.statcan.gc.ca/daily-quotidien/120531/dq120531e-eng.htm

The Secretariat for the Intersectoral Healthy Living Network in partnership with the F/P/T Healthy Living Task Group and the F/P/T Advisory Committee on Population Health and Health Security (ACPHHS). (2006). The integrated Pan-Canadian healthy living strategy 2005." Retrieved from www.phac-aspc.gc.ca/hl-vs-strat/pdf/hls_e.pdf

The Stanford DECIDE Drug Education Curriculum, Garfield Company, CA.

Watson, P., & Tharp, R. (1993). *Self-directed behavior: Self-modification for personal adjustment*. Pacific Grove, CA: Brooks/Cole, 13.

World Health Organization. (1947). Constitution of the World Health Organization. *Chronicles of the World Health Organization*. Switzerland: Geneva.

World Health Organization. (2013). Health topics: Health promotion. Retrieved from www.who.int/topics/health_promotion/en/

CHAPTER 2

Afifi, M. (2007). Gender differences in mental health, *Singapore Medical Journal, 48*(5), 385.

Astin, A. et al. (2004). Spirituality in higher education: A national study of college students' search for meaning and purpose, Higher Education Research Institute, Graduate School of Education & Information Studies, UCLA. Retrieved from www.spirituality.ucla.edu

Astin, A. W., Astin, H. S., & Lindholm, J. A. (2011). *Cultivating the spirit: How college can enhance students' inner lives*. Retrieved from http://books.google.ca/books?hl=en&lr=&id=Em_4lwmKB74C&oi=fnd&p-g=PR7&dq=spirituality+Astin&ots=60otVm_S0h&sig=aAOosh-0GjlbHBEonXX_wZuMSM3g#v=onepage&q=spirituality%20Astin&f=false

Astin, J. A., Shapiro, S. L., Eisenberg, D. M., & Forys, K. L. (2003). Mind–body medicine: State of the science, implications for practice. *Journal of the American Board of Family Practice, 16*, 131–147.

Barbiero, G., Berto, R., & Pasini, M. (2011). Biophilia in practice: Children perceive the restorative value of nature and this improves performance in attention test. *University Research Catalogue*. Retrieved from http://www.univr.it/main?ent=catalogoaol&id=383411&page=dettaglioPubblicazione

Bishop, J., et al. (2004). Mindfulness: A proposed operational definition. *Clinical Psychology, 11*, 230–241.

Blanchflower, D. G., Oswald, A. J., & Stewart-Brown, S. (2012). Is psychological well-being linked to the consumption of fruits and vegetables? *Social Indicators Research.* doi:10.1007/s11205-012-0173-y.

Canadian Mental Health Association, B.C. Division. (2005). Mental health and substance use disorders: Key issues. Retrieved from www.cmha.bc.ca/files/7-mi_substance_use.pdf

Canadian Mental Health Association. (2009a). Benefits of good mental health. Retrieved from http://www.cmha.ca/bins/print_page.asp?cid=2-267-1320&lang=1

Canadian Mental Health Association. (2009b). Men and mental illness. Retrieved from http://www.cmha.ca/bins/print_page.asp?cid=3-726&lang=1

Canadian Mental Health Association. (2009c). Post traumatic stress disorder. Retrieved from www.cmha.ca/bins/print_page.asp?cid=3-94-97&lang=1

Canadian Mental Health Association. (2013). Fast facts about mental illness. Retrieved from http://www.cmha.ca/media/fast-facts-about-mental-illness/

Canadian Mental Health Association. (n.d.). Youth and suicide. Retrieved from www.cmha.ca/bins/print_page.asp?cid=3-101-104&lang=1

CBS This Morning. (1996). How to choose a therapist. July 24–26.

Charities Aid Foundation. (2014). World Giving Index 2014: A global view of giving trends. Retrieved from www.cafonline.org/PDF/World-GivingIndex2012WEB.pdf.

Cohen-Katz, J., Wiley, S., Capuano, T., Baker, D. M., Deitrick, L., & Shapiro, S. (2005). The effects of mindfulness-based stress reduction on nurse stress and burnout, part II: A quantitative and qualitative study. *Holistic Nurse Practice, 1*, 26–35.

Davidson, R., Maxwell, J. S., & Shackman, A. J. (2004). The privileged status of emotion in the brain. *Proceedings of the National Academy of Sciences of the United States of America, 101*, 33.

Diener, E., & Seligman, M. E. P. (2004). Beyond money: Toward an economy of well-being. *Psychological Science in the Public Interest, 5*, 1–31.

Dovidio, J. F., Hewstone, M., Glick, P., & Esses, V. M. (2010). *The SAGE handbook of prejudice, stereotyping and discrimination*, London, England: SAGE Publications, Ltd.

Elkins, D. (1998). *Beyond religion—A personal program for building a spiritual life outside the walls of traditional religion.* Wheaton, IL: Quest Books.

Epperson, C. N., Steiner, M., Hartlage, S. A., Eriksson, E., Schmidt, P. J., Jones, I., & Yonkers, K. A. (2012). Premenstrual dysphoric disorder: Evidence for a new category for DSM-5. *American Journal of Psychiatry, 169*(5), 465–475.

Fredrickson, B. (2000). Cultivating positive emotions to optimize health and well-being. *Prevention and Treatment 3*, article 0001a.

Gertz, K. R. (1990). Mood probe: Pinpointing the crucial differences between emotional lows and the gridlock of depression. *Self, 165–168, 204.*

Gottman, J. M., & Silver, N. (1999). *The seven principles of making marriage work.* New York: Crown Publishers Inc.

Grady, D. (1992). Think right, stay well. *American Health, 11*, 50–54.

Igoumenou, A. (2010). Relationship between depression and cancer. *Psychiatrike, 21*(3), 205–216.

Kalat, J. W. (1996). Treatment of psychologically troubled people. In Plotnik, R., *Introduction to psychology* (4th ed.). Pacific Grove, CA: Brooks/Cole, 648–678.

Karen, K. et al. (2006). *Mind/body health: The effects of attitudes, emotions, and relationships* (3rd ed.). San Francisco: Benjamin Cummings.

Kilpatrick, M. W. (2008). Exercise, mood, and psychological well-being: A practitioner's guide to theory, research and application. *ACSM's Health & Fitness Journal, 12*(5), 14–20.

Kluger, J. (2005). The funny thing about laughter. *Time, 165*(3), A25–A29.

Kraut, R., Patterson, M., Lundmark, V., Kiesler, S., Mukophadhyay, T., & Scherlis, W. (1998). Internet paradox. A social technology that reduces social involvement and psychological well-being? *American Psychologist, 53*(9), 1017–1031.

Langlois, K. A., Samokhvalov, A. V., Rehm, J., Spence, S. T., & Connor Gorber, S. K. (2011). Health state descriptions for Canadians: Mental illnesses. Statistics Canada, catalogue no. 82-619-MIE2005002. Ottawa: Statistics Canada.

Lazarus, R. (1991). *Emotion and adaptation.* New York: Oxford Press.

Lemonick, M. (2005). The biology of joy. *Time, 165*(3), A12–A14.

Levesque-Bristol, C., Knapp, T. D., & Fisher, B. J. (2010). The effectiveness of service-learning: It's not always what you think. *Journal of Experiential Education, 33*(3), 208–224. doi:10.5193/JEE33.3.208

Mood Disorders Society of Canada. (2009). Quick facts: Mental illness and addiction in Canada. Retrieved from: www.mooddisorderscanada.ca/documents/Media%20Room/Quick%20Facts%203rd%20Edition%20Referenced%20Plain%20Text.pdf

National Mental Health Association. (1988). *Mental health.* Alexandria, VA: National Mental Health Association, 3–4.

National Sleep Foundation. (2007). NSF's 2007 Sleep in America Poll: Stressed-out American women have no time for sleep. Retrieved from www.sleepfoundation.org

National Sleep Foundation. (2011). How much sleep do we really need? Retrieved from www.sleepfoundation.org/article/how-sleep-works/how-much-sleep-do-we-really-need

Nordqvist, J. (2012). What is rapid eye movement? *Medical News Today,* July 17, 2012. Retrieved from www.medicalnewstoday.com/articles/247927.php

O'Connell, A., & O'Connell, V. (1992). *Choice and change: Psychology of holistic growth, adjustment, and creativity.* Englewood Cliffs, NJ: Prentice Hall.

Pausch, R., & Zaslow, J. (2008). *The last lecture.* New York: Hyperion, 180.

Peterson, C., & Seligman, M. (2004). *Character strengths and virtues.* London: Oxford University Press.

Polzer Casarez, R. L., & Engebretson, J. C. (2012). Ethical issues of incorporating spiritual care into clinical practice. *Journal of Clinical Nursing, 21*, 2099–2107. doi:10.1111/j.1365-2702.2012.04168.x

Richardson, C. R., Faulkner, G., McDevitt, J., Skrinar, G. S., Hutchinson, D. S., & Piette, J. D. (2005). Integrating physical activity into mental health services for persons with serious mental illness. *Psychiatric Services, 56*(3), 324–331.

Ritter, C. (1988). Social supports, social networks, and health behaviors. In D. Gochman (Ed.). *Health behavior: Emerging research perspectives.* New York: Plenum.

Royal Commission on Aboriginal Peoples. (1995). *Special report on suicide among Aboriginal People.* Ottawa: Minister of Supply and Services.

Schlaepfer, T. E., & Nemeroff, C. B. (2012). *Neurobiology of psychiatric disorders.* Amsterdam, Netherlands: Elsevier.

Schmalz, D. L., Deane, G. D., Birch, L. L., & Krahnstoever Davison, K. (2007). A longitudinal assessment of the links between physical activity and self-esteem in early adolescent non-Hispanic females. *Journal of Adolescent Health, 41*(6), 559–565.

Segal, Z., et al. (2001). *Mindfulness-based cognitive therapy for depression: A new approach to preventing relapse*. New York: Guilford Publications.

Seligman, M. (1990). *Learned optimism*. New York: Knopf.

Statistics Canada. (2012). Suicides and suicide rate by age and sex group. Retrieved from www.statcan.gc.ca/tables-tableaux/sum-som/l01/cst01/hlth66a-eng.htm

Statistics Canada. (2013a). Canadian community health survey: Mental health, 2012. Retrieved from www23.statcan.gc.ca/imdb/p2SV.pl?Function=getSurvey&SDDS=5015

Statistics Canada. (2013b). Suicide prevention. Retrieved from http://hc-sc.gc.ca/fniah-spnia/promotion/suicide/index-eng.php

Statistics Canada. (2014a). Perceived mental health (very good or excellent). Retrieved from www.statcan.gc.ca/tables-tableaux/sum-som/l01/cst01/health111b-eng.htm

Statistics Canada. (2014b). Perceived mental health (fair or poor). Retrieved from www.statcan.gc.ca/tables-tableaux/sum-som/l01/cst01/health110d-eng.htm

Tacon, A. M., McComb, J., Caldera, Y., & Randolph, P. (2003). Mindfulness meditation, anxiety reduction, and heart disease: A pilot study. *Family and Community Health, 26*(1), 25–33.

The Free Dictionary by Farlex. (n.d.). Retrieved from http://medical-dictionary.thefreedictionary.com/psychoneuroimmunology

Thompson Rivers University. (2013). Spiritual health. Retrieved from www.tru.ca/wellness/spiritual.html

Weiss, M., Nordlie, J. W., & Siegel, E. P. (2005). Mindfulness-based stress reduction as an adjunct to outpatient psychotherapy. *Psychotherapy and Psychosomatics, 74*(2), 108–112.

Whalen, D. (n.d.). Seasonal affective disorder (SAD) prepared for the Canadian Mental Health Association. Retrieved from www.cmhanl.ca/pdf/Seasonal%20Affective%20Disorder%20(SAD)2.pdf

World Health Organization. (2013). Suicide prevention (SUPRE). Retrieved from www.who.int/mental_health/prevention/suicide/suicideprevent/en/

Yang, Y. C., Boen, C., Gerken, K., Li, T., Schorpp, K., & Mullan Harris, K. (2016). Social relationships and physiological determinants of longevity across the human life span. *Proceedings of the National Academy of Sciences*, 201511085. doi: 10.1073/pnas.1511085112

Zimbardo, P., Weber, A., & Johnson, R. (2000). *Psychology*. Boston: Allyn & Bacon, 403.

CHAPTER 3

Akhshabi, M., Khalatbari, J., Givarian, H., & Salehi, M. (2013). The relationship between identity components and hardiness among university students. *Life Science Journal, 10*(2s), 203–205.

Bressert, S. (2006). The impact of stress. Psychology Central. Retrieved from http://psychcentral.com/lib/2006/the-impact-of-stress/

Canadian Mental Health Association. (2009). Coping with stress. Retrieved from www.cmha.ca/bins/print_page.asp?cid=2-28-30&lang=1

Dold, C. (2004, May). The new yoga. *Health*, 73–77.

Dungy, T. (2010). *The mentor leader*. Carol Stream, IL: Tyndale House.

Eliot, R. (1984). *Is it worth dying for?* New York: Bantam Books, 225.

Eliot, R. (1994). *From Stress to Strength: How to Lighten Your Load and Save Your Life*. New York: Bantam Books.

Friedman, M., & Rosenman, R. H. (1974). *Type A behavior and your heart*. New York: Knopf.

Geukes, K., Mesagno, C., Hanrahan, S. J., & Kellmann, M. (2013). Performing under pressure in private: Activation of self-focus traits. *International Journal of Sport and ExercisePsychology, 11*, 11–23.

Holmes, T., & Rahe, R. (1967). The Social Readjustment Rating Scale. *Journal of Psychosocial Research, 11*, 213–217.

Hystad, S. W., Eid, J., & Laberg J. C. (2011). Psychological hardiness predicts admission into Norwegian military officer schools. *Military Psychology, 23*, 381–389.

Hystad, S. W., Eid, J., Laberg, J. C., Johnsen, B. H., & Bartone, P. T. (2009). Academic stress and health: Exploring the moderating role of personality. *Scandinavian Journal of Educational Research, 53*(5), 421–429.

Koolhaas, J. M., Bartolomucci, A., Buwalda, B., de Boer, S. F., Flügge, G., Korte, S. M., ... Fuchs, E. (2011). Stress revisited: A critical evaluation of the stress concept. *Neuroscience & Biobehavioral Reviews, 35*(5), 1291–1301.

Lazarus, R. (1985). The trivialization of distress. In J. Rosen & L. Solomon (Eds.), *Preventing health risk behaviors and promoting coping with illness*. Hanover, NH: University Press of New England, 279–298.

McKinnon, M. (2014). Canadian digital, social and mobile statistics on global scale. *Canadian Internet Business Newsletter*. http://canadiansinternet.com/canadian-digital-social-mobile-statistics-global-scale-2014/

Morris, C. (1993). *Understanding psychology*. Englewood Cliffs, NJ: Prentice Hall, 447–448.

Ragland, R., & Brand, R. (1989). Distrust, rage may be toxic: Cores that put type A person at risk. *Journal of the American Medical Association, 261*, 813, 814.

Selye, H. (1974). *Stress without distress*. New York: Lippincott, 28–29.

Shellenbarger, S. (2003). Multitasking makes you stupid: Studies show pitfalls of doing too much at once. *Wall Street Journal*, February 27, D1.

Tavakolia, M. (2010). A positive approach to stress, resistance, and organizational change. *Procedia - Social and Behavioral Sciences Volume 5*, 2010, 1794–1798.

The Free Dictionary by Farlex. (n.d.). Retrieved from www.thefreedictionary.com/psychoneuroimmunology

Trueba, A. F., & Ritz, T. (2013). Stress, asthma, and respiratory infections: Pathways involving airway immunology and microbial endocrinology. *Brain, Behavior, and Immunity, 29*, 11–27.

Ware, S. G., & Young, R. M. (2010). *Modeling narrative conflict to generate interesting stories*. Proceedings of the Sixth AAAI Conference on Artificial Intelligence and Interactive Digital Entertainment, 210–215.

Weil, M., & Rosen, L. (2004). Technostress: Are you a victim of technosis? Retrieved from www.technostress.com/tstechnosis.htm

Yan, B., & Zeng, Y. (2011). Design conflict: Conceptual structure and mathematical representation. *Journal of Integrated Design and Process Science, 15*(1), 7–89.

Zielinski, D. (2004). Techno-stressed? *Presentations, 18*(2), 28–34.

FOCUS ON SPIRITUAL HEALTH

Brantley, J. (2011). *Mindfulness, kindness, compassion and equanimity*. Retrieved from www.dukehealth.org/health_library/health_articles/mindfulnesskindnesscompassion

Chiesa, A., & Serretti, A. (2009). Mindfulness-based stress reduction for stress management in healthy people: A review and meta-analysis. *Journal of Alternative and Complementary Medicine, 15*(5), 593–600.

Cotton, S., Puchalski, C. M., Sherman, S. N., Mrus, J. M., Peterson, A. H., Feinberg, J., ... Tsevat, J. (2006). Spirituality and religion in patients with HIV/AIDS. *Journal of General Internal Medicine, 21*(S5), S1–S2.

Environmental Protection Agency (EPA). (2010). *Environmental stewardship*. Retrieved from www.epa.gov/stewardship

Franke, R., Ruiz, S., Sharkness, J., DeAngelo, L., & Pryor, J. P. (2010). *Findings from the 2009 Administration of the College Senior Survey (CSS): National Aggregates," Higher Education Research Institute*. Retrieved from www.heri.ucla.edu/publications-brp.php

Jahnke, R., Larkey, L., Rogers, C., Etnier, J., & Lin, F. (2010). A comprehensive review of health benefits of Qigong and Tai Chi. *American*

Journal of Health Promotion, 24(6), e1–e25. Retrieved from www.ncbi.nlm.nih.gov/pubmed/20594090

Koenig, H. G. (2008). *Medicine, religion and health: Where science and spirituality meet.* Philadelphia: Templeton Foundation Press.

National Cancer Institute (NCI). (2010). *Spirituality in cancer care.* Retrieved from www.cancer.gov/cancertopics/pdq/supportivecare/spirituality/patient

National Cancer Institute. (2011). *General information on spirituality.* Retrieved from www.cancer.gov/cancertopics/pdq/supportivecare/spirituality/Patient/page1

Oman, D., Shapiro, S., Thoreson, C., Plante, T., & Flinders, T. (2008). Meditation lowers stress and supports forgiveness among college students: A randomized controlled trial. *Journal of American College Health, 56*(5), 425–431.

Peterson, J. L., Johnson, M. A., & Tenzek, K. E. (2010). Spirituality as a life line: Women living with HIV/AIDS and the role of spirituality in their support system. *Journal of Interdisciplinary Feminist Thought, 4*(1).

Pew Research Center. (2008). *Pew forum on religion & public life, U.S. religious landscape survey religious beliefs and practices: Diverse and politically relevant.* Washington, DC. Retrieved from http://religions.pewforum.org/reports

Reese, H. (2011). Candle meditation. Retrieved from www.project-meditation.org/a_mt2/candle-meditation.html

Seaward, B. (2012). *Managing stress: Principles and strategies for health and well-being,* 7th ed. Sudbury, MA: Jones and Bartlett.

University of Maryland Medical Center. (2009). *Spirituality.* Retrieved from www.umm.edu/altmed/articles/spirituality-000360.htm

U.S. Department of Health and Human Services, National Institutes of Health, National Center for Complementary and Alternative Medicine. (NCCAM). (2009). Research spotlight: Meditation may increase empathy. Retrieved from http://nccam.nih.gov/research/results/spotlight/060608.htm

U.S. Department of Health and Human Services, National Institutes of Health, National Center for Complementary and Alternative Medicine. (2011). Exploring the science of complementary and alternative medicine: Third strategic plan: 2011–2015. *NIH Publication No. 11-7643, D458.* Retrieved from http://nccam.nih.gov/about/plans/2011/

Wells, R. E., Phillips, R. S., Schachter, S. C., & McCarthy, E. P. (2010). Complementary and alternative medicine use among U.S. adults with common neurological conditions. *Journal of Neurology, 257*(11), 1822–31. doi:10.1007/s00415-010-5616-2

Winter, U., Hauri, D., Huber, S., Jenewein, J., Schnyder, U., & Kraemer, B. (2009). The psychological outcome of religious coping with stressful life events in a Swiss sample of church attendees. *Psychotherapy and Psychosomatics, 78*(4), 240–244.

Zohar, D. (1997). *ReWiring the corporate brain: Using the new science to rethink how we structure and lead organizations.* San Francisco: Berrett Koehler.

CHAPTER 4

American Academy of Orthopedic Surgeons. (1991). *Athletic training and sports medicine,* 2nd ed. Park Ridge, IL, AAOS.

American Alliance for Health, Physical Education, Recreation and Dance. (1999). *Physical education for lifelong fitness: The physical best teacher's guide.* Champaign, IL: Human Kinetics, 78–79.

Andreoli, A., Celi, M., Volpe, S. L., Sorge, R., & Tarantino, U. (2012). Long-term effect of exercise on bone mineral density and body composition in post-menopausal ex-elite athletes: A retrospective study. *European Journal of Clinical Nutrition, 66,* 69–74. doi:10.1038/ejcn.2011.104

Batt, M. E. (2011). Medial tibial stress syndrome. *British Journal of Sports Medicine, 45*(2). doi:10.1136/bjsm.2010.081570.9

Bauer, U. E., Briss, P. A., Goodman, R.A., & Bowman, B. A. (2014). Prevention of chronic disease in the 21st century: Elimination of the leading preventable causes of premature death and disability in the USA. *The Lancet, 384*(9937), 45–52.

Behm, D. G., & Chaouchi, A. (2011). A review of the acute effects of static and dynamic stretching on performance. *European Journal of Applied Physiology, 111*(11), 2633–2651. doi: 10.1007/s00421-011-1879-2.

Behm, D. G., & Kibele, A. (2007). Effects of differing intensities of static stretching on jump performance. *European Journal of Applied Physiology, 101*(5), 587–594.

Biber Brewer, R., & Gregory, A. J. M. (2012). Chronic lower leg pain in athletes. *Sports Health, 4*(2), 121–127. doi: 10.1177/1941738111426115

Blair, S. N., Kohl III, H. W., Paffenbarger, R. S., Clark, D. G., Cooper, K. H., & Gibbons, L. W. (1989). Physical fitness and all-cause mortality: A prospective study of healthy men and women. *Journal of the American Medical Association, 262*(17), 2395–2401.

Bouchard, C., Shephard, R. J., Stephens, T., Sutton, J. R., & McPherson, B. D. (1988). Exercise, fitness, and health: The consensus statement. In C. Bouchard, R. J. Shephard, T. Stephens, J. R. Sutton & B. D. McPherson (Eds.). *Exercise, fitness, and health: A consensus of current knowledge.* Champaign, IL: Human Kinetics, 4–7.

Brody, D. M. (1987). Running injuries: Prevention and management. *Clinical Symposia, 39*(3), 1–36.

Canadian Broadcasting Corporation (CBC). (2015). Article, 15 September. Available at www.cbc.ca/news/canada/montreal/quebec-doctors-can-now-prescribe-exercise-1.3215821

Canadian Society for Exercise Physiology (CSEP). (2012a). *Canadian physical activity guidelines, Canadian sedentary behaviour guidelines.* Retrieved from www.csep.ca/cmfiles/guidelines/csep_guidelines_handbook.pdf

Canadian Society for Exercise Physiology (CSEP). (2012b). *Physical activity guidelines for special populations.* Retrieved from www.csep.ca/en/guidelines/physical-activity-guidelines-for-special-populations

Canadian Society for Exercise Physiology. (2003). *The Canadian physical activity, fitness & lifestyle approach (CPAFLA): CSEP health & fitness program's health-related appraisal and counselling strategy,* 3rd ed. Ottawa: Canadian Society for Exercise Physiology.

Cardoso Jr., C. G., Gomides, R. S., Queiroz, A. C. C., Pinto, L. G., da Silveira Lobo, F., Tinucci, T., ... de Moraes Forjaz, C. L. (2010). Acute and chronic effects of aerobic and resistance exercise on ambulatory blood pressure. *Clinics, 65*(3), 317–325. doi:10.1590/S1807-59322010000030001

Colley, R., Garriguet, D., Jannsen, I., Craig, C., Clarke, J., & Tremblay, M. (2011). Physical activity of Canadian children and youth: Accelerator results from the 2007 and 2009 Canadian health measures survey. *Statistics Canada, 22*(1), 15–23. Retrieved from www.ncbi.nlm.nih.gov/pubmed/21510586

Dunlop, J. W. C., Hartmann, M. A., Bréchet, Y. J., Fratzl, P., & Weinkamer, R. (2009). New suggestions for the mechanical control of bone remodeling. *Calcification Tissue International, 85*(1), 45–54.

Eichner, E. R. (1993, January). Infection, immunity, and exercise: What to tell patients? *Physician and Sportsmedicine,* 125–135.

Erie, J. C. (1991, November). Eye injuries: Prevention, evaluation, and treatment. *Physician and Sportsmedicine,* 108–122.

Ewing Garber, C., Blissmer, B., Deschenes, M. R., Franklin, B. A., Lamonte, M. J., Lee, I-M., ... Swain, D. P. (2011). Quantity and quality of exercise for developing and maintaining cardiorespiratory, musculoskeletal, and neuromotor fitness in apparently healthy adults: Guidance for prescribing exercise. *Medicine & Science in Sport & Exercise, 43*(7), 1334–1359.

Felson, D. T., Zhang, Y., Anthony, J. M., Naimark, A., & Anderson, J. J. (1992). Weight loss reduces the risk of symptomatic knee osteoarthritis in women: The Framingham Study. *Annals of Internal Medicine, 116,* 535–539.

Fox, E., Bowers, R., & Foss, M. (1989). *The physiological basis for exercise and sport.* Dubuque, IA: Brown and Benchmark.

Froehlich Chow, A. & Humbert, L. (2013). Perceptions of early years caregivers: Factors influencing the promotion of physical activity opportunities in rural care centres. *The International Society for Child Indicators. 7,* 57–73.

Garber, C. E., Blissmer, B., Deschenes, M. R., Franklin, B. A., Lamonte, M. J., Nieman, D. C., & Swain, D. P. (2011). American College of Sports Medicine position stand. Quantity and quality of exercise for developing and maintaining cardiorespiratory, musculoskeletal, and neuromotor fitness in apparently healthy adults: Guidance for prescribing exercise. *Medicine and Science in Sports and Exercise, 43*(7), 1334–1359. doi:10.1249/MSS.0b013e318213fefb

Gleeson, M. (2007). Immune function in sport and exercise. *Journal of Applied Physiology, 103*(2), 693–699.

Government of Canada. (2016). *Sedentary lifestyles contributing to sleep deprivation among children and youth.* Retrieved from http://news.gc.ca/web/article-en.do?nid=1085719&tp=1

Hafen, B. Q., & Karren, K. J. (1992). *Prehospital emergency care and crisis intervention,* 4th ed. Englewood Cliffs, NJ: Prentice-Hall.

Hallal, P. C., & Lee, I. (2013). Prescription of physical activity: an undervalued intervention. *The Lancet, 381*(9864), 356–357. http://dx.doi.org/10.1016/S0140-6736(12)61804-2.

Health Canada: Physical Activity Unit. (2004). Helpful definitions. Retrieved from www.hc-sc.gc.ca/hppb/fitness/definitions.html

Helmrich, S. P., Ragland, D. R., & Paffenbarger, Jr., R. S. (1994). Prevention of non-insulin-dependent diabetes mellitus with physical activity. *Medicine and Science in Sports and Exercise, 26,* 824–830.

Herzberg, G. R. (2004). Aerobic exercise, lipoproteins, and cardiovascular disease: Benefits and possible risks. *Canadian Journal of Applied Physiology, 2*(6), 800–807.

Hilliard-Robertson, P. C., Schneider, S. M., Bishop, S. L., & Guilliams, M. E. (2003). Strength gains following different combined concentric and eccentric exercise regimens. *Aviation, Space and Environmental Medicine, 74*(4), 342–347.

Hitchcock, H. (2011). How long does it take muscles to recover after training? Retrieved from www.livestrong.com/article/444183-how-long-does-it-take-muscles-to-recover-after-weight-training/

International Physical Literacy Association. (2015). Canada's physical literacy consensus statement. Retrieved from www.physicalliteracy.ca/sites/default/files/Consensus-Handout-EN-WEB_1.pdf

Kell, R. T., Bell, G., & Quinney, A. (2001). Musculoskeletal fitness, health outcomes, and quality of life. *Sports Medicine, 31*(12), 863–873.

Knuttgen, H. C., & Kraemer, W. J. (1987). Terminology and measurement in exercise performance. *Journal of Applied Sport Science Research, 1,* 1–10.

Kovar, P. A., Allegrante, J. P., MacKenzie, C. R., Peterson, M. G., Gutin, B., & Charlson, M. E. (1992). Supervised fitness walking in patients with osteoarthritis of the knee: A randomized, controlled trial. *Annals of Internal Medicine, 116,* 529–534.

Kraemer, W. J., & Ratamess, N. A. (2004). Fundamentals of resistance training: Progression and exercise prescription. *Medicine and Science in Sports and Exercise, 36*(4), 674–688.

Lewicki, R., Tchórzewski, H., Denys, A., Kowalska, M., & Golińska, A. (1987). Effect of physical exercise on some parameters of immunity in conditioned sportsmen. *International Journal of Sports Medicine, 08*(5), 309–314: doi:10.1055/s-2008-1025675

Lobelo, F., & de Quevedo, I. G. (2014). The evidence in support of physicians and health care providers as physical activity role models. *American Journal of Lifestyle Medicine, 1.*55982761352012E15. doi:10.1177/155982761352012.

Mackenzie, B. (2000). Training principles. Retrieved from www.brianmac.co.uk/trnprin.htm

Messier, S. P., Mihalko, S. L., Legault, C., Miller, G. D., Nicklas, B. J., DeVita, P., ... & Williamson, J. D. (2013). Effects of intensive diet and exercise on knee joint loads, inflammation, and clinical outcomes among overweight and obese adults with knee osteoarthritis: the IDEA randomized clinical trial. *Jama, 310*(12), 1263–1273.

Molloy, L. A. (2012). Managing chronic plantar fasciitis: When conservative strategies fail. *Journal of the American Academy of Physical Assistants.* Retrieved from http://journals.lww.com/jaapa/pages/default.aspx

Moreira, A., Delgado, L., Moreira, P., & Haahtela, T. (2009). Does exercise increase the risk of upper respiratory tract infections? *Oxford Journals Medicine British Medical Bulletin, 90*(1), 111–131.

Paffenbarger, R., Hyde, R., Wing, A., & Hsieh, C. (1986). Physical activity, all cause mortality, longevity of college alumni. *New England Journal of Medicine, 314,* 605–613.

Patel, A. V., Bernstein, L., Deka, A., Feigelson, H. S., Campbell, P. T., Gapstur, S.M., ..., & Thun, M.J. (2010). Leisure time spent sitting in relation to total mortality in a prospective cohort of US adults. *American Journal of Epidemiology, 172*(4), 419–429. doi: 10.1093/aje/kwq155.

Pelletier, C., Dai, S., Roberts, K. C., Bienek, A., Onysko, J., & Pelletier, L. (2012). Diabetes in Canada: Facts and figures from a public health perspective. *Chronic Diseases and Injuries in Canada, 33*(1), 53–54.

Powers, S. K., Dodd, S. L., Thompson, A. M., & Condon, C. C. (2006). *Total fitness and wellness,* Cdn. ed. Toronto: Pearson.

Quinn, E. (2013). Stretching and flexibility for sports: Learning the difference between flexibility stretching and warming up for sports. Retrieved from http://sportsmedicine.about.com/od/flexibilityandstretching/a/Flexibility.htm

Right to Play. (n.d.). *Sport and health: Preventing disease and promoting health.* Retrieved from www.righttoplay.com/canada/our-impact/Documents/Final_Report_Chapter_2.pdf

Robson-Ansley, P., Howatson, G., Tallent, J., Mitcheson, K., Walshe, I., Toms, C., ... Ansley, L. (2012). Prevalence of allergy and upper respiratory tract symptoms in runners of London marathon. Retrieved from www.setantacollege.com/wp-content/uploads/Journal_db/Prevalence%20of%20Allergy%20and%20Upper%20Respiratory%20Tract%20Symptoms.pdf

Roig, M., O'Brien, K., Kirk, G., Murray, R., McKinnon, P., Shadgan, B., & Reid, W. D. (2008). The effects of eccentric versus concentric resistance training on muscle strength and mass in healthy adults: A systematic review with meta-analysis. *British Journal of Sports Medicine, 43*(8), 556–568. doi:10.1136/bjsm.2008.051417

Sallis, R. (2015). Exercise is medicine: a call to action for physicians to assess and prescribe exercise. *The Physician and Sportsmedicine, 43*(1), 22–26.

Spence, J. C., & Humphries, B. (2001). The effect of resistance training on bone strength in women: A quantitative review. *Alberta Centre for Active Living, 8*(5). Retrieved from www.centre4activeliving.ca/publications/research-update/2001/sept-bone-strength.htm

Spence, J. C., Plotnikoff, R. C., & Mummery, W. K. (2002). The awareness and use of Canada's Physical Activity Guide to Healthy Living. *Canadian Journal of Public Health, 93*(5), 394–396.

Spence, J. C., Plotnikoff, R. C., Rovniak, L. S., Martin Glinis, K. A., Rodgers, W., & Lear, S. A. (2006). Perceived neighbourhood correlates of walking among participants vising the 'Canada on the Move' website. *Canadian Journal of Public Health, 97,* S39–S44.

Stamford, B. (1993, March). Tracking your heart rate for fitness. *Physician and Sportsmedicine, 21*(3), 227–228.

Statistics Canada. (2008). Physical activity level, changes between 1994/1995 and 2004/2005, by age group. Retrieved from www40.statcan.ca/cbin/fl/cstprintflag.gci

Statistics Canada. (2013). Directly measured physical activity of Canadian children and youth, 2012 and 2013. *Health Fact Sheet.* Statistics Canada Catalogue no. 82-625-X. www.statcan.gc.ca/pub/82-625-x/2013001/article/11807-eng.htm.

Stupar, M., Côté, P., French, M. R., & Hawker, G. A. (2010). The association between low back pain and osteoarthritis of the hip and knee: A population-based cohort study. *Journal of Manipulative and Physiological Therapeutics, 33*(5), 349–354.

Third Report of the National Cholesterol Education Program Expert Panel on Detection, Evaluation, and Treatment of High Blood Cholesterol in Adults. (2001). *Journal of the American Medical Association, 285*(19), 1–19.

Thompson, A. M., Campagna, P. D., Rehman, L. A., Murphy, R. J. L., Rasmussen, R. L., & Ness, G. W. (2005). Physical activity and body mass index in grade 3, 7, and 11 Nova Scotia students. *Medicine & Science in Sports & Exercise, 37*(11), 1902–1908.

Thompson, A. M., Humbert, M. L., & Mirwald, R. L. (2003). A longitudinal study of the impact of childhood and adolescent physical activity experiences on adult physical activity perceptions and behaviours. *Qualitative Health Research, 13*(3), 358–377.

Thompson, A. M., McHugh, T. L., Blanchard, C. M., Campagna, P. D., Durant, M. A., Murphy R. J. L., ... Wadsworth, L. A. (2009). Physical activity of children and youth in Nova Scotia from 2001/02 and 2005/06. *Preventive Medicine, 49,* 407–409.

Thompson, D. L. (2005). VO$_{2max}$: The basics: Part 1. *ACSM's Health & Fitness Journal, 9*(3), 5.

Thornton, J. S. (1990, January). Hypothermia shouldn't freeze out cold-weather athletes. *Physician and Sportsmedicine,* 109–113.

Tremblay, M. S., Warburton, D. E. R., Janssen, I., Paterson, D. H., Latimer, A. E., Rhodes, R. E., & Duggan, M. (2011). New Canadian physical activity guidelines. *Applied Physiology, Nutrition & Metabolism, 36,* 36–46.

Tudor-Locke, C. E., Bell, R. C., & Meyers, A. M. (2000). Revisiting the role of physical activity and exercise in the treatment of type II diabetes. *Canadian Journal of Applied Physiology, 25*(6), 466–492.

Vonhof, J. (2011). *Fixing your feet: Prevention and treatment for athletes,* 5th ed. Retrieved from http://books.google.ca/books?hl= en&lr=&id=7gpb8nlQjKkC&oi=fnd&pg=PP6&dq=In+addition,+it+is+ crucial+to+replace+footwear+regularly+(some+suggest+after+running+ approximately+1000+kilometres)+to+ensure+that+the+shock+ absorbency+is+still+effective.&ots=XUi-Dcd86Y&sig=WC0mp4J5_h- rU7-P4cdLeh5oNos#v=onepage&q&f=false

Warburton, D. E. R., Katzmarzyk, P. T., Rhodes, R. E., & Shephard, R. J. (2007). Evidence-informed physical activity guidelines for Canadian adults. *Canadian Journal of Public Health, 98,* S16–S68.

Warburton, D. E. R., Whitney Nicol, C., & Bredin, S. S. D. (2006a). Prescribing exercise as preventive therapy. *Canadian Medical Association Journal, 174*(7), 961–974. Erratum. (2008). *178*(6), 731–732.

Warburton, D. E. R., Whitney Nicol, C., & Bredin, S. S. D. (2006b). Health benefits of physical activity: The evidence. *Canadian Medical Association Journal, 174*(6), 801–809.

Wasserman, R. C., & Buccini, R. V. (1990). Helmet protection from head injuries among recreational bicyclists. *American Journal of Sports Medicine, 18,* 96–97.

Wood, P. D. (1994). Physical activity, diet, and health: Independent and interactive effects. *Medicine and Science in Sports and Exercise, 26,* 838–843.

World Health Organization. (2003). Health and development through physical activity and sport. WHO/NHM/NPH/PAH/O3.2. Geneva: WHO Document Production Services.

CHAPTER 5

Albanes, D. (2009). Vitamin supplements and cancer prevention: Where do randomized controlled trials stand? *Journal of the National Cancer Institute, 101*(2), 2–4.

American Dietetic Association. (n.d.). Retrieved from www.eatright.org

American Medical Association. (2004). Diagnosis and management of foodborne illness: A primer for physicians and other health care professionals. Retrieved from www.ama-assn.org/ama/org

Aristoy, M-C., & Toldra, F. (2012). *Handbook of analysis of active compounds in functional foods:* Chapter 1: Essential amino acids.

Retrieved from http://books.google.ca/books?hl=en&lr=&id= 9yLrG9OgfM8C&oi=fnd&pg=PA3&dq=essential+amino+acids&ots= S_buQuPXyf&sig=cwncmS6JUned_Qq2I64GPZP8RQw#v= onepage&q=essential%20amino%20acids&f=false

Bjelakovic, G., Nikolova, D., Gluud, L. L., Simonetti, R. G., & Gluud, C. (2007). Mortality in randomized trials of antioxidant supplements for primary and secondary prevention: Systematic review and meta-analysis. *Journal of the American Medical Association, 297*(8), 842–857.

Blanchflower, D. G., Oswald, A. J., & Stewart-Brown, S. (2012). Is psychological well-being linked to the consumption of fruits and vegetables? *Social Indicators Research.* doi:10.1007/s11205-012-0173-y

Boffetta, P., et al. (2010). Fruit and vegetable intake and overall cancer risk in the European Prospective Investigation into Cancer and Nutrition (EPIC). *Journal of the National Cancer Institute, 102*(8), 529–537.

Brandt, K., Leifert, C., Sanderson, R., & Seal, C. J. (2011). Agroecosystem management and nutritional quality of plant foods: the case of organic fruits and vegetables. *Critical Reviews in Plant Sciences,30*(1–2), 177–197.

Canadian Food Inspection Agency. (2012). Causes of food poisoning. Retrieved from www.inspection.gc.ca/food/information-for-consumers/fact-sheets/food-poisoning/eng/1331151916451/ 1331152055552

Centers for Disease Control and Prevention. (2002). Food borne illnesses. Retrieved from www.cdc.gov

Clarke, R., Halsey, J., Lewington, S., Lonn, E., Armitage, J., Manson, J. E., ... B-Vitamin Treatment Trialists' Collaboration. (2010). Effects of lowering homocysteine levels with B vitamins on cardiovascular disease, cancer, and cause-specific mortality: Meta-analysis of 8 randomized trials involving 37,485 individuals. *Archives of Internal Medicine,170,* 1622–1631.

Coghlan, A. (2010). Engineered maize toxicity claims roundly rebuffed. *New Scientist, 2744.*

Conrad, S. (n.d.). Current perspectives on understanding fat. *Fact Sheet for Canadian Council of Food and Nutrition.* Retrieved from www.cfcn.ca/ in_action/fact_sheets.asp

Cook, N. R., Albert, C. M., Gaziano, J. M., Zaharris, E., MacFadyen, J., Danielson, E., ... Manson, J. E. (2007). A randomized factorial trial of vitamins C and E and beta-carotene in the secondary prevention of cardiovascular events in women. *Archives of Internal Medicine, 167,* 1610–1618.

CSPI. (2012). Federal bill proposes to implement sodium reduction strategy for Canada. Retrieved from http://cspinet.org/canada/pdf/cspi. comment.sodiumreductiostrategyforcanadaact.pdf

Dietitians of Canada. (2006). Vitamin D—Many Canadians may not be getting enough. Retrieved from www.dietitians.ca/news/media

Dietitians of Canada. (2010). Food sources of iron. Retrieved from www.dietitians.ca/Nutrition-Resources-A-Z/Factsheets/Minerals/ Food-Sources-of-Iron.aspx

Dietitians of Canada. (2013). How to stay hydrated. Retrieved from www.dietitians.ca/Nutrition-Resources-A-Z/Factsheets/ Miscellaneous/Why-is-water-so-important-for-my-body— Know-when-.aspx

Dietitians of Canada. (2016). Hormones and antibiotics in food production. Retrieved from https://www.eatrightontario.ca/en/Articles/ Farming-Food-production/Hormones-and-antibiotics-in-food-production.aspx

Forge, F. (2004). Organic farming in Canada: An overview. Retrieved from www.parl.gc.ca/content/LOP/ResearchPublications/ prb0029-e.pdf

Garzon, D. L., Kempker, T., & Piel, P. (2011). Primary care management if food allergy and food intolerance. *The Nurse Practitioner: The American Journal of Primary Health Care, 36*(12), 34–40.

Haseen, F. M., Cantwell, M., O'Sullivan, J. M., & Murray, L. J. (2009). Is there a benefit from lycopene supplementation in men with prostate cancer? A systematic review. *Prostate Cancer Prostatic Disease, 12*(4), 325–332.

Health Canada. (2010). Food and nutrition, sodium reduction strategy for Canada. H164-121/2010E ISBN. Retrieved from www.hc-sc.gc.ca/fn-an/nutrition/sodium/related-info-connexe/strateg/reduct-strat-eng.php#a21

Health Canada. (n.d.a). Food and nutrition, Canada's food guides from 1942 to 1992. Retrieved from www.hc-sc.gc.ca/fn-an/food-guide-aliment/hist/fg_history-histoire_ga_e.html#process

Health Canada. (n.d.b). *Eating well with Canada's food guide.* Ottawa: Minister of Supply and Services, HC Pub: 4651; Cat. H164-38/1-2007E; ISBN: 0-662-44467-1. Retrieved from www.healthcanada.gc.ca/foodguide

Health Canada. (2015). Food and nutrition, trans fat. Retrieved from http://hc-sc.gc.ca/fn-an/nutrition/gras-trans-fats/index-eng.php

Institute of Medicine of the National Academies. (2005). Dietary, functional, and total fiber. *Dietary Reference Intakes for Energy, Carbohydrate, Fiber, Fat, Fatty Acids, Cholesterol, Protein, and Amino Acids.* Washington, DC: The National Academies Press, 2005, 339–421. Available at www.nap.edu/openbook.php?isbn=0309085373

Jatoi, A., Burch, P., Hillman, D., Vanyo, J. M., Dakhil, S., Nikcevich, D., ... North Central Cancer Treatment Group. (2007). A tomato-based, lycopene-containing intervention for androgen-independent prostate cancer: Results of a phase II study from the North Central Cancer Treatment Group. *Urology, 69,* 289–294.

Kang, J. H., & Grodstein, F. (2008). Plasma carotenoids and tocopherols and cognitive function: A prospective study. *Neurobiological Aging, 29*(9), 1394–1403.

Laidlaw, S. (2007, October). Growing interest in sports nutrition could fuel new market for milk. *Milk Producer,* 25–30.

Lin, J., Cook, N. R., Albert, C., Zaharris, E., Gaziano, J. M., Van Denburgh, M., ... Manson, J. E. (2009). Vitamins C and E and beta carotene supplementation and cancer risk: A randomized controlled trial. *Journal of the National Cancer Institute, 101*(1), 14–23.

Louis, P. F. (2012). Six signs you may have gluten sensitivity. Retrieved from www.naturalnews.com/038170_gluten_sensitivity_symptoms_intolerance.html

Mah, S. (n.d.). Current perspectives on trans fat. *Fact Sheet for Canadian Council of Food and Nutrition.* Retrieved from www.cfcn.ca/in_action/fact_sheets.asp

Malina, R. M., Bouchard, C., & Bar-Or, O. (2004). *Growth, maturation and physical activity,* 2nd ed. Champaign, IL: Human Kinetics.

Maughan, R. J., & Shirreffs, S. M. (2010). Development of hydration strategies to optimize performance for athletes in high-intensity sports and in sports with repeated intense efforts. *Scandinavian Journal of Medicine and Science in Sports, 20*(S2), 59.

Morris, P., Motarjemi, Y., & Kaferstein, F. (1997). Emerging food-borne diseases. *World Health, 50,* 16–22.

Parasuraman, R., & Venkat, K. K. (2010). Crystal-induced kidney disease in 2 kidney transplant recipients. *American Journal of Kidney Disease, 55*(1), 192–197. doi:10.1053/j.ajkd.2009.08.012.

RT Question More. (2013). US makes first step toward banning trans fat. Retrieved from http://rt.com/usa/trans-fat-ban-first-step-388/

Siekmeier, R., Steffen, C., & Marz, W. (2007). Role of oxidants and antioxidants in atherosclerosis: Results of in vitro and in vivo investigations. *Journal of Cardiovascular Pharmacology and Therapeutics, 12,* 265–262.

Slatore, C. G., Littman, A. J., Au, D. H., Satia, J. A., & White, E. (2008). Long-term use of supplemental multivitamins, vitamin C, vitamin E, and folate does not reduce the risk of lung cancer. *American Journal of Respiratory and Critical Care Medicine, 177,* 524–530.

Smith-Spangler, C., Brandeau, M. L., Hunter, G., E., Bavinger, J. C., Pearson, M., Eschback, P. J., ...Bravata, D. M. (2012). Are organic foods safer or healthier than conventional alternatives?A systematic review. *Annals of Internal Medicine,157*(5), 348–66. doi:10.7326/0003-4819-157-5-201209040-00009

Thompson, J., Manore, M., & Sheeska, J. (2007). *Nutrition: A functional approach,* Cdn. ed. Toronto: Pearson Benjamin Cummings.

Tremblay, A., & Chaput, J-P. (2008). About unsuspected potential determinants of obesity. *Applied Physiology, Nutrition, and Metabolism, 33*(4), 791–796.

Vatanparast, H., Dolega-Cieszkowski, J. H., & Whiting, S. J. (2009). Many adult Canadians are not meeting current calcium recommendations from food and supplement intake. *Applied Physiology, Nutrition, and Metabolism, 3*(2), 191–196.

World Cancer Research Fund/American Institute for Cancer Research. (2007). *Food, nutrition, physical activity, and the prevention of cancer: A global perspective.* Washington DC: AICR.

World Health Organization. (n.d.). 20 questions on genetically modified foods. Retrieved from www.iatp.org/files/20_Questions_on_Genetically_Modified_GM_Foods.htm

CHAPTER 6

Anonymous. (n.d.). Top 50 models. Retrieved from http://models.com/rankings/ui/Top50

Baker, S. T., Jerums, G., Prendergast, L. A., Panagiotopolous, S., Strauss, B. J., & Proietto, J. (2012). Less fat reduction per unit weight loss in type 2 diabetic compared with nondiabetic obese individuals completing a very-low-calorie diet program. *Metabolism, 61*(6), 873–882.

Bravata, D. M., Sanders, L., Huang, J., Krumholz, H.M., Olkin, I., Gardner, C. D., & Bravata D. M. (2003). Efficacy and safety of low-carbohydrate diets. *Journal of the American Medical Association, 289*(14), 1837–1850.

Brownell, K. (1993). Comments on the latest study on yo-yo diets by Steven N. Blair of the Institute for Aerobics Research in Dallas. Paper presented at the annual research meeting of the American Heart Association. Monterey, CA, January.

Bulimia Anorexia Nervosa Association (Canada). (n.d.). Retrieved from www.bana.ca

Colley, R., Garriguet, D., Jannsen, I., Craig, C., Clarke, J., & Tremblay, M. (2011). Physical activity of Canadian children and youth: Accelerator results from the 2007 and 2009 Canadian health measures survey. *Statistics Canada, 22*(1), 1–9.

Conner, W. E. & Conner, S. L., (2004). Should a low fat, high-carb diet be recommended for everyone? *New England Journal of Medicine, 350,* 1691–1692.

DeNoon, D. J. (2010). Sit at leisure, die at haste. *WebMD Health News,* July 23.

Durnin, J. V. G. A., & Womersley, J. (1974). Body fat assessed from total body density and its estimation from skinfold thickness: Measurements on 481 men and women aged from 16 to 72 years. *British Journal of Nutrition, 320,* 77–97.

Elmer-Dewitt, P. (1995). Fat times. *Time,* January 16, 60.

Flint, A. J., Rexrode, K. M., Hu, F. B., Glynn, R. J., Caspard, H., Manson, J. E., ... Rimm, E. B. (2010). Body mass index, waist circumference, and risk of coronary heart disease: A prospective study among men and women. *Obesity Research in Clinical Practice, 4*(3), e171–e181. doi:10.1016/j.orcp.2010.01.001

Foster, G. D., Wyatt, H. R., Hill, J. O., McGuckin, B. G., Brill, C., Mohammed, B. S., ... Klein, S. (2003). A randomized trial of low carbohydrate diet for obesity. *New England Journal of Medicine, 348*(21), 2082–2090.

French, S., & Jeffery, R. (1994). Consequences of dieting to lose weight: Effects on physical and mental health. *Health Psychology, 13*(3), 195–212.

Gronke, S., Muller, G., Hirsch, J., Fellert, S., Andreou, A., Haase, T., ... Kuhnlein, R. P. (2007). Dual lipolytic control of body fat storage and mobiliztion in drosophila. *PLoS Biology, 5*(6), e137. doi: 10.1371/journal.pbio.0050137

Hagobian, T. A., & Braun, B. (2010). Physical activity and the hormonal regulation of appetite: Sex differences and weight control. *Exercise and Sport Science Reviews, 38*(1), 25–30.

Harvard Women's Health Watch. (1996, May). Treating eating disorders. *Harvard Women's Health Watch*, 4–5.

Health Canada. (2003). *Canadian guidelines for body weight classifications in adults*. Retrieved from www.hc-sc.gc.ca/hpfb-dgpsa/onpp-bppn/weight_book_tc_e.html

Health Canada. (n.d.). *Eating well with Canada's food guide*. Ottawa: Minister of Supply and Services, HC Pub, 4651; Cat. H164-38/1-2007E; ISBN: 0-662-44467-1. Retrieved from www.healthcanada.gc.ca/foodguide

Hofker, M., & Wijmenga, C. (2009). A supersized list of obesity genes. *Nature Genetics, 41*(2), 139–140.

Horm, J., & Anderson, K. (1993). Who in America is trying to lose weight? *Annals of Internal Medicine, 119*, 672–676.

Hruschka, D. J., Brewis, A. A., Wutich, A., & Morin, B. (2011). Shared Norms and Their Explanation for the Social Clustering of Obesity. *American Journal of Public Health, 101*(S1), S295–S300.

Jackson, A. S., & Pollock, M. L. (1978). Generalized equations for predicting body density of men. *British Journal of Nutrition, 40*, 497–504.

Jackson, A. S., & Pollock, M. L. (1980). Generalized equations for predicting body density of women. *Medicine and Science in Sports and Exercise, 12*, 175–192.

Jacobs, E. J., Newton, C. C., Wang, Y., Patel, A. V., McCullough, M. L., Campbell, P. T., … Gapstur, S. M. (2010). Waist circumference and all-cause mortality in a large US cohort. *Archives of Internal Medicine, 170*(15), 1293–1301. doi:10.1001/archinternmed.2010.201

Jones, J. M., Bennett, S., Olmsted, M. P., Lawson, M. L., & Rodin. G. (2001). Disordered eating attitudes and behaviours in teenaged girls: A school-based study. *Canadian Medical Association Journal, 165*(5), 547–552.

Katzmarzyk, P. T. (2002). The Canadian obesity epidemic, 1985–1998. *Canadian Medical Association Journal, 166*(8), 1039–1040.

Kaye, W. H., Fudge, J. L., & Paulus, M. (2009). New insights into symptoms and neurocircuit function of anorexia nervosa. *Nature Reviews, 10*, 573–584.

Lichman, S., Pisarska, K., Berman, E. R., Pestone, M., Dowling, H., Offenbacker, E., …Heymsfield, S. B. (1992). Discrepancy between self-reported and actual caloric intake and exercise in obese subjects. *New England Journal of Medicine, 327*, 1894–1897.

Lissner, L., Odell, P., D'Agostino, R., Stokes, J., Kreger, B., Belanger, A., & Brownell, K. (1991). Variabilities in body weight and health outcomes in the Framingham study. *New England Journal of Medicine, 324*, 1839–1844.

Loos, L., & Bouchard, C. (2003). Obesity—Is it a genetic disorder? *Journal of Internal Medicine, 254*, 401–425.

Lydecker, J. A., Pisetsky, E. M., Mitchell, K. S., Thornton, L. M., Kendler, K. S., Reichborn-Kjennerud, T., … Mazzeo, S. E. (2012). Association between co-twin sex and eating disorders in opposite sex twin pairs: Evaluations in North American, Norwegian, and Swedish samples. *Journal of Psychosomatic Research, 72*(1), 73–77.

Malina, R. M., Bouchard, C., & Bar-Or, O. (2004). *Growth, maturation and physical activity*, 2nd ed. Champaign, IL: Human Kinetics.

Mayo Clinic. (2005). Special report: Weight control. Retrieved from www.mayoclinic.com

National Eating Disorder Information Centre. (2008). Help for family and friends. Retrieved from www.nedic.ca/giveandgethelp/helpforfriendsfamily.shtml

National Institutes of Health. (2008). Very low-calorie diets. Retrieved from http://win.niddk.nih.gov/publications/PDFs/verylowcaldietsbw.pdf

North American Association for the Study of Obesity (NAASO), The Obesity Society. (2007). *Obesity, bias, and stigmatization*. Retrieved from www.naaso.org/information/weight_bias.asp

Obesity Network of Canada. (2009). Obesity as a disability. Retrieved from http://www.obesitynetwork.ca/list.aspx?gp=32&list=66&item=322

Ontario Ministry of Health. (n.d.). Why exercise is vital to health. Retrieved from www.mhp.gov.on.ca/en/active-living/exercise.asp

Polotsky, A. J., & Santero, N. (2010). The role of body weight in menstrual disturbances and ammenorhea, Chapter 8. Retrieved from http://books.google.ca/books?hl=en&lr=&id=4836MLk-PoIYC&oi=fnd&pg=PA127&dq=amenorrhea+low+body+-fat&ots=3Wonwb1RDd&sig=xjatby8DZG3Aht_0xSgFMy-JTxPI#v=onepage&q=amenorrhea%20low%20body%20fat&f=false

Raftis, A. (2010). Anorexia nervosa in adolescence and adults – causes, consequences and methods of treatment. *Journal of the American College of Nutrition, 29*(4), 437.

Raine, K. D. (2005). Determinants of healthy eating in Canada: An overview and synthesis. *Canadian Journal of Public Health, 96*(3), S8–S14.

Rankinen, T., Zuberi, A., Chagnon, Y. C., Weisnagel, S. J., Argyropoulos, G., Walts, B., … Bouchard, C. (2006). The human obesity gene map: 2005 update. *Obesity, 14*, 529–644.

Reeder, B. A., Senthilselvan, A., Després, J-P., Angel, A., Liu, L., Wang, H., & Rabkin, S. W. (1997). The association of cardiovascular disease risk factors with abdominal obesity in Canada. *Canadian Medical Association Journal, 157*, S39–S45.

Robison, J., Hoerr, S. L., Strandmark, J., & Marvis, B. (1993). Obesity, weight loss, and health. *Journal of the American Dietetic Association, 93*, 448.

Samaha, F. F., Iqbal, N., Seshadri, P., Chicano, K. L., Daily, D. A., McGrory, J., … Stern, L. (2003). A low-carbohydrate as compared with a low-fat diet in severe obesity. *New England Journal of Medicine, 348*(21), 2074–2081.

Sloan, A., & Weir, J. (1970). Nomogram for prediction of body density and total fat from skinfold measurements. *Journal of Applied Physiology, 28*, 221–222.

Speakman, J. R., Levitsky, D. A., Allison, D. B., Bray, M. S., de Castro, J. M., Clegg, D. J., … Westerterp-Plantenga, M. S. (2011). Set points, settling points and some alternative models: Theoretical options to understand how genes and environments combine to regulate body adiposity. *Disease Models & Mechanisms, 4*, 733–745. doi:10.1242/dmm.008698

Statistics Canada. (2014a). Body mass index, overweight or obese, self-reported, adults by sex. CANSIM, table 105-0501 and Catalogue no. 82-221-X. Retrieved from www.statcan.gc.ca/tables-tableaux/sum-som/l01/cst01/health82b-eng.htm

Statistics Canada. (2014b). Body mass index, overweight or obese, self-reported, youth by sex. CANSIM, table 105-0501 and Catalogue no. 82-221-X. Retrieved from www.statcan.gc.ca/tables-tableaux/sum-som/l01/cst01/health83b-eng.htm

Stunkard, A. (1985). *Psychiatric update: American Psychiatric Association*. New York: Harper and Row, 87.

Thompson, J., Manore, M., & Sheeshka, J. (2007). *Nutrition: A functional approach*, Cdn. ed. Toronto: Pearson Benjamin Cummings.

Tremblay, A., & Chaput, J-P. (2008). About unsuspected potential determinants of obesity. *Applied Physiology, Nutrition, and Metabolism, 33*(4), 791–796.

Tremblay, M. S., & Willms, J. D. (2000). Secular trends in the body mass index of Canadian children. *Canadian Medical Association Journal, 163*, 1429–1433.

Wadsworth, L. A., & Berenbaum, S. (2001). Textual analyses of nutrition messages on prime time television. *Canadian Home Economics Journal, 51*, 13–18.

Wadsworth, L. A., & MacQuarrie, A. (2002). Nutrition messages on Saturday morning children's television: 1989–1998. *Canadian Journal of Dietetic Practice and Research, 63*, S105.

Wang, G-J., Geliebter, A., Volkow, N. D., Telang, F. W., Logan, J., Jayne, M. C., … Fowler, J. S. (2011). Enhanced striatal dopamine release during food stimulation in binge eating disorder. *Obesity, 19*(8), 1601–1608. doi:10.1038/oby.2011.27

Williams, D., Baskin, D., & Schwartz, M. (2006). Leptin regulation of anorexic responses to glucagon-like peptide-1 receptor stimulation. *Diabetes, 55*(12), 3387–3393.

Wilson, G. (1993). Relation of dieting and voluntary weight loss to psychological functioning and binge eating. *Annals of Internal Medicine, 119*, 727–730.

FOCUS ON BODY IMAGE

Ahmed, I., Genen, L., & Cook, T. (2010). Psychiatric manifestations of body dysmorphic disorder. *Medscape*. Retrieved from http://emedicine.medscape.com/article/291182-overview

American Psychiatric Association. (2010). *DSM-5 development: proposed revision: 307.1 Anorexia nervosa,* Updated October 2010. Retrieved from http://www.dsm5.org/ProposedRevisions/Pages/proposedrevision.aspx?rid=24

Beals, K., & Hill, A. (2006). The prevalence of disordered eating, menstrual dysfunction, and low bone mineral density among U.S. collegiate athletes. *International Journal of Sport Nutrition and Exercise Metabolism, 16*(3), 1–23.

Bratrud, S. R., Parmer, M. M., Whitehead, J. R., & Eklund, R. C. (2010). Social physique anxiety, physical self-perceptions and eating disorder risk: A two-sample study. *Pamukkale Journal of Sport Sciences, 1*(3), 1–10.

Eating Disorder Institute. (2009). *What are neurotransmitters and how do they influence the development of eating disorders?* Retrieved from www.eatingdisorder-institute.com/?tag=neurotransmitters

Feusner, J. D., Townsend, J., Bystritsky, A., McKinley, M., Moller, H., & Bookheimer, S. (2009). Regional brain volumes and symptom severity in body dysmorphic disorder. *Psychiatry Research, 172*(2), 161–167.

Fitzsimmons-Craft, E. E., Harney, M. B., Brownstone, L. M., Higgins, M. K., & Bardone-Cone, A. M. (2012). Examining social physique anxiety and disordered eating in college women. The roles of social comparison and body surveillance. *Appetite, 59*(3), 796–805. doi:10.1016/j.appet.2012.08.019

Forsberg, S., & Lock, J. (2006). The relationship between perfectionism, eating disorders and athletes: A review. *Minerva Pediatrica, 58*(6), 525–534.

Franco, K. N. (2011). *Cleveland Clinic Center for Continuing Education: Eating disorders.* Retrieved from www.clevelandclinicmeded.com/medicalpubs/diseasemanagement/psychiatry-psychology/eating-disorders

Guidi, J., Pender, M., Hollon, S. D., Zisook, S., Schwartz, F. H., Pedrelli, P., ... Petersen, T. J. (2009). The prevalence of compulsive eating and exercise among college students: An exploratory study. *Psychiatry Research, 165*(1–2), 154–162.

Mayo Clinic Staff. (2010). *Body dysmorphic disorder.* Retrieved from www.mayoclinic.com/health/body-dysmorphic-disorder/DS00559

Mirasol Eating Disorder Recovery Centers. (2010). *Eating disorder statistics.* Retrieved from www.mirasol.net/eating-disorders/information.php#statistics

Mülazimoğlu-Balli, O., Koka, C., & Aşçi, F. H. (2010). An examination of social physique anxiety with regard to sex and level of sport involvement. *Journal of Human Kinetics, 26*, 115–122.

National Alliance on Mental Illness. (2010). *Bulimia nervosa.* Retrieved from www.nami.org/template.cfm?Section=by_illness&template=/ContentManagement/ContentDisplay.cfm&ContentID=65839

National Association of Anorexia Nervosa and Associated Disorders. (n.d.). *Eating disorders: General information.* Retrieved from www.anad.org/get-information/about-eating-disorders/general-information

National Association of Anorexia Nervosa and Associated Disorders. (2011). *Binge eating disorder.* Retrieved from www.anad.org/get-information/about-eating-disorders/binge-eating-disorder/

Public Health Agency of Canada. (2011). What are eating disorders? *The Human Face of Mental Health and Mental Illness in Canada 2006.* Retrieved from www.phac-aspc.gc.ca/publicat/human-humain06/10-eng.php

Ronco, L. (2007). The female athlete triad: When women push their limits in high-performance sports. *American Fitness, 25*(2), 22–24.

Silverman, M. (n.d.). What is muscle dysmorphia? Massachusetts General Hospital. Retrieved from https://mghocd.org/what-is-muscle-dysmorphia

Statistics Canada. (2002). Mental health and well-being, Canadian Community Health Survey (CCHS), Cycle 1.2. Retrieved from www23.statcan.gc.ca/imdb-bmdi/document/3226_DLI_D1_T22_V2-eng.pdf

Statistics Canada. (2012). Overweight and obese adults (self-reported), 2011. Retrieved from www.statcan.gc.ca/pub/82-625-x/2012001/article/11664-eng.htm

Swami, V., Frederick, D. A., Aavik, T., Alcalay, L., Allik, J., Anderson, D., ...Zivcic-Becirevic, I. (2010). The attractive female body weight and female body dissatisfaction in 26 countries across 10 world regions: Results of the International Body Project I. *Personality and Social Psychology Bulletin, 36*(3), 309–325.

Thompson, A. M., & Chad, K. E. (2002). The relationship of social physique anxiety to risk for developing an eating disorder in young females. *Journal of Adolescent Health, 31*(2), 183–189.

Tylka T. L. (2013). Evidence for the Body Appreciation Scale's measurement equivalence/invariance between U.S. college women and men. *Body Image, 10*(3), 415–418. doi:10.1016/j.bodyim.2013.03.005

University of Kansas Student Health. (n.d.). *Body image myths and misconceptions.* Retrieved from http://hawkhealth.ku.edu/?q=node/20

University of the West of England. (2011). *30% of women would trade at least one year of their life to achieve their ideal body weight and shape.* Retrieved from http://info.uwe.ac.uk/news/UWENews/news.aspx?id=1949

Waldron, J. J. (2011). When building muscle turns into muscle dysmorphia. *Association for Applied Psychology.* Retrieved from http://appliedsportpsych.org/Resource-Center/health-and-fitness/articles/muscledysmorphia

Webb, J. B., Warren-Findlow, J., Chou, Y. Y., & Adams, L. (2013). Do you see what I see? An exploration of inter-ethnic ideal body size comparisons among college women. *Body Image, 10*(3), 369–739. doi:10.1016/j.bodyim.2013.03.005

Womenshealth.gov. (2009). Body image. Retrieved from www.womenshealth.gov/bodyimage/

CHAPTER 7

Acevedo, B. P., & Aron, A. (2009). Does a long-term relationship kill romantic love? *Review of General Psychology, 13*(1), 59–65. doi:10.1037/a0014226

Allahdadi, K. J., Tostes, R. C. A., & Webb, R. C. (2009). Female sexual dysfunction: Therapeutic options and experimental challenges. *Cardiovascular and Hematology Agents in Medical Chemistry, 7*(4), 260–269.

American Academy of Pediatrics. (2013). Different types of families: A portrait gallery. Retrieved from www.healthychildren.org/English/family-life/family-dynamics/types-of-families/Pages/Different-Types-of-Familes-A-Portrait-Gallery.aspx

Baron, R. A., & Byrne, D. (1994). *Social psychology.* Boston: Allyn & Bacon, 318.

Baskerville, T. A., & Douglas, A. J. (2010). Dopamine and oxytocin interactions underlying behaviors: Potential contributions to behavioral disorders. *CNS Neuroscience Therapy, 16*(3), e92–123. doi:10.1111/j.1755-5949.2010.00154.x

Brehm, S. S. (1992). *Intimate relationships.* New York: McGraw-Hill, 4–5.

Burggraf Torppa, C. (2010). Gender issues: Communication differences in interpersonal relationships, Family and Consumer Sciences, Ohio State University Extension. Retrieved from http://ohioline.osu.edu/flm02/pdf/fs04.pdf

Caputo, J., Hazel, H. C., & McMahon, C. (1994). *Interpersonal communication*. Boston: Allyn & Bacon, 224.

Clark, W., & Crompton, S. (n.d.). Till death do us part? The risk of first and second marriage dissolution. Retrieved from www.statcan.gc.ca/pub/11-008x/2006001/9198-eng.htm/

Comfort, A. (1972). *The joy of sex*. New York: Simon and Schuster, 14.

Common Law Relationships. (n.d.). Retrieved from www.commonlawrelationships.ca/

Darling, C., & Davidson, J. (1986). Enhancing relationships: Understanding the feminine mystique of pretending orgasm. *Journal of Sex and Marital Therapy, 12*(19), 182–196.

Dijkstra, P., Barelds, D. P. H., & Groothof, H. A. K. (2010). An inventory and update of jealousy-evoking partner behaviours in modern society. *Clinical Psychology & Psychotherapy, 17*(4), 329–345. doi:10.1002/cpp.668

Fisher, H. (1993). *Anatomy of love: The natural history of monogamy, adultery, and divorce*. New York: Norton.

Friedman, R., & Downey, J. (1994). Homosexuality. *New England Journal of Medicine, 33*, 923–928.

Furukawa, A. P., Patton, P. E., Amato, P., Li, H., & Leclair, C. M. (2012). Dyspareunia and sexual dysfunction in women seeking fertility treatment. *Fertility and Sterility, 98*(6), 1544–1548.e2. doi:10.1016/j.fertnstert.2012.08.011

Hatfield, E. (1988). Passionate and companionate love. In R. J. Sternberg & M. Barnes (Eds.), *The psychology of love*. New Haven: Yale University Press, 191–217.

Hatfield, E., Bensman, L., & Rapson, R. L. (2011). A brief history of social scientists' attempts to measure passionate love. *Journal of Personal and Social Relationships*. Retrieved from http://spr.sagepub.com/content/29/2/143.short

Herek, G. M., & McLemore, K. A. (2013). Sexual prejudice. *Annual Review of Psychology 64*, 309–333.

Hendricks, S., & Hendricks, C. (1992). *Liking, loving, and relating*, 2nd ed. Pacific Grove, CA: Brooks/Cole.

Kagerbauer, S. M., Martin, J., Schuster, T., Blobner, M., Kochs, E. F., & Landgraf, R. (2013). Plasma oxytocin and vasopressin do not predict neuropeptide concentrations in the human cerebrospinal fluid. *Journal of Neuroendocrinology, 25*(7), 668–673. doi:10.1111/jne.12038

Kippenberger, S., Havlíček, J., Bernd, A., Thaçi, D., Kaufmann, R., & Meissner, M. (2012). 'Nosing around' the human skin: What information is concealed in skin odour? *Experimental Dermatology, 21*(9), 655–659. doi:10.1111/j.1600-0625.2012.01545.x

Klausner, K., & Hasselbring, B. (1990). *Aching for love: The sexual drama of the adult child*. New York: Harper and Row.

Lassri, D., & Shahar, G. (2012). Self-criticism mediates the link between childhood emotional maltreatment and young adults' romantic relationships. *Journal of Social and Clinical Psychology, 31*(3), 289–311.

Malina, R. M., Bouchard, C., & Bar-Or, O. (2004). *Growth, maturation and physical activity*, 2nd ed. Champaign, IL: Human Kinetics.

Manusov, V., & Harvey, J. (Eds). (2001). *Attribution, communication behavior and close relationships*. New York: Cambridge University Press.

Martin, C. L., & Ruble, D. N. (2010). Patterns of gender development. *Annual Review of Psychology, 61*, 353–381. doi:10.1146/annurev.psych.093008.100511

MayoClinic.com. (2003). Nurture relationships: A healthy habit for healthy aging. *Mayo Foundation for Medical Education and Research* (MFMER). Retrieved from www.mayohealth.org

McIntyre, K. (2013). Happily married couples consider themselves healthier, says MU expert: Medical professionals should consider how marital quality affects patients' health. *University of Missouri, News Bureau*. Retrieved from http://munews.missouri.edu/news-releases/2013/0213-happily-married-couples-consider-themselves-healthier-says-mu-expert/

McLoughlin, C. (2003). Science of love—cupid's chemistry. *The Naked Scientists Online*. Retrieved from www.thenakedscientist.com/HTML/Columnists/clairemcloughlincolumn1.htm

Medline Plus. (2010). *Inhibited sexual desire*. Retrieved from www.nlm.nih.gov/medlineplus/ency/article/001952.htm

Moylan, C. A., Herrenkohl, T. I., Sousa, C., Tajima, E. A., Herrenkohl, R. C., & Russo, M. J. (2010). The effects of child abuse and exposure to domestic violence on adolescent internalizing and externalizing behavior problems. *Journal of Family Violence, 25*(1), 53–63.

National Cancer Institute. (n.d.). *Menopausal hormonal therapy and cancer*. Retrieved from www.cancer.gov/cancertopics/factsheet/Risk/menopausal-hormones

National Institute of Aging. (2008). *Health and aging: Menopause*. Retrieved from www.nia.nih.gov/health/publication/menopause

National Kidney and Urological Diseases Information Clearinghouse. (n.d.). *Erectile dysfunction*. Retrieved from http://kidney.niddk.nih.gov/kudiseases/pubs/impotence/index.htm

Options for Sexual Health. (2012). *Intimacy and relationships*. Retrieved from www.optionsforsexualhealth.org/sexual-health/sexuality/intimacy-and-relationships

Pfizer Labs. (2010). Viagra®. Retrieved from www.pfizer.com/files/products/uspi_viagra.pdf

Rosario, M. & Schrimshaw, E. (2014). Theories and etiologies of sexual orientation. *APA Handbook of Sexuality and Psychology 1*, 555–596.

Rowland, D., McMahon, C. G., Abdo, C., Chen, J., Jannini, E., Waldinger, M. D., & Young Ahn, T. (2010). Disorders of orgasm and ejaculation in men. *The Journal of Sexual Medicine, 7*(4), 1668–1686. doi:10.1111/j.1743-6109.2010.01782.x

Sairam, K., Kulinskaya, E., Hanbury, D., Boustead, G., & McNicholas, T. (2002). Oral sildenafil (Viagra) in male erectile dysfunction: Use, efficacy and safety profile in an unselected cohort presenting to a British district general hospital. *BioMedCentral, 18*, 2–4. Retrieved from www.ncbi.nlm.nih.gov/pubmed/12006106

Snapp, C., & Leary, M. (2001). Hurt feelings among new acquaintances: Moderating effects of interpersonal familiarity. *Journal of Social and Personal Relationships, 18*(3), 1344–1350.

Statistics Canada. (2002). Changing conjugal life in Canada. *The Daily*, July 11.

Statistics Canada. (2012). *Population by marital status and sex*. Retrieved from www.statcan.gc.ca/tables-tableaux/sum-som/l01/cst01/famil01-eng.htm

Tannen, D. (1990). *You just don't understand: Women and men in conversation*. New York: Ballantine.

Tennov, D. (1989). *Love and limerence*. Chelsea, MI: Scarborough House, 45–50.

The Canadian Encyclopedia. (2012). Marriage and divorce. Retrieved from www.thecanadianencyclopedia.com/articles/marriage-and-divorce

The Vanier Institute of the Family. (n.d.). *Our approach to family*. Retrieved from www.vanierinstitute.ca/definition_of_family

Toufexis, A., & Gray, P. (1993). What is love? The right chemistry. *Time*, 47–52.

Turner, J., & Rubinson, L. (1993). *Contemporary human sexuality*. Englewood Cliffs, NJ: Prentice Hall, 457.

Uberg, K. Goldstein, M., & Toro, P. (2005). Supportive relationships as a moderator of the effects of peer drinking on adolescents. *Journal of Research on Adolescents, 15*(1), 1–20.

White, A. M., Philogene, G. S., Fine, L., & Sinha, S. (2009). Social support and self-reported health status of older adults in the United States. *American Journal of Public Health, 99*(10), 1872–1878. doi:10.2105/AJPH.2008.146894

Whiteman, S. D., Becerra Bernard, J. M., & Jensen, A. C. (2010). *Sibling influence in human development*. New York, NY Springer Publishing. Retrieved from http://books.google.ca/books?hl=en&lr=&id=eJ3E03ShScsC&oi=fnd&pg=PR1&dq=sibling+development+implications+for+mental+health+practitioners&ots=-YtZ1HUhw_&sig=inRT2FUlmooq4tAm32dy_o_eqY4

CHAPTER 8

Bruner, B., Chad, K., & Chizen, D. (2006). Effects of exercise and nutritional counseling in women with polycystic ovary syndrome. *Applied Journal of Physiology, Nutrition, and Metabolism, 31*(4), 384–391.

Bulletti, C., Coccia, M. E., Battistoni, S., & Borini, A. (2010). Endometriosis and infertility. *Journal of Assisted Reproductive Genetics, 27,* 441–447. doi:10.1007/s10815-010-9436-1

Canadian Institute for Health Information. (2010). *Abortion in Canada.* Retrieved from http://abortionincanada.ca/stats/annual-abortion-rates/

Canadian Women's Health Network. (2013). *Polycistic ovary syndrome (PCOS).* Retrieved from www.cwhn.ca/en/node/44804

Centers for Disease Control and Prevention. (2011a). *Facts about Down syndrome.* Retrieved from www.cdc.gov/ncbddd/birthdefects/downsyndrome.html

Centers for Disease Control and Prevention. (2011b). *Pelvic inflammatory disease (PID) – CDC fact sheet.* Retrieved from www.cdc.gov/std/pid/stdfact-pid.htm

Chadwick, K. D., Burkman, R. T., Tornesi, B. M., & Mahadevan, B. (2011). Fifty years of "the pill": Risk reduction and discovery of benefits beyond contraception, reflections, and forecast. *Toxicological Science, 125*(1), 2–9. doi:10.1093/toxsci/kfr242

Chaillet, N., Dubé, E., Dugas, M., Francoeur, D., Dubé, J., Gagnon, S., & Dumont, A. (2007). Identifying barriers and facilitators towards implementing guidelines to reduce caesarean section rates in Quebec. *Bulletin of the World Health Organization, 85*(10), 733–820.

Childbirth by Choice Trust. (1995). *Abortion in Canada today: The situation province by province.* Retrieved from www.faslink.org/Childbirth%20By%20Choice%20Trust.htm

Cornell, C. (2011). The real cost of raising a child. *Money Sense Magazine.* Retrieved from www.moneysense.ca/2011/08/10/the-real-cost-of-raising-kids/

Davies, G. A. L., Wolfe, L. A., Mottola, M. F., & MacKinnon, C. (2003). Joint SOGC/CSEP clinical practice guideline: Exercise in pregnancy and the postpartum period. *Canadian Journal of Applied Physiology, 28*(3), 329–341. Retrieved from www.csep.ca/cmfiles/publications/scholarly/Joint_SOGC_CSEP_Guidelines.pdf

Government of Canada. (2013). *Infertility.* Retrieved from http://healthycanadians.gc.ca/health-sante/pregnancy-grossesse/fert-eng.php

Greydanus, D. E., & Shearin, R. B. (1990). *Adolescent sexuality and gynecology.* Philadelphia: Lea & Febiger, 107.

Harms, R. W. (2012). How long do sperm live after ejaculation? Retrieved from www.mayoclinic.com/health/pregnancy/AN00281

Hatcher, R., Trussell, J. Nelson, A. L., Cates Jr., W., Stewart, F., & Kowal, D. (2007). *Contraceptive technology,* 19th rev. ed. New York, NY: Contraceptive Technology Communications.

Human Resources and Skills Development Canada. (2012). *Parental leave.* Retrieved from www.hrsdc.gc.ca/eng/labour/employment_standards/federal/leave/maternity_types.shtml

Kong, A., Frigge, M. L., Masson, G., Besenbacher, S., Sulem, P., Magnusson, G., ... & Wong, W. S. (2012). Rate of de novo mutations and the importance of father/'s age to disease risk. *Nature, 488*(7412), 471–475.

Liao, P. V., & Dollin, J. (2012). Half a century of the oral contraceptive pill: Historical review and view to the future. *Canadian Family Physician, 58*(12), e757–e760.

Maguire, K., & Westhoff, C. (2011). The state of hormonal contraception today: Established and emerging noncontraceptive health benefits. *American Journal of Obstetrics & Gynecology. Supplement to October 2011,* S1–S8. Retrieved from www.musaeduca.cl/site/lib/revistas/Octubre2011/Thestateofhormonalcontraceptiontodayestablishedandemergingnoncontraceptivehealthbenefits.pdf

May, P. A., & Gossage, J. P. (n.d.). Maternal risk factors for fetal alcohol spectrum disorders: Not as simple as it might seem. *Alcohol Research &*

Health, 34(1). Retrieved from http://pubs.niaaa.nih.gov/publications/arh341/15-26.htm

MedlinePlus. (2013a). *Toxic shock sydrome.* Retrieved from www.nlm.nih.gov/medlineplus/ency/article/000653.htm

MedlinePlus. (2013b). *Miscarriage.* Retrieved from www.nlm.nih.gov/medlineplus/ency/article/001488.htm

Moschos, E., & Twickler, D. M. (2011). Intrauterine devices in early pregnancy: Findings on ultrasound and clinical outcomes. *American Journal of Obstetrics & Gynecology, 204*(427), e1–e6.

Mount Sinai Hospital. (n.d.). *Amniocentisis.* Retreived from www.mountsinai.on.ca/care/pdmg/tests/amnio

OvaScience. (2013). *About infertility.* Retrived from www.ovascience.com/technology/about-infertility.aspx

Planned Parenthood. (n.d.). Chronology of court cases: Dr. Morgentaler and others. Retrieved from http://girlsactionfoundation.ca/en/en/member/planned_parenthood_federation_canada

Planned Parenthood. (2013a). *Birth control pills.* Retrieved from www.plannedparenthood.org/health-topics/birth-control/birth-control-pill-4228.htm

Planned Parenthood. (2013b). *Morning-after pill (Emergency contraception).* Retrieved from www.plannedparenthood.org/health-topics/emergency-contraception-morning-after-pill-4363.asp

Planned Parenthood. (2013c). *IUD.* Retrieved from www.plannedparenthood.org/health-topics/birth-control/iud-4245.htm

Planned Parenthood. (2013d). *Temperature method.* Retrieved from www.plannedparenthood.org/health-topics/birth-control/temperature-method-22143.htm

Public Health Agency of Canada. (2009). *Breastfeeding and Infant Nutrition.* Retrieved from www.phac-aspc.gc.ca/hp-ps/dca-dea/stages-etapes/childhood-enfance_0-2/nutrition/

Public Health Agency of Canada. (2012). *Joint statement on safe sleep: Preventing sudden infant deaths in Canada.* Retrieved from www.phac-aspc.gc.ca/hp-ps/dca-dea/stages-etapes/childhood-enfance_0-2/sids/jsss-ecss-eng.php

Schmidt, K. (1992, December 14). The dark legacy of fatherhood. *U.S. News and World Report,* 94–95.

Sharpe, R. M. (2012). Sperm count and fertility in men: A rocky road ahead. *EMBO Reports,* 1–6. Retrieved from www.sciencemediacentre.org/wp-content/uploads/2012/12/Sharpe12-EMBO-Reports.pdf

Statistics Canada. (2009). *Live births and fetal deaths (stillbirths), by geography — Type of birth (single or multiple).* Retrieved from http://www.statcan.gc.ca/pub/84f0210x/2009000/t025-eng.pdf

Statistics Canada. (2012). *Infant mortality rates by province and territory (both sexes).* Retrieved from www.statcan.gc.ca/tables-tableaux/sum-som/l01/cst01/health21a-eng.htm

Statistics Canada. (2013). *Does Statistics Canada collect this information?* Retrieved from www.statcan.gc.ca/help-aide/collection-eng.htm

Sunnybrook and Women's Health Sciences Centre. (n.d.). Decision-making about unplanned pregnancy. *Sexual Health Centre.* Retrieved from www.womenshealthmatters.ca

U.S. Department of Health and Human Services. (1990). *The health benefits of smoking cessation: A report of the surgeon general.* Washington, DC: United States Public Health Service, Office on Smoking and Health.

FOCUS ON SEXUALLY TRANSMITTED INFECTIONS (STIs)

American College of Obstetricians and Gynecologists (ACOG). (2008). *How to prevent sexually transmitted diseases.* ACOG Education Pamphlet AP009. Washington, DC: American College of Obstetricians and

Gynecologists, 2008. Retrieved from www.acog.org/publications/patient_education/bp009.cfm

American Social Health Association. (2011). *Sexual health: prevention tips.* Retrieved from www.ashastd.org/sexualhealth/reduce_risk_prevention_tips.cfm

Centers for Disease Control and Prevention, Division of STD Prevention, National Center for HIV/AIDS, Viral Hepatitis, STD, and TB Prevention. (2010). *Sexually transmitted diseases surveillance, 2009: STDs in women and infants.* Retrieved from www.cdc.gov/std/stats09/womenandinf.htm

Centers for Disease Control and Prevention. (2011). *STD treatment guidelines 2010: Epididymitis.* Retrieved from www.cdc.gov/std/treatment/2010/epididymitis.htm

Kinstler, L. (2012). "Everyone's doing it": Defining campus hookup culture. *The Bowdoin Orient*, December 7, 2012. Retrieved from http://bowdoinorient.com/article/7821

MedlinePlus. (2011). Pelvic inflammatory disease (PID). Retrieved from www.nlm.nih.gov/medlineplus/ency/article/000888.htm

Public Health Agency of Canada. (2012). *STI and hepatitis C statistics.* Retrieved from www.phac-aspc.gc.ca/sti-its-surv-epi/surveillance-eng.php

Public Health Agency of Canada. (2013a). *Pelvic inflammatory disease (PID), Canadian guidelines on sexually transmitted infections—updated January 2010.* Retrieved from www.phac-aspc.gc.ca/std-mts/sti-its/cgsti-ldcits/section-4-4-eng.php

Public Health Agency of Canada. (2013b). *Epididymitis, Canadian guidelines on sexually transmitted infections—updated January 2010.* Retrieved from www.phac-aspc.gc.ca/std-mts/sti-its/cgsti-ldcits/section-4-2-eng.php

The Canadian Press. (2011). Sexually transmitted infections: Rates increase among universities-aged population. *The Huffington Post.* Retrieved from www.huffingtonpost.ca/2011/11/11/sexually-transmitted-infections-university-_n_1088144.html

U.S. National Library of Medicine. (2010, August). Epididymitis. Last review. Retrieved from www.ncbi.nlm.nih.gov/pubmedhealth/PMH0002258/

CHAPTER 9

Babor, T. F., Higgins-Biddle, J. C., Saunders, J. B., & Monteiro, M. G. (1993). *Alcohol use disorders identification test: Guidelines for use in primary care*, 2nd ed. World Health Organization. Retrieved from www.addictionsandrecovery.org/addiction-self-test.htm

Barrett, S. P., Meisner, J. R., & Stewart, S. H. (2008). What constitutes prescription drug misuse? Problems and pitfalls of current conceptualizations. *Current Drug Abuse Reviews, 1,* 255–262.

Boynton Health. (2016). *Alcohol, tobacco, and other drugs.* Retrieved from www.bhs.umn.edu/alcohol-drugs/absorption-rate-factors.htm

Canada.com. (n.d.). *Top 10 prescribed drugs in B.C.* Retrieved from www.canada.com/vancouversun/news/story.html?id=6be1752d-b5dd-4214-be9c-2bf5e228ed41

Canadian Centre on Substance Abuse. (2013). *First do no harm: Responding to Canada's prescription drug crisis.* Retrieved from www.ccsa.ca/Eng/Priorities/Prescription-Drug-Misuse/Canada-prescription-drug-strategy/Pages/default.aspx.

Canadian Institute for Health Information. (2012). Drug spending continues to slow. Retrieved from www.cihi.ca/cihi-ext-portal/internet/en/document/spending+and+health+workforce/spending/spending+by+category/release_03may12

Canadian Institute for Health Information. (2015). Canadians spent $28.8 billion on prescription drugs in 2014. https://www.cihi.ca/en/types-of-care/pharmaceutical-care-and-utilization/canadians-spent-288-billion-on-prescription-drugs

Canadian Partnership for Responsible Gambling. (2014). Canadian gambling digest 2012–2013. Retrieved from www.cprg.ca

Centre for Addiction and Mental Health. (2004). *What is OxyContin.* Retrieved from www.camh.net/About_Addiction_Mental_Health/Drug_and_Addiction_Information/oxycontin

Chan, N-L. (2013). Drug nutrient interactions. *Journal of Parenteral and Enteral Nutrition.* doi:10.1177/0148607113488799

CNN Health. (2012). *Experts: Alcohol enemas 'extremely dangerous.'* Retrieved from www.cnn.com/2012/09/26/health/alcohol-enemas/index.html

Cook, B., & Hausenblas, H. A. (2008). The role of exercise dependence for the relationship between exercise behavior and eating pathology: Mediator or moderator? *Journal of Health Psychology, 13*(4), 495–502.

Doweiko, H. F. (1993). *Concepts of chemical dependency.* Pacific Grove, CA: Brooks/Cole.

Fabian, T. (2013). Aging changes and pharmacotherapy principles. In M. D. Miller & L-K. K. Solai (Eds.), *Geriatric psychiatry.* Retrieved from http://books.google.ca/books?hl=en&lr=&id=mHM5QdFS5b-0C&oi=fnd&pg=PA79&dq=the+elderly+often+experience+more+-placebo+and+side+effects+with+their+prescription+and+over-the--counter+drug+use+than+other+populations&ots=wNNUkDzQb-c&sig=0yPgXoU0xDwJmQMlZQLprQJ8ies#v=onepage&q&f=false

Gambling as Addiction. (2005). Gambling as addiction. *Science, 307*(5708), 349. Retrieved from www.sciencemag.org/cgi/content/summary

Go Ask Alice. (n.d.). *Vodka tampons.* Retrieved from http://goaskalice.columbia.edu/vodka-tampons

Guzman, F. (2013). *Pharmacodynamics: Cross tolerance definition.* Retrieved from http://pharmacologycorner.com/pharmacodynamics-cross-tolerance-definition/

Hanson, G. R., Venturelli, P. J., & Fleckenstein, A. E. (2012). *Drugs and society*—11th ed. Retrieved from http://books.google.ca/books?id=HCvrhJuBuWAC&pg=PA613&lpg=PA613&dq=set+and+setting+definition+drugs&source=bl&ots=grMSdffr-fE&sig=6AK0P8BFlObxjW8VVntY0cZBNsI&hl=en&sa=X&ei=Nr2fUfWBFLOqyQG1r4AQ&ved=0CFcQ6AEwCTgK#v=onepage&q=set%20and%20setting%20definition%20drugs&f=false

Hoffinan, R. S., & Weinhouse, G. L. (2013). *Management of moderate and severe alcohol withdrawal symptoms.* Retrieved from www.uptodate.com/contents/management-of-moderate-and-severe-alcohol-withdrawal-syndromes

Johnson, V. (1986). *Intervention: Helping someone who doesn't want help.* Minneapolis, MN: Johnson Institute, 16–35.

Kerr, T., Small, W., Moore, D., & Wood, E. (2007). A micro-environmental intervention to reduce the harms associated with drug-related overdose: Evidence from the evaluation of Vancouver's Safer Injection Facility. *International Journal of Drug Policy, 18*(1), 37–45.

Kuhn, M. A. (2002). Herbal remedies, drug-herbal interactions. *Critical Care Nurse, 22*(2), 22–35.

LifeRing Canada. (2011). LifeRing: Alcohol and drug peer support groups. Retrieved from www.liferingcanada.org/philosophy-and-ideas

Marshall, K. (2011). Gambling 2011, Statistics Canada Catalogue no. 75-001-X: *Perspectives on Labour and Income.* Retrieved from www.statcan.gc.ca/pub/75-001-x/2011004/article/11551-eng.pdf

MedlinePlus. (2013). *Delirium tremens.* Retrieved from www.nlm.nih.gov/medlineplus/ency/article/000766.htm

Morrison, C., & Gore, H. (2010). The relationship between excessive Internet use and depression: A questionnaire-based study of 1,319 young people and adults. *Psychopathology, 43*(2), 121–126.

Nakken, C. (1988). *The addictive personality.* Center City, MN: Hazelden, 23.

National Institute of Drug Abuse. (2010). *Drugs, brain, and behavior: The science of addiction.* Retrieved from www.drugabuse.gov/publications/science-addiction/drugs-brain

Pharmainfo.net. (n.d.). Drug interactions—Antagonism. Retrieved from www.pharmainfo.net/vijayaratna/blog/drug-interactions-antagonism

Placebo Effect. (2012). *Placebo effect: A beginner's guide.* Retrieved from www.placeboeffect.com/placebo-effect/

Responsible Gambling Council, Canadian Partnership for Responsible Gambling. (2012). *Canadian Gambling Digest 2010–2011.* Retrieved from www.cprg.ca/articles/2010-11%20Canadian%20Gambling%20 Digest.pdf

Single, E., Rehm, J., Robson, L., & Truong, M. V. (2000). The relative risks and etiologic fractions of different causes of death and disease attributable to alcohol, tobacco, and illicit drug use in Canada. *Canadian Medical Association Journal, 162*(12), 1669–1675.

Sussman, S., & Sussman, A. N. (2011). Considering the definition of addiction. *International Journal of Environmental Research in Public Health, 8*(10), 4025–4038. doi:10.3390/ijerph8104025

The Annenburg Public Policy Center. (2005). Card playing trend in young people continues. *Press Release,* September 25, 2005. Retrieved from www.annenbergpublicpolicycenter.org

The Center for Internet Addiction. (2010). *The growing epidemic.* Retrieved from www.netaddiction.com

The Free Dictionary by Farlax. (n.d.). Retrieved from http://medical-dictionary.thefreedictionary.com/addiction

Turner, N. E., MacDonald, J., & Somerset, M. (2007). Life skills, mathematical reasoning and critical thinking: A curriculum for the prevention of problem gambling. *Journal of Gambling Studies, 24*(3), 367–380.

U.S. Food and Drug Administration. (2013). Combating misuse and abuse of prescription drugs: Q&A with Michael Klein, Ph.D. Retrieved from www.fda.gov/ForConsumers/ConsumerUpdates/ucm220112.htm

Vickers, A., Zollman, C., & Lee, R. (2001). Herbal medicine. *Western Journal of Medicine, 175*(2), 125–128. Retrieved from www.ncbi.nlm.nih.gov/pmc/articles/PMC1071505/

Welte, J. W., Barnes, G. M., Wieczorek, W. F., & Tidwell, M. C. (2004). Gambling participation and pathology in the United States. *Addictive Behaviors, 29*(5), 983–989.

CHAPTER 10

Abdelaziz, M. M., Kamalanathan, A. N., & John, C. M. (2011). Holiday heart syndrome. *Saudi Journal of Internal Medicine, 1*(2), 1432 H–2011 G.

Addiction Research Foundation. (n.d.). Statistical Information Service. Retrieved from www.camh.ca/en/hospital/about_camh/newsroom/for_reporters/Pages/addictionmentalhealthstatistics.aspx

Booyse, F. M., Pan, W., Grenett, H. E., Parks, D. A., Darley-Usmar, V. M., Bradley, K. M., & Tabengwa, E. M. (2007). Mechanism by which alcohol and wine polyphenols affect coronary heart disease risk. *Annals of Epidemiology, 17,* S24–S31.

Canadian Centre on Substance Abuse. (n.d.). *Canada's low risk drinking guidelines.* Retrieved from www.ccsa.ca/Eng/Priorities/Alcohol/Canada-Low-Risk-Alcohol-Drinking-Guidelines/Pages/default.aspx

Centre for Addiction and Mental Health. (2003). *Do you know … Alcohol, other drugs and driving.* Retrieved from www.camh.net/About_Addiction_Mental_Health/Drug_and_Addiction_Information/alchohol_drugs_driving_dyk.html.

Centre for Addiction and Mental Health. (2011). *Caffeine.* Retrieved from www.camh.ca/en/hospital/health_information/a_z_mental_health_and_addiction_information/Caffeine/Pages/default.aspx

Centre for Addiction and Mental Health. (2012). Do you know … Tobacco. Retrieved from www.camh.ca/en/hospital/health_information/a_z_mental_health_and_addiction_information/tobacco/Pages/tobacco_dyk.aspx

CNN Health. (2012). *Experts: Alcohol enemas 'extremely dangerous'.* Retrieved from www.cnn.com/2012/09/26/health/alcohol-enemas/index.html

Consumer Reports. (2012, December). The buzz on energy-drink caffeine: Caffeine levels per serving for the 27 products we checked ranged from 6 milligrams to 242 milligrams per serving. Retrieved from www.consumerreports.org/cro/magazine/2012/12/the-buzz-on-energy-drink-caffeine/index.htm#

CTV Montreal News. (2013). *Liquid rush: Do energy drinks pose a health risk?* Retrieved from http://montreal.ctvnews.ca/liquid-rush-do-energy-drinks-pose-a-health-risk-1.1196559

Davis, J. L. (2013). *Drink less for strong bones.* Retrieved from www.webmd.com/osteoporosis/features/alcohol

Flegal, K., MacDonald, N., & Hébert, P. C. (2011). Binge drinking: All too prevalent and hazardous. *Canadian Medical Association Journal, 183*(4), 411. doi:10.1503/cmaj.110029

Foxcroft, D. R., Ireland, D., Lister-Sharp, D. J., Lowe, G., & Breen, R. (2013). Longer-term primary prevention for alcohol misuse in young people: A systematic review. *Addiction, 98,* 397–411.

George, T. P. (2007). Alcohol use and misuse. *Canadian Medical Association Journal, 176*(5), 621–622.

Go Ask Alice. (n.d.). *Vodka tampons.* Retrieved from http://goaskalice.columbia.edu/vodka-tampons

Goldberg, I. J., Mosca, L., Piano, M. R., & Fisher, E. A. (2001). AHA science advisory: Wine and your heart: A science advisory for healthcare professionals from the Nutrition Committee, Council on Epidemiology and Prevention, and Council on Cardiovascular Nursing of the American Heart Association. *Circulation, 103,* 472–475.

Goodwin, F. K., & Gause, E. M. (1990). Alcohol, drug abuse, and mental health administration. *Prevention Pipeline, 3,* 19.

Graham, T. E., Battram, D. S., Deta., F., El-Sohemy, A., & Thong, F. S. L. (2008). Does caffeine alter muscle carbohydrate and fat metabolism during exercise? *Applied Physiology, Nutrition, and Metabolism, 33*(6), 1311–1318.

Handwerk, B. (2009). *Coffee may cause hallucinations.* Retrieved from http://news.nationalgeographic.com/news/2009/01/090114-caffeine-hallucinations.html

Health Canada. (2007). *Nicotine.* Retrieved from www.hc-sc.gc.ca/hc-ps/tobac-tabac/res/news-nouvelles/nicotine-eng.php

Health Canada. (2008). *Canadian addiction survey, a national survey of Canadians' use of alcohol and other drugs: Focus on gender.* Ottawa: Health Canada.

Health Canada. (2013). *Canada's low-risk alcohol drinking guidelines.* Canadian Centre on Substance Abuse. Retrieved from www.hc-sc.gc.ca/hc-ps/drugs-drogues/stat/_2012/summary-sommaire-eng.php#s7a

Hsu, C. (2012, August 16). Clubbers downing "Red Bull and Vodka" are 600% more likely to suffer heart palpitations, *Medical Daily.* Retrieved from www.medicaldaily.com/articles/11548/20120816/red-bull-alcohol-monster-energy-drinks-club-heart-palpitations.htm

Kinney, J., & Leaton, G. (1991). *Loosening the grip: A handbook of alcohol information,* 4th ed. St. Louis: Times Mirror/Mosby.

Lewis, M. A., Blayney, J. A., Lostutter, T. W., Granato, H., Kilmer, J. R., & Lee, C. M. (2011). They drink how much and where? Normative perceptions by drinking contexts and their association to college students' alcohol consumption. *Journal of the Study of Alcohol and Drugs, 72,* 844–853.

Mangat, D. (2011). *Drunkorexia: Dying to drink,* Retrieved from www.excal.on.ca/sportshealth/health/drunkorexia-dying-to-drink/

Mental Health Canada. (n.d.). *Children of alcoholics: Are they different?* Retrieved from www.mentalhealthcanada.com/article_detail.asp?lang=e&id=19

National Eating Disorder Association. (n.d.). NEDA, feeling hope. Retrieved from www.nationaleatingdisorders.org/

National Institute on Alcohol Abuse and Alcoholism. (2010). *Beyond hangovers: Understanding alcohol's impact on your health.* Retrieved from http://pubs.niaaa.nih.gov/publications/Hangovers/beyondHangovers.htm

National Library of Medicine. (2013). *Xanthine derivatives.* Retrieved from http://livertox.nlm.nih.gov/XanthineDerivatives.htm

O'Connor, A. M. (2006). Ottawa decision support framework to address decisional conflict. Retrieved from decisionaid.ohri.ca/docs/develop/odsf.Pdf

Perkinson, R. R. (2011). Type 1 and type 2 alcoholism. Retrieved from www.health.am/psy/more/type-1-and-type-2-alcoholism/

Public Health Agency of Canada. (2016). *The chief public health officer's report on the state of public health in Canada, 2015: Alcohol consumption in Canada.* Retrieved from http://healthycanadians.gc.ca/publications/department-ministere/state-public-health-alcohol-2015-etat-sante-publique-alcool/index-eng.php

quit 4 life. (n.d.). *Zyban (Buprorion) and varenicline (Champix') information sheets.* Southern Health, NHS Foundation Trust. Retrieved from www.quit4life.nhs.uk/Zyban_and_Champix_info_sheet.pdf

Ray, O. & Ksir, C. (1990). *Drugs, society, and human behavior.* St. Louis: Times Mirror/Mosby.

Rehm, J., Ballunas, D., Brochu, S., Fischer, B., Gnam, W., Patra, J., … Taylor, B. (2006). *The costs of substance abuse in Canada 2002.* Ottawa: Canadian Centre on Substance Abuse.

Reid, J. L., Hammond, D., Burkhalter, R., & Ahmed, R. (2012). *Tobacco use in Canada: Patterns and trends, 2012 edition.* Waterloo, ON: University of Waterloo, Propel Centre for Population Health Impact.

Sheps, S. G. (2012). *Does drinking alcohol affect your blood pressure?* Retrieved from www.mayoclinic.com/health/blood-pressure/AN00318

Sifferlin, A. (2013). What's in your energy drink? *Time.* Retrieved from healthland.time.com/2013/02/04/whats-in-your-energy-drink/

Single, E., Rehm, J., Robson, L., & Truong, M. V. (2000). The relative risks and etiologic fractions of different causes of death and disease attributable to alcohol, tobacco, and illicit drug use in Canada. *Canadian Medical Association Journal, 162*(12), 1669–1675.

Single, E., Robson, L., Xie, X., & Rehm, J. (1996). *The costs of substance abuse in Canada.* Ottawa: Canadian Centre on Substance Abuse.

Stade, B., Ungar, W. J., Stevens, B., Beyene, J., & Koren, G. (2006). The burden of prenatal exposure to alcohol: Measurement and cost. *Journal of Fetal Alcohol Syndrome International, 4*, 1–14.

Statistics Canada. (2011). Impaired driving in Canada, 2011. Retrieved from http://www.statcan.gc.ca/pub/85-002-x/2013001/article/11739-eng.htm

Statistics Canada. (2012a, March 26). Control and sale of alcoholic beverages. *The Daily.* Retrieved from www.statcan.gc.ca/daily-quotidien/150504/dq150504a-eng.htm

Statistics Canada. (2012b, July 25). Leading causes of death 2009. *The Daily.* Retrieved from http://www.statcan.gc.ca/daily-quotidien/120725/dq120725b-eng.pdf

Statistics Canada. (2012c, June 19). Canadian Community Health Survey, 2011. *The Daily.* Retrieved from http://www.statcan.gc.ca: Catalogue no. 11-001-X

Statistics Canada. (2013). Heavy Drinking. Retrieved from www.statcan.gc.ca/pub/82-625-x/2015001/article/14183-eng.htm

Statistics Canada. (2014a). Control and sale of alcoholic beverages, for the year ending March 31, 2014. Retrieved from www.statcan.gc.ca/daily-quotidien/150504/dq150504a-eng.htm

Statistics Canada. (2014b). Canadian Community Health Survey, 2014. Retrieved from http://www.statcan.gc.ca/pub/82-625-x/2015001/article/14190.htm#n3

Tamburri, R. (2012, August 29). Heavy drinking a problem at most Canadian campuses: Report. *University Affairs.* Retrieved from www.universityaffairs.ca/heavy-drinking-a-problem-at-most-canadian-campuses-report.aspx

Tarnopolsky, M. A. (2008). Effect of caffeine on the neuromuscular system—potential as an ergogenic aid. *Applied Physiology, Nutrition, and Metabolism, 33*(6), 1284–1289.

The Canadian Lung Association. (2012). *Smoking and tobacco: Secondhand smoke.* Retrieved from www.lung.ca/protect-protegez/tobacco-tabagisme/second-secondaire/index_e.php

Thompson, J., Manore, M., & Sheeska, J. (2007). *Nutrition: A functional approach,* Cdn. ed. Toronto: Pearson Benjamin Cummings.

Tunnicliffe, J. M., Erdman, K. A., Reimer, R. A., Lun, V., & Shearer, J. (2008). Consumption of dietary caffeine and coffee in physically active populations: Physiological interactions. *Applied Physiology, Nutrition, and Metabolism, 33*(6), 1301–1310.

Tunnicliffe, J. M., & Shearer, J. (2008). Coffee, glucose homeostasis, and insulin resistance: Physiological mechanisms and mediators. *Applied Physiology, Nutrition, and Metabolism, 33*(6), 1290–1300.

U.S. DHHS/Office on Smoking and Health. (1994). Psychological risk factors for initiating tobacco use. *Preventing Tobacco Use among Young People. A Report of the Surgeon General.* Atlanta: Author.

van Dam, R. M. (2008). Coffee consumption and risk of type 2 diabetes, cardiovascular disease, and cancer. *Applied Physiology, Nutrition, and Metabolism, 33*(6), 1269–1283.

Wagnerberger, S., Kanuri, G., & Bergheim, I. (2012). Alcohol drinking patterns and nutrition in alcoholic liver disease. In I. Shimizu (ed.) *Trends in alcoholic liver disease research—Clinical and scientific aspects.* Retrieved from http://cdn.intechopen.com/pdfs/25876/InTech-Alcohol_drinking_patterns_and_nutrition_in_alcoholic_liver_disease.pdf

World Health Organization. (2011). Alcohol. Retrieved from www.who.int/mediacentre/factsheets/fs349/en/index.html

World Health Organization. (2013). *Why tobacco is a public health priority.* Retrieved from www.who.int/tobacco/health_priority/en/

CHAPTER 11

Addiction Research Foundation. (1991). *Drug abuse update: Drugs and driving.* Spring.

Canadian Centre on Substance Abuse. (n.d.). Substance abuse policy in Canada, presentation to the House Standing Committee on Health. Retrieved from www.lop.parl.gc.ca/content/lop/researchpublications/942-e.htm

Canadian Centre on Substance Abuse and the Centre for Addiction and Mental Health. (2002). The first 20 years. Retrieved from www.ccsa.ca/Resource%20Library/ccsa0115362008.pdf

Canadian Foundation for Drug Policy. (1997). *Canada drug legislation update.* Ottawa: Author.

Canadian Public Health Association. (n.d.). *What is methadone and how does it work?* Retrieved from www.cpha.ca/en/portals/substance/prevention/faq05.aspx

Cas Palmera. (2010a). *Nicknames, street names and slang for methamphetamine.* Retrieved from http://casapalmera.com/nicknames-street-names-and-slang-for-methamphetamine/

Cas Palmera. (2010b). *Nicknames, street names and slang for heroine.* Retrieved from http://casapalmera.com/nicknames-street-names-and-slang-for-heroin/

Cas Palmera. (2010c). *Nicknames, street names and sang for ecstasy.* Retrieved from http://casapalmera.com/nicknames-street-names-and-slang-for-mdmaecstasy/

Cas Palmera. (2012). *Street names of cocaine.* Retrieved from http://casapalmera.com/street-names-of-cocaine/

Centre for Addiction and Mental Health (CAMH). (n.d.a). Do you know … Cocaine. Retrieved from www.camh.net/About_Addiction_Mental_Health/Drug_and_Addiction_Information/cocaine_dyk.html

Centre for Addiction and Mental Health. (n.d.b). Do you know … Ecstasy. Retrieved from http://www.camh.net/About_Addiction_Mental_Health/Drug_and_Addiction_Information/ecstasy_dyk.html

Centre for Addiction and Mental Health. (n.d.c). Do you know … Anabolic steroids. Retrieved from http://www.camh.net/About_Addiction_Mental_Health/Drug_and_Addiction_Information/anabolic_steroids_dyk.html

Centre for Addiction and Mental Health (CAMH). (2004). Do you know … Amphetamines. Retrieved from www.camh.net/About_Addiction_Mental_Health/Drug_and_Addiction_Information/amphetamines_dyk.html

Centre for Addiction and Mental Health (CAMH). (2005a). Do you know … Methamphetamines. Retrieved from www.camh.net/About_Addiction_Mental_Health/Drug_and_Addiction_Information/methamphetamine_dyk.html

Centre for Addiction and Mental Health (CAMH). (2005b). Do you know … Cannabis. Retrieved from www.camh.net/

About_Addiction_Mental_Health/Drug_and_Addiction_Information/cannabis_dyk.html

Centre for Addiction and Mental Health (CAMH). (2006). About cocaine. Retrieved from http://www.camh.ca/en/hospital/Documents/www.camh.net/About_Addiction_Mental_Health/Drug_and_Addiction_Information/about_cocaine.pdf

Day, A. M., Metrik, J., Spillane, N. S., & Kahler, C. W. (2013). Working memory and impulsivity predict marijuana-related problems among frequent users. *Drug and Alcohol Dependence, 131*(0), 171–174.

Drug Guide. (2013). *Morphine.* Retrieved from www.drugfree.org/drug-guide/morphine

Drug Library. (n.d.). *Mescaline.* Retrieved from www.druglibrary.eu/library/books/recreationaldrugs/mescaline.htm

Drug Overdose. (2013). *Ridding your vocabulary of codeine street names.* Retrieved from www.drug-overdose.com/codeine_street_names.htm

Foundation for a Drug-Free World. (2013). *The truth about LSD.* Retrieved from drugfreeworld.org/drugfacts/lsd/street-names-for-lsd.html

Health Canada. (2009a). *Health concerns: Cocaine and crack cocaine.* Retrieved from www.hc-sc.gc.ca/hc-ps/drugs-drogues/learn-renseigne/cocaine-eng.php#b

Health Canada. (2009b). *Psilocyben (magic mushrooms).* Retrieved from www.hc-sc.gc.ca/hc-ps/drugs-drogues/learn-renseigne/psilocybin-eng.php

Health Canada. (2009c). *Ecstasy.* Retrieved from www.hc-sc.gc.ca/hc-ps/drugs-drogues/learn-renseigne/ecstasy-eng.php

Health Canada. (2012). *Canadian alcohol and drug use monitoring survey.* Retrieved from www.hc-sc.gc.ca/hc-ps/drugs-drogues/stat/_2012/summary-sommaire-eng.php#s6

Health Canada. (2013). *Medical use of marihuana.* Retrieved from www.hc-sc.gc.ca/dhp-mps/marihuana/index-eng.php

HealthLinkBC. (2013). *Anabolic steroid use.* Retrieved from www.healthlinkbc.ca/kb/content/special/za1277.html

Hui, A. (2013). Canadian teens lead developed world in cannabis use: Unicef report. *Globe and Mail,* April 15, 2013. Retrieved from www.theglobeandmail.com/news/national/canadian-teens-lead-developed-world-in-cannabis-use-unicef-report/article11221668/

Mathias, R. (1996). Marijuana impairs driving-related skill and workplace performance. *NIDA Notes, 11*(1), 6.

McMillen, M. (2013). 'Bath salts' drug trend: Expert Q & A. *Mental Health Center.* Retrieved from www.webmd.com/mental-health/features/bath-salts-drug-dangers

National Institute on Drug Abuse. (1989). NIDA capsules: Designer drugs, *August,* 17–21.

Rhodes, T., Stoneman, A., Hope, V., Hunt, N., Martin, A., & Judd, A. (2006). Groin injecting in the context of crack cocaine and homelessness: From 'risk boundary' to 'acceptable risk.' *International Journal of Drug Policy, 17,* 164–170.

Statistics Canada. (2015). *Canadian tobacco, alcohol and drugs survey: Summary of results for 2013.* Ottawa, ON: Author. Retrieved from http://healthycanadians.gc.ca/science-research-sciences-recherches/data-donnees/ctads-ectad/summary-sommaire-2013-eng.php

Tropp Sneider, J., Gruber, S. A., Rogowska, J., Silveri, M. M., & Yurgelun-Todd, D. A. (2013). A preliminary study of functional brain activation among marijuana users during performance of a virtual maze task. *Journal of Addiction, Volume 2013,* Article ID 461029, 12 pages.

United Nations Office on Drugs and Crime (UNODC). (2012). World Drug Report 2012. Retrieved from www.unodc.org/unodc/en/data-and-analysis/WDR-2012.html

Vancouver Coastal Health. (n.d.). *Supervised injection sites.* Retrieved from http://supervisedinjection.vch.ca/home/

Visser, J. (2012). Highly addictive drug blamed for cannibal attack in Miami a growing threat in Maritime Canada. *The National Post,* May 30, 2012. Retrieved from http://news.nationalpost.com/2012/05/30/highly-addictive-drug-blamed-for-cannibal-like-attack-a-growing-threat-in-maritime-canada/

World Health Organization. (n.d.). *Other psychoactive substances.* Retrieved from www.who.int/substances_abuse/facts/psychoactives/en/print.html

Zilkowsky, D. (2001). Canada's National Drug Strategy. Forum on Correction Research: Focusing on Alcohol and Drugs. January 2001, *13*(3), 1–4. Retrieved from www.csc-scc.gc.ca/research/forum/e133/133a_e.pdf

FOCUS ON IMPROVING YOUR SLEEP

American Academy of Sleep Medicine. (2006). Narcolepsy. *AASM.* Retrieved from www.aasmnet.org/Resources/FactSheets/Narcolepsy.pdf

American Academy of Sleep Medicine. (2008). *A sleep study may be your best investment for long-term health.* Retrieved from www.sleepeducation.com/Article.aspx?id=1083

American College Health Association. (2011). *American College Health Association–National College Health Assessment II (ACHA–NCHA II): Reference group data report fall 2010.* Baltimore: American College Health Association.

Banks, S., & Dinges, D. F. (2007). Behavioral and physiological consequences of sleep restriction. *Journal of Clinical Sleep Medicine, 3*(5), 519–528.

Bear, M. F., Connors, B. W., & Paradiso, M. A. (2007). *Neuroscience: Exploring the brain,* 3rd ed. Baltimore: Lippincott Williams & Wilkins, 600.

Bollinger, T., Bollinger, A., Oster, H., & Scolbach, W. (2010). Sleep, immunity and circadian clocks: A mechanistic model. *Gerontology, 56*(6), 574–580. doi:10.1159/000281827

Canadian Association of College and University Student Services (CACUSS) and Canadian Mental Health Association British Columbia. (2013). Mental health and well-being in post-secondary education: A literature and environmental scan to support planning and action in Canada. Retrieved from www.cacuss.ca/about/currentProjects/MentalHealth_report.htm

Cappuccio, F., Cooper, D., Lanfranco, D., & Miller, M. (2011). Sleep duration predicts cardiovascular outcomes: A systematic review and meta-analysis of prospective studies. *European Heart Journal.* doi:10.1093/eurheart

Cappuccio, F. P., D'Elia, L., Strazzullo, P., & Miller, M. A. (2010). Quantity and quality of sleep and incidence of type 2 diabetes: A systematic review and meta-analysis. *Diabetes Care, 33*(2), 414–420. doi:10.2337/dc09-1124.

Cappuccio, F., Lanfranco, D., Strazzula, P., & Miller, M. A. (2010). Sleep duration and all-cause mortality: A systematic review and meta-analysis of prospective studies. *Sleep, 33*(5), 585–592.

Cappuccio, F. P., Taggart, F. M., Kandala, N. B., Currie, A., Peile, E., Stranges, S., & Miller, M. A. (2008). Meta-analysis of short sleep duration and obesity in children and adults. *Sleep, 31,* 619–626.

Centers for Disease Control and Prevention. (2012). Sleep and sleep disorders. Retrieved from www.cdc.gov/sleep/

Chen, J. C., Brunner, R. L., Ren, H., Wassertheil-Smoller, S., Larson, J. C., Levine, D. W., … Stefanick, M. L. (2008). Sleep duration and risk of ischemic stroke in postmenopausal women. *Stroke, 30*(12), 3185–3192.

Cohen, S., Doyle, W. J., Alper, C. M., Janicki-Deverts, D., & Turner, R. B. (2009). Sleep habits and susceptibility to the common cold. *Archives of Internal Medicine, 169*(1), 62–67.

Eichenbaum, H. (2007). To sleep, perchance to integrate. *Proceedings of the National Academy of Sciences of the United States of America, 104*(18), 7317–7318.

Ellenbogen, J. M., Hulbert, J. C., Jiang, Y., & Stickgold, R. (2009). The sleeping brain's influence on verbal memory: Boosting resistance to interference. *PLoS ONE, 4*(1), e4117.

Genzel, L., Dresler, M., Wehrle, R., Grözinger, M., & Steiger A. (2009). Slow wave sleep and REM sleep awakenings do not affect sleep dependent memory consolidation. *Sleep, 32*(3), 302–310.

Gregory, A. M., Rijsdijk, F. V., Lau, J. Y., Dahl, R. E., & Eley, T. C. (2009). The direction of longitudinal associations between sleep problems and depression symptoms: A study of twins aged 8 and 10 years. *Sleep, 32*(2), 189–199.

Hairston, K., Bryer-Ash, H., Norris, J., Haffner, S., Bowden, D. W., & Wagenknecht, L. E. (2010). Sleep duration and five-year fat accumulation in a minority cohort: The IRAS family study. *Sleep, 33*(3), 289–295.

Hasler, G. (2004). The association between short sleep duration and obesity in young adults: A 13 year prospective study. *Sleep, 27*, 661–665.

Lanfranchi, R., Prince, F., Filipini, D., & Carrier, J. (2010). Sleep deprivation increases blood pressure in healthy normotensive elderly and attenuates the blood pressure response to orthostatic challenges. *Sleep, 34*(3), 335–339.

Law, D. (2007). Exhaustion in university students and the effect of coursework involvement. *Journal of American College Health, 55*(4), 239–245.

National Institute of Neurological Disorders and Stroke. (2011). *Restless legs syndrome fact sheet.* Retrieved from: www.ninds.nih.gov/disorders/restless_legs/detail_restless_legs.htm

National Sleep Foundation. (n.d.). *Depression and sleep.* Retrieved from www.sleepfoundation.org/article/sleep-topics/depression-and-sleep

National Sleep Foundation. (2008). *Longer work days leave Americans nodding off on the job.* Press Release, March 3.

National Sleep Foundation. (2009). *Obesity and sleep.* Retrieved from: www.sleepfoundation.org/article/sleep-topics/obesity-and-sleep

National Sleep Foundation. (2010). *2010 sleep in America poll: Highlights and key findings.* Retrieved from www.sleepfoundation.org/sites/default/files/nsaw/NSF%20Sleep%20in%20%20America%20-Poll%20-%20Summary%20of%20Findings%20.pdf

National Sleep Foundation. (2011). Annual Sleep in America Poll Exploring Connections with Communications Technology Use and Sleep. Retrieved from www.sleepfoundation.org/media-center/press-release/annual-sleep-america-poll-exploring-connections-communications-technology-use-

Nielsen, L., Danielson, T., & Serensen, A. (2011). Short sleep duration as a possible cause of obesity: Critical analysis of the epidemiological evidence. *Obesity Reviews, 12*(2), 78–92.

Okun, M. L., Coussons-Read, M., & Hall, M. (2009). Disturbed sleep is associated with increased C-reactive protein in young women. *Brain, Behavior, and Immunity, 23*(3), 351–354.

Patel, S. R., Zhu, X., Storfer-Isser, A., Mehra, R., Jenny, N. S., Tracy, R., & Redline, S. (2009). Sleep duration and biomarkers of inflammation. *Sleep, 32*(2), 200–204.

Roth, T. (2004). Expert column—stress, anxiety, and insomnia: What every PCP should know. *Current Perspectives in Insomnia, 4.* Retrieved from http://cme.medscape.com

Sabanayagam, C., & Shankar, A. (2010). Sleep duration and cardiovascular disease: Results from the National Health Interview Survey. *Sleep, 33*(8), 1037–1042.

Sheth, B. R., Janvelyan, D., & Khan, M. (2008). Practice makes imperfect: Restorative effects of sleep on motor learning. *PLoS ONE, 3*(9), e3190.

Sleep Disorders Guide. (n.d.). *Sleep apnea statistics.* Retrieved from www.sleepdisordersguide.com/sleepapnea/sleep-apnea-statistics.html

Spiegel, K., Tasali, E., Penev, P., & Cauter, E. (2004). Brief communication: Sleep curtailment in healthy young men is associated with decreased leptin levels, elevated ghrelin levels, and increased hunger and appetite. *Annals of Internal Medicine, 141,* 846–850.

Thatcher, P. V. (2008). University students and the 'all-nighter': Correlates and patterns of students' engagement in a single night of total sleep deprivation. *Behavioral Sleep Medicine, 6*(1), 16–31.

Tracy, J. (2008, September 30). Colleges calling sleep a success prerequisite, *Boston Globe*, p. A1.

CHAPTER 12

Alberta Cancer Foundation. (2013). *The tomorrow project: Will you lend a hand to end cancer.* Retrieved from www.in4tomorrow.ca/

American Cancer Society. (1994). *Cancer facts and figures 1994.* Atlanta: American Cancer Society.

American Cancer Society. (2005). *Cancer facts and figures 2005.* Atlanta: American Cancer Society.

American Cancer Society. (2013). *Endometrial (uterine) cancer.* Retrieved from www.cancer.org/cancer/endometrialcancer/detailedguide/endometrial-uterine-cancer-risk-factors

Barrow, M. (1992). *Heart talk: Understanding cardiovascular diseases.* Gainsville, FL: Cor-Ed Publishing.

Bender, J. L., Hohenandel, J., Wong, J., Katz, J., Ferris, L. E., Shobbrook, C., ... Jadad, A. R. (2008). What patients with cancer want to know about pain: A qualitative study. *Journal of Pain Symptom Management, 35*(2), 177–187.

Bernstein, L., Henderson, B. E., Hanisch, R., Sullivan-Halley, J., & Ross, R. K. (1994). Physical exercise and reduced risk of breast cancer in young women. *Journal of the National Cancer Institute, 86*(18), 1403–1408.

Brinton, L. A., Richesson, D. A., Gierach, G. L., Lacey Jr, J. V., Park, Y., Hollenbeck, R. R., & Schatzkin, A. (2003). Prospective evaluation of risk factors for male breast cancer. *Journal of the National Cancer Institute, 100*(20), 1477–1481.

Calle, E. E., Rodriguez, C., Walker-Thurmond, K., & Thun, M. J. (2003). Overweight, obesity, and mortality from cancer in a prospectively studied cohort of U.S. adults. *New England Journal of Medicine, 348*(17), 1625–1638.

Canadian Cancer Society. (2008a). *Know your breasts and signs and symptoms of breast cancer.* Retrieved from www.cancer.ca/en/cancer-information/cancer-type/breast/signs-and-symptoms/?region=bc

Canadian Cancer Society. (2008b). *Four new genes for colorectal cancer identified.* Retrieved from www.cancer.ca/Canada-wide/About%20us/Media%20centre/CW-Media%20releases/CW

Canadian Cancer Society. (2012). *A pap test could save your life.* Retrieved from www.cancer.ca/~/media/cancer.ca/CW/publications/A%20pap%20test%20could%20save%20your%20life/Cervical-Pap-test-EN-Jul2012.pdf

Canadian Cancer Society. (2013a). *Human papilloma virus.* Retrieved from www.cancer.ca/en/cancer-information/cancer-101/what-is-a-risk-factor/viruses-bacteria-and-other-infectious-agents/hpv/?region=ns

Canadian Cancer Society. (2013b). *Risk factors for colorectal cancer.* Retrieved from www.cancer.ca/en/cancer-information/cancer-type/colorectal/risks/?region=on#Fibre

Canadian Cancer Society. (2013c). *Ovarian cancer statistics.* Retrieved from www.cancer.ca/en/cancer-information/cancer-type/ovarian/statistics/?region=on

Canadian Cancer Society. (2013d). *Signs and symptoms of leukemia.* Retrieved from www.cancer.ca/en/cancer-information/cancer-type/leukemia/signs-and-symptoms/?region=on

Canadian Cancer Society/National Cancer Institute of Canada. (2006). *Canadian cancer statistics 2006.* Toronto: CCS/NCIC.

Canadian Cancer Society's Steering Committee on Cancer Statistics. (2012). *Canadian cancer statistics 2012.* Toronto: Canadian Cancer Society.

Canadian Cancer Society's Steering Committee on Cancer Statistics. (2015). Canadian cancer statistics 2015. Toronto: Canadian Cancer

Society. Retrieved from www.cancer.ca/~/media/cancer.ca/CW/cancer%20information/cancer%20101/Canadian%20cancer%-20statistics/Canadian-Cancer-Statistics-2015-EN.pdf.

Canadian Cancer Statistics. (2015). Special topic: Predictions of the future burden of cancer in Canada. Retrieved from www.cancer.ca/~/media/cancer.ca/CW/cancer%20information/cancer%20101/Canadian%20cancer%20statistics/Canadian-Cancer-Statistics-2015-EN.pdf

Canadian Institute for Health Information. (2003). *Health care in Canada 2003.* Ottawa: Canadian Institute for Health Information.

Canadian Nuclear Safety Commission. (2013). *Radiation and incidence of cancer around Ontario nuclear power plants from 1990 to 2008 (The RADI-CON study).* Retrieved from www.nuclearsafety.gc.ca/eng/reading-room/healthstudies/radicon-study/index.cfm

Carolinas Medical Center Northeast. (2011). *Neurosciences/stroke.* Retrieved from www.carolinashealthcare.org/cmc-northeast-neurosciences-stroke

Centers for Disease Control and Prevention. (2013). *Stroke facts.* Retrieved from www.cdc.gov/stroke/facts.htm

Centers for Disease Control and Prevention. (2015). *High blood pressure facts.* Retrieved from www.cdc.gov/bloodpressure/facts.htm

Crane, T. E., Khulpateea, B. R., Alberts, D. S., Basen-Engquist, K., & Thomson, C. A. (2014). Dietary intake and ovarian cancer risk: A systematic review. *Cancer Epidemiology Biomarkers & Prevention, 23*(2), 255–273. JOUR. Retrieved from http://cebp.aacrjournals.org/content/23/2/255.abstract

Genest, J., McPherson, R., & Frohlich, J. (2009). Canadian Cancer Society/Canadian guidelines for the diagnosis and treatment of dyslipidemia and prevention of cardiovascular disease in the adult - 2009 recommendations. *Canadian Journal of Cardiology, 10*, 567–579.

Gilmour, H. (2008). Depression and risk of heart disease. Statistics Canada: Catalogue 82-003-XPE, *Health Reports, 19*(3).

Health Canada. (1997). *Heart disease and stroke in Canada, 1997, a report prepared in collaboration with Health Canada, the Laboratory Centre for Disease Control, Statistics Canada, and the University of Saskatchewan.* Ottawa: Heart and Stroke Foundation of Canada, June, 42.

Heart and Stroke Foundation. (2012). *Heart and Stroke Foundation warns: Too many Canadians risk death or disability by not calling 9-1-1 at the first sign of stroke.* Retrieved from http://www.heartandstroke.com/site/apps/nlnet/content2.aspx?b=3485819&c=ikIQLcMWJtE&ct=11782217

Heart and Stroke Foundation. (2008). Has election fever put you under pressure? World Heart Day is Sunday, September 28, press release, 2008. Retrieved from www.heartandstroke.com/site/apps/nlnet/content2.aspx?c=ikIQLcMWJtE&b=3485819&ct=5992163

Heart and Stroke Foundation. (2009). *Anatomy of the heart.* Retrieved from www.heartandstroke.com/site/c.ikIQLcMWJtE/b.3532069/k.4265/Heart_disease__Anatomy_of_the_Heart.htm

Heart and Stroke Foundation. (2011). *Atherosclerosis.* Retrieved from www.heartandstroke.com/site/c.ikIQLcMWJtE/b.3484059/k.2FED/Heart_disease__Atherosclerosis.htm

Heart and Stroke Foundation. (2012). *Getting your blood pressure in check.* Retrieved from www.heartandstroke.com/site/c.ikIQLcMWJtE/b.3484023/

Heart and Stroke Foundation. (2013). *Heart disease, stroke, and healthy living.* Retrieved from www.heartandstroke.com/site/c.ikIQLcMWJtE/b.2796497/k.BF8B/Home.htm

James, P., Oparil, S., Carter, B. L., Cushman, W. C., Dennison-Himmelfarb, C., Handler, J.... Narva, E. O. (2014). Evidence-based guideline for the management of high blood pressure in adults: Report from the panel members appointed to the eighth joint national committee (JNC 8). *Journal of American Medical Association, 311*(5), 507–20. doi:10.1001/jama213.284427

Knudson, A. G. (1986). Genetics of human cancer. *Annual Review of Genetics, 20*, 231–251.

Krontirus, T. G. (1983). The emerging genetics of human cancer. *New England Journal of Medicine, 309*, 404–409.

Mayo Clinic. (2012). *Arteriosclerosis/atherosclerosis.* Retrieved from www.mayoclinic.com/health/arteriosclerosis-atherosclerosis/DS00525/DSECTION=causes

Milan, A. (2011). *Mortality: Causes of death, 2007, Statistics Canada.* Retrieved from www.statcan.gc.ca/pub/91-209-x/2011001/article/11525-eng.htm

Mozaffarian, D., Benjamin, E. J., Go, A., S., Arnett, D. K., Blaha, M. J., Cushman, M.... Turner, M. B (2015). Heart disease and stroke statistics. *Centers for Disease Control and Prevention, High Blood Pressure Facts.* Retrieved from www.cdc.gov/bloodpressure/facts.htm

National Cancer Institute of Canada. (n.d.). *Breast cancer.* Retrieved from www.ncic.cancer.ca/About%20us20and%20news/Cancer%20statistics/Breast%20cancer

National Heart, Lung, and Blood Institute. (1995). *Heart memo: The cardiovascular health of women.* Bethesda, MD: NHLBI, 5.

Peto, J. (2001). Cancer epidemiology in the last century and next decade. *Nature, 411*, 390–395.

Public Health Agency of Canada. (2012). *Breast cancer.* Retrieved from www.phac-aspc.gc.ca/cd-mc/cancer/breast_cancer-cancer_du_sein-eng.php

Reeder, B. A., Senthilselvan, A., Després, J-P, Angel, A., Liu, L., Wang, H., & Rabkin, S. W. (1997). The association of cardiovascular disease risk factors with abdominal obesity in Canada. *Canadian Medical Association Journal, 157*, S39–S45.

Risch, H. A., Jain, M., Marrett, L. D., & Howe, G. R. (1994). Dietary fat intake and risk of epithelial ovarian cancer. *Journal of the National Cancer Institute, 86*(18), 1409–1415.

Rosendorf, C., Lackland, D. T., Allison, M., Aronow, W. S., Black, H. R., Blumenthal, R. S.... White, W. B. (2015). Treatment of hypertension in patients with coronary artery disease: a scientific statement from the American Heart Association, American College of Cardiology, and American Society of Hypertension. *Journal of the American College of Cardiology, 65*(18), 1998–2038.

Rutten-Jacobs, L. Arntz, R. M., Maaijwee, N. A., Schoonderwaldt, H. C., Dorresteijn, L. D., van Dijk, E. J., & de Leeuw, F. E. (2015). Cardiovascular disease is the main cause of long-term excess mortality after ischemic stroke in young adults. *Hypertension, 65*(3), 670–675.

Scott, S. (2007). Essential hypertension: Treatment without medications (Part 2 of 2). *ACSM's Health & Fitness Journal, 11*(8), 37–39.

Stanford School of Medicine. (2011). *Warning signs of stroke.* Retrieved from http://stanfordmedicine.org/about/

Statistics Canada. (2010). Heart health and cholesterol levels of Canadians, 2007 to 2009. Retrieved from www.statcan.gc.ca/pub/82-625-x/2010001/article/11136-eng.htm

Statistics Canada. (2012). *Leading causes of death, by sex (both sexes).* Retrieved from www.statcan.gc.ca/tables-tableaux/sum-som/l01/cst01/hlth36a-eng.htm

Statistics Canada. (2013). *High blood pressure, by age group and sex (percent).* Retrieved from www.statcan.gc.ca/tables-tableaux/sum-som/l01/cst01/health03b-eng.htm

Women's Heart Foundation. (2007). *Warning signs of stroke.* Retrieved from www.womensheart.org/content/Stroke/stroke_warning_signs.asp

World Cancer Research Fund/American Institute for Cancer Research. (2009). *Policy and action for cancer prevention. Food, nutrition, and physical activity: A global perspective.* Washington, DC: AICR.

World Health Organization. (2008). 10 facts on the global burden of disease. Retrieved from www.who.Int/features/factfiles/global_burden/en/index.html

World Health Organization. (2012). *Infections cause one in six of all cancers worldwide: IARC (International Agency for Research on Cancer).* Retrieved from www.iarc.fr/en/media-centre/iarcnews/pdf/TLO-INF-May2012-Eng.pdf

World Health Organization. (2013). *Cardiovascular diseases (CVDs)*. Retrieved from www.who.int/mediacentre/factsheets/fs317/en/index.html

CHAPTER 13

AIDS.GOV. (2012). *What is AIDS?* Retrieved from http://aids.gov/hiv-aids-basics/hiv-aids-101/what-is-hiv-aids/

Allen, J. (1994). Oh, my aching head. *Life*, 66–76.

Baker, L. J., & O'Brien, P. M. S. (2012). Potential strategies to avoid progestogen-induced premenstrual disorders. *Menopause International, 18*(2), 73–76. doi:10.1258/mi.2012.012016

BC Center for Disease Control. (2012). *Shingles*. Retrieved from www.bccdc.ca/dis-cond/a-z/_s/Shingles/default.htm

Canadian Cancer Society's Steering Committee on Cancer Statistics. (2012). *Canadian cancer statistics 2012*. Toronto, ON: Canadian Cancer Society.

Canadian Diabetes Association. (2012). *Diabetes and you*. Retrieved from www.diabetes.ca/diabetes-and-you/

Centers for Disease Control and Prevention. (n.d.). *Asthma's impact on the nation: Data from the CDC National Asthma Control Program*. Retrieved from www.cdc.gov/asthma/impacts_nation/AsthmaFactSheet.pdf

Crohn's and Colitis Foundation of Canada. (n.d.). *Ulcerative colitis*. Retrieved from www.ccfc.ca/site/c.ajIRK4NLLhJ0E/b.6349431/

Fields-Gardner, C., & Campa, A. (2010). American dietetics a position of the American Dietetic Association: Nutrition intervention and human immunodeficiency virus infection. *Journal of the American Dietetic Association, 110*(7), 1105–1119.

Health Canada. (n.d.a). *Sexual and reproductive health day*. Retrieved from www.hc-sclgclca/ahc-asc/minist/messages/2008_02_12-eng.php

Health Canada. (n.d.b). Canadian diabetes strategy. Retrieved from www.hc-sc.gc.ca/english/media/releases/1999/99135ebk3.htm

Health Canada. (1999). *Canadian sexually transmitted disease surveillance report*. Retrieved from www.publications.gc.ca/collections/collection_2016/aspc-phac/HP3-1-26-S6-eng.pdf

Health Canada. (2006). *Chlamydia*. Retrieved from www.hc-sc.gc.ca/hl-vs/iyh-vsv/diseases-maladies/chlamyd-eng.php

Health Canada. (2008). Seniors and aging—Osteoarthritis. Retrieved from www.hc-sc.gc.ca/hl-vs/iyh-vsv/diseases-maladies/seniors-aines-ost-art-eng.php

Health Canada. (2010). *Summary report on the findings of the oral health component of the Canadian health measures survey 2007–2009*. Retrieved from www.fptdwg.ca/assets/PDF/CHMS/CHMS-E-summ.pdf

Health Canada. (2011). Arthritis awareness month.Retrieved from www.hc-sc.gc.ca/ahc-asc/minist/messages/_2011/2011_09_01a-eng.php

Health Canada. (2012). Tuberculosis. Retrieved from www.hc-sc.gc.ca/hl-vs/iyh-vsv/diseases-maladies/tubercu-eng.php

HealthLinkBC. (2013). *Breast lumps*. Retrieved from www.healthlinkbc.ca/kb/content/special/hw51015spec.html

Kadian, S., & O'Brien, S. (2012). Classification of premenstrual disorders as proposed by the international society for premenstrual disorders. *Menopause International, 18*(2), 43-47. doi:10.1258/mi.2012.012017

Mayo Clinic. (2012). *Premenstrual syndrome: Causes*. Retrieved from www.mayoclinic.com/health/premenstrual-syndrome/DS00134/DSECTION=causes

MedicineNet.com. (n.d.). *Pubic lice (crabs)*. Retrieved from www.medicinenet.com/pubic_lice_crabs/article.htm

Montgomery, L. (n.d.). *Migraine*. Retrieved from http://prc.canadianpaincoalition.ca/en/migraine.html

National Headache Foundation (NFH). (2004). *NFH headache fact sheet*. Retrieved from www.headaches.org

National Institute of Allergy and Infectious Diseases. (2005). *HIV infection and AIDS: An overview*. Retrieved from www.niaid.nih.gov/factsheets/hivinf.htm

Nelson, K., Williams, C., & Graham, N. (2001). *Infectious disease epidemiology: Theory and practice*. Gaithersburg, MD: Aspen Publishers, 17–39.

Public Health Agency of Canada. (1996). *Canada communicable disease report, 22*(18).

Public Health Agency of Canada. (2011a). *Epstein-Barr virus, pathogen safety data sheet: Infectious substances*. Retrieved from www.phac-aspc.gc.ca/lab-bio/res/psds-ftss/epstein-barr-eng.php

Public Health Agency of Canada. (2011b). *Hepatitis B infection in Canada: Brief report*. Retrieved from www.phac-aspc.gc.ca/id-mi/hepatitisBCan-hepatiteBCan-eng.php

Public Health Agency of Canada. (2011c). *Reported cases and rates of gonorrhea by age group and sex, 1980 to 2009*. Retrieved from www.phac-aspc.gc.ca/std-mts/sti-its_tab/gonorrhea_pts-eng.php

Public Health Agency of Canada. (2011e). Diabetes in Canada: Facts and figures from a public health perspective. Retrieved from www.phac-aspc.gc.ca/cd-mc/publications/diabetes-diabete/facts-figures-faits-chiffres-2011/chap4-eng.php

Public Health Agency of Canada. (2012a). Vaccine Safety. Retrieved from www.phac-aspc.gc.ca/im/vs-sv

Public Health Agency of Canada. (2012b). *Mumps*. Retrieved from www.phac-aspc.gc.ca/im/vpd-mev/mumps-eng.php

Public Health Agency of Canada. (2012c). *Summary estimates of HIV prevalence and incidence in Canada, 2011*. Retrieved from www.phac-aspc.gc.ca/aids-sida/publication/survreport/estimat2011-eng.php

Public Health Agency of Canada. (2013a). *Asthma*. Retrieved from www.phac-aspc.gc.ca/cd-mc/crd-mrc/asthma-asthme-eng.php

Public Health Agency of Canada. (2013b). *Canadian guidelines on sexually transmitted infections—Updated January 2010*. Retrieved from www.phac-aspc.gc.ca/std-mts/sti-its/cgsti-ldcits/section-4-4-eng.php

Public Health Agency of Canada. (2013c). *Measles*. Retrieved from www.phac-aspc.gc.ca/im/vpd-mev/measles-rougeole-eng.php

Public Health Agency of Canada. (2015a). *Chlamydia and lymphogranuloma venereum in Canada: 2003–2012. Summary report*. Retrieved from www.phac-aspc.gc.ca/publicat/ccdr-rmtc/15vol41/dr-rm41-02/surv-1-eng.php

Public Health Agency of Canada. (2015b). *Gonorrhea in Canada: 2003–2012*. Retrieved from www.phac-aspc.gc.ca/publicat/ccdr-rmtc/15vol41/dr-rm41-02/surv-2-eng.php

Public Health Agency of Canada. (2015c). *Summary: Estimates of HIV incidence, prevalence and proportion undiagnosed in Canada, 2014*. Retrieved from http://healthycanadians.gc.ca/publications/diseases-conditions-maladies-affections/hiv-aids-estimates-2014-vih-sida-estimations/index-eng.php

Rotermann, M., Langlois, K. A., Severini, A., & Totten, S. (2013). Prevalence of chlamydia trachomatis and herpes simplex virus type 2: Results from the 2009 to 2011 Canadian health measures survey. Retrieved from www.statcan.gc.ca/pub/82-003-x/2013004/article/11777-eng.htm

Shulman, T., Phair, J., & Sommers, H. (1992). *The biological and clinical basis of infectious disease*. Philadelphia: W. B. Saunders.

Society of Obstetricians and Gynecologists of Canada (SOGC). (2008). Guidelines for the management of herpes simplex virus in pregnancy. *SOGC Clinical Practice Guideline*, No. 208. Retrieved from www.sogc.org/guidelines/documents/gui208CPG0806.pdf

Trubnikov, M., Yan, P., & Archibald, C. (2014). Estimated prevalence of hepatitis C virus infection in Canada, 2011. *Canada Communicable Disease Report, 40-19*. Available at www.phac-aspc.gc.ca/publicat/ccdr-rmtc/14vol40/dr-rm40-19/surveillance-b-eng.php

Wong, T., & Sutherland, D. (2002). Canadian STI national goals and phase specific strategies. *Sexually Transmitted Infections, 78*, i189–i190.

World Health Organization. (1999). *Report on infectious disease: Removing obstacles to health development*. World Health Organization. Retrieved from www.who.int/infectious-disease-report/index-rpt99.html

World Health Organization. (2013a). *Epilepsy*. Retrieved from www.who.int/topics/epilepsy/en/

World Health Organization. (2013b). *Headache disorders*. Retrieved from www.who.int/mediacentre/factsheets/fs277/en/

World Health Organization. (2015a). *Global tuberculosis report 2015*. Retrieved from www.who.int/tb/publications/global_report/gtbr2015_executive_summary.pdf

World Health Organization. (2015b). *HIV/AIDS*. Retrieved from www.who.int/mediacentre/factsheets/fs360/en/

World Health Organization. (2015c). *Measles*. Retrieved from www.who.int/mediacentre/factsheets/fs286/en/

FOCUS ON DIABETES

American Diabetes Association. (2010). *Top 10 benefits of being active*. Retrieved from www.diabetes.org/food-nutrition-lifestyle/fitness/fitness-management/top-10-benefits-being-active.jsp

American Heart Association. (2009). *Metabolic syndrome*. Retrieved from www.americanheart.org/presenter.jhtml?identifier=4756

Anderson, J. W., Baird, P., Davis, Jr., R. H., Ferreri, S., Knudtson, M., Koraym, A., . . . Williams, C. L. (2009). Health benefits of dietary fiber. *Nutrition Reviews, 67*(4), 188–205. doi:10.1111/j.1753-4887.2009.00189

Aronsohn, R. S., Whitmore, H., Van Cauter, E., & Tasali, E. (2010). Impact of untreated obstructive sleep apnea on glucose control in type 2 diabetes. *American Journal of Respiratory and Critical Care Medicine, 182*(2), 507–513. doi:10.1164/rccm.200909-1423OC

Brekke, H. K., Jansson, P. A., & Lenner, R. A. (2005). Long term effects of lifestyle intervention in type 2 diabetes relatives. *Diabetes Research and Clinical Practice, 70*, 225–234.

Cappuccio, F. P., D'Elia, L., Strazzullo, P., & Miller, M. A. (2010). Quantity and quality of sleep and incidence of type 2 diabetes: A systematic review and meta-analysis. *Diabetes Care, 33*(2), 414–420. doi:10.2337/dc09-1124.

Centers for Disease Control and Prevention. (2005). *National diabetes fact sheet: General information and national estimates on diabetes in the United States, 2005*. Atlanta: U.S. Department of Health and Human Services, Centers for Disease Control and Prevention.

Centers for Disease Control and Prevention. (2011). *National diabetes fact sheet: National estimates and general information on diabetes and prediabetes in the United States, 2011*. Atlanta: U.S. Department of Health and Human Services, Centers for Disease Control and Prevention.

Chita, Y., & Steptoe, A. (2010). Greater cardiovascular responses to laboratory mental stress are associated with poor subsequent cardiovascular risk status: A meta-analysis of prospective evidence. *Hypertension, 55*(4), 1026–1032. doi:10.1161/HypertensionAHA.1098.146621.

Das, U., & Rao, A. (2007). Gene expression profile in obesity and type 2 diabetes mellitus. *Lipids in Health and Disease, 6*, 35.

de Munter, J. S., Hu, F. B., Spiegelman, D., Franz, M., & van Dam, R. M. (2007). Whole grain, bran, and germ intake and risk of type 2 diabetes: A prospective cohort study and systematic review. *PLoS Medicine, 4*(8), e261.

Dedoussis, G. V., Kaliora, A. C., & Panagiotakos, D. B. (2007). Genes, diet, and type 2 diabetes mellitus: A review. *Review of Diabetic Studies, 4*(1), 13–24.

Fan, Y. et al. (2009). Dynamic changes in salivary cortisol and secretory immunoglobulin: A response to acute stress. *Stress and Health, 25*(2), 189–194.

Hall, M. H., Muldoon, M. F., Jennings, J. R., Buysse, D. J., Flory, J. D., & Manuck, S. B. (2008). Self-reported sleep duration is associated with the metabolic syndrome in midlife adults. *Sleep, 31*(5), 635–643.

Knutson, K. L., Spiegel, K., Penev, P., & van Cauter, E. (2007). The metabolic consequences of sleep deprivation. *Sleep Medicine Reviews, 11*(3), 163–178.

Kriska, A. M., Hawkins, M., & Richardson, C. R. (2008). Physical activity and the prevention of type II diabetes. *Current Sports Medicine Reports, 7*(4), 182–184.

Lankinen, M., Schwab, U., Erkkilä, A., Seppänen-Laakso, T., Hannila, M. L., Mussalo, H., . . . Oresic, M. (2009). Fatty fish intake decreases lipids related to inflammation and insulin signaling—a lipidomics approach. *PLoS One, 4*(4), e5258. doi:10.1371/journal.pone.0005258

Linus Pauling Institute. (2010). *Glycemic index and glycemic load*. Retrieved from http://lpi.oregonstate.edu/infocenter/foods/grains/gigl.html

National Heart Lung and Blood Institute. (2010). *What is metabolic syndrome?* Retrieved from www.nhlbi.nih.gov/health/dci/Diseases/ms/ms_whatis.html

National Institute of Diabetes and Digestive and Kidney Diseases. (2008). Diabetes prevention program. Retrieved from www.niddkrepository.org/studies/dppos/

New Mexico Health Care Takes on Diabetes. (2008). Pre-diabetes is a precursor to diabetes. *Diabetes Resources, 10*(2). Retrieved from http://nmtod.com/diabetesresources.html

Pouwer, F., Kupper, N., & Adriaanse, M. C. (2010). Does emotional stress cause type 2 diabetes mellitus? A review from the European Depression In Diabetes (EDID) Research Consortium. *Discovery Medicine, 9*(45), 112–118.

Puustinen, P., Koponen, H., Kautiainen, H., Mäntyselkä, P., & Vanhala, M. (2011). Psychological distress predicts the development of metabolic syndrome: A prospective population-based study. *Psychosomatic Medicine, 73*, 158–165. doi:10.1097/PSY.0b013e3182037315.

Statistics Canada. (2013). Diabetes by age group and sex (percent). Retrieved from www.statcan.gc.ca/tables-tableaux/sum-som/l01/cst01/health53b-eng.htm

Tremblay, M. S., Warburton, D. E. R., Janssen, I., Paterson, D. H., Latimer, A. E., Rhodes, R. E., & Duggan, M. (2011). New Canadian physical activity guidelines. *Applied Physiology, Nutrition & Metabolism, 36*, 36–46.

CHAPTER 14

Baan, R., Grosse, Y., Straif, K., Secretan, B., El Ghissassi, F., Bouvard, V., . . . Cogliano, V. (2009). A review of human carcinogens—Part F: Chemical agents and related occupations. *The Lancet Oncology, 10*(12), 1143–1144. Retrieved from www.thelancet.com/journals/lanonc/article/PIIS1470-2045(09)70358-4/fulltext.

Brook, B. (2012). Could nuclear fission energy etc., solve the green house problem? The affirmative case. *Energy Policy. 42*, 4–8.

Canadian Centre for Occupational Health and Safety. (2007). Noise: Non-auditory effects. Retrieved from www.ccohs.ca/oshanswers/phys_agents/non_auditory.html

Canadian Centre for Occupational Health and Safety. (2010). *Pesticides: Health effects*. Retrieved from www.ccohs.ca/oshanswers/chemicals/pesticides/health_effects.html

Canadian Centre for Occupational Health and Safety. (2011). Indoor air quality: General. Retrieved from www.ccohs.ca/oshanswers/chemicals/iaq_intro.html

Canadian Environmental Assessment Agency. (n.d.). *Introduction and features: Canadian environmental assessment act*. Retrieved from www.ceaa-acee.gc.ca/013/intro_e.htm.

Canadian Lung Association. (2012). *Pollution and air quality*. Retrieved from www.lung.ca/protect-protegez/pollution-pollution/outdoor-exterior/pollutants-polluants_e.php

Canadian Nuclear Association. (2009). *Nuclear facts: What about radiation is harmful?* Retrieved from www.cna.ca/wp-content/uploads/13-NuclearFacts-whataboutradiation.pdf

Caplan, R. (1990). *Our earth, ourselves*. New York: Bantam.

Environment Canada. (n.d.a). *Canadian environmental protection act, 1999 (CEPA, 1999)*. Retrieved from www.ec.gc.ca/CEPARegistry/the_act/

Environment Canada. (n.d.b). *Agreements*. Retrieved from www.ec.gc.ca/cleanair-airpur/Agreements-WS475C5F00-1_En.htm

Environment Canada. (n.d.c). *Canadian 1996 NOx/VOC Science assessment, executive summary*. Retrieved from www.ec.gc.ca/air/acid-rain_e.html

Environment Canada. (1995). *Toxic substances management policy*. Ottawa: Government of Canada.

Environment Canada. (2010). *Groundwater contamination*. Retrieved from www.ec.gc.ca/eau-water/default.asp?lang=En&n=6A7FB7B2-1#Sec2

Environment Canada. (2012). *Acid Rain*. Retrieved from www.ec.gc.ca/air/default.asp?lang=En&n=7E5E9F00-1

Flavin, C. (1990). Slowing global warming. In L. R. Brown, A. B. Durning, H. F. French, C. Flavin, J. L. Jacobson, M. D. Lowe, . . . J. E. Young (eds.). *State of the world*. Washington, DC: Worldwatch Institute.

French, H. F. (1990). Clearing the air. In L. R. Brown, A. B. Durning, H. F. French, C. Flavin, J. L. Jacobson, M. D. Lowe, . . . J. E. Young (eds.). *State of the world*. Washington, DC: Worldwatch Institute.

Griffin Jr., R. (1991). Introducing NPS water pollution. *EPA Journal, 17*, 6–9.

Haub, C., & Kaneda, T. (2014). 2014 World Population Data Sheet. Retrieved from www.prb.org/pdf14/2014-world-population-data-sheet_eng.pdf

Health Canada. (1997). *Health and environment handbook*. 125–126. Retrieved from http://publications.gc.ca/collections/Collection/H46-2-98-211E-4.pdf

Health Canada. (2009). *Food and nutrition: Environmental contaminants*. Retrieved from www.hc-sc.gc.ca/fn-an/securit/chem-chim/environ/index-eng.php

Health Canada. (2012). *Formaldehyde*. Retrieved from www.hc-sc.gc.ca/ewh-semt/air/in/poll/construction/formaldehyde-eng.php#a2

Health Canada. (2013). *Lead and human health*. Retrieved from www.hc-sc.gc.ca/hl-vs/iyh-vsv/environ/lead-plomb-eng.php#a2

Moeller, D. W. (1992). *Environmental health*. Cambridge, MA: Harvard University Press, 31.

Nadakavukaren, A. (1990). *Man and environment: A health perspective*. Prospect Heights, IL: Waveland, 412–414.

Statistics Canada. (2012). Deaths. *The Daily*, Thursday, May 31, 2012. Retrieved from www.statcan.gc.ca/daily-quotidien/120531/dq120531e-eng.htm

Thompson, L., El-Solh, S., & McGuire, O. (2006). *Benzene in Canadian gasoline: Report on the effect of the benzene in gasoline regulations 2006*. Retrieved from www.ec.gc.ca/cleanair-airpur/caol/OGEB/bnz06_eng.html

U.S. Environmental Protection Agency. (2002). *The inside story: A guide to indoor air quality*. EPA Document # 402-K-93-007. Retrieved from http://epa.gov/iaq/pubs/insdet.html

U.S. Environmental Protection Agency. (2007). *Chloroform*. Retrieved from www.epa.gov/ttnatw01/hlthef/chlorofo.html

U.S. Environmental Protection Agency. (2012). Effects of acid rain— Human health. Retrieved from www.epa.gov/acidrain/effects/health.html

World Health Organization. (n.d.a). *Public health and the environment: Health through a better environment*. Retrieved from www.who.int/phe/en/

World Health Organization. (n.d.b). *10 facts on preventing disease through healthy environments*. Retrieved from www.who.int/features/factfiles/environmental_health/environmental_health_facts/en/index.html

World Health Organization. (2002). Polychlorinated dibenzodioxins, polychlorinated dibenzofurans, and coplanar polychlorinated biphenyls. In *Safety evaluation of certain food additives and contaminants*. Geneva: World Health Organization WHO Food Additives Series, No. 48. Available at www.inchem.org/documents/jecfa/jecmono/v48je20.htm).

World Health Organization. (2003). *Polychlorinated biphenyls: Human health aspects*. Geneva: World Health Organization, International Programme on Chemical Safety. Concise International Chemical Assessment Document 55. Available at www.inchem.org/documents/cicads/cicads/cicad55.htm

World Health Organization. (2009a). *World population prospects: The 2008 Revision*. Retrieved from www.who.int/pmnch/topics/2008_populationstats/en/

World Health Organization. (2009b). *10 facts about water scarcity*. Retrieved from www.who.int/features/factfiles/water/en/

World Health Organization. (2013b). *Children's environmental health, air pollution*. Retrieved from www.who.int/ceh/risks/cehair/en/

World Health Organization. (2013c). Q&As: Environmental health. Retrieved from www.who.int/topics/environmental_health/qa/en/index.html

World Health Organization. (2014). Dioxins and their effect on human health. Retrieved from www.who.int/mediacentre/factsheets/fs225/en/

CHAPTER 15

Alam, S. (2014). Youth court statistics in Canada 2013-2014. *Canadian Centre for Justice Statistics*. Retrieved from http://www.statcan.gc.ca/pub/85-002-x/2015001/article/14224-eng.pdf

Benson, D., Charlton, C., & Goodhart, F. (1992). Acquaintance rape on campus: A literature review. *Journal of American College Health, 40*, 158.

Berkowitz, A. (1992). College men as perpetrators of acquaintance rape and sexual assault: A review of the literature. *Journal of American College Health, 40*, 177.

Brennan, S. (2012a). *Youth court statistics in Canada 2010/2011*. Retrieved from www.statcan.gc.ca/pub/85-002-x/2012001/article/11645-eng.htm

Brennan, S. (2012b). *Victimization of older Canadians, 2009*. Retrieved from www.statcan.gc.ca/pub/85-002-x/2012001/article/11627-eng.htm

Brennan, S. (2013). *Police-reported crime statistics in Canada, 2011*. Retrieved from www.statcan.gc.ca/pub/85-002-x/2012001/article/11692-eng.htm#a8

Brennan, S., & Taylor-Butts, A. (n.d.). Sexual assault in Canada. *Canadian Centre for Justice Statistics, Statistics Canada*. Retrieved from www.statcan.gc.ca/pub/85f0033m/85f0033m2008019-eng.htm.

Canadian Women's Foundation. (n.d.). Fact sheet: Moving women out of violence. Retrieved from www.canadianwomen.org/sites/canadianwomen.org/files/PDF-FactSheet-StopViolence-Jan2013.pdf

Canadian Women's Foundation. (2016). The facts about violence against women. Retrieved from www.canadianwomen.org/facts-about-violence

Clifford, A. C., Doran, C. M., & Tsey, K. (2013). A systematic review of suicide prevention interventions targeting indigenous peoples in Australia, United States, Canada and New Zealand. *BMC Public Health, 13*, 463. Retrieved from www.biomedcentral.com/content/pdf/1471-2458-13-463.pdf

Dauvergne, M., & De Socio, L. (2009). *Firearms and violent crime*. Retrieved from www.statcan.gc.ca/pub/85-002-x/2008002/article/10518-eng.htm

Department of Justice Canada. (2009). *Family violence: Department of Justice Canada overview paper*. Retrieved from http://canada.justice.gc.ca/eng/pi/fv-vf/facts-info/fv-vf/index.html

Gagné, P., & Desparois, L. (1995). Male erotomania: A type of dangerous sexual harassment. *Canadian Journal of Psychiatry, 40*(3), 136–141.

Health Canada. (n.d.). *Abuse and neglect of older adults*. Cat. No. H72-22/6-1998E.

Health Canada. (1993). *Dating and violence: Fact sheet*. Retrieved from www23.statcan.gc.ca/imdb/p2SV.pl?Function=getSurvey&SDDS=3896&Item_Id=1712.

Health Canada. (2009). *It's your health: Suicide prevention*. Retrieved from www.hc-sc.gc.ca/hl-vs/alt_formats/pacrb-dgapcr/pdf/iyh-vsv/diseases-maladies/suicide-eng.pdf

Health Canada. (2013). *First Nations and Inuit health: Mental health and wellness*. Retrieved from www.hc-sc.gc.ca/fniah-spnia/promotion/mental/index-eng.php

Joerger, A., et al. (1992). Why men batter: Why women stay. *Community Safety Quarterly, 5*, 22–23.

Malina, R. M., Bouchard, C., & Bar-Or. O. (2004). *Growth, maturation and physical activity*, 2nd ed. Champaign, IL: Human Kinetics.

McLeod, L. (1980). *Wife battering in Canada: The vicious circle*. Ottawa: Canadian Advisory Council on the Status of Women.

Miller, A. (1992). Newly recognized shattering effects of child abuse. *Empathic Parenting*, 1 & 2.

Morrison, K. A. (2008). Differentiating between physically violent and non-violent stalkers: An examination of Canadian cases. *Journal of Forensics Science, 53*(3), 742–751.

Pan, H., Malone, J., & Tyree, A. (1994). Physical aggression in early marriage: Pre-relationship and relationship effects. *Journal of Consulting Psychology, 62*(3), 594–602.

Parkinson, D., & Claire, Z. (2013). The hidden disaster: Domestic violence in the aftermath of natural disaster. Retrieved from https://ajem.infoservices.com.au/items/AJEM-28-02-09

Patel, D. (1980). *Dealing with interracial conflict: Policy alternatives*. Montreal: Institute for Research on Public Policy.

Perreault, S., & Brennan, S. (2015). Criminal victimization in Canada, 2009. Retrieved from www.statcan.gc.ca/pub/85-002-x/2010002/article/11340-eng.htm

Public Health Agency of Canada. (1986). Ottawa charter for health promotion. Retrieved from www.phac-aspc.gc.ca/ph-sp/docs/charter-chartre/pdf/charter.pdf

Royal Canadian Mounted Police. (2010). *Homicide in Canada, 2007 Statistics Canada, juristat*. Retrieved from www.rcmp-grc.gc.ca/pubs/fire-feu-eval/t2a-eng.htm

Royal Canadian Mounted Police. (2012). The effect of family violence on children—Where does it hurt? Retrieved from www.rcmp-grc.gc.ca/cp-pc/chi-enf-abu-eng.htm

Royal Canadian Mounted Police. (2013). *Facts and figures: January – March 2013: Canadian firearms program*. Retrieved from www.rcmp-grc.gc.ca/cfp-pcaf/facts-faits/index-eng.htm

Schneider, T. (1992). Rape prevention. *Community Safety Quarterly*, 8–13.

Sinha, M. (2012). *Family violence in Canada: A statistical profile, 2010: Statistics Canada*. Retrieved from www.statcan.gc.ca/pub/85-002-x/2012001/article/11643-eng.htm

Solicitor General. (n.d.). Family violence: Not a private problem. *RCMP Policy*, Public Education Doc. 1966.

Statistics Canada. (1995). Selected violations against the person, by gender of victim and accused, 1995.*Canadian Crime Statistics*. Retrieved from www.statcan.gc.ca/pub/85-002-x/85-002-x2008001-eng.pdf

Statistics Canada. (2012). *Suicides and suicide rate, by sex and by age group*. Retrieved from http://www.statcan.gc.ca/tables-tableaux/sum-som/l01/cst01/hlth66a-eng.htm

Statistics Canada. (2013). *Homicide survey, number of solved homicides, by type of accused-victim relationship, Canada, annual (number)*. Retrieved from www5.statcan.gc.ca/cansim/pick-choisir?lang=eng&p2=33&id=2530006

Statistics Canada. (2015a). *Family violence in Canada: A statistical profile 2013*. Retrieved from www.statcan.gc.ca/pub/85-002-x/2014001/article/14114-eng.pdf

Statistics Canada. (2015b). *Police-reported crime statistics in Canada, 2014*. Retrieved from www.statcan.gc.ca/pub/85-002-x/2015001/article/14211-eng.pdf

Suderman, M., & Jaffe, P. (1996). *Preventing violence: School and community-based strategies*, Health Canada.

Thompson, M. P., Koss, M. P., Kingree, J. B., Goree, J., & Rice, J. (2011). A prospective mediational model of sexual aggression among college men. *Journal of Interpersonal Violence, 26*(13), 2716–2734. doi:10.1177/0886260510388285

Trocomé, N., Fallon, B., MacLaurin, B., Daciuk, J., Felstiner, C., Black, T., . . .Cloutier, R. (2005). *Canadian incidence study of reported child abuse and neglect—2003: Major findings*. Ottawa: Minister of Public Works and Government Services Canada.

van Dijk, J. J. M., Mayhew, P., & Killias, M. (1990). *Experiencing crime across the world*. Deventer, the Netherlands: Kluwer Law and Taxation Publishers, 38.

West, N. (1992). Crimes against women. *Community Safety Survey, 5*, 1.

Whittaker, M. (1992). The continuum of violence against women: Psychological and physical consequences. *Journal of American College Health, 40*, 151.

Wilson, G., et al. (1996). *Abnormal psychology*. Boston, MA: Allyn & Bacon.

World Health Organization. (2010). Child maltreatment. *Fact Sheet Nᵒ 150*, August. www.who.int/mediacentre/factsheets/fs150/en/index.html

World Health Organization. (2013a). *Violence prevention alliance: Definition and typology of violence*. Retrieved from www.who.int/violenceprevention/approach/definition/en/

World Health Organization. (2013b). *Injuries and violence prevention*. Retrieved from www.who.int/violence_injury_prevention/violence/en/

CHAPTER 16

Canadian Association of Naturopathic Doctors. (2013). *What is naturopathic medicine?* Retrieved from www.cand.ca/index.php?78&L=0

Canadian Institute for Health Information. (n.d.). *Health care in Canada 2010*. Retrieved from www.cihi.ca/cihi-ext-portal/internet/en/document/health+system+performance/indicators/performance/release_16dec10

Canadian Institute for Health Information. (2013). *Regulated Nurses: Canadian Trends, 2007 to 2011*. Retrieved from www.cihi.ca/free_products/Regulated_Nurses_EN.pdf

Canadian Institute for Health Information. (2014a). *Health workforce: Number of doctors in Canada*. Retrieved from www.cihi.ca/en/spending-and-health-workforce/health-workforce/number-of-doctors-in-canada-is-rising-but-average

Canadian Institute for Health Information. (2014b). *Regulated nurses: Canadian trends*. Retrieved from www.cihi.ca/en/spending-and-health-workforce/health-workforce/supply-of-nurses-in-canada-declines-for-first-time-in

Canadian Institute for Health Information. (2016). *National health expenditures: How much does Canada spend on health care?* Retrieved from https://www.cihi.ca/en/spending-and-health-workforce/spending/national-health-expenditure-trends/nhex2015-topic1

Commission on the Future of Health Care in Canada. (n.d.). Romanow report proposes sweeping changes to Medicare, November 28, 2002. Retrieved from www.hc-sc.gc.ca/english/care/romanow/hcc0403.html.

Evans, K. G. (n.d.). *Consent: A guide for Canadian physicians*, 4th ed. Retrieved from www.cmpa-acpm.ca/cmpapd04/docs/resource_files/ml_guides/consent_guide/com_cg_informedconsent-e.cfm

Health Canada. (n.d.). *Health care system*. Retrieved from www.hc-sc.gc.ca/hcs-sss/index_e.html

Health Canada. (1999). *Toward a healthy future: Second report on the health of Canadians, a public policy report developed by the Federal, Provincial and Territorial Advisory Committee on Population Health (ACPH) in collaboration with Health Canada, Statistics Canada, the Canadian Institute for Health Information and a project team from the Centre for Health Promotion, University of Toronto*. Ottawa: Health Canada, 136.

Health Canada. (2011). *Healthy Canadians: A federal report on comparable health indicators 2010*. Retrieved from www.hc-sc.gc.ca/hcs-sss/pubs/system-regime/2010-fed-comp-indicat/index-eng.php#f1

Health Canada. (2012). *Canada's health care system*. Retrieved from www .hc-sc.gc.ca/hcs-sss/pubs/system-regime/2011-hcs-sss/index-eng.php#a1

Health Canada. (2015). *Natural and non-prescription health products*. Retrieved from http://hc-sc.gc.ca/dhp-mps/prodnatur/index-eng.php

Mayo Clinic. (n.d.). *Massage therapy*. Retrieved from www.mayoclinic .org/massage-therapy/

Mayo Clinic Staff. (2009). *Gebak supplements: What to know before you buy*. Retrieved from www.mayoclinic.com/health/herbalsupplements/SA00044

Mayo Clinic. (2012). *Acupuncture*. Retrieved from www.mayoclinic. com/health/acupuncture/MY00946

National Center for Complementary and Alternative Medicine. (n.d.). *Get the facts: 10 things to know about evaluating medical resources on the web*. Retrieved from www.nccam.nih.gov

National Center for Complementary and Alternative Medicine. (2010). *Kava*. Retrieved from http://nccam.nih.gov/health/kava

Newfoundland and Labrador Massage Therapy Association. (n.d.). *Frequently asked questions about massage therapy*. Retrieved from www.nlmta. ca/res/index.html

Public Health Agency of Canada. (n.d.). *Canadian health network: Health system*. Retrieved from www.canadian-health-network.ca/ servlet/ContentServer?cid=1047418085892&pagename=CHN-RCS%2FPage%2FGTPageTemplate&c=Page&lang=En

Public Health Agency of Canada. (2008). *Complimentary and alternative health*. Retrieved from www.phac-aspc.gc.ca/chn-rcs/cah-acps-eng.php

Sims, T., & Tsai, J. L. (2015). Patients respond more positively to physicians who focus on their ideal affect. *Emotion, 15*(3), 303–318. Retrieved from http://psycnet.apa.org/index.cfm?fa=buy .optionToBuy&id=2014-42732-001

Statistics Canada. (2005). Health reports: Use of alternative health care, 2003. *The Daily*, March 15, 2005. Retrieved from www.statcan.gc.ca/daily-quotidien/050315/dq050315b-eng.htm

CHAPTER 17

Aiken, L. R. (1994). *Dying, death, and bereavement*, 3rd ed. Boston: Allyn & Bacon, 4.

Alzheimer Society of Canada. (2012). A new way of looking at the impact of dementia in Canada. Retrieved from www.alzheimer.ca/ ~/media/Files/national/Media-releases/asc_factsheet_new_data_ 09272012_en.ashx

American Academy of Pediatrics: Committee on Nutrition. (1999). Calcium requirements of infants, children, and adolescents. *Pediatrics, 104*(5), 1152–1157. Retrieved from http://pediatrics.aappublications.org/con-tent/104/5/1152.full

Badley, E. M., Canizares, M., Perruccio, A. V., Hogg-Johnson, S. & Gignac, M. A. (2015). Benefits gained, benefits lost: comparing baby boomers to other generations in a longitudinal cohort study self-rated health. *Milbank Q, 93*(1), 40–72. doi: 10.1111/1468-0009.12105.

Bettez, M., Tu, L. M., Carlson, K., Corcos, J., Gajewski, J., Jolivet, M., & Bailly, G. (2012). 2012 update: Guidelines for adult urinary incontinence. Collaborative consensus document for the Canadian uro-logical association. *Canadian Urology Association Journal, 6*(5), 354–363. Retrieved from www.cuaj.ca/cuaj-jauc/vol6-no5/12248.pdf

Canadian Medical Association. (1987). Guidelines for the diagnosis of brain death. *Canadian Medical Association Journal, 136*, 200A.

Canadian Society for Exercise Physiology. (2013). Canadian physi-cal activity guidelines and Canadian sedentary behaviour guidelines. Retrieved from www.csep.ca/english/view.asp?x=949

Doka, K. J. (1989). *Disenfranchised grief: Recognizing hidden sorrow*. Lexington, MA: Lexington Books.

Hayslip, B., & Panek, P. (1992). *Adult development and aging*. New York: Harper and Row, 21.

Health Canada. (1999a). *Toward a healthy future: Second report on the health of Canadians, a public policy report developed by the Federal, Provincial and*

Territorial Advisory Committee on Population Health (ACPH) in collaboration with Health Canada, Statistics Canada, the Canadian Institute for Health Information and a project team from the Centre for Health Promotion, Univer-sity of Toronto. Ottawa: Health Canada, 166.

Health Canada. (1999b). *Statistical snapshot #5: More women than men*. Division of Aging and Seniors. Retrieved from www.statcan.gc.ca/ pub/89-503-x/2010001/article/11475-eng.htm

Health Canada. (2008). *Seniors and aging: Osteoporosis*. Retrieved from www.hc-sc.gc.ca/hl-vs/iyh-vsv/diseases-maladies/seniors-aines-ost-eng.php

Hoover, M., & Retermann, M. (2012). Statistics Canada: Seniors' use of and unmet needs for home care, 2009. Retrieved from www.statcan .gc.ca/pub/82-003-x/2012004/article/11760-eng.htm

International Osteoporosis Foundation. (2013). Facts and stats. Retrieved from www.iofbonehealth.com/sites/default/files/ osteoporos_int-2010vitamin_d_iof_position_statement.pdf

Jeangsawang, N., Malathum, P., Panpakdee, O., Brooten, D., & Nitya-suddhi, D. (2012). Comparison of outcomes of discharge planning and post-discharge follow-up care, provided by advanced practice, expert-by experience, and novice nurses, to hospitalized elders with chronic healthcare conditions. *Pacific Rim International Journal of Nursing Research, 16*(4), 343–360. Retrieved from http://forum.tci-thaijo.org/index.php/ PRIJNR/article/viewFile/5574/4844

Kamerman, J. B. (1988). *Death in the midst of life*. Englewood Cliffs, NJ: Prentice Hall, 71.

Kastenbaum, R. J. (1995). *Death, society, and human experience*, 5th ed. Boston: Allyn & Bacon, 95.

Kübler-Ross, E. (1969). *On death and dying*. New York: Macmillan, 113.

Malina, R. M., Bouchard, C., & Bar-Or, O. (2004). *Growth, maturation and physical activity*, 2nd ed. Champaign, IL: Human Kinetics.

Mayo Clinic. (2011). *Urinary incontinence*. Retrieved from www.mayoclinic.com/health/urinary-incontinence/DS00404/ DSECTION=causes

National Advisory Council on Aging. (n.d.). 1999 and beyond— Challenges of an aging Canadian society. Retrieved from http://ncoa.org/

National Council on Aging. (n.d.). *Half of older Americans report they are sexually active, 4 in 10 want more sex, says new survey*. Retrieved from http://ncoa.org/mews/archives.sexsurvey.htm

National Research Council, Food and Nutrition Board. (1989). *Rec-ommended Dietary Allowances, 10th ed., a report of the subcommittee on the 10th edition of the FDA's dietary allowances*. Washington, DC: National Academy Press.

Ontario Human Rights Commission. (n.d.). *Ageism and age dis-crimination (fact sheet)*. Retrieved from www.ohrc.on.ca/en/ ageism-and-age-discrimination-fact-sheet

Osteoporosis Canada. (2012). *What is osteoporosis?* Retrieved from www.osteoporosis.ca/osteoporosis-and-you/what-is-osteoporosis/

Oxford English Dictionary. (1969). Death. Oxford: Oxford University Press, 72, 334, 735.

Philadelphia Corporation for Aging. (2013). Older adults and sexuality. *Health Matters, 14*, 14. Retrieved from www.pcacares.org/

Public Health Agency of Canada. (2010). *The Chief Public Health Officer's Report on The State of Public Health in Canada 2010*: Chapter 3: The health and well-being of Canadian seniors. Retrieved from www.phac-aspc.gc.ca/cphorsphc-respcacsp/2010/fr-rc/cphorsphc-respcacsp-06-eng.php

Ramage-Morin, P. L., & Garriguet, D. (2013). *Nutritional risks among older Canadians, Statistics Canada*. Retrieved from www.statcan.gc.ca/pub/82-003-x/2013003/article/11773-eng.htm

Statistics Canada. (2012). *Population by sex and age group, 2012*. Retrieved from www.statcan.gc.ca/tables-tableaux/sum-som/l01/cst01/ demo10a-eng.htm

Statistics Canada. (2013). Perceived mental health by age group and sex. Retrieved from www.statcan.gc.ca/tables-tableaux/sum-som/l01/cst01/health110b-eng.htm

Statistics Canada. (2015). Population estimates: By sex and age group, 2015. Retrieved from www.statcan.gc.ca/daily-quotidien/150929/dq150929b-eng.htm

Thompson, J., Manore, M., & Sheeska, J. (2007). *Nutrition: A functional approach,* Cdn. ed. Toronto: Pearson Benjamin Cummings.

Worden, J. W. (2001). *Grief counseling and grief therapy: A handbook for the mental health practitioner,* 3rd ed. New York: Springer.

FOCUS ON FINANCIAL HEALTH

BusinessDictionary.com. (n.d.). *Financial health.* Retrieved from www.businessdictionary.com/definition/financial-health.html

Capital Wellness. (2010). *The 7 dimensions of wellness: Financial wellness.* Retrieved from http://capitalwellness.ca/7dimension.asp

InvestorWords.com. (n.d.). *Financial health.* Retrieved from www.investorwords.com/6812/financial_health.html

Krisher, B. (2011). *Financial stress and mental health: Basic tools for counsellors.* Retrieved from www.kgdebt.ca/financial-stress-mental-health-tools-counsellors/

Movenblog. (n.d.). *The behaviours that destroy your financial health (and how to avoid them).* Retrieved from http://lifehacker.com/5978123/the-behaviors-that-destroy-your-financial-health-and-how-to-avoid-them

Pryor, J. H., Eagan, K., Palucki Blake, L., Hurtado, S., Berdan, J., & Case, M. H. (2012). *The American freshman: National norms fall 2012.* Los Angeles: Higher Education Research Institute, UCLA.

Working Toward Wellness. (2010). *Mental health and financial health.* Retrieved from www.workingtowardwellness.ca/healthy_living/dealing-with-stress/resources/your-financial-health/mental-health-and-financial-health

INDEX

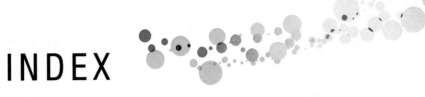

Eating Well with Canada's Food Guide, 164
Ebola virus, 374
eccentric muscle contraction, 95
e-cigarettes, 303
ecstasy, 324–325
ectopic pregnancy, 246–247
ED-NOS. See eating disorder not otherwise specified
	(ED-NOS)
ejaculation
	defined, 210
	premature, 216
	retarded, 216
elder abuse, 449–450
elderly, 483
	See also aging
electrocardiogram (ECG or EKG), 352
electroencephalogram, 493
electronic cigarettes. See e-cigarettes
ELISA test, for HIV/AIDS testing, 396
embolus, 345
embryo, 242
embryo freezing, 249
embryo transfer, 249
emergency contraceptive pills, 227
emotional abuse, 198
emotional availability, 192
emotional health
	defined, 4, 30
	pregnancy and, 235
	psychosocial health, 30–31
emotional stability, 37
emotions, 30
empathy, 190
emphysema, 399
Employee Assistance Program (EAP), 203
EMR. See exercise metabolic rate (EMR)
enabling factors, 9–10
endemic, 376
endogenous depression, 42
endometriosis, 248, 402
endometrium, 207
energy, defined, 122
energy drinks
	alcohol and, 307
	caffeine, 305, 306
environment
	cancer and, 358
	eating habits and, 159
	infectious diseases and, 373
	psychosocial health and, 34
environmental health
	air pollution. See air pollution
	defined, 4
	food quality, 434–435
	land pollution, 432
	managing, 436–437
	noise pollution, 432
	radiation, 432–434
	water pollution, 429–432
Environmental Protection Agency, 300
environmental stewardship, 83
environmental stress, 61
environmental tobacco smoke (ETS), 300
enzymes, 379
epidemics, 372
epidermis, 375
epididymis, 210

epididymitis, 257
epilepsy, 400–401
	See also seizure disorders
epinephrine, 58
Epstein-Barr virus, 406
erectile dysfunction, 215
	See also sexual arousal disorders
ergogenic drugs, 325
erogenous zones, 213
erotic touching, 213
Escherichia coli, 374
esophagus, 119
essential amino acids, 124
essential fat, 154
essential hypertension, 346
estrogen, 204, 207, 208
	cigarette smoking and, 486
	in contraceptives, 223, 224, 226, 227
	endometrial cancer and, 365
	menopause and, 208, 209, 486
	ovarian cancer and, 365
ethanol, 286
ethnicity
	cardiovascular disease, 351
	and osteoporosis, 486
ethyl alcohol, 286
ETS. See environmental tobacco smoke (ETS)
eustress, 54
euthanasia, 500
exclusiveness, 194
exercise
	See also physical activity
	compulsive, 185–186
	determining type of, 93
	flexibility, 102
	frequency, 91
	intensity, 91–93
	pregnancy recommendations for, 240–241
	stretching, 97
	time, 93
exercise disorders, 185–186
exercise metabolic rate (EMR), 157
exhaustion phase of GAS, 59
exhibitionism, 214
exogenous depression, 42
expectorants, 275
experience, openness to, 37
external female genitals, 205
external influences, on psychosocial health, 34
external male genitals, 209
extroversion, 37
eye disease, diabetes and, 415
eyesight and aging, 487

F

FAE. See fetal alcohol effects (FAE)
faith, 32
fallopian tubes, 207
falls, 456
	See also injuries
false claims, 464
FAM. See fertility awareness methods (FAM)
family
	alcoholism and, 294, 295, 296
	behaviour change and, 15–16
	body image and, 179

SNS. *See* sympathetic nervous system (SNS)

snuff, 298

social age, 482

social assumptions, sexual assault and, 451

social bias, against overweight, 165–166

social bonds, 31

social death, 495

social factors
    alcoholism and, 293–294
    cancer and, 358

social health
    defined, 4
    psychosocial health and, 31

social interactions, 68

socialization, 205

social network and weight, 166

social networking safety, 449

social physique anxiety (SPA), 181

Social Readjustment Rating Scale (SRRS), 59

social reinforcers, 18

social supports, 31

social worker, 49

Society of Obstetricians and Gynaecologists of Canada, 240

sociopsychological variables, 14

sodium, 131

solid waste, 432

solo practitioners, 475

soluble fibre, 125

somatic death, 492

specific absorption rate (SAR), 433

spermatogenesis, 210

spermicides, 227

spiritual health
    altruism, 83
    concepts, 76–77
    contemplation, 81
    defined, 4
    environmental stewardship, 83
    expanding mind, 80–81
    interactions with others, 31
    interconnectedness, 32
    meaningful purpose in life, 79
    meditation, 82–83
    mindfulness, 32, 81–82
    overview, 76
    physical health and, 79
    prayer, 83
    psychological counselling, 80
    psychological health and, 79–80
    quest for well-being, 31–32
    relationships, 78
    religion, concepts and characteristics, 77
    service learning, 34
    spiritual intelligence, 79
    stress and, 80
    taking time to reflect, 34
    values, 78
    volunteering, 33
    yoga, 80, 98–99

spiritual intelligence, 79

spirituality
    See also spiritual health
    addiction and, 267
    concept of, 76–77
    as a part of daily life, 32
    into practice, 33
    religion *vs.*, 77

spiritual resurgence, 33

spontaneous remission, 464

sports drinks, 136

SRRS. *See* Social Readjustment Rating Scale (SRRS)

standardized extracts, 472

staphylococcal infections, 374–375

starches, 125

starvation, 167

static stretching, 97
    flexibility, 102

Statistics Canada
    abortion and, 234
    on sexual assault, 450
    on suicide, 46, 443
    Violence Against Women survey, 446

sterilization
    defined, 232
    female, 232–233
    male, 233–234

steroids, 325–326

STI. *See* sexually transmitted infections (STI)

stillbirth, 247

stimulants, 275–276

St. John's wort, 472

stomach, 121

stopping negative thoughts, 19

storage fat, 154–155

streptococcal infections, 375

streptococci, 375

stress
    calcium depletion and, 134
    dealing with, 65–68
    defined, 54
    environmental, 61
    hair loss and, 56
    impaired immunity, 55
    individual response to, 350–351
    overview, 54
    post-secondary students and, 63–65
    psychosocial sources of, 59–61
    self-concept and, 61–62
    self-imposed stress, 61–63
    sources of, 59–63
    weight gain, 56

stress incontinence, 487

stress inoculation, 18–19

stress management
    alternative techniques, 72
    crying, 68
    dealing with stress, 65–68
    emotional responses and, 68
    laughing, 68
    mental action, 69–70
    physical action, 70–71
    physical activity and, 90
    social interactions and, 68
    spiritual health and, 80
    support groups and, 69
    time management, 71

stressor, 54
    assessing, 65
    recognizing and changing responses to, 66

stretching exercises, 97

stroke, 345–346
    aneurysm, 345
    defined, 345
    embolus, 345

turmeric *(Curcuma longa)*, 269
Twain, Mark, 8
12-step program, 267
Twiggy, 166
type 1 diabetes, 402, 413, 414
  See also diabetes
type 2 diabetes, 90, 402, 413–414
  See also diabetes
Type A Behavior and Your Heart (Friedman and
    Rosenman), 62
Type A personality, 62, 63
Type B personality, 62
Type C personality, 63
typical-use effectiveness rate
  of condoms, 223
  of contraceptive sponge, 230
  defined, 223
  of diaphragm with spermicidal cream or jelly, 229
  of oral contraceptives, 226
  of withdrawal method, 231

U

ulcerative colitis, 403
ultrafast computed tomography (CT), 353
ultrasound, prenatal testing and screening, 243
ultraviolet B (UV-B) radiation, 131, 426
Uniform Crime Reporting survey, 440
unintentional injuries, 456
United Nations
  on family types, 192–193
  on overpopulation, 421
  on violence against women, 445
unsaturated fats, 126
urethral opening, 205
urgency incontinence, 487
urinary incontinence, 487
urinary tract infections (UTI), 391–392
urination, diabetes and, 414
U.S. Environmental Protection Agency, 425
uterine cancer, 365–366
uterus, 207
UTI. *See* urinary tract infections (UTI)
UVB radiation. *See* ultraviolet B (UV-B) radiation

V

vaccination, 380–382, 383
vaccines, HPV, 390
vacuum aspiration abortion, 234, 235
vagina, 205
vaginal intercourse, 213–214
vaginal opening, 205, 207
vaginismus, 216
vaginitis, 391
values, spiritual health and, 78
Vancouver
  anti-Chinese and Japanese riot (1907), 444
  seasonal affective disorder (SAD), 44
Vancouver Coastal Health, 326
Vanier Institute of the Family, 192
variable resistance, 95
variant sexual behaviour, 214
varicella-zoster virus, 378
vas deferens, 210
vasectomy, 233–234
  See also male sterilization
vasocongestion, 211

vasopressin, 195
VDT. *See* video display terminals (VDT)
vegetarianism, 135–136
vegetarians, 135
veins, 342
venereal warts, 389–391
  risk of, 389
  treatment for, 389, 391
ventricles, 341
very low-calorie diets (VLCD), 160
Viagra, 215
victimization
  consequences of, 452
  rate of, 440
  sexual. *See* sexual assault
  unintentional injuries and, 456
victimology, 36
video display terminals (VDT), 407
violence
  alcohol and, 285
  against children, 447–449
  cycle of violence theory, 445–446
  defined, 440
  domestic, 446–447. *See also* domestic violence
  of hate, 444–445
  health and, 455–456
  homicide, 441–442
  against men, 449
  against older adults, 449–450
  social networking, 449
  suicide, 442–443
  against women, 445–446
  youth, 444
Violence Against Women survey, 446
Violence Protection Alliance of the World Health
    Organization, 440
Virtual Hospice, 500
virulent organism, 372
viruses
  chicken pox, 378
  common cold, 376–377
  defined, 376
  Ebola, 374
  hepatitis, 377–378
  human immunodeficiency virus. *See* HIV/AIDS
  human papilloma viruses (HPV),
    360, 389, 390
  incubation periods, 376
  infectious mononucleosis, 377
  influenza, 377
  measles, 378–379
  mumps, 378
  slow-acting, 376
  varicella-zoster, 378
  West Nile, 374
vitamin(s), 128–131
  antioxidants, 128, 130–131
  defined, 128
  fat-soluble, 128, 130
  vitamin D, 131
  water-soluble, 128, 129
vitamin D
  aging and, 491
  calcium and, 134
  cancers and, 131
  dietary reference intakes, 131
  UVB radiation, 131